THE PATHOLOGY AND SURGERY OF THE VEINS OF THE LOWER LIMB

TO OUR WIVES

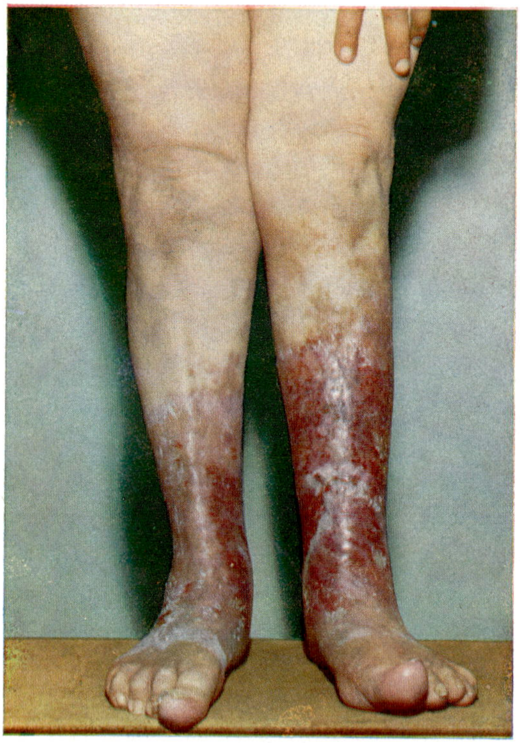

Plaster Dermatitis — *see* page 70.

THE PATHOLOGY AND SURGERY OF THE VEINS OF THE LOWER LIMB

HAROLD DODD, Ch.M.(L'pool), F.R.C.S.(Eng.)
Emeritus Surgeon to St. Mary's Hospital (London) Group, Royal London Homeopathic Hospital, King George Hospital, Ilford and Royal Hospital, Richmond

FRANK B. COCKETT, M.S.(Lond.), F.R.C.S.(Eng.)
Surgeon to St. Thomas's Hospital, London

with a Foreword by
R. R. Linton, M.D.
Boston, Massachusetts

Second edition

CHURCHILL LIVINGSTONE
EDINBURGH LONDON AND NEW YORK
1976

CHURCHILL LIVINGSTONE
Medical Division of Longman Group Limited

Distributed in the United States of America by Longman Inc., 19 West 44th Street, New York, N.Y. 10036 and by associated companies, branches and representatives throughout the world.

First edition 1956
Second edition 1976

ISBN 0 443 01292 X

Library of Congress Cataloging in Publication Data

Dodd, Harold
The pathology and surgery of the veins of the lower limb.
1. Varicose veins. 2. Thromboembolism.
3. Extremities, Lower—Blood vessels—Surgery.
I. Cockett, Frank Bernard, joint author. II. Title.
(DNLM: 1. Vascular diseases. 2. Veins—Surgery. 3. Leg—Surgery. WG600 D639p)
RC695.D6 1976 617′.414′07 75-599

Printed in Great Britain

Foreword

It is a pleasure and an honor I deeply appreciate to be asked to write the foreword for the new edition of *The Pathology and Surgery of the Veins of the Lower Limb*, now twenty years since I did it for the first edition. It was a landmark in bringing to the attention of the medical profession a most excellent and comprehensive book dealing with this branch of vascular surgery, something that had never before been so well accomplished. The new edition now carries on in the same excellent manner bringing the subject up to date.

This new edition opens with an interesting historical resume of anatomists, physiologists, physicians and surgeons who have contributed much in the past and the present to give a better understanding of the diseased condition of the veins of the lower extremity, and describes some of the more important methods of treatment.

Without question a better understanding of the surgical anatomy, applied physiology and the pathologic conditions, that is given by the authors has resulted in great advances in the treatment of venous diseases of the lower extremity. The newer methods are brought up to date for the diagnosis of thromboembolic disease including the use of I^{125}, ultrasound with the transcutaneous Doppler unit, and angiography of the leg veins and the pulmonary arteries.

Emphasis is expressed again regarding the importance of a thorough knowledge of the etiology, the physiology, and the surgical anatomy of these blood vessels. In addition the effect of these blood vessels in the diseased state is discussed from simple varicose veins to the more complicated thromboembolic and post-thrombotic states of the lower limb. This enables one to understand the rationale of the various forms of treatment of the diseases of these blood vessels, which in my opinion is not comprehended even today much better than it was almost two centuries ago by the great majority of physicians and surgeons.

The methods of treating the most serious condition, thromboembolic disease, are well documented. Of special interest, also, are the prophylaxis and the therapy of the different types of iliofemoral and deep venous thrombosis, and the post-thrombotic changes in the lower extremities. An excellent discussion is also given of the congenital venous anomalies. The subject of simple varicose veins is discussed with the recommendation that the best form of treatment is the surgical removal of these blood vessels, and in addition the interruption of the incompetent communicating or perforating veins.

As in the previous edition great emphasis is placed on the late changes that develop in the skin and subcutaneous tissues in the 'gaiter' area of the ankle because of the decompensation of the lower leg venous pump due to incompetence of the communicating or perforating veins in this region, both on the internal and the external aspects of the ankle. The authors emphasize the important role that they play in the etiology of the chronic venous ulcers of the distal third of the lower extremity. They stress that the interruption of these veins is the most important surgical procedure that will help in obtaining a cure of these distressing and disabling problems of the veins of the lower extremity. Considerable emphasis is also placed on the new 'Cockett' syndrome with reference to the etiology and the treatment of this condition with its lower limb complications and sequelae.

Without question it is my recommendation that those who are interested in the etiology and treatment of these very common types of peripheral vascular diseases, namely those that involve the veins of the lower limbs, should carefully read this excellent book with much benefit.

Boston, Mass. 1976

R. R. Linton

Preface

It is twenty years since the first edition of this book appeared. During this period there has been such a rapid increase in our knowledge of all aspects of venous disease, that we have had to rewrite it almost completely.

Much of the old material has been pruned and shortened and several new chapters have appeared, particularly on physiology and congenital malformations, the newer diagnostic methods, and the more recent work on thrombo-embolism and its management.

As before, we have written with the practical aspects of the subject in mind. No finer training ground for surgery is to be found than in dealing with venous conditions. The diagnosis of the exact venous fault needs clinical skill and thoroughness. The operative procedures, though often considered trivial, are actually a testing exercise in exact dissection and good surgical technique, which when mastered largely overcome the difficulties of more extensive operations. The after care of the patient is of great interest and importance. It is therefore for the young trainee surgeon that we hope this book will hold a special message. However, the manifestations of diseases of the veins, especially the deep veins, are seen and have to be treated by every sort of doctor from general practitioner to dermatologist or consulting physician, and in the sections on thrombosis, embolism, and ulceration of the leg, its diagnosis and treatment, we hope that they also will find matter of interest.

Since the last edition, an immense amount of literature on venous problems has blossomed. It is difficult for the average surgeon to evaluate this, and find his way through many conflicting papers and reports to a sensible system of management of a patient. We have specially tried to provide guidance here, summarising the results of research and setting out practical régimes of management, based on this. Adequate references have been provided to give those interested a 'lead' to the relevant recent literature.

Particular care has been taken with the section on venous anatomy as this subject receives scant attention elsewhere. It is not possible to operate on varicose veins, or to understand thrombosis and the post-thrombotic syndrome, without precise anatomical knowledge.

It is a pleasure to express our appreciation for the generous assistance of our friends and colleagues—particularly those who have contributed special new sections of the book and whose names appear on the contributors' page. One of us (F. B. Cockett) has had the stimulating experience of working for many years in close contact with Professor Henry Barcroft, Professor J. B. Kinmonth, Professor Norman Browse and Dr Michael Lea Thomas. The experience, help and encouragement of these colleagues, who have between them contributed so much to the understanding of vascular problems over the years, is gratefully acknowledged. Bob Linton has once again, after twenty years, contributed our foreword, so marking our long and fruitful association with him which started in 1954.

We must also thank Mrs Monica Fain for deciphering our handwriting and repeated

typing of the manuscript. Similar appreciation is due to Major W. G. Leaper, M.V.O.
Finally, we must thank the staff of our publishers for their patience and co-operation in overcoming many production difficulties.
We acknowledge the gracious permission of Her Majesty the Queen to photograph the Leonardo da Vinci originals in the Royal Collection at Windsor Castle.

London, 1976

H. Dodd
F. B. Cockett

Contributors

Anning, S. T., T.D., M.D., F.R.C.P., Consultant Physician, Department of Dermatology, Leeds General Infirmary.

Norman L. Browse, M.D., F.R.C.S., Professor of Vascular Surgery, St. Thomas's Hospital, London, S.E.1.

Desmond N. Croft, M.A., D.M., B.Ch.(Oxon), M.R.C.P., Physician, and Physician to Department of Nuclear Medicine, St. Thomas's Hospital, London, S.E.1.

John Ludbrook, M.D., Ch.M.(N.Z.), F.R.C.S., F.R.A.C.S., Professor of Surgery, University of Adelaide; the visiting specialist in surgery, Royal Adelaide Hospital; Consultant in Surgery to the Queen Elizabeth, Adelaide Children's and Queen Victoria Hospitals.

Michael Lea Thomas, M.A., M.B., B.Chir.(Cantab), F.R.C.P.(London), F.R.C.R., D.M.R.D., Vascular Radiologist, St. Thomas's Hospital, London, S.E.1.

David Negus, D.M., F.R.C.S., Senior Surgical Registrar, St. Thomas's Hospital, London, S.E.1.

Contents

Part I
History, Anatomy and Physiology

Fig. 1.1 Superficial venous pressures at rest and at exercise in the erect position.

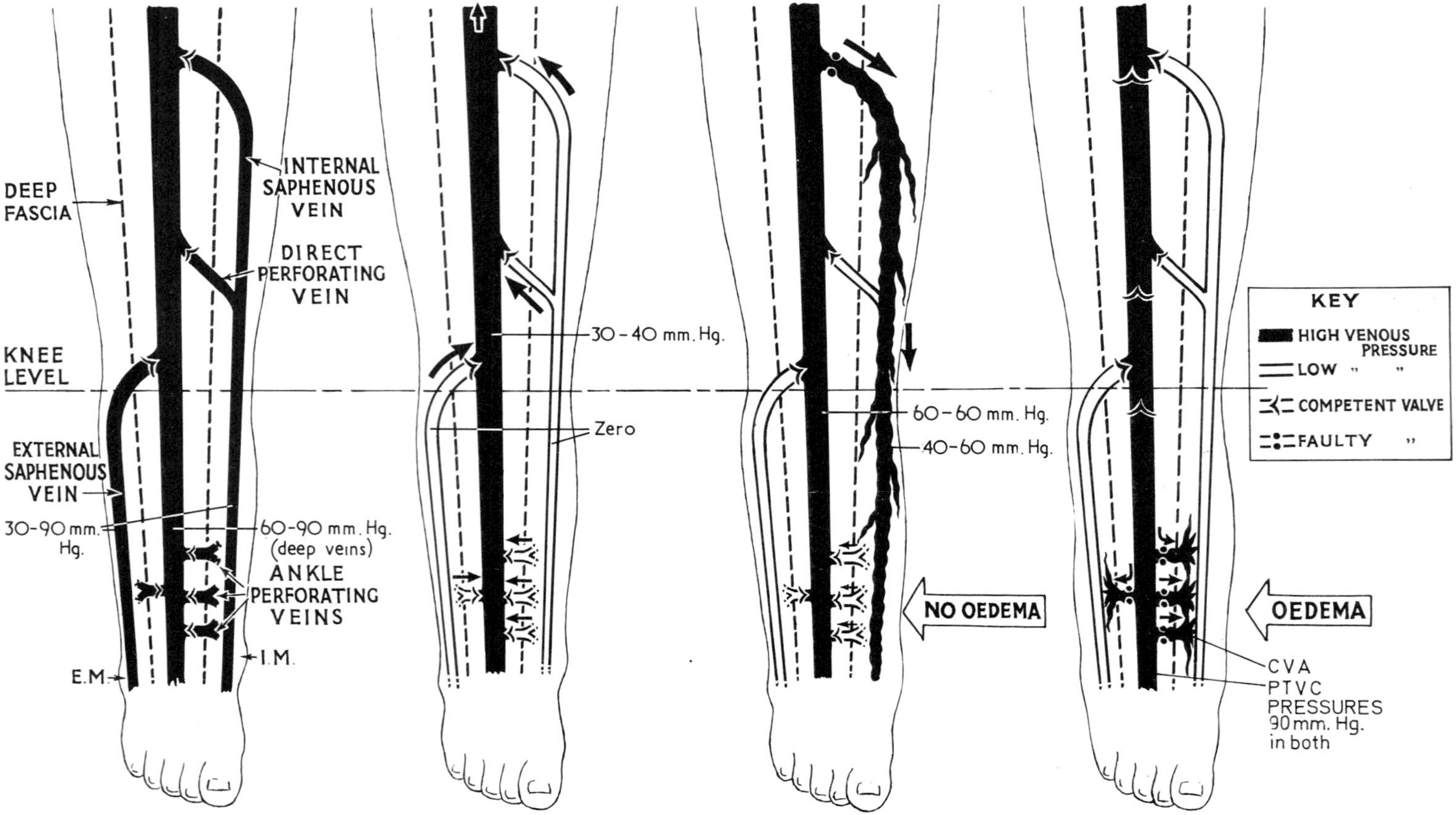

Normal veins
Standing at rest
Superficial venous
hypertension present

Normal veins
Leg exercising
No superficial
venous hypertension

Incompetent long saphenous
vein
Competent ankle perforators
Leg exercising
Slight diffused superficial
venous hypertension

Incompetent ankle
perforators only
Leg exercising
Severe local superficial
venous hypertension

1. Introduction

Varicose veins are one of the commonest ailments of Western peoples; probably one in five women and one in fifteen men over the age of forty-five have them. Gunnar Bauer (1950) says, 'It has been estimated that there are ten times as many sufferers from chronic venous disease of the lower extremities as from arterial disease with leg symptoms.'

Varicose veins are so numerous that only by every general surgeon having special knowledge and training in them and their associated complications, and accepting his share of their care, can the community's need in this respect be met. The reward is prompt, much lasting comfort is bestowed on individuals and their families, often working efficiency is restored. The operations for varicose veins are exacting, but the technical skill acquired is valuable in more major procedures.

We would say that every 'bad' leg can be materially improved by systematic diagnosis and planned treatment.

The actual finite cause of varicose veins is still unknown, but the more exact knowledge of the anatomy of the venous system of the leg, and the physiological mechanism whereby venous blood returns to the heart against gravity has provided clearer understanding of the pathology and of the disorders that medical men are called upon to treat.

Venous valvular failure and superficial venous hypertension

Perhaps the most important of these studies has been on the behaviour of the venous pressure of the superficial and deep veins of the lower limbs in the erect position during rest and exercise and on the function of the muscular venous pump. They have brought forth a clear and simple concept of the basic physiological mechanism at fault in varicose veins (Fig. 1.1).

The fundamental fact to grasp is that the venous drainage of the superficial tissues in the erect exercising leg is inwards to the deep veins via the various perforating or communicating veins. While exercising, the pressure in the main deep venous trunks is high, but the pressure in normal superficial veins gradually falls to nearly zero. In other words the blood in the superficial veins is sucked inwards to the deep veins of the limb during muscular movement and from these it is squeezed up towards the heart. What prevents this high pressure in the deep veins from being transmitted to the superficial veins during exercise? The answer is that at every point where a superficial vein joins a deep vein (great saphenous, small saphenous and all the communicating or perforating veins) there is a valve which prevents the reflux of blood from the deep to the superficial system. These valves prevent the hypertension in the deep veins from being transmitted to the superficial veins.

The primary cause of the development of the varicosis in the superficial veins lies in the destruction of the strategic valves in the perforating veins. This allows the normal high venous pressure developing within the musculofascial sheath during muscular activity to pass out and be exerted on the poorly supported superficial veins, resulting in an ambulatory venous hypertension in the affected group of superficial veins. This sustained venous hypertension in the superficial veins during movement and standing results in their gradual stretching, enlargement, and tortuosity; a process which goes on steadily over the years, until the original valvular leak is found and stopped by surgery. In fact the surgical aim in venous defects and their complications is *to diagnose the site of the high pressure 'leak' from the deep veins into the superficial veins and to close it by ligation at its source.*

The comparative degree of superficial venous hypertension

There is one further fundamental point. The ambulatory venous pressure which is transmitted outwards by a leak high in the limb, as at the saphenofemoral junction, is less than that which is transmitted out by a faulty perforating vein at the ankle level. Further, the leak at the saphenofemoral junction is into a large vein, the internal saphenous, with its numerous and considerable tributaries which can 'disseminate' the pressure readily and widely. The leak at the lower leg level, by the ankle perforating veins, is by a short wide vein or veins which drain fairly directly into an adjacent capillary bed. Hence for these reasons the effect of a pressure leak at the ankle level is likely to be more destructive than one from higher in the limb. This concept is of great importance in understanding the pathology of ankle ulceration.

The cause of venous valvular failure

Thrombosis is an important and probably the most common cause of valve destruction in the perforating veins in the lower part of the limb. But we are still uncertain what exactly causes the highest saphenous valve to become incompetent or destroyed in an early case of great saphenous incompetence.

Heredity undoubtedly plays a great part in the genesis of varicose veins. Whether a particular anatomical arrangement of valves, which predisposes to the throwing of great strain on the highest saphenous valve is inherited, or whether it is an actual weakness of the vein wall, it is impossible to say. Both factors probably play a part.

Definition

A varicose vein is one which has permanently lost its valvular efficiency. Venous distension and dilation, especially in the erect position, exaggerates this valvular incompetence. Even when some patients are horizontal, their varicose veins do not shrink as do healthy ones. As a result of continuous dilatation under pressure in the course of time a varicose vein becomes elongated, tortuous, pouched, thickened, inelastic and friable.

The term 'varicosity' is applied generally to those superficial vessels so affected in the lower limbs, but similar changes may also occur in veins in the anal canal, as haemorrhoids, and less often in the termination of the left spermatic cord as a varicocele. Other rare varices arise elsewhere, e.g. in the broad ligament, and in cases of portal hypertension at the lower end of the oesophagus.

Varicosities in the lower limbs by far outnumber all similar venous disorders and the purpose of this monograph is to describe these and their allied disorders.

REFERENCES

Bauer, G. (1950) *Angiology*, **1**, 229.

2. The Historical Aspects

S. T. ANNING, T.D., M.A., M.D. (Camb.), M.R.C.P.

The study of medical history enables the growth of knowledge and the development of certain concepts to be traced. This is well demonstrated by consideration of the historical aspects of varicose veins, venous thrombosis and ulceration of the leg, for from early times these conditions have been described and theories as to their cause expounded. In miniature the evolution of medical thought through the ages can be illustrated.

The papyrus of Ebers (c. 1550 B.C.) mentions varicose veins and the author advises against operation for this condition (Major, 1954). Hippocrates (460–377 B.C.) associated ulcers on the legs with enlarged veins and wrote: 'In the case of an ulcer, it is not expedient to stand; more especially if the ulcer be situated in the leg.' He believed that the Scythians, as a result of horse-riding, were afflicted with varicosity of the veins because their feet were always hanging down from their mounts. He also noted that varicose veins of the legs do not occur before puberty. Hippocrates described the use of compressive bandages and is sometimes quoted as advising small punctures in varicose veins which should not be opened freely 'for generally large ulcers are the consequence of the incisions'. However, this last advice appears in *De Ulceribus*, a book which is not now accepted as part of the authentic Hippocratic collection.

Varicose veins are illustrated on a votive table from the Asklepieion in Athens (Fig. 2.1) and an early account of a patient with this condition, which appears in Plutarch's *Lives*, is that of Caius Marius, the Roman tyrant who died in 86 B.C. He underwent operation for his varicose veins:

Marius is praised for both temperance and endurance, of which latter he gave a decided instance in an operation of surgery. For having, as it seems, both his legs full of great tumours, and disliking the deformity, he determined to put himself into the hands of an operator; when, without being tied, he stretched out one of his legs, and silently, without changing countenance, endured most excessive torments in the cutting, never either flinching or complaining; but when the surgeon went to the other, he declined to have it done, saying, 'I see the cure is not worth the pain.' (Clough, 1859.)

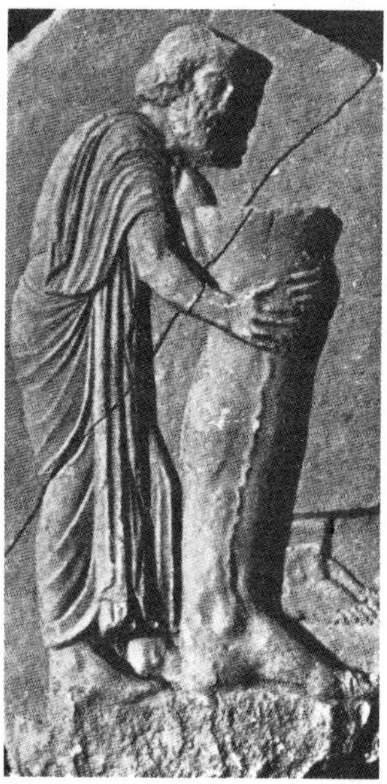

Fig. 2.1 Votive relief. Man holding a huge leg showing varicose veins. From the Asklepicion, Athens, now in the National Museum, Athens. (Laignel-Levastine *Histoire de la Médicine*, I. Paris, 1936. Albin Michel éditeur, 22 Rue Huyghens, Paris.)

Much was written about these conditions in Roman times. Aurelius Cornelius Celsus (25 B.C.–A.D. 50) advised the use of plasters for leg ulcers and linen roller bandages. Varicose veins were to be treated by exposure followed by avulsion with a blunt hook or by a touch of the cautery.

Claudius Galen (A.D. 130–200) also tore out varicose veins with a blunt hook. He applied wine to leg ulcers and was opposed to frequent changes of the dressing. Juvenal, almost his contemporary, mentioned about A.D. 115 that the 'soothsayer [with so much standing about] will soon be troubled with varicose veins'.

The first to ligate varicose veins seems to have been the Byzantine physician Aetius of Amida on the Tigris (502–575). Paulus Aegineta (607–690) also performed this operation but preferred to carry out ligation of veins on the inner part of the thighs 'where they generally arise'.

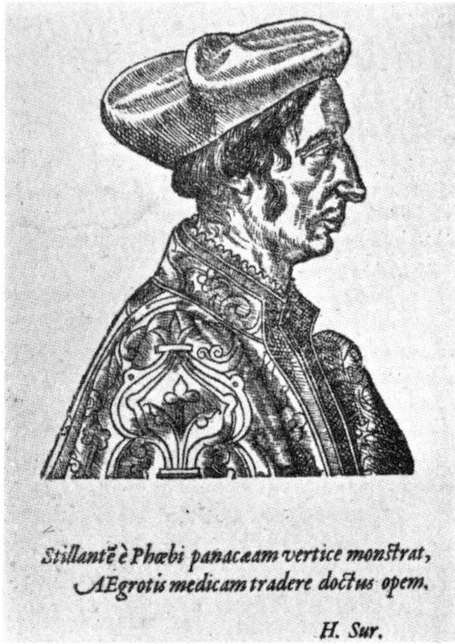
Stillantē è Phœbi panacæam vertice monſtrat,
Ægrotis medicam tradere doctus opem.
H. Sur.

Fig. 2.2 Jean Fernel (1506–1588). From the reverse of the title-page of his *Therapeutices universalis seu medendi rationis, libri septem.* Frankfurt, 1574.

THE HUMORAL THEORY

Galen's theory of humours, taken from Hippocrates, together with his idea of the to-and-fro movement of blood with its various spirits, dominated medical thought for fifteen centuries. Varices were attributed to the weight of stagnant 'gross' blood on the walls of veins. Haly Abbas (d. 994) believed that they were filled with a black bile and occurred in those who worked hard and stood long. Being outside the main venous channels the deleterious humours were thought to be side-tracked and safe unless pressed back by bandaging. They might then lead to madness or other disasters. (Cf. Hippocrates' aphorism: 'Varicose veins or haemorrhoids appearing in a case of madness put an end to it.')

The cause of the thickening of the blood which led to varices was considered by Fernel (1604) (Fig. 2.2) in his book *Pathologia*. He wrote: 'It [the varix] comes also from a blow, from a contusion, from excessive effort, from hard work and much travelling; sometimes from "plethora" as in most pregnant women.' Child-bearing and 'standing too much before kings' were believed by Marianus Sanctus of Barletta (1555) to be the chief causes of varicose veins and another surgeon, Paré (Fig. 2.3), writing in 1579 on the aetiology of varicose veins said: 'The matter of them is usually melancholy blood, for varices often grow in men of a melancholy temper, and which usually feed on gross meats, or such as breed gross and melancholy humours. Also women with child are commonly troubled with them, by reason of the heaping together of their suppressed menstrual evacuation. The precedent causes are a vehement concussion of the body, leaping, running, a painful journey on foot, a fall, the carrying of a heavy burden, torture or racking. . . . It is best not to meddle with such as are inveterate; for of such being cured there is to be feared a reflux of the melancholly bloud to the noble parts, whence there may be imminent danger of malign ulcers, a cancer, madness or suffocation' (Paré). Pigeaux, as late as 1843, wrote of a cook who several times had abortions because

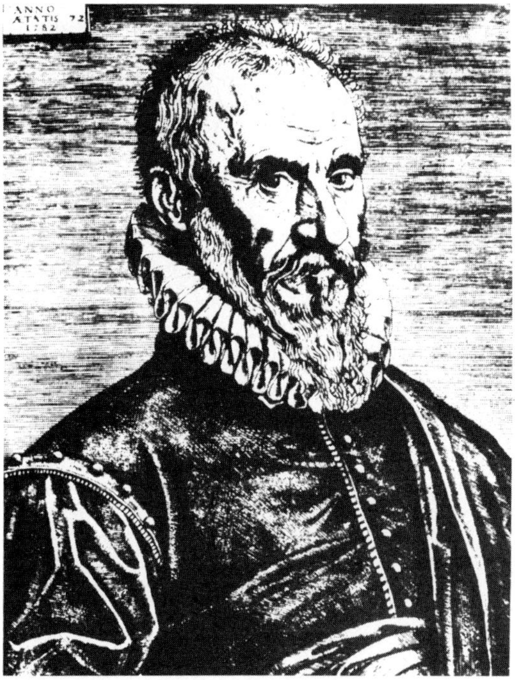

Fig. 2.3 Ambroise Paré (1510–1590).

her varicose veins were bandaged during pregnancies.

Fernel (1604) referred to oedematous ulcers caused by the collection of corrupt humours and Vicary (1536) (Fig. 2.4) noted that 'the Legges . . . when they are offended or wounded, are very perillous, because unto them runneth a great quantity of humors', and he added that they are 'troublesome and curious to heale'. Based on the humoral theory the view was held that it would be risky to cure a leg ulcer, though Hippocrates, Celsus, Galen, Aetius of Amida and Paulus Aegineta had no such inhibitions. However, Avicenna (980–1037) believed that ulcers in old people should not be healed and if healed should be broken down. Even in the eighteenth century Le Dran (1731) in France and Heister (1768) in Germany took a similar view and considered the ulcer to be a drain for humours which, if not expelled, would cause serious illness. Sharp in 1758 wrote that 'in old people the cure is often dangerous'. Benjamin Bell (1789), however, was prepared to believe that, with a small degree of caution, the cure of every ulcer may be attempted. As late as 1801 Home could write: 'If a patient of a gouty habit has an ulcer on the leg . . . any attempt to heal the ulcer is improper' and Buchan (1822) expressed himself forcibly on this subject:

> If an ulcer conduces to the patient's health, from whatever cause it proceeds, it ought not to be healed; but if on the contrary, it wastes the strength, and consumes the patient by a slow fever, it should be healed as soon as possible.
>
> We would earnestly recommend a strict attention to these particulars to all who have the misfortune to labour under this disorder, particularly persons in the decline of life; as we have frequently known people throw away their lives by want of it, while they were extolling and generously rewarding those whom they ought to have looked upon as their executioners.

In 1859 Hunt remarked that many patients still believed that the ulcer was salutary, and that it could not be healed without risk of damage to the general health, though he referred to it as an unfounded and now almost obsolete prejudice. Nevertheless, even today in country districts old women may be found who firmly believe in the danger of healing leg ulcers.

Derived from the humoral theory was the idea of menstrual ulcers. 'Many', wrote Barbette (1675), 'by a Suppression of the Menstruals fall into a melancholy Madness, as we have twice observed. Many great Diseases, as a Cachexy, Dropsie, Cardialgy, Swoonding, Palpitation of the Heart, Madness, Gout, Dizziness, Falling-sickness, Apoplexy, etc. do proceed from a Suppression of the Menstruals'. Moreover, the menstrual blood, collecting in the legs during pregnancy becomes stagnant and, in order to allow its escape, ulceration follows. Writers in the seventeenth and eighteenth century (e.g. Ettmüller, 1688) continued to believe that menstrual blood is 'gross' and collects in the legs during pregnancy causing varicose veins and ulcers. Astruc (1761) seems to have been the first to state clearly that menstrual blood is not a collection of bad humours. Even in the

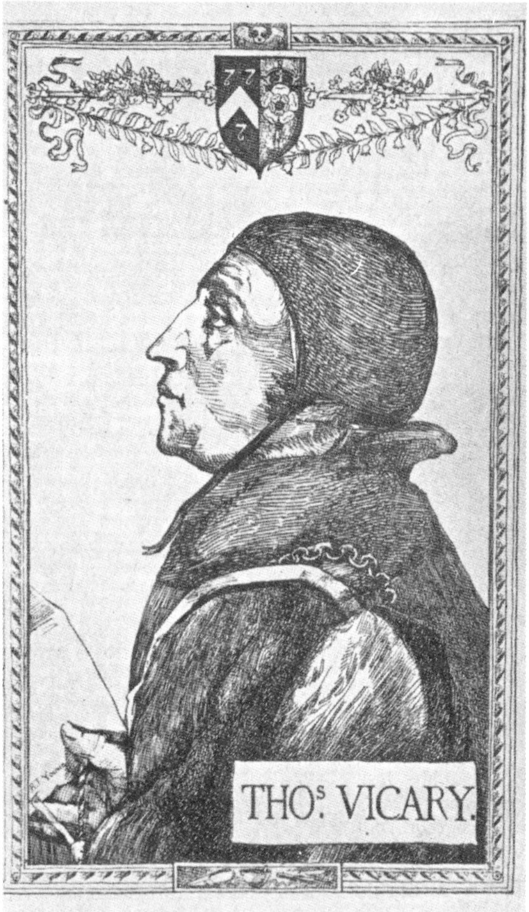

Fig. 2.4 Thomas Vicary (1495–1561). From an impression in the Wellcome Collection of an etching after the picture by Holbein representing the Union of the Barbers and Surgeons.

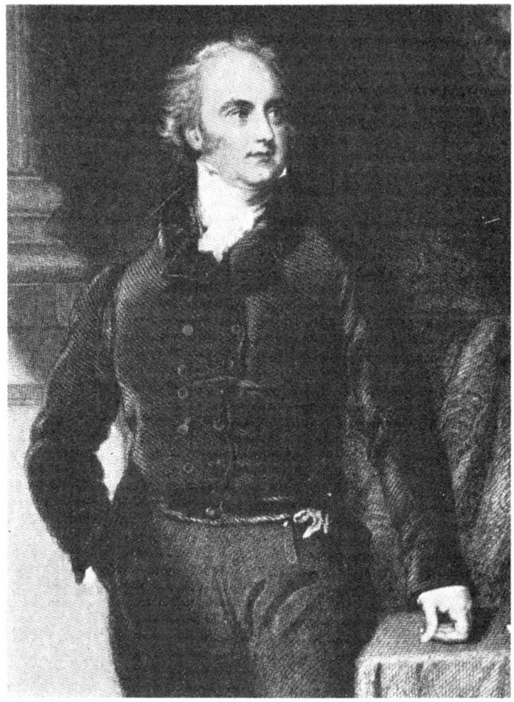

Fig. 2.5 Sir Astley Paston Cooper (1768–1841). From the engraving by W. H. Mote after a portrait by T. Lawrence. Engraving in the Wellcome Historical Medical Museum.

first half of last century Sir Astley Cooper (1824) (Fig. 2.5) and Critchett (1849) wrote of menstrual ulcers related to amenorrhoea from any cause, and prior to the investigations of Davis (1822), post-partum venous thrombosis was explained in terms of the humoral theory.

The lochia were considered to be bad humours whose retention often occurs during puerperal fever, and is likely to cause trouble. In 1603, Roderiguez a Castro published his work *De Universa Mulierum Morborum Medicina*. He not only considered the swollen and livid legs of pregnant women but made observations concerning swellings of the lower extremities in the puerperium: 'vidimus crurum tumores post partum contingere, si lochia minus copiosa procedant'.* He considered that immoderate drinking after childbirth precipitated the trouble and made the important observation that it might occur after copious bleeding.

In this country post-partum thrombosis was first described in 1676 by Richard Wiseman, Sergeant-Chirurgian to Charles II (Fig. 2.6). In a chapter on *Abscesses and Corrosive Ulcers Arising From Distempers of*

* After childbirth we observe swelling of the legs to occur when the lochia flow less copiously.

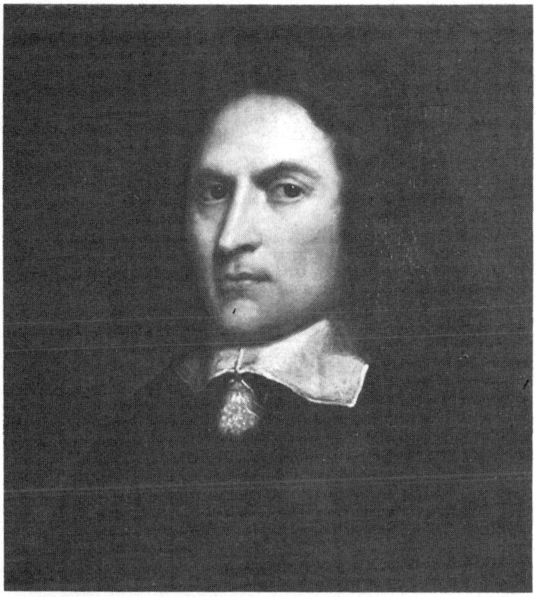

Fig. 2.6 Richard Wiseman (1622–1676).

the Uterus in Child-bed, he relates the following history:

> An Apothecary's wife, living in my Neighbourhood in the Old Bailey, after a hard Child-bed labour was seized with a Fever, and great pain in her right Thigh, from the Groin and Hip downward to the Knee, swelling the Member round, without inflammation or discolouring the skin.

Wiseman did not speculate about the causes of the condition and, although familiar with venous thrombosis, did not relate the two.

Another theory to explain the swelling of the limb in phlegmasia dolens was put forward by Puzos (1759) and owed much to the idea of humours. He considered that milk is formed in women during pregnancy, as well as after delivery, and is directed principally to the uterus in the former, and to the breasts later. When the *foetus in utero* or the infant at the breast cannot consume the whole of the milk that is formed, the excess escapes in the excretions or collects in certain parts of the body and particularly in the lower limbs.

In 1784 Charles White who was 'man-midwife extraordinary to the Manchester Lying-in Hospital' published a tract on the swelling in one or both of the lower extremities during the puerperium. He wrote that it is not owing to any defect of the lochia as it happens to those who have the most regular discharge', 'nor to a deposit of milk as it happens under every circumstance attending that secretion'. He thought 'that the proximate cause of this disorder is an obstruction, detention and accumulation of lymph in the limb', brought about by rupture of the lymphatics from pressure of the 'foetus's head' during labour (a mechanical cause) and he did not believe that it occurred under other conditions than parturition.

The credit must go to Davis of Queen Charlotte's Hospital for first appreciating that the veins were the seat of the trouble. He published in 1822 a remarkable paper on *The Proximate Cause of Phlegmasia Dolens* which he showed to result from a 'violent inflammation of one or more of the principal veins within and in the immediate neighbourhood of the pelvis'. Phlegmasia dolens following typhus fever (Ferriar, 1810) and injury (Hodgson, 1815) were described. Trousseau (1865) gave a masterly lecture on the subject (Fig. 2.7).

THE MECHANICAL THEORY

However, a fundamental blow to the humoral theory had been struck when Harvey wrote of his discovery of the circulation of the blood (1628) (Fig. 2.8). He had reached his conclusions after studying the valves in veins, appreciating that, in a vessel containing valves, a to-and-fro movement of blood is not possible.

Wiseman (1676) realised that valvular incompetence results from dilatation of a vein and, although the association of varicose veins and leg ulcers had been noted by Hippocrates, he seems to have been the first to consider that ulcers might be the direct result of a circulatory defect and used the term 'varicous ulcer'.

It is noteworthy that many eighteenth century writers on leg ulcers, such as Underwood (1783), Bell (1789), Baynton (1797), and

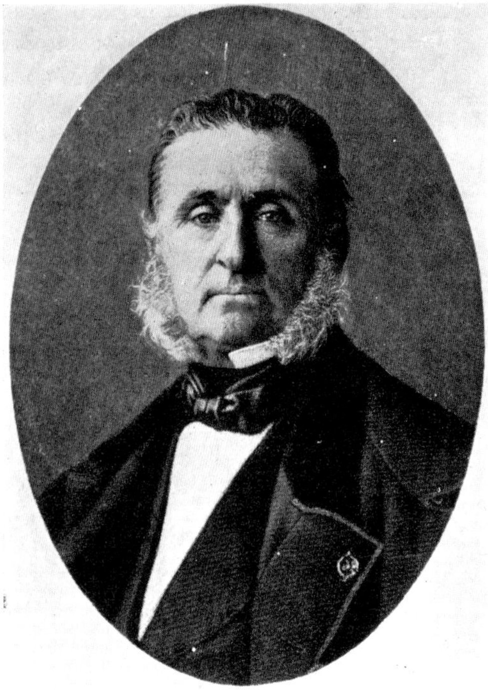

Fig. 2.7 Armand Trousseau (1801–1867). From a lithograph.

The mechanical theory was applied to ulcers. Thus Sharp in 1758 wrote: 'The Indisposition of these Sores is in some measure owing to the Gravitation of the Humours downwards', and in 1797 Baynton declared that the disease arises 'from the unfavourable situation of the parts which are placed at a remote distance in the human machine from the fountain of life and heat, and are obliged to return the venous blood and lymph to the heart under some peculiarly unfavourable and disadvantageous circumstances'. Two years later Whately had written that 'when the body is erect, the blood and lymph return from the extremities contrary to their gravity, in a column of several feet'.

During the nineteenth century, however, the emphasis was on varicose veins as the cause of leg ulcers and the term 'varicose ulcer', scarcely used since Wiseman's day, became established. Home (1801) believed an ulcer was more difficult to heal if there were varicose veins and Hodgson (1815) wrote of ulcers 'which are generally situated near the ankle, and are remarkably intractable. They appear to depend', he thought, 'upon the

Whately (1799), made no reference to varicose veins as a cause. New ideas were growing. Probably chiefly influenced by Newton's *Principia* (1687) and by Morgan's book on *The Philosophical Principles of Medicine* (1725), which was based on it, there were many adherents to the iatromechanical doctrines which viewed the body as a machine with pumps, tubes and valves, and with levers of bones and joints activated by muscles. For example, Quincy (1722) in the preface to his *Lexicon Physico-Medicum* wrote: 'And because what is brought from Physicks and Mechanicks takes up so much room here, it may be necessary to inform the Reader, that there is no Knowledge in Medicine but by such means.' We have seen that White's theory of the cause of phlegmasia dolens was mechanical and Dionis (1708) attributed the varicose veins in pregnant women to the pressure of the uterus on the iliac veins.

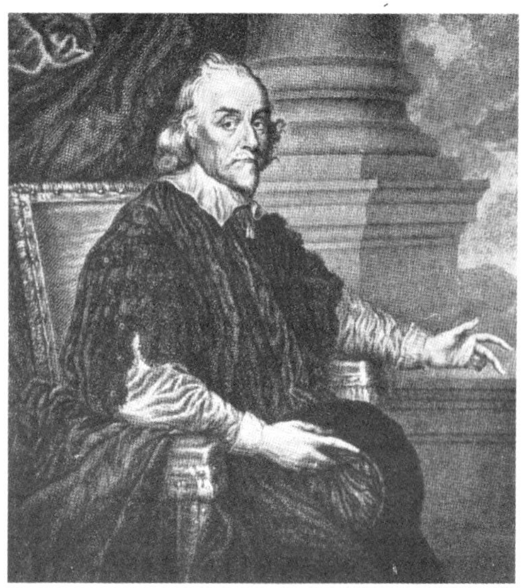

Fig. 2.8 William Harvey (1578–1657). From the line engraving by J. Hall after the picture in the Royal College of Physicians.

varicose conditions of the veins, for when the latter is relieved, the ulcers are as readily cured as ulcers in general'. Many writers of the nineteenth century—Brodie (Fig. 2.9), Cooper, Critchett, Hilton (Fig. 2.10), Hunt, Scott and others—stressed the importance of varicose veins, but Gay (Fig. 2.11) and Spender, both writing in 1868, believed that venous thrombosis also played an important part and Gay pointed out that severe varicosity may exist without ulceration. Indeed, Gay denied the validity of the doctrine of the varicose ulcer and thought, like Chapman (1853), that the term should be discarded.

THE PATHOPHYSIOLOGICAL APPROACH

Gay's work appears to have been the first scientific investigation of these conditions in this country, though in France, Verneuil (1855) had made careful observations and dissections. Gay pointed out that with superficial varicosity there may be other serious lesions affecting both arteries and veins, deep

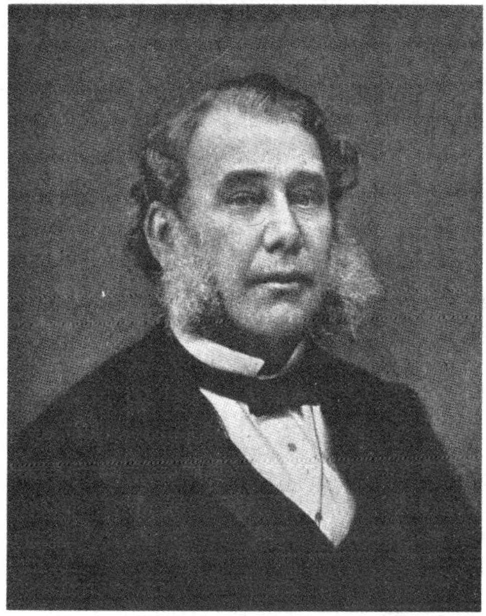

Fig. 2.10 John Hilton (1804–1878).

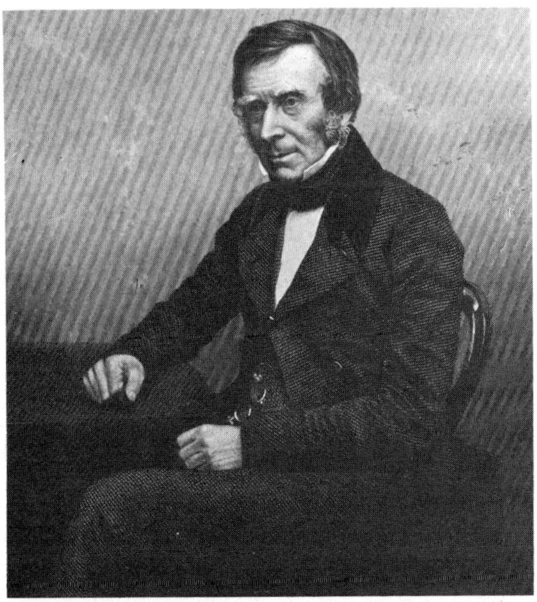

Fig. 2.9 Sir Benjamin Brodie (1783–1862).

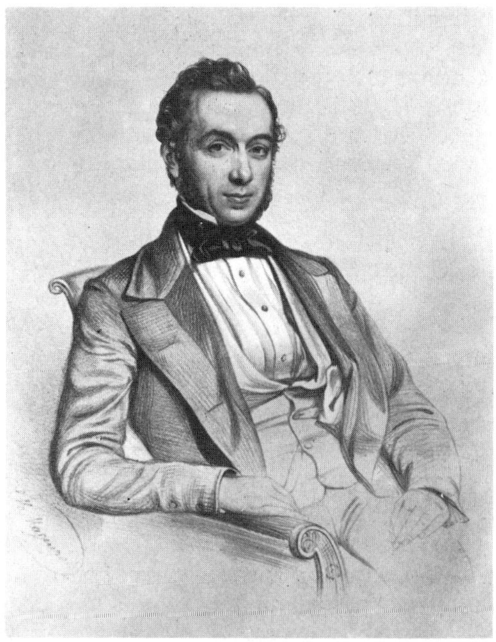

Fig. 2.11 John Gay (1812–1885).

and superficial, which cannot be ignored, and he considered that:

> Ulceration is not a direct consequence of varicosity, but of other conditions of the venous system with which varicosity is not infrequently a complication, but without which neither one of the allied skin affections °induration and bronzing[5] is met with, conditions which involve obstruction of the trunk veins, deep and superficial, either from impediments on the venous side, or incompetency on the arterial, or from both causes combined.

The truth of these statements has become manifest in the last decade, during which the importance of deep venous thrombosis and arterial disease in the aetiology of leg ulcers has become more generally appreciated. Interest is now taken in the circulation of blood through the limb as a whole. The effect of muscular contraction in assisting the flow of venous blood, especially from the lower limb, was understood by Harvey (1628) and Lower (1670) but until recently the concept of a 'leg muscle pump' has attracted little attention.

Rational treatment is based on aetiology. Different theories attempting to explain the cause of a disease inevitably have their influence on therapy even though much of it is empirical. This is clearly seen when the subject of treatment is approached historically.

TREATMENT

In considering the historical aspects of treatment we shall deal primarily with leg ulcers and must take into account four methods: treatment by compression of the limb, local treatment of the ulcer, the surgical treatment of varicose veins, and the general treatment of the patient.

Compression

The value of firm compression of the leg was appreciated early and we have mentioned that linen roller bandages were used by Celsus. Henri de Mondeville (Fig. 2.12), writing between 1306 and 1320, thought that a

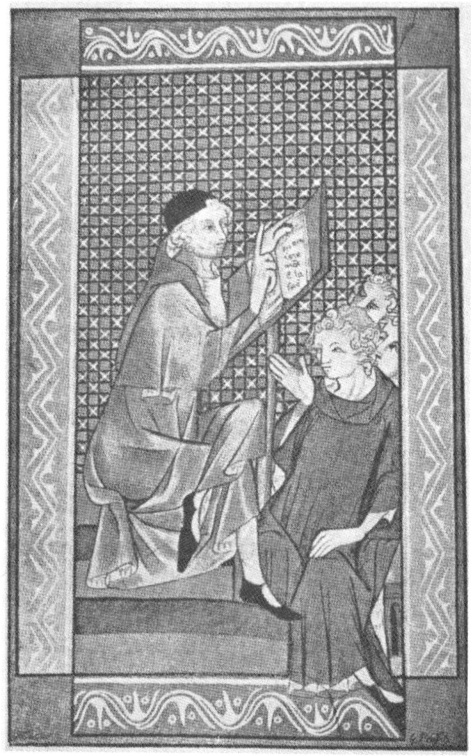

Fig. 2.12 Hènri de Mondeville (1260–1320) lecturing to his pupils. From a manuscript of his *Chirurgia* (1314), in the Bibliothèque Nationale, Paris.

bandage embracing the whole limb was advantageous because it 'drives back the evil harmful humours infiltrated in the leg and the ulcer' and 'it, moreover, prevents and stops the flow of humours tending to come'. Guy de Chauliac (1363) (Fig. 2.13) used diachylon plaster bandages very similar to those employed by Marianus Sanctus of Barletta (1555), Baynton (1797), Brodie (1846) and by doctors nowadays. Ambroise Paré, taken prisoner in the campaign of 1553 when acting as surgeon to Henri II, cured the leg ulcer of Lord Vaudeville, his captor, though it had been present six or seven years. After local treatment he 'roule the Leg beginning at the foote, and finishing at the knee, not forgetting a little bolster upon the Varicous veine'. He also used local compression with a lead plate

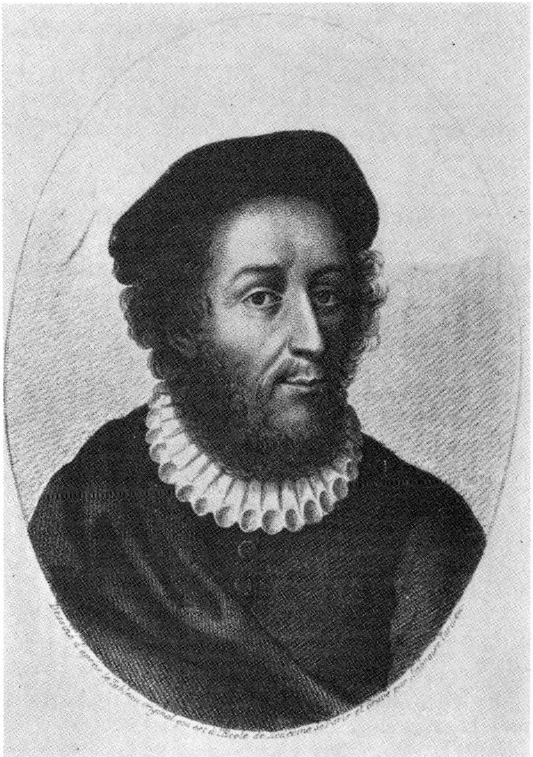

Fig. 2.13 Guy de Chauliac (1298–1368). From the engraving by Ambroise Tardieu after the picture in the Ecole de Médicine, Paris.

but insisted on rest in bed 'which is commanded by Hippocrates'.

Wiseman (1676) introduced a new method of compressing the leg affected by leg ulcers—a laced stocking usually made of soft leather such as dog skin (Fig. 2.14). This became widely used both in this country and on the Continent. Petit (1790) preferred this method as the degree of compression can be varied by the lacing. Wiseman also mentioned bandaging but it does not seem to have been in general use—certainly not in 1771 when Else wrote: 'About two years and a half ago, in a conversation with Dr Huck upon this subject, he told me, that Mr Battiscombe, apothecary, in Half-moon-street, Piccadilly, had a very speedy method of curing sore legs; one remarkable instance of which he had lately seen, and had heard of others. The case which had fallen within his knowledge was that of a servant-maid, who had laboured under a very bad painful ulcer of the leg for twelve or fourteen years, and had come out of two hospitals without her cure. Dr Huck said, that he did not know the whole of Mr Battiscombe's method, but that he believed the principal part of it consisted in the application of a tight bandage. He said that Mr Battiscombe first applied a linen rag, moistened with a liquor, which was probably tincture of myrrh: that over this he applied a thin plate of lead, and then a roller very tight from the toes to above the knee . . . I immediately recollected, that Mr Battiscombe had cured a grenadier and an officer's servant, of ulcers in the legs, which I thought would be difficult to heal without rest, and therefore advised them to go into an hospital . . . Mr Martin, my colleague in St

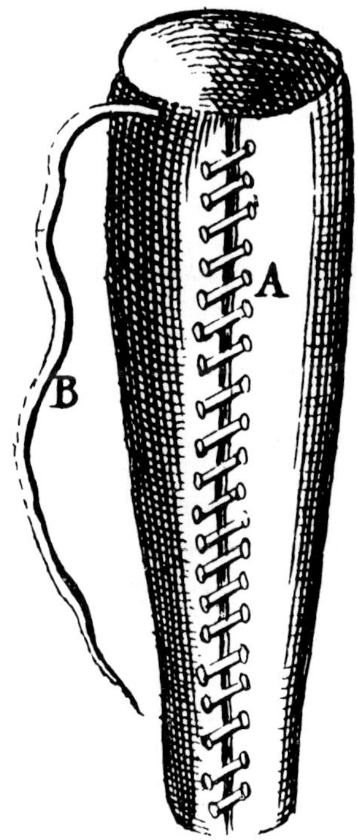

Fig. 2.14 Richard Wiseman's leather stocking (*from Heister 1768*).

Thomas's Hospital, and I, determined to try what bandage would do in old ulcers of the legs, without administering any internal medicine, and find it so exceedingly efficacious, that I believe it will seldom fail where there is no carious bone.' He thought that a tight roller bandage applied from the toes to the knee was much better than a laced stocking.

Underwood (1783) wrote on the treatment of ulcers without rest and used 'Welch flannel' for bandaging as he found it elastic. In the nineteenth century Brodie, Hunt and Spender gave excellent accounts of the treatment of ulcers by bandaging, and Cooper (1824) believed that compression allows the venous valves to recover their lost action. Two important advances in recent times have been the introduction of the elastic adhesive bandage by Dickson Wright (1930) and the combination of firm massage and elastic webbing bandages to reduce oedema and induration (Bisgaard, 1948).

Local treatment

From the time of Celsus details are known of local applications used in the treatment of leg ulcers. Though methods have altered the principles of treatment have changed little. In place of the wine applied to ulcers by Galen we use other antiseptics and, though Paré and surgeons after him placed lead plates over ulcers, silver foil is now being used (Milberg and Tolmach, 1954). Critchett in 1849 covered ulcers with the lining membrane of egg-shells and in 1950 Troensegaard-Hansen used amnion. The eighteenth-century surgeon cleansed the ulcer of slough by a digestive application and in 1954 Spier and Cliffton used plasminogen and streptokinase.

Nevertheless, the growing use of the microscope and the advance of bacteriology had a great influence on the local treatment of leg ulcers. From the time of Lister the control of micro-organisms on the surface of leg ulcers by means of antiseptics became of increasing interest. Inevitably an ulcer becomes secondarily infected with various organisms commonly present on the skin but there is rarely any relationship between the type of infection or the number of bacteria in the ulcerated area and the slowness or rapidity with which the ulcer heals. As Dickson Wright (1930) showed, a leg ulcer will heal although infected if the oedema is abolished; local treatment is of secondary importance. 'But', to quote from Le Clerc (1723), 'as all these methods are sometimes useless and as there are some ulcers which need the hand of the surgeon, Celsus also teaches in particular a method of curing them by operation'.

Surgical treatment of varicose veins

We have mentioned that Celsus and Galen tore out varicose veins after they had been exposed and that Aetius of Amida seems to have been the first to use ligation. Paulus Aeginata gave careful directions for this operation.

> Wherefore, having washed the man, and applied a ligature round the upper part of the thigh, we are to direct him to walk about, and when the vein becomes distended we are to mark its situation with writing ink or collyrium, to the extent of three fingers' breadth or a little more, and having placed the man in a reclining posture with his leg extended, we apply another ligature above the knee; and where the vein a scalpel, but not to a greater depth than the thickness of the skin, lest we divide the vein; and having separated the lips of the wound with hooks, and dissected away the membranes with crooked specilla, like those used in the operation for hydrocoele, and laid bare the vein, and freed it all round, we loose the ligatures from the thigh, and having raised the vessel with a blind hook, and introduced under it a needle having a double thread we cut the double of it, and opening the vein in the middle with a lancet, evacuate as much blood as may be required. Then having tied the upper part of the vessel with one of the ligatures, and stretched the leg, we evacuate the blood in the limb by compression with the hands. Then having tied the lower part of the vein, we may either cut out the portion intermediate between the ligatures, or suffer it to remain until it drops out of its own accord with the ligatures; then we have to put a dry pledget into the wound, and apply over it an oblong compress soaked in wine and oil, and secure them with a bandage, and accomplish the cure by the treatment applicable in cases of suppuration.

The descriptions of the operative procedures of later writers are remarkably similar. Though nowadays ligation of the internal saphenous vein in the thigh is usually associated with the name of Friedrich Trendelenburg (1844–1924) (Fig. 2.15), Paré had practised the operation in the sixteenth century, followed 200 years later by Rima (1777–1843).

But ligation alone was not sufficient for adherents of the humoral theory. The 'gross' blood must be removed. Thus Fabricius ab Aquapendente (1533–1619) (Fig. 2.16) tied the vein above and below the varix, and, having evacuated its contents by puncturing the latter, obliterated the cavity by compression.

Paré, however, clearly recognised the presence of thrombophlebitis in a superficial varicose vein when he wrote:

> They often swell with congealed and dryed bloud, and cause pain which is increased by going and compression. Such like varices are to be opened by dividing the veine with a Lancet, and then the blood must be pressed out, and evacuated by pressing it upwards and downwards; which I have oft-times done, and that with happy success to the Patient, whom I have made to rest for some dayes, and have applyed convenient medicine.

But he also wrote that 'a Varix is therefore cut or taken away so to intercept the passage of the bloud and humours mixed together therewith, flowing to an ulcer seated beneath' (Paré).

Dionis (1708), like Fabricius, recommended, as one method of treating varices, that the vein should be punctured, the blood removed and compression applied. Heister in 1739 believed that the worst of the varices should be opened 'by a longitudinal Incision with the Scalpel, or a Lancet: then taking away about eight or ten Ounces of the grumous and viscid Blood' (Heister, 1768). Petit (1790) also insisted on the efficacy of puncturing varices with a lancet. During the bleeding the limb was gently massaged so as 'to press out the thick black blood'. As James wrote in 1743:

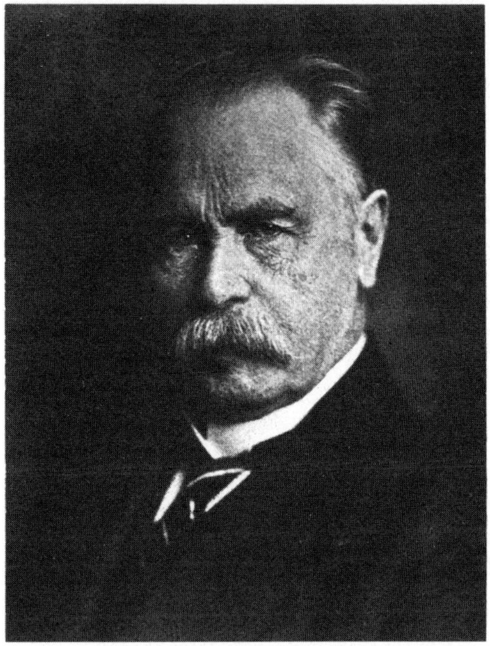

Fig. 2.15 Friedrich Trendelenburg (1844–1925).

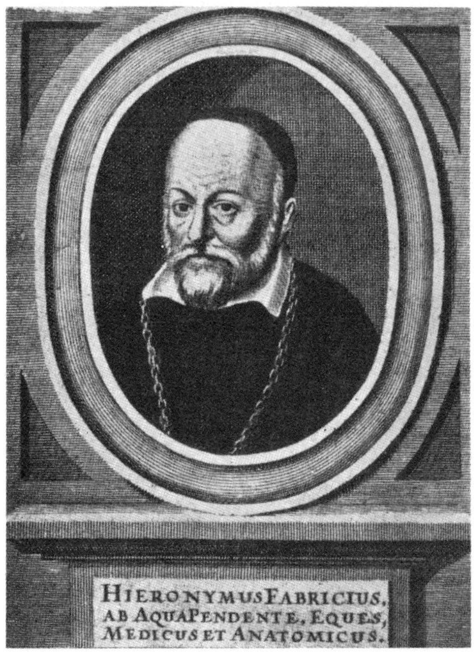

Fig. 2.16 Hieronymus Fabricius ab Aquapendente (c. 1533–1619). From the line-engraving after the anonymous picture in the Padua Anatomy School.

> The smaller Kinds of Varices usually create but little Uneasiness; and are, therefore, neglected by the Patient, as not requiring the Assistance of the Surgeon.
>
> In order, however, to prevent a small, and, at first, Inconsiderable Evil, from increasing by degrees, and growing formidable, to the great Detriment, and Annoyance of the Patient, it is adviseable to open a Vein, with all Speed, and take away a Quantity of Blood; and, after that, to prescribe a proper Regimen of Diet: This done, it will be convenient to secure the diseased Feet in the most careful and exact manner, with a repellent, or, as it is commonly called, expulsive Bandage.

In 1816 Brodie, because the necessity of withdrawing 'gross' blood had by this time disappeared, merely divided the varicose vein subcutaneously with a bistoury. However, in the past, the surgical treatment of varicose veins does not seem to have been popular and Wiseman (1676), with Caius Marius in mind, wrote: 'I have never met with one Patient that cared to hear of the Cure by Ligature, nor indeed have I seen any great reason for it.'

Apart from the question of the patient's suffering during the operation, the complication of sepsis made it highly dangerous. Cooper (1824) stated that no fewer than eight cases terminating fatally after ligature had come to his knowledge and Chapman (1864) wrote:

> One of these accidents, it is said, happened in the practice of Sir Astley himself, some months after he had roundly declared that a surgeon who performed such an operation deserved to have a ligature applied round his own neck.

Home (1801), Hodgson (1815), Brodie (1816) and other authors also stressed the dangers of ligation, dangers which were diminished by the advent of antiseptic surgery following the teaching of Lister, and which were almost eradicated when the importance of asepsis became recognised.

Percutaneous ligation was introduced, and discarded, in the nineteenth century though an author in 1943 described it as his own invention. Davat (1833) passed several needles through the skin and affected vein and then tied figure-of-eight ligatures around both ends of each needle. This resulted in an inflammatory reaction in the vein and finally in its obliteration. Erichsen (1853) employed a slightly different method. He wrote:

> The most convenient way of obliterating the varicose veins, in my opinion, and that which I always employ, consists in compressing the vessel at several points, by passing a hare-lip pin underneath it, laying a piece of wax-bougie upon the vessel, and then applying the twisted suture around the pin and over the bougie.

Popliteal ligation must briefly be mentioned. Hodgson (1815) had written: 'For the purpose of diminishing the length, and consequently the weight of the column, it has been proposed to obliterate a portion of the dilated vein by the application of a ligature.' Parona (1894), endeavouring to apply the theory of Verneuil (1855) that the deep veins are responsible for the superficial varices, ligated the popliteal vein to cut off the hydrostatic pressure of the column in the femoral vein from the varicose veins below. In recent years popliteal ligation has again been advocated by Bauer (1948).

Hodgson (1815) had noticed that coagulation of blood in veins 'terminated in a spontaneous cure of varices'. 'The vessel was ultimately obliterated, and the blood was conveyed through collateral vessels.' A means of producing this coagulation at will was sought and 'galvanopuncture' was used in Italy (Chapman, 1864). The injection of substances directly into a vein to produce thrombosis was, as Boyd (1948) said, 'fortunately delayed until the introduction of the hypodermic syringe by Francis Rynd in 1845'. Chapman (1864) wrote that 'attempts have been made to obliterate varicose veins by injecting the perchloride of iron into them; and a French author, M. Pravaz, reports very favourably of its action'. He describes complications arising from this treatment, which until recently had a considerable vogue.

Another development, reminiscent of Celsus with his blunt hook, is the stripping operation.

Keller (1905) removed the internal saphenous vein by passing through the vein a wire loop or probe with a ligature attached. This was tied to the end of the vein and on pulling it the vein was extirpated. Mayo (1906) and Babcock (1907) used strippers with which the divided vein was pulled out.

General treatment

It has long been appreciated that the general treatment of the patient with a leg ulcer must not be neglected. Octavius Horatianus directed such a one to avoid the bath, the fire, the sun, cold air, loud cries, intoxication, venery and passion.

Inevitably the humoral theory had an influence on general treatment, an influence which persisted into the eighteenth century; an example of which is the enthusiasm of physicians of that period for bleeding their patients. Heister (1768) had written in 1739: 'To prevent the Disorder from running to any great length . . . it may be proper to bleed the Patient' and he advised 'Abstinence and a strict Regimen in Diet'.

Petit (1790) stressed the importance of general remedies, diet and rest in bed, and Hunter (1835) (Fig. 2.17) considered that a horizontal posture, with temperance, should be the first thing advised in sore legs, especially in poor people suffering from bad living, much exercise and cold, who benefit from the rest, food and warmth when in hospital. However, Chapman (1853) took a different view and wrote: 'Porter in moderation is almost always necessary in hospital cases, and in confirmed spirit drinkers no experienced surgeon would venture to prohibit altogether the accustomed stimulus.'

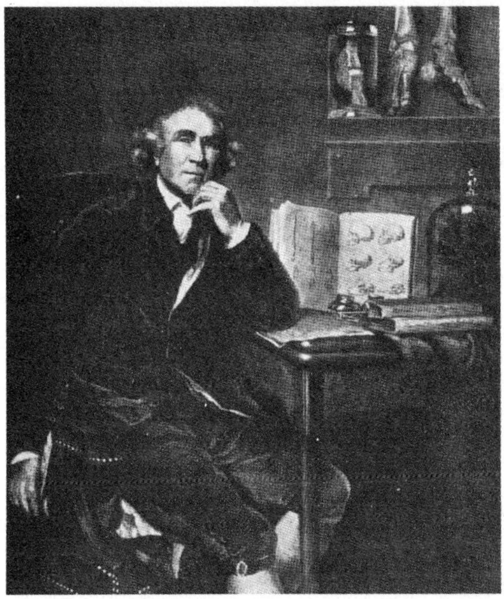

Fig. 2.17 John Hunter (1728–1793). From the painting in the Royal College of Surgeons of England by Reynolds.

CONCLUSION

The history of varicose veins and leg ulcers has been traced and we have noted the influence of the humoral and mechanical theories, and the pathophysiological approach to the subject both on views concerning the aetiology of these conditions and on methods of treatment.

Samuel Butler (1835–1902) wrote: 'The history of art is the history of revivals.' It might well have been said of the history of medicine.

REFERENCES

Allen, E. V., Barker, N. W. & Hines, E. A., Jun. (1946) *Peripheral Vascular Diseases*. Philadelphia: Saunders.

Astruc, J. (1761–65) *Traité des Maladies des Femmes*. Paris, Cavelier.

Avicenna. *De ulcerib. Lib. IV*. Quoted by Underwood (1783).

Babcock, W. W. (1907) A new operation for the extirpation of the varicose veins of the leg. *New York med. J.*, **86**, 153.

Barbette, P. (1675) *The Practice of The Most Successful Physitian Paul Barbette*. With notes of F. Deckers. London: Brome.

Bauer, G. (1948) The aetiology of leg ulcers and their treatment by resection of the popliteal veins. *J. int. Chir.*, 937.
Baynton, T. (1797) *A New Method of Treating Old Ulcers of the Legs.* Bristol: Biggs.
Bell, B. (1789) *A Treatise on the Theory and Management of Ulcers.* Edinburgh: Elliot.
Bisgaard, H. (1948) *Ulcers and Eczema of the Leg Sequels of Phlebitis, etc.* Copenhagen: Munksgaard.
Boyd, A. M. (1948) Discussion on primary treatment of varicose veins. *Proc R. Soc. Med.*, **41**, 631.
Brodie, B. C. (1816) Observations on the treatment of varicose veins of the legs. *Med.-chir. Trans.*, **7**, 195.
Brodie, B. C. (1846) *Lectures Illustrative of Various Subjects in Pathology and Surgery.* London: Longmans.
Buchan, W. (1822) *Domestic Medicine; or a Treatise on the Prevention and Cure of Diseases.* London: Lewis.
Celsus, A. C. Trans. James Grieve (1756) *Of Medicine in Eight Books.* London: Wilson and Durham.
Chapman, H. T. (1853) *Treatment of Obstinate Ulcers and Cutaneous Eruptions on the Leg without Confinement*, 2nd edn. London: Churchill.
Chapman, H. T. (1864) *Varicose Veins: their Nature, Consequences, and Treatment*, 2nd edn. London: Churchill.
Chauliac, G. De (1363) Trans. E. Nicaise (1890) *La Grande Chirurgie de Guy de Chauliac.* Paris: Alcan.
Clough, A. H. (1859) Dryden's Trans. *Plutarch's Lives.* Vol. III, 53. London: Sampson Low.
Cooper, A. (1824) *The Lectures of Sir Astley Cooper Bart., on the Principles and Practice of Surgery.* London: Thomas.
Critchett, G. (1849) *Lectures on the Cause and Treatment of Ulcers of the Lower Extremity.* London: Churchill.
Davat (1883) Cited by Allen, Barker, and Hines (1946).
Davis, D. D. (1822) The proximate cause of phlegmasia dolens. *Med.-chir. Trans.*, **12**, 419.
Dionis, P. (1708) *Cours d'Opérations de Chirurgie.* Brussels: Les frères t'Serstevens et Claudinot.
Else, J. (1771) Account of a successful method of treating sore legs. *Med. Obsns.*, **4**, 347.
Erichsen, J. (1853) *The Science and Art of Surgery.* London: Walton.
Ettmülleri, M. (1688) *Opera Omnia.* Frankfort: Zunneri.
Fabricius ab Aquapendente. *Opera Chirurgica.* Cited by Hodgson, J. (1815).
Fernel, J. (1604) *Universa Medicina, Ambiani Pathologiae.* Coloniae Allobrogum.
Ferriar, J. (1810) *An affection of the lymphatic vessels hitherto misunderstood.* Medical Histories and Reflections, Vol. III.
Galen, C. (1562) *Ad scripti libri*, p. 34. Venice: Vincentium Valgrisium.
Gay, J. (1868) On varicose diseases of the lower extremities. *The Lettsomian Lectures of 1867.* London; Churchill.
Harvey, W. (1628) Ed. G. Keynes (1928). *Exercitatio anatomica de motu cordis.* London: Nonesuch Press.
Heister, L. (1768) *A General System of Surgery.* (Author's preface: Helmstadt, 1739.) 8th edn. London: Whiston.
Hilton, J. (1861) A course of lectures on pain and the therapeutic influence of mechanical and physiological rest. *Lancet*, **2**, 245.
Hippocrates. Ed. F. Adams (1849) *The Genuine Works of Hippocrates.* London: Sydenham Soc.
Hodgson, J. (1815) *A Treatise on the Diseases of Arteries and Veins.* London: Underwood.
Home, E. (1801) *Practical Observations on the Treatment of Ulcers on the Leg, Considered as a Branch of Military Surgery*, 2nd edn. London: Bulmer.
Hull, J. (1800) *Essay on Phlegmas alba dolens.* Manchester: Dean.
Hunt, T. (1859) *A Guide to the Treatment of Diseases of the Skin: with Suggestions for their Prevention*, 4th edn. London: Richards.
Hunter, J. Ed. J. F. Palmer (1835) *The Works of John Hunter, F.R.S.* London: Longman *et al.*
James, R. (1743). *A Medicinal Dictionary.* London: Osborne.
Juvenal. Trans. G. G. Ramsey (1918) *The Loeb Classical Library.* Satire VI. London: Heinemann.
Keller, W. L. (1905) A new method of extirpating the internal saphenous and similar veins in varicose conditions; a preliminary report. *New York med. J.*, **82**, 385.
Le Clerc, D. (1723). *Histoire de la Médecine.* Amsterdam: Depens.
Le Dran, H.-F. (1731) *Observations de Chirurgie.* Vol. I. Paris: Osmont.
Lower, R. (1670). *Tractatus de corde item de motu et colore sanguinis et chyli in eum transitu*, 2nd edn. London: Allestry.
Major, R. H. (1954). *A History of Medicine.* Vol. I. Oxford: Blackwell.
Marianus Sanctus Barolitanus (1555) In *Chirurgia: de chirurgia scriptores optimi.* Zürich: Gessner.
Mayo, C. H. (1906) Treatment of varicose veins. *Surg. Gynec. Obstet.*, **2**, 385.
Milberg, I. L. & Tolmach, J. A. (1954). Treatment of chronic leg ulcers with absorbable gelatin sponge (Gelfoam) powder. *J. Amer. med. Ass.*, **155**, 1219.
Mondeville, H. de. Trans. E. Nicaise (1893) *Chirurgie de Maitre Henri de Mondeville composée de 1306 à 1320.* Paris: Alcan.
Morgan, T. (1725). *Philosophical Principles of Medicine.* London: Darby and Browne.
Paré, A. Ed. T. Johnson (1649) *The Workes of that Famous Chirurgian Ambrose Parey.* London: Cotes and Du Gard.
Parona (1894). Cited by Warwick, W. T. (1931).
Paulus Aeginata. Ed. F. Adams (1844–47). *The Seven Books of Paulus Aeginata.* London: Sydenham Soc.
Petit, J. L. (1790) *Traité des Maladies Chirurgicales.* Vol. II. Paris: Mequignon.
Pigeaux, A.-L. J. (1843) *Traité Pratique des Maladies des Vaisseaux. Contenant des Recherches Historiques Spéciales.* Paris: Labé et Rouvier.

Puzos, N. (1759). *Traité des Accouchemens.* Paris: Deslandes.
Quincy, J. (1722) *Lexicon Physico-Medicum,* 2nd edn. London: Bell *et al.*
Roderiguez a Castro (1603) *De universa muliebrium morborum Medicina.* Hamburg. Cited by Hull (1800).
Scott, J. (1828) *Surgical Observations on the Treatment of Chronic Inflammation in Various Structures; Particularly as Exemplified in the Diseases of the Joints.* London: Longman *et al.*
Sharp, S. (1758) *A Treatise on the Operations of Surgery,* 7th edn. London: Tonson.
Spender, J. K. (1868) *A Manual of the Pathology and Treatment of Ulcers and Cutaneous Diseases of the Lower Limbs.* London: Churchill.
Spier, I. R. & Cliffton, E. E. (1954). Local ambulatory treatment of chronic leg ulcers with hyaluronidase, plasminogen, and antibiotics. *Surg. Gynec. Obstet.,* **98**. 667.
The Medical Works of Hippocrates. Ed. J. Chadwick & W. N. Mann (1950). Oxford: Blackwell.
Trendelenburg, F. (1891) *Beitr. Klin. Chir.,* **7**, 195.
Troensegaard-Hansen, E. (1950) Amniotic grafts in chronic skin ulceration. *Lancet,* **1**, 859.
Trousseau, A. (1865) Phlegmasia alba dolens. In *Clinique Médicale de l'Hotel-Dieu de Paris,* 2nd edn. Vol. III. Paris: Baillière.
Underwood, M. (1783) *A Treatise upon Ulcers of the Legs.* London: Mathews.
Verneuil, A. (1855) Du siége réel et primitif des varices des membres inferieurs. *Gaz. méd. Paris,* **10**, 524.
Vicary, T. (1636) *The Englishman's Treasure.* London: Alsop and Fawcet.
Warwick, W. T. (1931) *The Rational Treatment of Varicose Veins and Varicocele.* London: Faber and Faber.
Whately, T. (1799) *Practical Observations on the Cure of Wounds and Ulcers on the Legs without Rest.* London: Cadell and Davies.
White, C. (1784) *An Inquiry into the Nature and Cause of the Swelling in One or Both of the Lower Extremities, which Sometimes Happens to Lying-in Women.* Warrington.
Wiseman, R. (1676) *Several Chirurgical Treatises.* London: Royston and Took.
Wright, A. Dickson (1930) Treatment of varicose ulcers. *Brit. med. J.,* **2**, 996.

3. The Surgical Anatomy of the Veins of the Lower Limb

The anatomy of the arterial system is relatively constant; that of the venous system is subject to individual variation. This chapter will be concerned with presenting the basic pattern, and no attempt will be made to include every minor divergence. To do so would not only be tedious but would obscure important surgical points.

The veins of the extremity will be considered under the following headings:

1. The structure of the vein wall
2. The peripheral veins:
   (a) The superficial veins
   (b) The deep veins (inter- and intra-muscular)
   (c) The valves of these veins
   (d) The perforating veins, which connect 'a' and 'b'.
3. The iliac veins and inferior vena cava.

STRUCTURE OF THE VEIN WALL

The walls of the veins, like those of the arteries, are composed of three coats, the external or adventitia, the middle or media and the internal or intima. In the smallest veins these three coats are difficult to distinguish. The main difference between veins and arteries lies in the comparative weakness of the muscular middle coat in the former.

The external coat consists mainly of collagen fibres, largely longitudinal. In the larger veins it contains bundles of longitudinal, smooth muscle. The adventitia contains tiny blood vessels (vasa vasorium) and sympathetic nerve fibrils.

The middle muscular coat varies considerably between veins of different calibre. In venules (diameter between 0·2 and 1·0 mm) it is thin and composed almost exclusively of smooth muscle. In the small and medium sized veins (diameter 1 to 9 mm), it consists of connective tissue with smooth muscle fibres usually arranged circumferentially but sometimes longitudinal in the innermost part. Muscle fibres are well developed in the main superficial veins of the leg, the long and short saphenous, which have considerable contractile power. The media is less well developed in the smaller tributaries of these veins, which are consequently more liable to dilate and become tortuous and varicose in response to sustained high intravascular pressures.

In the large veins, which include the upper femoral and the iliac veins, the smooth muscle is much reduced and in the inferior vena cava is entirely lacking. In these veins the adventitia to some extent takes over the function of the media and their contractile power is more limited than that of the medium sized veins.

The internal coat or intima consists of endothelial cells which, in the medium sized and large veins, is supported on a subendothelial layer of connective tissue. This layer is lacking in the venules and small veins. An internal elastic lamina is present in the subendothelial layer of the larger veins. Special endothelial cells produce 'activator' which converts plasminogen into plasmin, and is responsible for fibrinolysis (see Chap. 14).

Unlike arteries, veins possess valves which direct blood flow towards the heart. Most valves have two leaflets consisting of folds of the intima reinforced centrally with connective tissue; the free edge of the leaflets lie in the direction of blood flow.

THE PERIPHERAL VEINS

The peripheral veins are considered under four headings: the superficial, the deep (inter- and intra-) muscular, valves and perforating veins.

The superficial venous system

The superficial veins lie in the subcutaneous fat where they are observable in three strata. First, the thin-walled subcuticular vessels or venules, which form a considerable plexus under the skin. In varicosis venules in the skin become visible. These venules join to make a network of larger subcutaneous veins of moderate size, and are the veins which form most of the prominent superficial varices following incompetence of the main trunks. The third layer consists of the main trunks of the long and short saphenous veins *which lie on the deep fascia*.

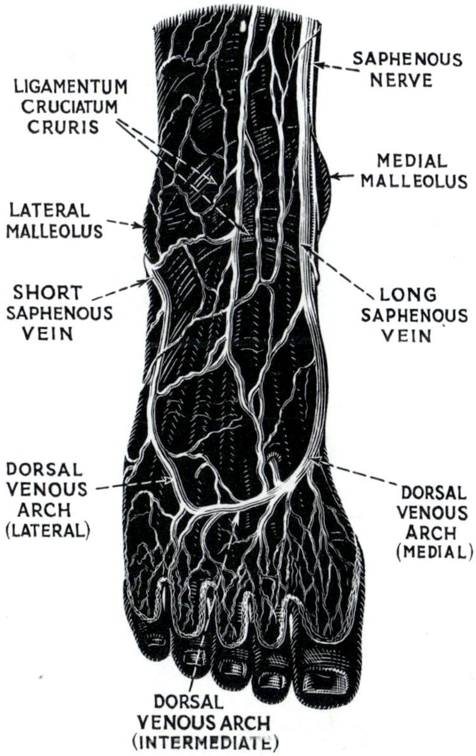

Fig. 3.1 Venous drainage of foot and ankle.

DRAINAGE FROM THE TOES AND FOOT (Fig. 3.1)

Each toe has four digital veins, two dorsal and two plantar. The dorsal digital veins join in the toe clefts to form the dorsal metatarsal veins which unite to form a dorsal venous arch. The dorsal arch is linked with medial and lateral marginal veins which run along the inner and outer borders of the foot. Ultimately the medial part of the dorsal venous arch is continued upwards as the long saphenous vein. The lateral marginal vein, which is less well defined and smaller than its medial counterpart, communicates with the short saphenous vein by way of the venous plexus behind and below the external malleolus.

The small venae comites of the dorsalis pedis artery are of little functional significance.

The plantar digital veins form the four deep metatarsal veins which run between the metatarsal bones and unite to form the deep plantar venous arch, which lies in association with the deep plantar arterial arch.

The dorsal and plantar digital and metatarsal vein communicate with each other freely at the roots of the toes between the metatarsal bones. The plantar digital veins also communicate with the adjacent superficial vessels in the sole of the foot to form a plantar subcutaneous venous arch which has numerous connections extending backwards to the veins of the heel, and by twigs to the lateral and medial marginal veins.

The numerous perforating veins of the foot are valved in such a way that most venous drainage from the dorsum passes to the long and short saphenous veins at the ankle and from the plantar surface to the posterior tibial veins (Fegan and Pegum, 1968).

THE HEEL

Beneath the skin of the heel there is a considerable venous plexus, which communicates by many small channels with the deep and superficial veins of the sole, and with the dorsal and plantar cutaneous veins.

THE LONG OR INTERNAL SAPHENOUS VEIN (Figs. 3.2 and 3.3) (Syn. great or large saphenous vein or saphena magna)

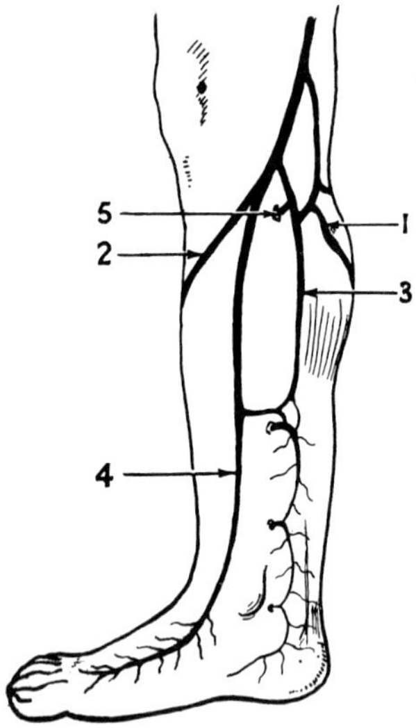

Fig. 3.2 The tributaries at or about knee level. 1. The connection with the external saphenous vein. 2. A tributary from the anterior surface of the leg. 3. The posterior arch tributary which also links the three internal ankle perforating veins. 4. The internal saphenous vein. 5. A constant direct communicating vein.

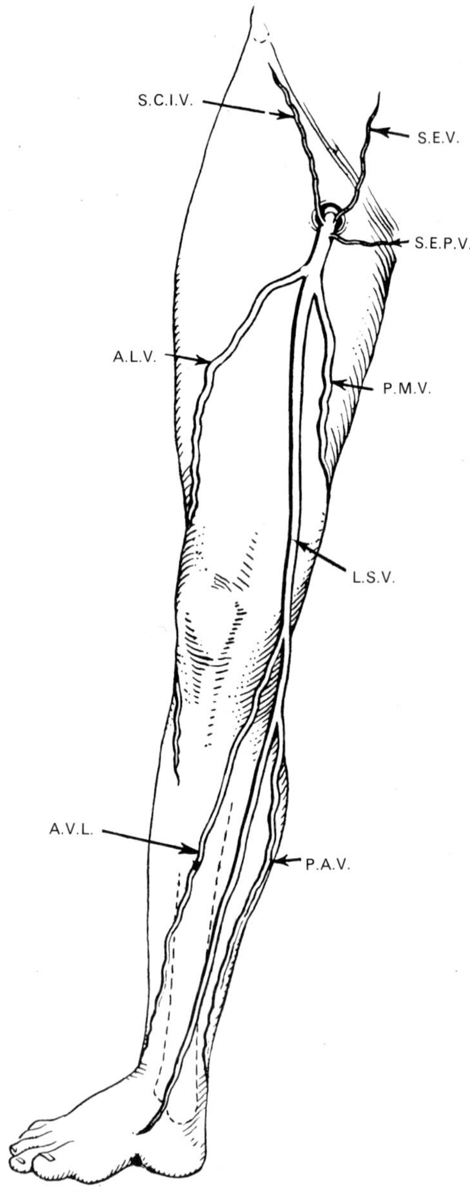

Fig. 3.3 The internal saphenous vein with its tributaries.
S.C.I.V. = Superficial circumflex iliac vein.
S.E.V. = Superficial epigastric vein.
S.E.P.V. = Superficial external pudic vein.
P.M.V. = Postero-medial vein.
L.S.V. = Long saphenous vein.
P.A.V. = Posterior arch vein.
A.V.L. = Anterior vein of leg.
A.L.V. = Antero-lateral vein of thigh.

The long saphenous vein is the longest vein in the body. It is formed by the union of veins from the inner part of the foot and the medial marginal vein and runs upwards for 1 to 1·5 inches in front of the medial malleolus of the tibia. It ascends the anterointernal part of the leg and thigh to end in the common femoral vein at the groin by going through the foramen ovale, an opening in the deep fascia. A thin prolongation of the femoral sheath passes down and ensheathes the last centimetre of the long saphenous vein and until this is dissected off, the foramen ovale is inconspicuous (the cribriform fascia).

At the ankle the position of the long saphenous vein is fairly constant, lying in the groove between the anterior border of the medial malleolus and the tendon of tibialis anterior. It extends obliquely backwards over the subcutaneous medial surface of the lower fourth of the tibia and along the medial border of this to the medial condyle of the femur and over the posteromedial aspect of the knee.

From here it climbs slightly forwards upon the anterointernal aspect of the thigh and into the foramen ovale to join the common femoral vein. It is occasionally duplicated from the knee to the groin and this can render it useless as an arterial substitute in operating to relieve femoral artery occlusion. Duplication may also result in inadequate removal of incompetent main channels in the surgery of varicose veins.

The landmark of the saphenofemoral junction

This is variously described. A reliable surface marking is 1 to 1·25 inches (2·5 to 3·25 cm) below and lateral to the pubic tubercle. (See Fig. 8.7). It is advisable to use this bony point as a surgical landmark, as the skin fold of the groin is unreliable, the saphenofemoral junction being below it in thin people and above it sometimes in the obese.

The long saphenous vein and the deep fascia

The relation of the long saphenous vein to the deep fascia is of surgical importance. In the lower two-thirds of the leg and in the upper two-thirds of the thigh the vein lies on and is closely applied to the deep fascia. As it crosses the knee joint it becomes more superficial and is often subcuticular. Because of its generally deep situation, the long saphenous vein is usually invisible except in spare, muscular limbs and when it is much enlarged.

The structures accompanying the long saphenous vein

In the foot and leg the saphenous nerve lies close beside the long saphenous vein. The nerve approaches the vein below the knee after piercing the fibromuscular roof of the adductor canal and going between the sartorius and gracilis muscles. The nerve is most closely applied to the vein in the lower two-thirds of the leg and here it is often injured in exploring or stripping the saphenous vein (see Fig. 8.20) (p. 127).

At the knee the saphenous branch of the descending genicular artery accompanies the long saphenous vein. This artery may become an important collateral vessel following thrombotic obstruction of the femoral artery in the adductor canal.

In the thigh twigs of the medial femoral cutaneous nerve run in the vicinity of the vein, although they are not closely applied to it.

Throughout its length the long saphenous vein is accompanied by lymphatic trunks draining the dorsum of the foot and the anterior and medial aspects of the leg and thigh. These end in the superficial group of inguinal lymph nodes (see Fig. 16.21) (p. 244).

Tributaries and communications of the long saphenous vein

Below the ankle this vein is fed by the medial marginal vein whose tributaries have already been described.

In the leg the long saphenous vein has few tributaries. There is a constant small connection between it and the upper of the three internal ankle perforating veins (Fig. 3.2), and there may be one or two small tributaries from the anterior aspect of the leg joining it in its lower third. Occasionally there is a small connection with the venous arch joining the internal ankle perforating veins. There is a free anastomosis between a tributary or tributaries of the short saphenous vein and the venous arch connecting the internal ankle perforating vein, by a vein running behind the tendo achilles. By this means the long and short saphenous system are connected in the lower third of the leg. These tributaries however are small and vary in number and size.

Around the knee the long saphenous vein receives no constant major tributary below the knee, but at this level it usually receives three large vessels or groups of vessels (Figs 3.2 and 3.3). These are: (1) *a calf group* which drain an area of the calf posteriorly. These veins connect with (and may occasionally replace), the short saphenous system behind the knee joint; (2) an *anterior vein of the leg* which winds up diagonally from the dorsum of the foot, ankle and anterior surface of the leg to join below the knee. It also links occasionally with a perforating vein at the middle of the anterior tibial compartment of the leg (Fig. 3.11); (3) the *posterior arch vein* which arises behind the medial malleolus of the ankle. This vein is large and constant and is formed by the union of the venous arches which connect the three ankle perforating veins. Above the upper perforating vein it passes up the medial surface of the leg to join the long saphenous vein at the inner aspect of the knee. Just below this junction it connects with the calf group of veins and therefore indirectly with the short saphenous system, and at the same level there is usually a perforating vein which joins it to the posterior tibial vein. (Fig. 3.2).

The posterior arch vein is of historical interest (sixteenth century) as it was depicted accurately by Leonardo da Vinci in one of his anatomical drawings (Fig. 3.4), and is often called Leonardo's vein.

In *the thigh* several small tributaries are received but the two largest are the posteromedial and anterolateral veins which join it close to its termination (Fig. 3.3).

The posteromedial vein is of considerable size and is formed in part by a small vein which arises from the short saphenous vein just before it enters the popliteal vein in the popliteal fossa. This vein runs up the posterior aspect of the thigh under the deep fascia. It pierces this at the medial aspect of the thigh and passes subcutaneously diagonally upwards on the deep fascia to join the long saphenous vein between its upper third and its termination. The point of connection is variable and the posteromedial vein may occasionally enter the femoral vein independently just below the saphenofemoral junction. The posteromedial vein receives numerous small tributaries from the skin and subcutaneous tissue of the popliteal fossa and upper half of the inner thigh.

At operation it can be difficult to distinguish the posteromedial tributary from the long saphenous vein for both lie on the deep fascia. It is also the main channel for drainage of the short saphenous vein in the 15 per cent of cases in which the latter fails to join the popliteal vein.

The anterolateral vein (Fig. 3.3)

This vessel drains the anterolateral surface of the thigh. It curves diagonally upwards from the outer side of the leg, knee and thigh to join the long saphenous vein in its terminal few centimetres. Figure 8.15 illustrates some of the variations in the ending of this vein. It lies in the *superficial layer* of subcutaneous tissue and is therefore more superficial than the long saphenous vein and its posteromedial tributary, both of which are deeper and less often visible when varicose. When enlarged the anterolateral vein is apparent under the skin and is often erroneously described as a varicose long saphenous vein.

The 'Hunterian' perforators

In the middle or lower third of the thigh the long saphenous vein, or more usually one of its lesser tributaries, connects with the femoral vein in Hunter's canal by a rather long perforating vein (Fig. 3.20) (p. 37).

Terminal tributaries of the long saphenous vein

As well as the posteromedial and anterolateral vein, there are several other tributaries joining the termination of the long saphenous vein which are surgically important.

The superficial and deep external pudendal vein

These vessels drain the perineum, upper inner thigh and external genitalia, running horizontally outwards from these areas.

The superficial external pudendal vein lies in the superficial fascia and is constant, it may be duplicated or triplicated.

The deep external pudendal vein is only occasionally a tributary of the long saphenous vein itself. More usually it joins the medial aspect of either the common femoral vein or the saphenofemoral junction *within* the fossa ovalis. It is present in 75 per cent of patients at operation, but because of its deep situation may easily be overlooked, unless the saphenofemoral junction and the common femoral vein are adequately explored. It is occasionally joined by the posteromedial vein (see Fig. 8.15) (p. 122).

Incompetence and dilatation of the deep external pudendal veins is one of the factors

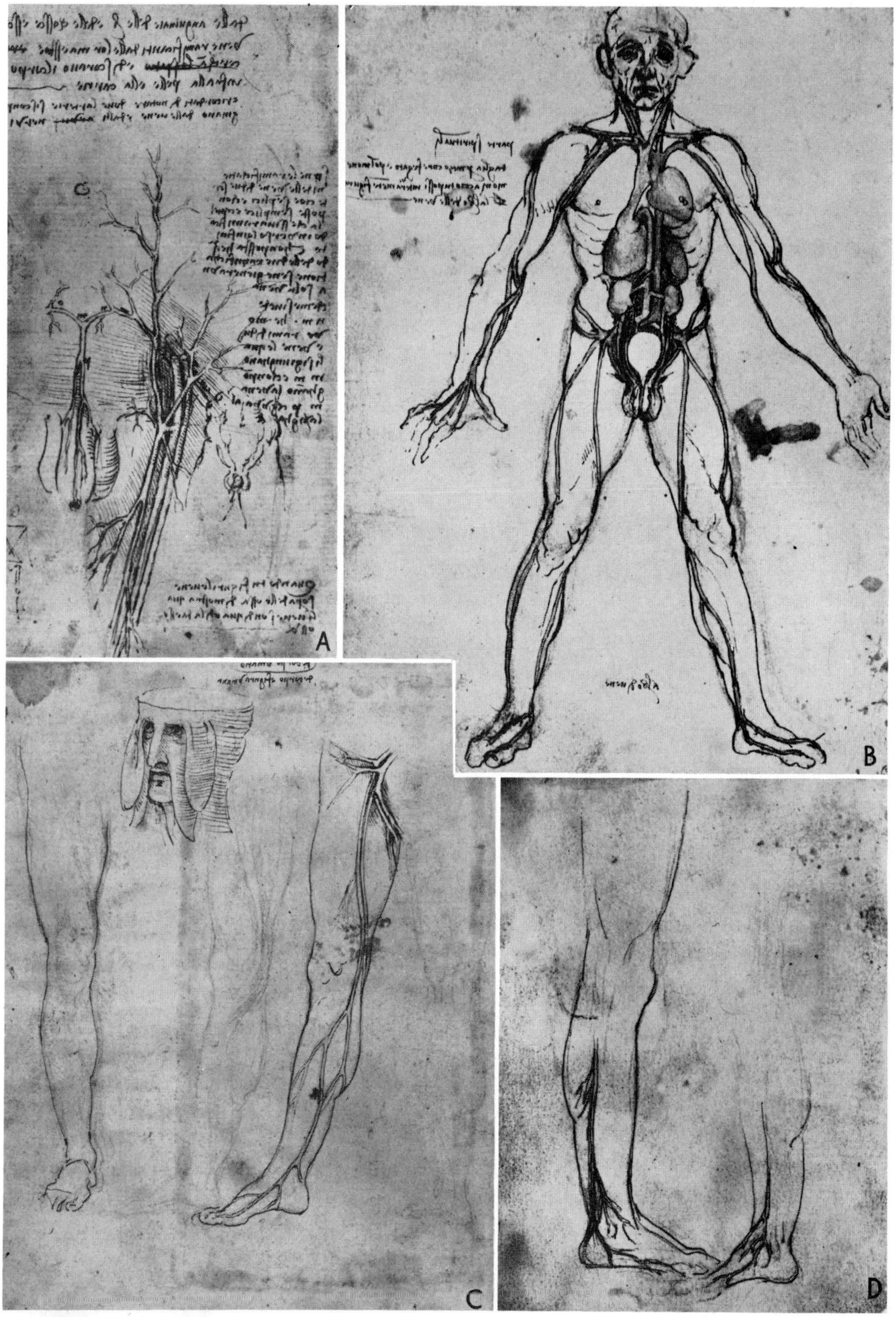

Fig. 3.4 Drawings of dissections of the veins of the leg by Leonardo da Vinci (1452–1514). A. Dissection of the origin of the great saphenous vein at the fossa ovale. B. An early drawing showing the great saphenous vein, its anterolateral tributary at the groin (compare Fig. 3.3) and the constant posterior arch vein arising just below the knee (compare Fig. 3.2). C. A drawing of the great saphenous vein in its entirety (compare Fig. 3.3). Note again that the posterior arch vein arising from the saphenous just below the knee, is clearly shown. D. A drawing of the lower end of the short saphenous vein (on the left) and the great saphenous vein (on the right) showing correctly their relationship to the external and internal malleoli. (These are photographs of the original drawings in the Royal Library at Windsor Castle and are reproduced here by gracious permission of Her Majesty the Queen.)

in the production of labial varices, which are a not uncommon complication of pregnancy.

The superficial epigastric vein

This vein passes vertically down from the subcutaneous tissue of the lower and central abdominal wall to enter the termination of the long saphenous vein. It connects with its fellow on the opposite side across the midline of the lower abdomen and also with the inguinoaxillary vein, thereby forming a connection with the axillary vein, which dilates to form impressive and important collateral channels in the event of obstruction or thrombosis of the subclavian, iliac veins or the inferior vena cava (Fig. 3.5.).

The superficial circumflex iliac vein

This drains the superficial tissue of the upper and outer aspects of the thigh and the lower and outer quadrant of the abdomen. It usually joins the termination of the long saphenous vein at the fossa ovalis, but may drain indirectly into the long saphenous vein by joining the superficial epigastric or anterolateral vein of the thigh and forming a large trunk.

The three tributaries, the superficial external pudendal, the superficial epigastric and the superficial circumflex iliac vein are always present but their manner of union with the long saphenous vein varies considerably as shown in Figures 3.5 and 8.15 (p. 122).

Duplication of the long saphenous vein

The surgical implications of this occasional findings have been discussed. Apparent doubling can be mimicked by the posteromedial tributary joining it at the foramen ovale, which vessel may be nearly as large as the long saphenous vein. Less often the anterolateral tributary may be straight and suggest a similar condition.

The superficial external pudendal artery (Fig. 3.5 and 3.6).

The relationship of this vessel to the long saphenous vein is of surgical importance. The artery passes subcutaneously inwards from the femoral artery to the subcutaneous tissues of the upper thigh, perineum and external

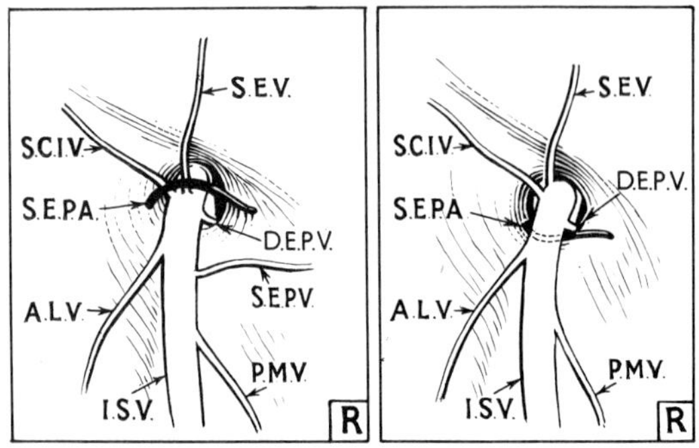

Fig. 3.5 Relationship of the superficial external pudic artery to the termination of the internal saphenous vein.

genitalia. It usually lies on the deep fascia in the curved lower free border of the foramen ovale, behind the long saphenous vein and just below the saphenofemoral junction. In about 30 per cent of patients it runs superficial to the termination of the long saphenous vein and therefore conceals the endings of the superficial epigastric and circumflex iliac veins. In these circumstances, it must be divided in order to expose these veins. Occasionally the superficial external pudendal artery may divide into two branches before reaching the saphenous vein. Both branches may pass deeply or superficially to the vein, or one may pass over and the other under it (Fig. 3.6).

Anomalous origin of the profunda femoris artery

A rare but important anomaly is a high origin of the profunda artery. It may arise

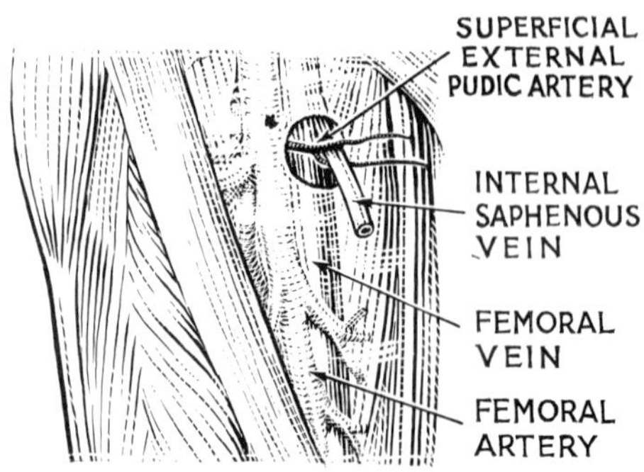

Fig. 3.6 The superficial external pudic artery bifurcating to enclose the internal saphenous vein.

from the common femoral artery immediately opposite or a little above the level of the foramen ovale. It then runs downwards and medially across the femoral vein either immediately *above* or *below* the sapheno-femoral junction (Fig. 3.7). In this abnormal and unexpected situation the artery may be mistaken for the femoral vein, and is liable to surgical injury, particularly during the operation of femoral venous thrombectomy.

Occasionally it leaves the common femoral artery at Poupart's ligament and at the foramen ovale, the common femoral vein lies between the profunda femoris artery medially and the femoral artery in its usual position laterally.

Summary. The long or internal saphenous vein extends from the medial side of the foot to the groin. Basically it has two pairs of tributaries, one pair joining it at the knee, and the other at the foramen ovale. The former consists of the posterior arch and the anterior vein of the leg, and the latter of the posteromedial and anterolateral veins of the thigh. They are subcutaneous and therefore visible when varicose. Varicosity of the long saphenous system causes one or more of these subordinate vessels to become prominent, tortuous and visible.

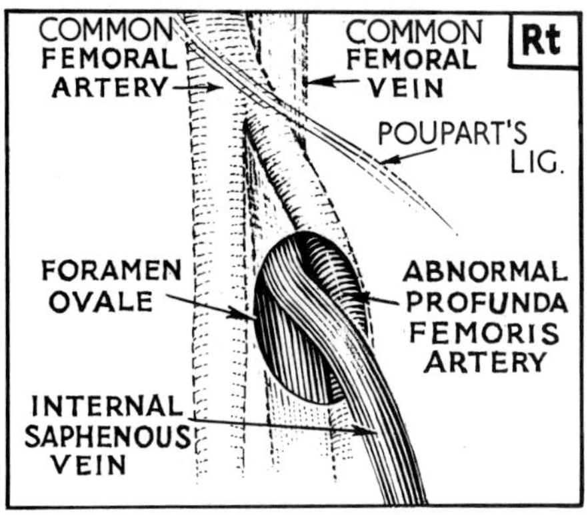

Fig. 3.7 Abnormally high origin of profunda femoris artery crossing the femoral vein and the termination of the internal saphenous vein.

THE SHORT OR EXTERNAL SAPHENOUS VEIN (Syn. small or lesser saphenous vein)

Development of the short saphenous vein represents the post-axial vein of the lower limb of the foetus which terminates in the internal iliac vein by way of the popliteal and inferior gluteal veins (see Chap. 11).

The short saphenous vein arises at the outer border of the foot behind the lateral malleolus of the ankle. It is formed by the union of the lateral marginal vein with numerous small veins draining the outer side of the heel. It passes upwards between the tendo achilles and the posterior edge of the lateral malleolus (in contrast to the long saphenous vein which lies *in front* of the medial malleolus). Two inches above the tip of the malleolus, the short saphenous vein is just lateral to the tendo achilles and from there it ascends straight up the centre of the calf to the popliteal fossa.

In the lower third of the calf it lies on the deep fascia and is covered only by skin and superficial fascia. In the middle third, it enters an intrafascial compartment in the aponeurotic investment of the gastrocnemius muscle, and in the upper third it finally penetrates the deep fascia and enters the popliteal space, lying between the heads of gastrocnemius.

The point of entry into the popliteal space is variable, being usually about 0·5 inch (1·25 cm) below the transverse skin crease behind the knee. Thus its fascial support and deep situation render the termination of this vein inconspicuous, even when it is markedly dilated and varicose. About an inch above the transverse skin crease behind the knee it turns deeply to join the popliteal vein, but this level varies considerably from 1 inch below the skin crease to 4 inches above it. Just before it ends it gives off a vein which ascends subfascially to the inner side of the thigh to join the long saphenous vein, either directly or by way of its calf group of tributaries (Fig. 3.9). A further tributary may also run directly up the middle of the thigh to the buttock. This represents a persisting post-axial vein (Fig. 3.8).

Variations in the termination of the short saphenous vein

Kosinski (1926) made 120 observations of

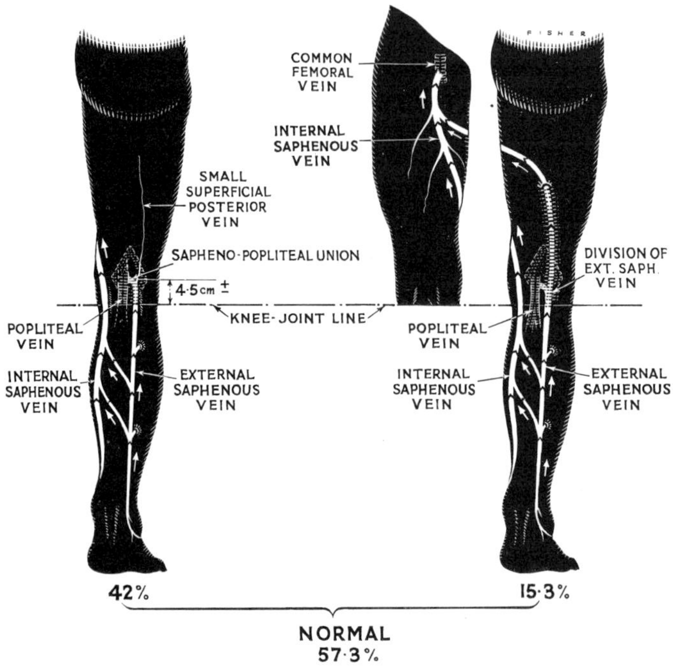

Fig. 3.8 Kosinski's variations of the external saphenous vein.

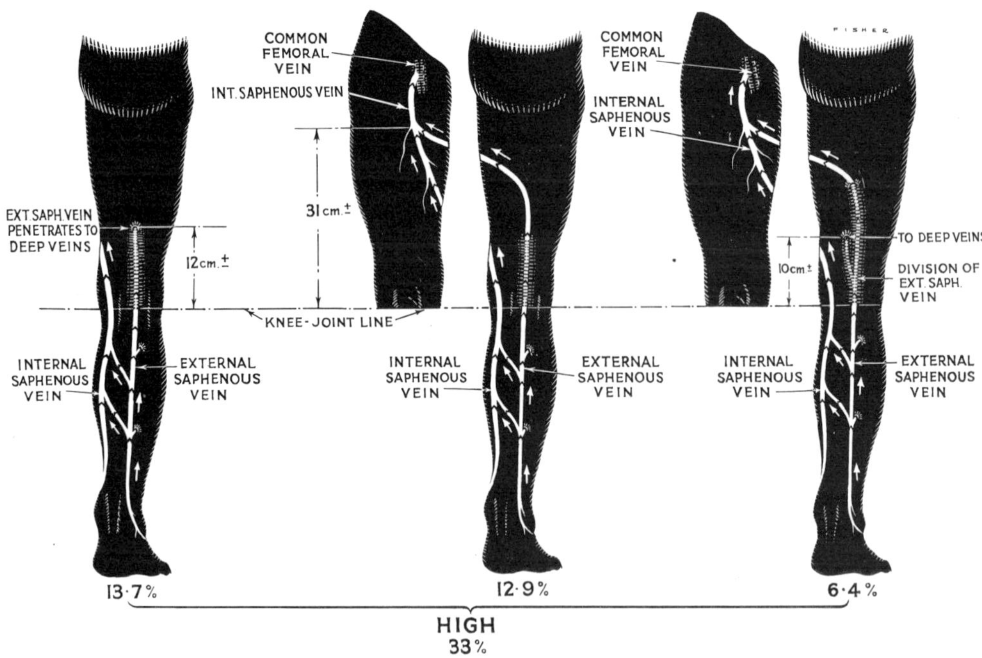

Fig. 3.9 Kosinski's variations of the external saphenous vein.

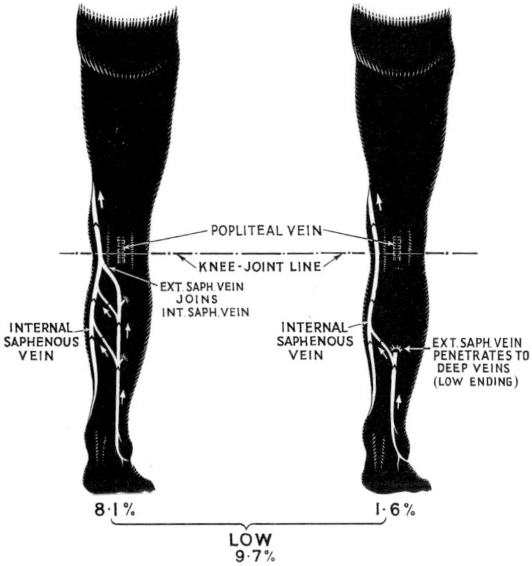

Fig. 3.10 Kosinski's variations of the external saphenous vein.

the short saphenous vein and found that there is considerable variation in its termination. It usually ends in one of three ways:

1. Normal (Fig. 3.8). In about 57 per cent it unites with the popliteal vein in the popliteal space a few centimetres above the level of the knee joint.
2. High (Fig. 3.9). A high termination occurs in about 33 per cent and the vessel ends in the centre of the thigh, either in the muscular veins, or by joining the long saphenous vein in its upper third, i.e. without entering the popliteal vein at all.
3. Low (Fig. 3.10). In about 9 per cent it joins the deep veins of the calf or the internal saphenous vein in the upper third of the leg.

Kosinski further subdivides these variations:

The normal (57·3 per cent). The external short saphenous vein unites directly with the popliteal vein in 42 per cent of cases. In 15 per cent it divides in the popliteal space into approximately equal branches, one of which joins the popliteal vein and the other ascends under the deep fascia of the centre of the posterior surface of the thigh. About the mid-thigh it becomes subcutaneous and turns medially and upwards to end in the upper third of the internal saphenous vein. (The antero-medial branch already described).

The *high termination* (33 per cent). In nearly 14 per cent the vein passes through the popliteal space unchanged and empties entirely into the deep veins of the lower third of the thigh. In about 13 per cent, the short saphenous vein joins the long saphenous in the upper third of the thigh without previous bifurcation. In 6.4 per cent these variations are combined, the short saphenous vein dividing in the popliteal space into equal divisions, one uniting with the deep veins of the lower third of the thigh; the other passing into the long saphenous vein, approximately in the upper third of the limb. In about 3 per cent the short saphenous vein also gives small twigs to the popliteal vein, and in 4·5 per cent there are connections between it and the muscular veins of the thigh.

The *low termination* (9·7 per cent). In 8 per cent of cases the short saphenous vein joins the long saphenous vein about knee-joint level. In other words the short saphenous vein may be replaced by a large tributary of the long saphenous vein ending at or below knee level. In 1·6 per cent of cases it joins the veins in the gastrocnemius muscle in the middle of the calf, its ending thus replacing the short perforating vein which normally joins the short saphenous vein at this point (Fig. 3.10).

Structures accompanying the short saphenous vein

In its lower third it is accompanied closely on its lateral side by the sural nerve, which must be preserved from injury during surgical operations. The short saphenous vein is also accompanied by lymphatic trunks which pass from the lateral aspect of the foot and end in the somewhat rare popliteal lymph nodes.

Tributaries (*See also* Fig. 7.7).

The short saphenous vein chiefly drains the lateral aspect of the heel and foot, but there are several communicating veins passing medially in the subcutaneous tissue over the tendo achilles to join the venous arches on the inside of the ankle which are connected to the three medial perforating veins. Thus it may have some part in draining the medial aspect of the ankle. This is clinically important because in this way the effects of incompetence of the short saphenous vein may be exerted on the inner as well as the outer tissues of the ankle. At the lower third of the leg it is joined on its outer side by a large and constant lateral ankle perforating vein which winds round the fibula to join the peroneal vein. The short saphenous vein also communicates with the soleus sinusoids and therefore indirectly with the posterior tibial and peroneal vein by an inconstant mid calf perforating vein.

Relationship of the short saphenous vein and the popliteal nerves

At the termination of the short saphenous vein in the popliteal fossa the medial popliteal nerve lies in close relation to it. The lateral popliteal nerve is in the outer part of the popliteal space, well removed from the vein, and is unlikely to be encountered during operation on the vein.

The deep veins of the lower limb

The main deep veins of the lower limb are the paired venae comitantes of the leg arteries, anterior and posterior tibial and peroneal. The popliteal and femoral veins are usually single conduits. They receive numerous tributaries from the surrounding muscles, corresponding roughly with the arteries.

THE ANTERIOR TIBIAL VENAE COMITES

These are the continuation of the dorsalis pedis veins. They run upwards between the tibia and fibula lying on the interosseous membrane anteriorly, closely overlaid by the anterior tibial group of muscles. At the upper fourth of the leg they turn posteriorly over the upper edge of the interosseous membrane close to the neck of the fibula to unite with the trunk formed by the union of the posterior tibial venae comites and the peroneal venae comites to constitute the popliteal vein at the lower border of popliteus muscle.

Tributaries

During their course they receive numerous tributaries from the anterior tibial group of muscles. At the lower end of the tibia a large tributary perforates the interosseous membrane to communicate with the origin of the peroneal vein in the posterior compartment of the leg. It is accompanied by the anterior perforating branch of the peroneal artery. About the middle of the leg a perforating vein sometimes joins it, after taking a rather long course and communicating with the anterior tributary of the long saphenous vein which passes over the front of the tibia and anterior tibial muscles (Fig. 3.11).

The anterior tibial vessels, because of their proximity to the neck of the fibula, may be involved in injuries to the upper end of this bone.

THE POSTERIOR TIBIAL AND PERONEAL VENAE COMITES

The medial and lateral plantar veins unite behind the medial malleolus to form the posterior tibial venae comites. These veins run upwards beside the posterior tibial artery and nerve lying on the tibialis posterior

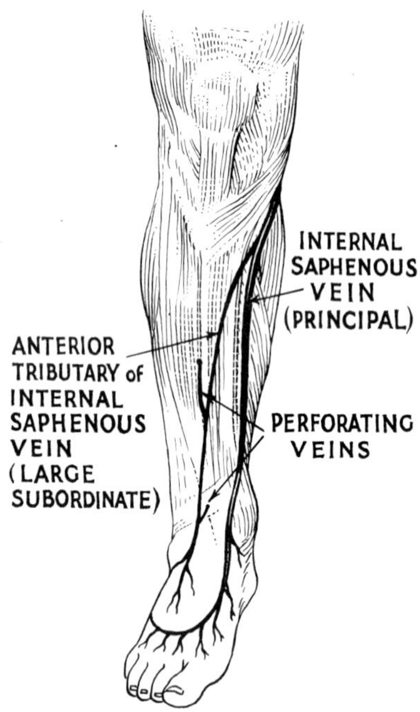

Fig. 3.11 Anterior perforating veins to the anterior tibial venae comites.

muscle, which separates them from the interosseous membrane and from the anterior tibial venae comites. (Fig. 3.12) The posterior tibial vessels lie in the posterior crural compartment and are covered superficially by a layer of fascia, soleus and gastrocnemius muscles. They receive numerous tributaries from these muscles of which the most important are the veins which form the soleus arcades. The posterior tibial vein also receives three direct perforating veins from the superficial tissue of the inner ankle. The posterior arch tributary of the long saphenous vein connects these vessels (Fig. 3.13).

THE PERONEAL VENAE COMITES

The peroneal veins are quite small in the distal third of the leg, and run deep to the flexor hallucis longus origin from the fibula in close relation to the interosseous membrane. In this region they receive a fairly constant large lateral perforating vein (Fig. 3.13), which, as it winds round the fibula, receives a tributary from the soleus muscle.

In the upper half of the leg, the peroneal veins emerge from under the flexor hallucis muscle belly to lie in the posterior compartment and here they receive several large, lax tributaries from the lateral aspect of the soleus muscle, which rapidly convert them

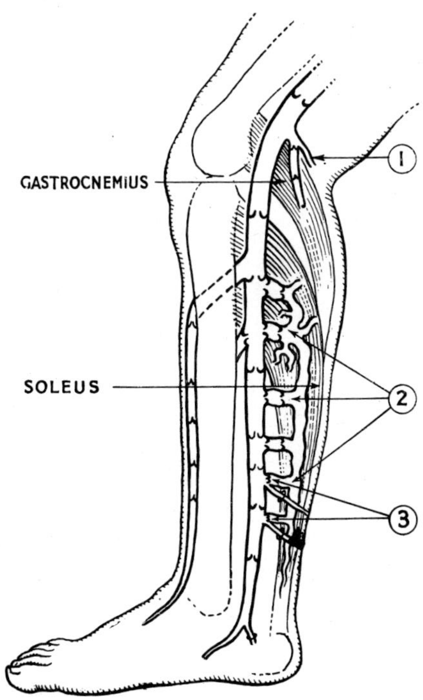

Fig. 3.12 Diagram of deep veins of leg. 1. Origin of gastrocnemial veins. 2. Venous sinuses in soleus. 3. Origin of upper and middle inner ankle perforating veins.

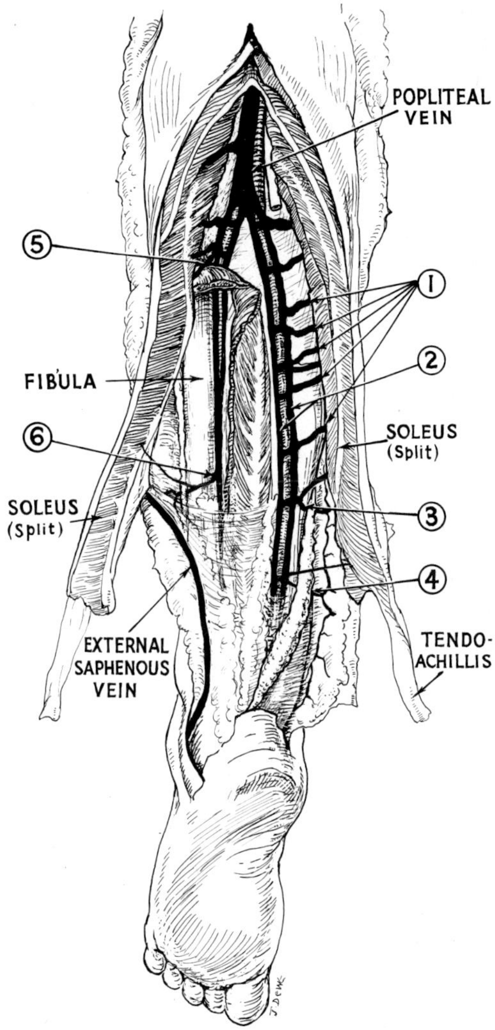

Fig. 3.13 Dissection of deep veins of posterior compartment of leg. 1. Veins draining soleus (tortuous). 2. Post tibial vena comites. 3. Upper internal perforating vein showing origin. 4. Middle perforating vein. 5. Peroneal vein (goes deep to flexor hallucis origin at this point). 6. Lateral perforating vein.

into large veins before they unite with the posterior tibial veins in the formation of the popliteal vein (Fig. 3.13). The posterior tibial and peroneal veins may communicate before their final confluence by means of a variable number of transversely running short veins in the upper third of the leg.

Venous drainage of soleus and gastrocnemius muscles

Since the first edition of this book the venous anatomy of these muscles has been further clarified by the corrosion cast technique developed by Tompsett (1959 and 1967) which has also been used by Cotton (1967). A few minutes spent studying these corrosion casts in the Anatomy Museum of the Royal College of Surgeons of England is worth a lot of time reading textbook accounts.

Figures 3.12 and 3.13 show the anatomy of the venous drainage of the calf muscles in diagrammatic form. Notice that the venous drainage of the soleus and gastrocnemius muscles, which constitute the greater bulk of the calf, differ in important aspects.

The soleus and its venous arcades and sinusoids

Most of the soleus muscle is drained by short thin veins of regular calibre which intercommunicate in an arborising pattern. The main vein forms arcades of variable length joining the posterior tibial and peroneal vein above and below at their extremities. These veins are profusely valved, the valves directing blood flow from the distal to the proximal part of the muscle and thence into the main venae comites. Soleal sinusoids occur as dilated segments of the venous arcades, they may measure up to 5 cm in length and up to 1 cm in diameter. Several short stubby veins may join to form one trunk or there may be only one large sausage shaped vessel. These sinusoids, which form the principal collecting chambers of the calf muscle pump, are generally devoid of valves, but they may be found at variable positions in the arcades. Tompsett's corrosion casts show the largest, sausage shaped sinusoids in the upper part of the calf, draining almost directly into the main calf veins just before their confluence to form the popliteal vein (Fig. 3.14).

THE SOLEAL VENOUS ARCADES AND THE PERFORATING VEINS

In the lower third of the leg the lower ends of the soleal arcades join the posterior tibial and peroneal veins. The main perforating veins penetrate the deep fascia to join the main venae comites at about the same level. Two medial perforating veins usually join the posterior tibial vein in close relation to the soleus arcade and the most proximal perforating vein may enter the lower end of the soleus vein just above its junction with the

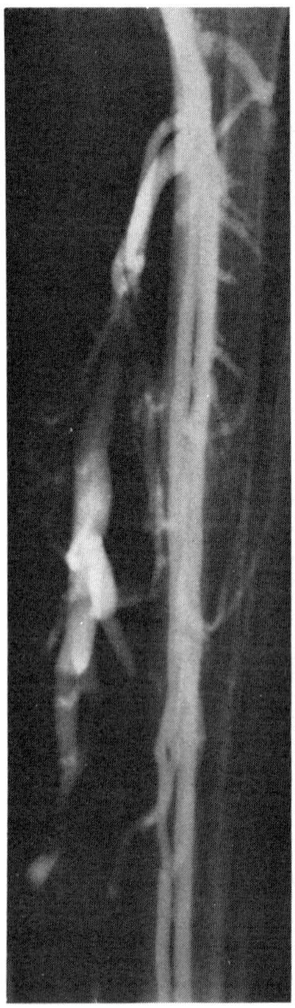

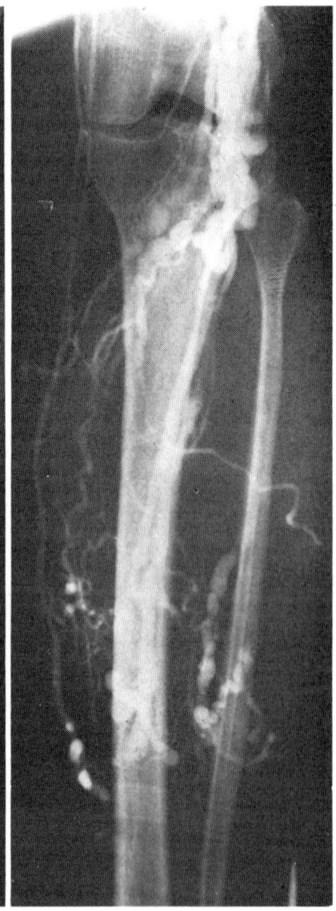

Fig. 3.14 Soleus sinusoids. Lateral phlebogram of a patient with large soleus sinusoids.

Fig. 3.15 Varicose gastrocnemial veins on a patient who had an incompetent re-canalised deep vein (proved by operation).

posterior tibial. Similarly the lateral ankle perforating vein enters the peroneal vein close to the lower end of the soleal arcade vein (Fig. 3.13).

This anatomical arrangement is probably responsible for the spread of thrombosis from the soleal sinusoids into the closely adjacent perforating veins. Subsequent recanalisation and valve incompetence in these vessels results in superficial ankle venous hypertension and later ulceration.

GASTROCNEMIUS MUSCLE

Each belly of the gastrocnemius muscle is drained by two large, valved veins which enter the popliteal vein in the lower part of the popliteal fossa. These veins are accompanied by an artery and nerve. Following post-thrombotic destruction of the valves in the popliteal and femoral veins, the gastrocnemius vein may dilate and become varicose (Fig. 3.15).

The deep fascia of the leg : calf-muscle pump

Before leaving the anatomy of this region an essential and unique point must be mentioned. The deep fascia of the leg invests the whole of the calf muscles closely, especially at its lower half where it becomes a tough aponeurosis which encloses the soleus muscle firmly. So intimate is this that when the fascia is cut during operation, the muscle immediately bulges through the incision. This arrangement constitutes an essential part of the 'calf-muscle pump'. The deep fascia, by restraining outward bulging of the muscle during its contraction, produces a high pressure within the muscle and on its deep surface during its contraction. This tension is exerted on the intra- and inter-muscular veins, in particular the soleus sinusoids, and forcibly expels the blood within them towards the heart. The mechanism of the muscle pump is dealt with in detail in Chapter 4 (Physiology).

THE POPLITEAL AND FEMORAL VEINS

Essentially the veins of the knee and thigh correspond to the arteries of these regions and consist of the popliteal vein and femoral vein, deep femoral (profunda femoris) and finally the common femoral vein.

The popliteal vein lies deeply in the popliteal fossa but is superficial to the popliteal artery which it crosses from its medial to its lateral aspect as it runs upwards. The tibial nerve is superficial to both and lies just beneath the popliteal fascia adjacent to the short saphenous vein and the flexure of the knee, but above and below this they become rapidly deeper.

Variations in the basic anatomical pattern of the popliteal and femoral vein are fairly common.

The anatomy of these veins as shown in Figure 3.16 A represents the basic normal but it is unusual for the popliteal and femoral veins to be represented by one single large trunk as shown in most anatomy books; Figure 3.16 B represents a common state of affairs where there is a main channel, with numerous venae comites, which are usually closely applied to the accompanying artery and intercommunicate in a plexiform manner. The popliteal and femoral veins may vary from an isolated single large channel as usually depicted to a plexus of intercommunicating venous channels, in which a single dominant channel can scarcely be discerned.

A further item of importance is in the region of the adductor (Hunter's) canal where the plexus of accompanying venae comites may be profuse, and there is a constant anatomosis with the profunda femoris system of veins. This connection provides an important collateral pathway when the superficial femoral vein is obstructed by thrombosis or surgical ligation. Finally, Figure 3.16 C represents a 12 per cent incidence, where the profunda vein is large and stems directly from the popliteal vein or popliteal venous plexus.

THE FEMORAL VEIN

The femoral vein ascends from the 'adductor canal' or opening into Hunter's subsartorial canal to the femoral (Scarpa's) triangle. It lies first posterolateral to the artery and then posterior to it and does not reach the medial side of the artery until it has been

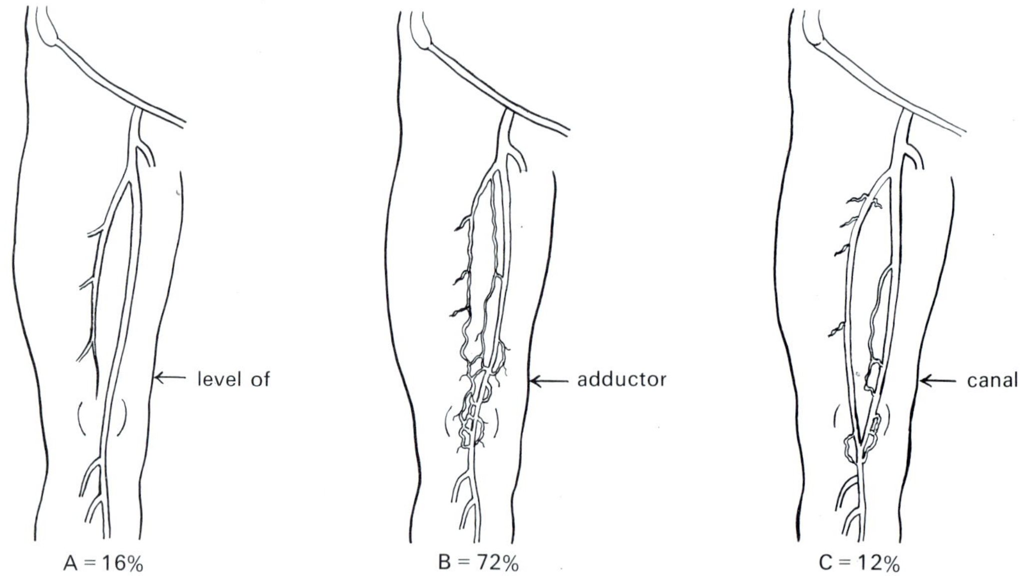

Fig. 3.16 Variation in the anatomy of the femoral and popliteal veins. These drawings present the numerous variations in the anatomy of the femoral and popliteal systems encountered in twenty-six dissections; the percentages indicate roughly the distributions of the various types. The noticeable thing is the variability in the anatomy. In group A there is one large main venous trunk, with relatively few small venae comitantes. In group B there is considerable reduplication of the main veins, as well as numerous small venae comitantes. In group C, the profunda vein travels down as a large channel to anastomose with the upper part of the popliteal vein.

joined by the profunda femoris vein to become the common femoral vein in the central part of the femoral triangle. These relations are of surgical importance in the operation of venous thrombectomy for ilio-femoral venous thrombosis. If the vein is approached too low it is often difficult to find. The common femoral artery must first be located, freed and retracted laterally.

THE PROFUNDA FEMORIS VEIN

Variations in the profunda vein have been described above. The vein lies in front of the corresponding artery and separates it from the adductor longus and the superficial femoral vein. The profunda femoris vein receives the venae comitantes of the muscular and perforating branches of its artery, and occasionally the circumflex femoral vein joins it instead of joining the common femoral vein direct. The profunda femoris vein is sometimes duplicated at its junction with the femoral vein. Our operative experience leads us to say that the union of the femoral and profunda femoris vein is 2 to 3 cm below the bifurcation of the common femoral artery.

THE COMMON FEMORAL VEIN

The common femoral vein lies medial to and slightly behind the common femoral artery. A number of tributaries enter either the superficial or common femoral vein, usually the latter. These are the medial and lateral circumflex iliac veins (venae comitantes of the arteries), the deep external pudendal vein, and a variable number of small muscular tributaries. The long saphenous vein joins the common femoral at the fossa ovalis and sometimes another superficial vein may enter independently. All these tributaries distend to act as collateral pathways in iliac vein thrombosis or obstruction.

The valves

THE VALVES OF THE DEEP VEINS

The valves of the leg veins are profuse and of great importance in the pump mechanism, whereby in the upright position, blood is returned to the heart against gravity. In the venous sinuses in the soleus muscle there are no valves, but in all the muscular veins, draining both the soleus and gastrocnemius muscles into the deep veins, valves are numerous. The posterior tibial and peroneal veins and the anterior tibial veins are closely valved, the valves being situated about every inch or so. In addition, all the perforating veins in the lower part of the calf, and all veins connecting the deep with the superficial veins in all parts of the lower limb are valved so that normally blood can only pass from the superficial to the deep veins and reflux outwards towards the skin is prevented.

The arrangement of valves in the large deep venous trunks, the popliteal, femoral, common femoral and iliac veins, is variable, but knowledge of this is important in considering the aetiology of both superficial varicose veins, and deep venous incompetence. This subject has been studied in recent years by Eger and Casper (1943), Powell and Lynn (1951), Basmajian (1952) and Cockett (1953).

In a series of dissections of the venous system of the lower limb from the inguinal ligament to popliteal fossa, the veins were opened and the number and site of the valves were studied. For the purpose of mapping out the valves, the limbs were divided into four lengths or segments shown in Figure 3.17. There was considerable variation in segment (b) as the level of origin of the profunda femoris vein varied considerably.

The findings were as follows (Fig. 3.17).

Segment A: Six out of 22 cases were valveless. The rest (i.e. 16) had 1 in this segment.

Segment B: No cases had a valve between the internal saphenous vein ending and the profunda origin.

Segment C: Eight cases had 4 or more valves. Twelve cases had 3 valves. Three cases had 2 valves. One case had 1 valve.

Segment D: Four cases had 3 or more valves. Eight cases had 2 valves. Eleven cases had 1 valve.

In one case only two valves were present in the whole vein from the inguinal ligament to the popliteal fossa. The greatest number of valves seen in the entire length was 9; the average number was 5. All the tributaries and particularly the muscular veins were frequently valved. All the valves were arranged to direct the flow into the deep vein and upwards (i.e. a centripetal stream). The most constant valve was that in the profunda femoris vein shortly before it joined the femoral vein to become the common femoral vein. The valve distribution is seen in Fig. 3.18 which is a photograph of a dissection. The highest femoral valve is where the

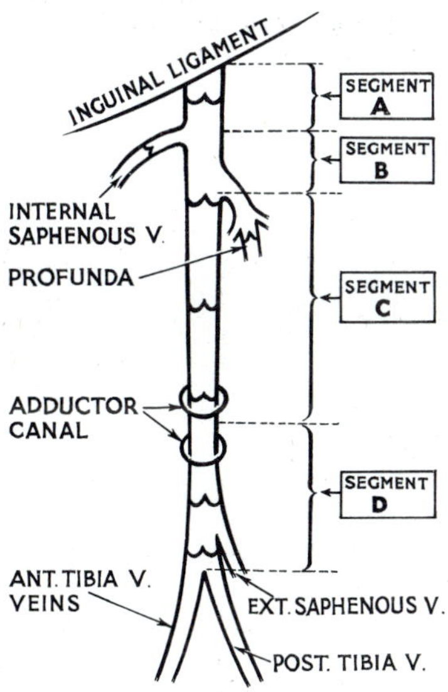

Fig. 3.17 Diagram of the arrangement of valves of the femoral and popliteal veins. A. The common femoral vein above the origin of the long saphenous vein. B. The common femoral vein between the origin of the long saphenous and the profunda veins. C. The femoral vein (or superficial femoral) between the origin of the profunda vein and the adductor ring, where the vein goes through the tendon of adductor magnus to reach the popliteal fossa. D. The popliteal vein.

profunda joins it, but the final profunda valve is an inch or more from its ending. This position of the valve explains why in many descending or retrograde phlebograms if the highest femoral valve is incompetent, the dye tends to flow into and fill the profunda system; its significance has been noted also by Boyd et al. (1953).

Valves were constantly present at the level of the adductor canal and in the mid-femoral region.

Many of these valves were tested for competence by injecting saline retrogradely down the vein. All effectively prevented the retrograde flow and were obviously sound.

We were unable to correlate the number of valves with the age of the patient in this small series, thus agreeing with the findings of Powell and Lynn (1951) based on 27 dissections.

Thus the emphasis is on the variations of normal anatomy. According to these results, from 2 to 9 valves maybe regarded as normal. Although complete absence of valves in the femoral and popliteal vein was not found in these dissections, there is venographic evidence that very rarely such cases occur (that is to say congenital absence of the valves as opposed to post-thrombotic destruction). Even in these cases all the valves in the muscular veins and in the deep veins of the calf appear to be present so that it is doubtful if even this congenital anomaly would lead to very striking symptoms. A knowledge of the variation of anatomy of these valves is important in the interpretation of venographs.

The classic work done by Eger and Casper (1943) on the valves of the external iliac and common femoral vein is illuminating, and reveals the potentiality of internal saphenous varicosis in nearly 40 per cent of people. These authors dissected out the valves of the external iliac and common femoral veins proximal to the saphenofemoral junction in 38 cadavers. Their results were as follows:

1. No vein contained more than one valve; thus in all persons only one barrier protects the internal saphenous vein from abdomino-thoracic pressures.

2. Bilateral absence of valves.
3 = 7·9 per cent

3. Unilateral absence of valves (Rt. 4, 10·4 per cent Lt. 7, 18·5 per cent)
11 = 28·9 per cent

4. Total absence on one or both sides.
14 = 36·8 per cent

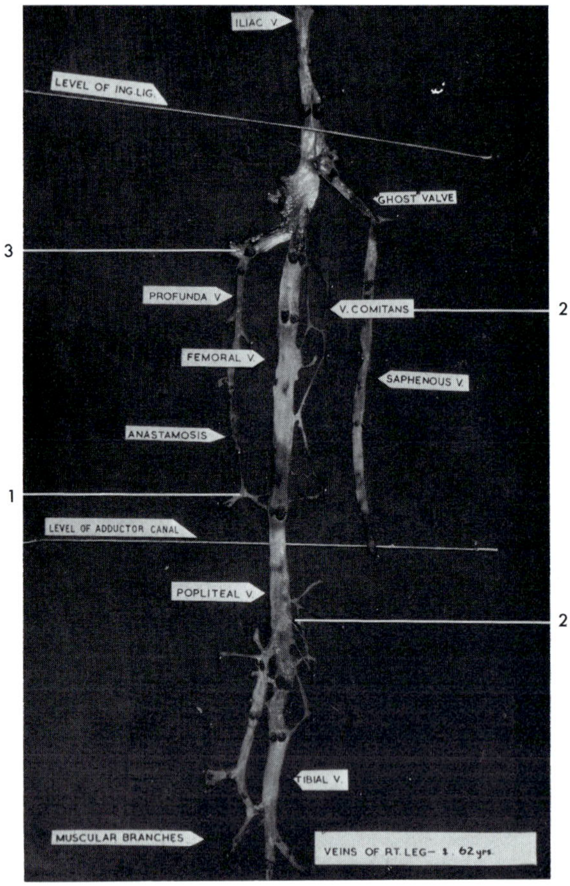

Fig. 3.18 Dissection of femoral and popliteal veins to show valves. This is a photograph of a dissection of the femoral and popliteal veins and their tributaries. The specimen was removed in toto from a post-mortem body, dissected free, opened and pinned out on a board. The valve cusps, were filled with a small plug of cotton wool soaked in methylene blue, to make them show up on a photograph. Note (1) The anastomosis of the profunda vein with the main femoral vein taking place by small branches at the level of the adductor canal. (This is a constant finding.) (2) The venae comitantes in both the femoral and the popliteal regions. (3) The situation of the first profunda valve.

Rt. ext. iliac vein valveless but one valve in common femoral vein. 21 = 55·2 per cent
Lt. ext. iliac vein valveless but one valve in common femoral vein. 20 = 52·6 per cent
Rt. femoral vein valveless but ext. iliac vein one valve. 4 = 10·4 per cent
Lt. femoral vein valveless but ext. iliac vein one valve 2 = 5·2 per cent

Recalling that the common iliac veins and inferior vena cava are valveless this study reveals that:

1. Normally the thoracoabdominal pressures on the veins of the lower limb are resisted by a single valve in the external iliac or common femoral veins.

2. The valve in the external iliac or femoral vein is absent bilaterally in 7·9 per cent and unilaterally in 28·9 per cent thus in these types (totalling 36·8 per cent) thoracoabdominal pressures are exerted directly on the highest valve of the internal saphenous vein, which is the possible reason for development of varicosities in this system.

3. The deep veins of the lower limbs in these 36·8 per cent of subjects are protected by the valves below the formation of the common femoral veins in the superficial and deep femoral veins (profunda veins).

In summary, the number of valves in the deep veins of the leg becomes progressively less from distal to proximal and there are none, or at best few, valves in the iliac veins. Valves direct blood from superficial to deep and from distal to proximal veins.

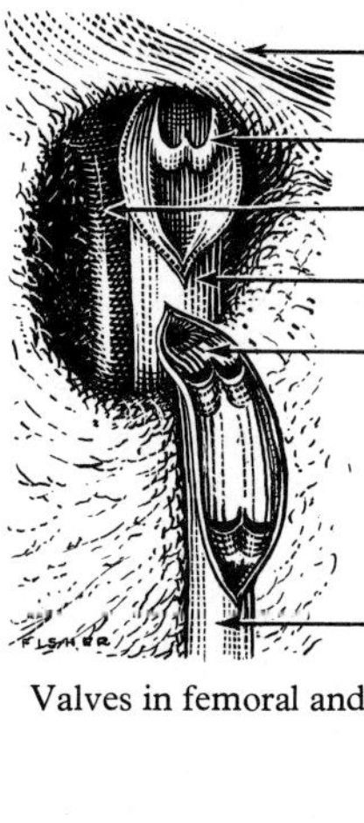

Fig. 3.19 Valves in femoral and internal saphenous veins.

The greater number of valves in the veins of the lower leg is consistent with the need to bear greater hydrostatic pressures than the more proximal veins. These leg veins are an essential component of the calf muscle pump (see Chap. 4).

THE VALVES OF THE SUPERFICIAL VEINS (Fig. 3.19) (*also* p. 135).

The valves of the long and short saphenous vein are important in the prevention of reflux and of varicose dilatation of the tributaries of these trunks. A study of the lumina of varicose saphenous veins removed at operation has shown that the valves can be divided into two types, major and ordinary.

Major valves consist of strong white cusps with firm thickened attachements to the vein wall, with obvious sinuses above them. They are conspicuous to the naked eye on opening the vein and are usually at the end of the venous trunks. We have occasionally seen one in the middle of the long saphenous vein below the point of entry of the posterior arch and anterior veins of the leg, i.e. at the level of the knee.

Ordinary valves are delicate structures. Their cusps are almost transparent; there is little or no change in the vein wall either in consistency or size of lumen where they are attached. They are not easily seen, but when a trickle of water is run on them centrifugally, the cusps float outwards, the water stream eddies and they become visible.

THE VALVES OF THE LONG SAPHENOUS VEINS

These are variously described by the anatomy books. The consensus of opinion is that there are 1 or occasionally 2 major valves in the terminal 2 to 3 cm and thereafter 10 to 20 lesser or ordinary valves to the ankle (Quain's Anatomy, 1892). Gray's Anatomy (1954) remarks that there are more in the leg than in the thigh. Whilst Beesley and Johnston (1939) state that there are 6 to 8 valves below the knee. Our inspections of stripped varicose long saphenous veins confirms the increased frequency below the knee.

In a personal communication, P. Warren, F.R.C.S., states that in his studies of apparently normal long saphenous veins from the knee to the groin the number of valves averaged 4·5 with a variation of 3 to 7.

THE VALVES OF THE SHORT SAPHENOUS VEIN

The short saphenous vein is rather more than half the length of the long saphenous trunk but it is more closely valved. It has a major valve at its termination (personal observation) and has 6 to 12 ordinary valves in its trunk to ankle (Quain's Anatomy). This follows the general rule regarding the valves of veins, that the more peripheral the vessel is, the more frequently it is valved.

The findings in varicose saphenous trunks will be touched on in Chapter 8. Our observations of the long and short saphenous veins removed at operation have shown the outstanding strength of their terminal valve. They are occasionally duplicated. Further, the valves in these defective veins are fewer than the textbooks state, especially in the internal saphenous vein.

Perforating or communicating veins

The perforating, or communicating veins normally carry blood from the superficial to the deep veins. They are of paramount importance in connection with varicose veins, and even more so with reference to ulcers of the lower third of the leg. Therefore they merit special consideration. In health they are so valved that they only permit blood to flow in one direction, i.e. from the superficial to the deep veins.

DIRECT AND INDIRECT COMMUNICATING VEINS

Le Dentu (1876) originally described perforating veins as direct or indirect. Perforating veins are direct when they pass straight from the superficial vein to the main deep veins or venae comites (i.e. the peroneal, posterior tibial, anterior tibial, popliteal or femoral). They are indirect when they pass from a superficial vein to a muscular vein within one of the large muscle bellies of the calf or thigh, and thence a further vessel connects with the main deep vein. According to Gay (1868) perforating veins usually start from subcutaneous veins of secondary size, i.e. tributaries of the saphenous trunks, and not from the main vessels. This statement is in accord with our own experience. Whilst the indirect perforating veins are small and irregularly distributed throughout the muscular part of the limb, the direct communicating veins are few, fairly large in size, and relatively constant in their anatomical position in the distal part of the leg.

THE DIRECT PERFORATING VEINS

The chief direct perforating veins are really the ends of the internal and external saphenous veins. Their terminal portions sometimes referred to as 'crooks'—like a shepherd's crook. They are best considered as perforating or communicating vessels between the superficial and deep systems which during the course of development have assumed importance in the normal superficial venous return from the leg.

They are, however, only part of a series of direct perforating veins, incompetence in any of which, by allowing a flow from the deep to the superficial veins will produce its special deleterious effect on the adjacent superficial circulation and tissues.

Each perforating vein above the ankle is valved at its union with its deep vein and also close to its perforation of the deep fascia.

PERFORATING VEINS IN RELATION TO THE INTERNAL SAPHENOUS SYSTEM

In the thigh. In the thigh there is a constant rather long perforating vein which begins in the internal saphenous vein or more usually one of its tributaries about the middle to lower third of the thigh, and ends in the segment of femoral vein below the deep femoral valve in Hunter's canal. This is shown in Figure 3.20 which is the normal size and position of the vein. Figure 3.21 shows what may occur when the valves in this perforating vein become incompetent which happens relatively rarely. This vein is occasionally duplicated.

In the leg. Just below knee level, a vein usually runs close to the posterior border of the tibia from the internal saphenous or its large tributary (posterior arch) to the posterior

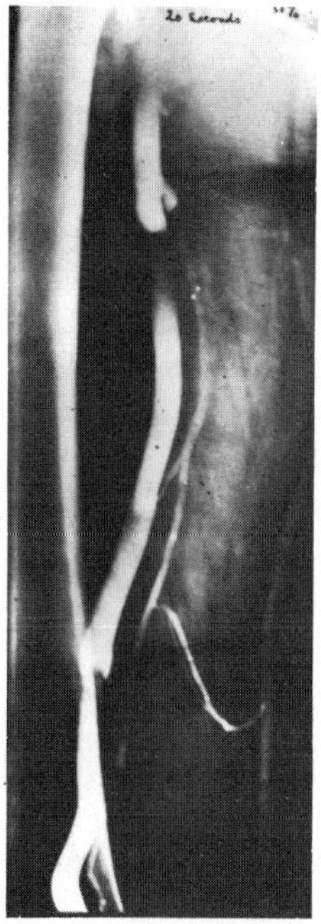

Fig. 3.20

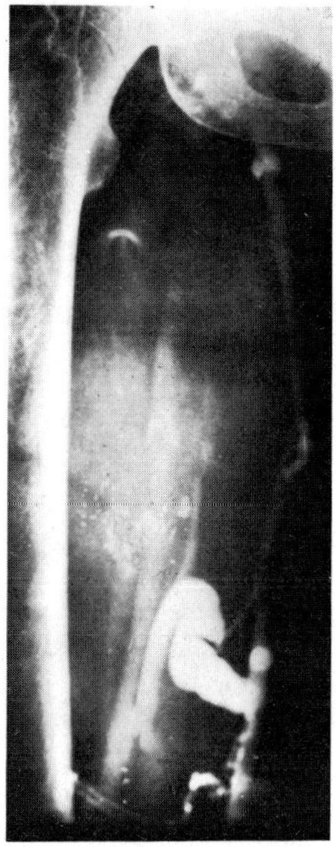

Fig. 3.21

Fig. 3.20 Normal femoral vein showing communicating vein at level of lower third of thigh.

Fig. 3.21 Venogram showing the same communicating vein as in Figure 3.20 when its valves became incompetent.

tibial veins. This is fairly constant and is shown in Figure 3.22.

In the lower half of the leg there are direct perforating veins of great clinical importance. These are known as the internal and external ankle perforating veins (Figs 3.23 to 3.29).

The internal ankle perforating veins. These three veins drain the lower and inner third of the leg; they penetrate the deep fascia and empty directly into the lower part of the posterior tibial venae comites. They are short and distinctive vessels, and there is some variation in their relative size from case to case (Fig. 3.22).

The upper one of the three is the most constant in its situation at about the junction of the lower and upper half of the leg at the posterior margin of the tibia (Figs 3.24 to 3.29). It constantly communicates with the long saphenous vein by a small tributary vein, but seldom directly. Occasionally it connects mainly with the long saphenous vein and merely gives a small tributary to the venous arch connecting it with the other two perforating veins (Fig. 3.28).

The middle perforator is fairly constant in position, usually about one hand's breadth above the tip of the internal malleolus and 0·5 inch to 1 inch *posterior* to the bony margin of the tibia.

The lowest perforator is just behind and below the internal malleolus situated over the surface marking of the posterior tibial artery and venae comites, and it is usually small in comparison with the other two, and is unimportant clinically.

There appears to be some reciprocity in size between the middle and upper of these veins. Thus, when the upper is large and well developed, the middle tends to be small, and vice versa (this is illustrated in Figs 3.23 to 3.29).

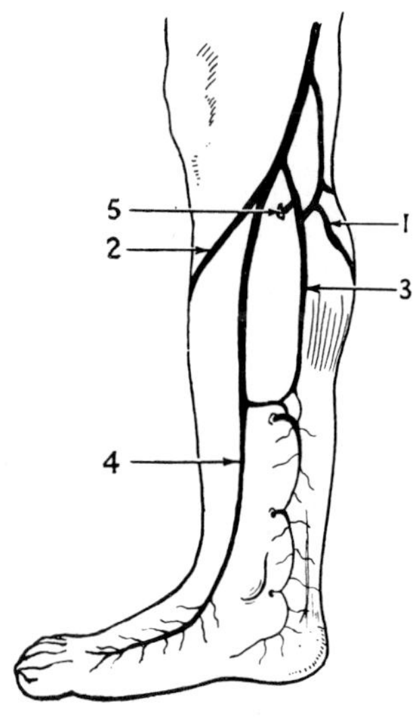

Fig. 3.22 The long saphenous vein and the internal ankle perforating veins. 1. The connection with the short saphenous vein. 2. A tributary from the anterior surface of the leg. 3. The posterior arch tributary which also links the three internal ankle perforating veins. 4. The internal saphenous vein. 5. A constant direct communicating vein.

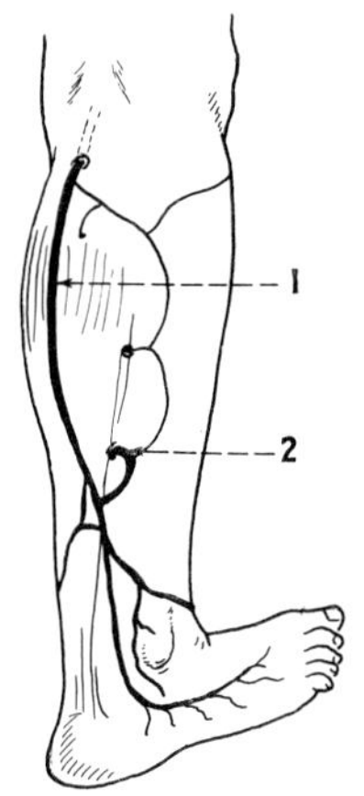

Fig. 3.23 The usual arrangement of the external ankle perforating veins. There is usually one large constant perforating vein (2) in the position shown 4 to 7 inches above the tip of external malleolus at the outer border of the tendo-Achillis. It usually connects with the external saphenous vein (1).

It can thus be appreciated that in the erect position the essential venous drainage of what is known clinically as the 'ulcer-bearing area' is taken directly into the deep veins, and not into the saphenous system. On the other hand, the effects of venous incompetence in the great or small saphenous systems can readily reach this area via their connections with the venous arches linking these perforating veins. It is into these thin-walled venous arches and the perforators that numerous small delicate vessels empty blood from the subcutaneous tissues of the ankle region.

The relation of the internal ankle perforating veins to the venous drainage of the soleus is interesting and important. A study should be made of Figures 3.24 to 3.26, which are photographs of detailed dissections of the upper and middle perforating veins on the inner side of the leg. These perforating veins enter the posterior tibial venae comites at the point where the lower end of the soleus arcade vein draining soleus joins the posterior tibial vein (Figs 3.27 and 3.28). Here too there is usually a large cross-communication between the two venae comites causing a venous pool. So here is a direct anatomical pathway for a thrombus spreading down the veins from soleus muscle to enter not only the posterior tibial veins, but also the perforating veins. The organisation and recanalisation of such a thrombus will destroy the valves of the obstructed vessels including those of the perforating vein. This occurrence in the acute state (i.e. spread of thrombus) has been seen by one of us many times at post mortem and we believe that this is probably the mechanism whereby the valves of the upper two perforating veins are destroyed rendering the vessels incompetent. The third and lowest perforating vein below and behind the malleolus has no such arrangement. It is not connected with any muscle: it is simply a direct small size tributary of the posterior tibial venae comites. Thus, there is no similar mechanism for the destruction of its valve. This is in accordance with our findings at operation. This third, lowest vein is usually small and we have seldom found it demonstrably incompetent. It probably plays little part in the aetiology of the ulcer syndrome.

This anatomical arrangement of the upper, and middle internal ankle perforators was noted and commented upon by Gay (1868). He remarked that at these points there appeared to be an alternative venous pathway direct from the soleus muscle to the superficial vein, which could be used if the deep veins were blocked.

DIRECT PERFORATING VEINS RELATED TO THE SHORT SAPHENOUS SYSTEM

There is one large constant external perforating vein whose origin has already been referred to in the position shown. (The common arrangement is shown in Fig. 3.23.) This vein joins the small saphenous vein or a tributary of it, after a characteristic looped course round the fibula at the junction of the lower and middle third of the calf on the lateral side. This vein is called the lateral, or external ankle perforating vein (Fig. 3.29); it is a direct perforating vein. As it penetrates the deep fascia it receives a tributary from the lower part of the soleus muscle and then winds

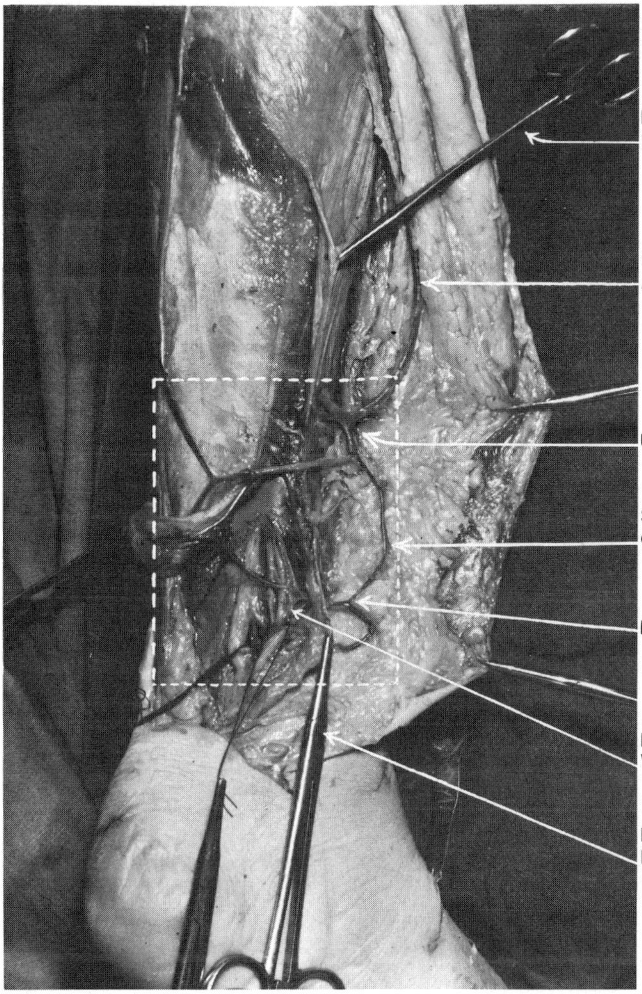

Fig. 3.24 Photograph of the dissection of an amputated leg, prepared by injecting black neoprene into the veins showing the detailed anatomy of the upper two ankle perforating veins on the inner side of the lower leg. The illustration shows the inner aspect of the lower leg dissected from behind. The upper and middle perforating veins are shown labelled. The fine venous arches connecting the perforators in the subcutaneous tissue are seen. The dotted square represents the 'close up view', Figs 3.25 and 3.26.

round the fibula to join the peroneal vein. This vessel is also significant from the point of view of ulceration of the lower third of the leg, as its valves can be destroyed by a thrombus spreading to it from the vein from the soleus muscle.

There is also a *'mid-calf'* perforating vein, draining directly into the soleus sinusoids in about 25 per cent of people. When present it also may be of clinical importance.

Direct perforating veins on the anterior aspect of the leg

About the middle of the leg from the anterior vein of the leg (a tributary of the long saphenous vein) (Fig. 3.11), a vein arises which perforates the deep fascia and pursues a long oblique course upwards to end in the anterior tibial venae comites. It is not usually large or of clinical significance.

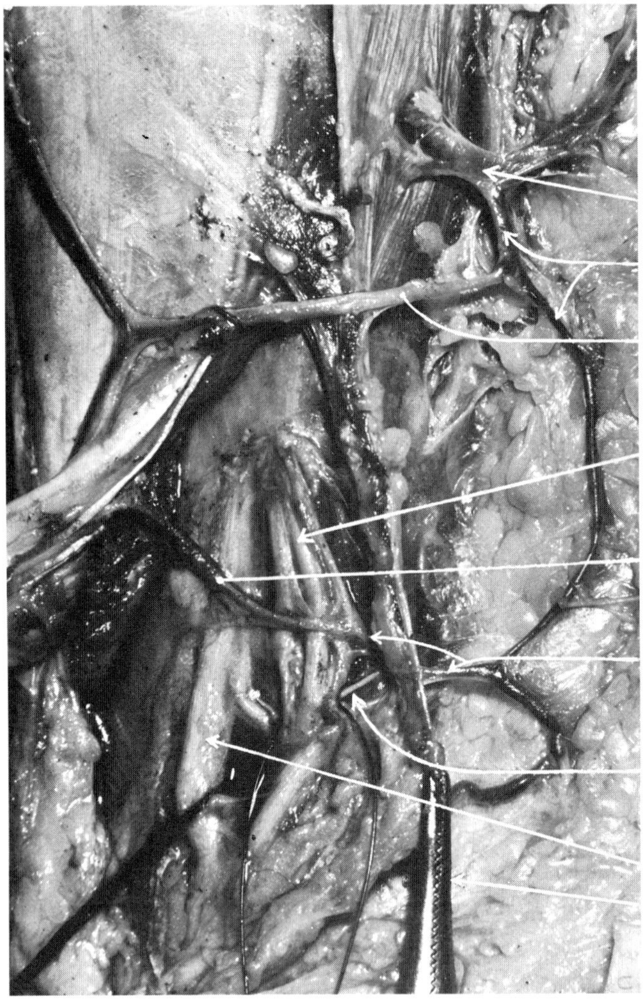

Fig. 3.25 This illustration shows the close-up (enclosed by the dotted lines in Fig. 3.24) of the region of the middle perforator. The artery forceps are holding up the deep fascia, and the vein is seen perforating it to enter the posterior tibial venae comites, and notice particularly how the vein from soleus joins in at the same point. This arrangement is also evident in the upper perforator (Fig. 3.26). The small perforating artery is well seen.

The lower ends of the anterior tibial and peroneal veins communicate with each other freely through the interosseous membrane just above the ankle forming a small venous plexus. The veins from the anterior aspect of the ankle and upper part of the dorsum of the foot, and the dorsalis pedis veins drain into this plexus. (This is the route whereby in venography an injection of diodone made into a vein of the dorsum of the foot passes deeply and outlines the peroneal and anterior tibial veins.)

The indirect perforating veins

There are a few small inconstant indirect perforating veins over the bellies of the gastrocnemius and soleus muscles and lower thigh. Most are too small to be capable of significant dilatation.

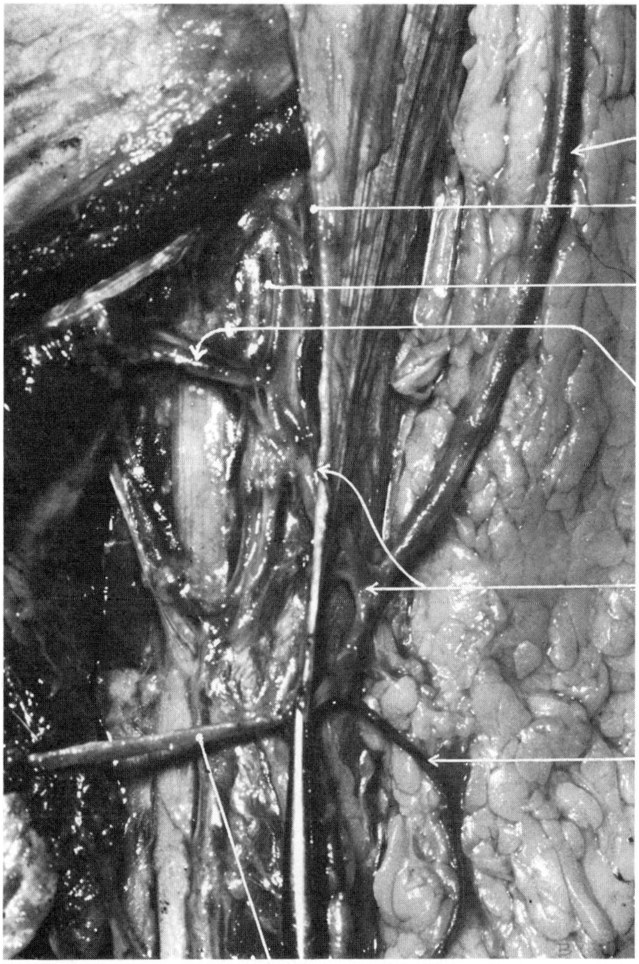

Fig. 3.26 Photograph of the further dissection of the same amputated leg, showing the detailed anatomy of the upper ankle perforating vein on the inner side of the lower leg, dissected to show its entry through the deep fascia into the posterior tibial venae comites.

Incompetent, indirect perforating veins differ from the larger, lower direct perforating veins in that although they are not responsible for induration or ulceration of the skin they do sometimes contribute to the formation of small superficial varices and they should be ligated in the treatment of these when present, but they are very rare.

The perforating veins of the foot between the superficial and deep systems are very numerous indeed (Fig. 3.30).

THE ILIAC VEINS AND INFERIOR VENA CAVA

An understanding of the anatomy of the iliac veins and their tributaries is important in the diagnosis and management of iliac vein thrombosis and of post-thrombotic venous obstruction (Fig. 3.31).

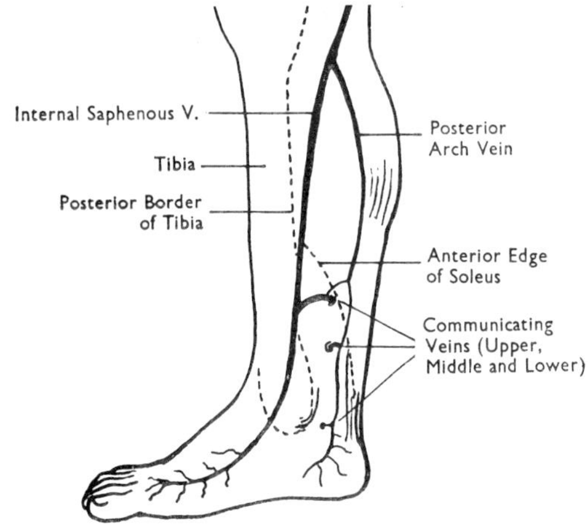

Fig. 3.27 Variation in the anatomy of the upper internal ankle perforating vein.

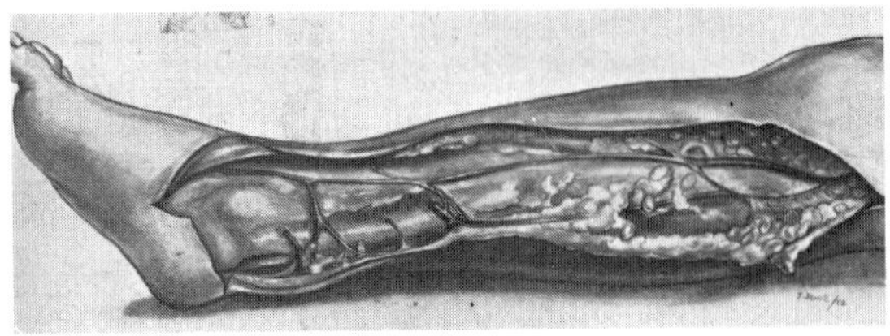

Fig. 3.28 Variations in the anatomy of the upper (large) and middle (small) ankle perforating veins.

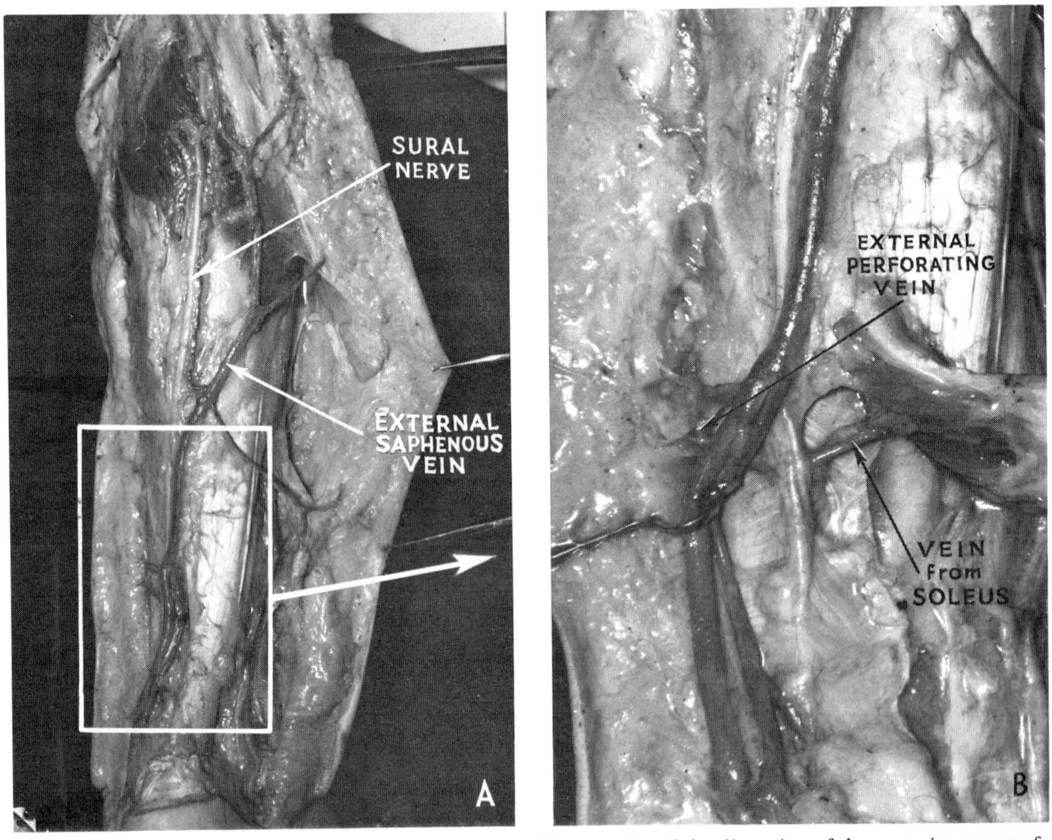

Fig. 3.29 Dissection of the external ankle perforating vein. Photographs of the dissection of the posterior aspect of an amputated leg, where veins had been injected with black neoprene. This shows the anatomy of the small saphenous vein and the external ankle perforating vein. A. General view of dissection. Note the anomaly of the upper part of the external saphenous vein (passes internally to join the internal saphenous vein). B. Close-up of the area of the external ankle perforator, with the soleus dissected up and held aside. The vein is seen perforating the deep fascia, when it immediately receives a large muscular tributary from soleus, before winding deeply round the inner aspect of the fibula to join the peroneal vein (not visible).

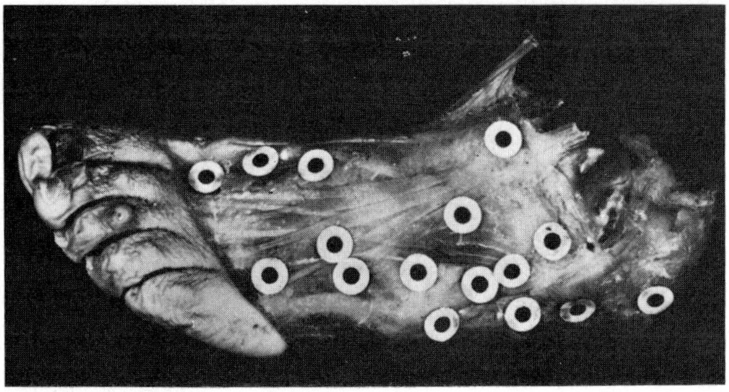

Fig. 3.30 Dissection of the foot showing the numerous sites of the perforating veins. Each perforating vein is marked by a paper marker. (By courtesy of D. A. W. Edwards.)

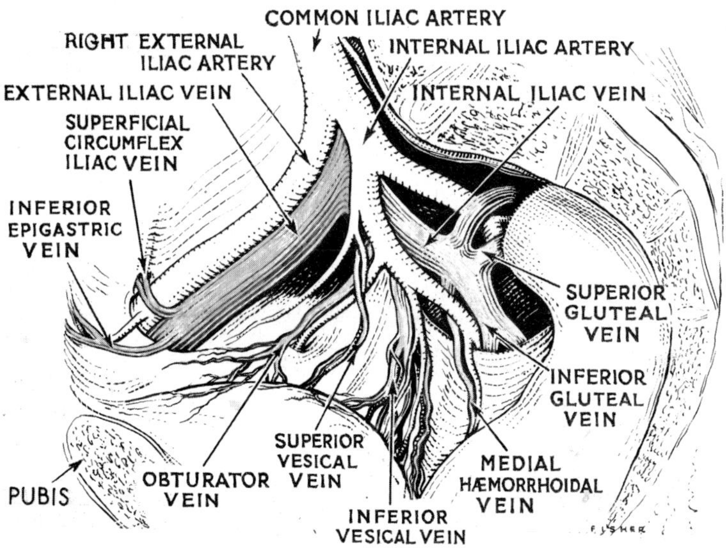

Fig. 3.31 Internal iliac vein and its tributaries.

The external iliac vein

This vein follows the line of the pelvic brim from the inguinal ligament to the sacroiliac joint, where it is joined inferomedially by the internal iliac vein emerging from the true pelvis.

TRIBUTARIES

The main tributaries of the external iliac vein are the inferior epigastric vein, which joins it anteriorly about 1 cm above the inguinal ligament, the deep circumflex iliac vein, and the pelvic vein, which connects the external iliac with the obturator vein in the obturator foramen. The deep epigastric and the pubic veins anastomose with their fellows of the opposite side, and also with the superficial external pudendal veins, tributaries of the long saphenous vein. They form important collaterals in common or external iliac vein obstruction.

The internal iliac vein

This large vein is formed in the floor of the true pelvic cavity by the union of the gluteal, internal pudendal and obturator veins which originate in the buttocks, thigh and perineum. The lateral sacral veins and the veins of the pelvic viscera (uterine veins) join it subsequently. The internal iliac vein ascends behind and slightly medial to the internal iliac artery to join the external iliac vein opposite the sacroiliac joint.

The superior and inferior gluteal veins enter the pelvis through the greater sciatic foramen. The internal pudendal vein drains the prostatic venous plexus, and the obturator veins begin in the upper part of the adductor region of the thigh. Its communication with the deep external pudendal vein makes a valuable anastomsis in external iliac venous obstruction.

The lateral sacral veins form connections with their opposite number through the sacral venous plexus. Similarly the middle rectal veins, inferior vesical, uterine and vaginal veins link with their opposites and also with the ovarian veins. Collateral pathways in external iliac vein obstruction are illustrated phlebographically in Figure 3.32, and diagrammatically in Figure 3.33.

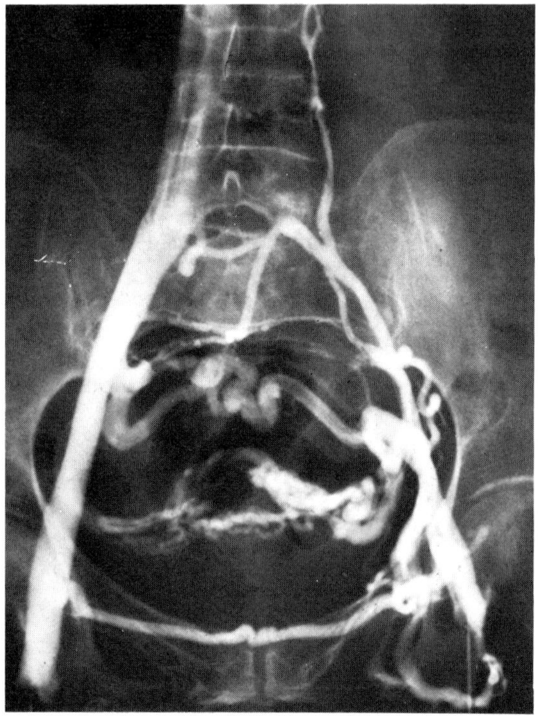

Fig. 3.32 Phlebogram showing post-thrombotic obstruction of the left common iliac vein. Pudendal, presacral and ascending lumbar collaterals are clearly seen.

The internal iliac vein may join the external iliac vein as two separate trunks, and occasionally may join the opposite external iliac vein.

THE COMMON ILIAC VEIN

This vein is a short, wide trunk which passes upwards from the sacroiliac joint to end on the right side of the fifth lumbar vertebrae by uniting with its fellow to form the inferior vena cava. This junction is one whole vertebra lower than the aortic bifurcation. The right common iliac vein and the inferior vena cava run in a more or less straight line from the pelvis upwards and the left common iliac vein joins it nearly at a right angle. Here, the left common iliac vein is forced forwards by the convexity of the low lumbar vertebrae and at the same time it is crossed anteriorly by the

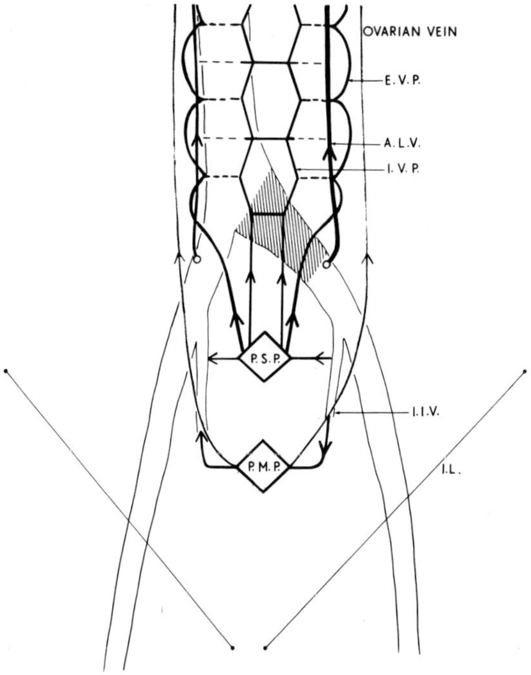

Fig. 3.33 Composite diagram of collateral veins in 11 patients with, common iliac vein obstruction (Group 2). Cross hatching indicates the extent of obstruction.

I.I.V. = Internal Iliac Vein
P.S.P. = Presacral Plexus
A.L.V. = Ascending Lumbar Vein
I.V.P. = Internal Vertebral Plexus
E.V.P. = External Vertebral Plexus
P.M.P. = Parametrial Plexus
Ovarian V. = Ovarian Vein
I.L. = Inguinal Ligament

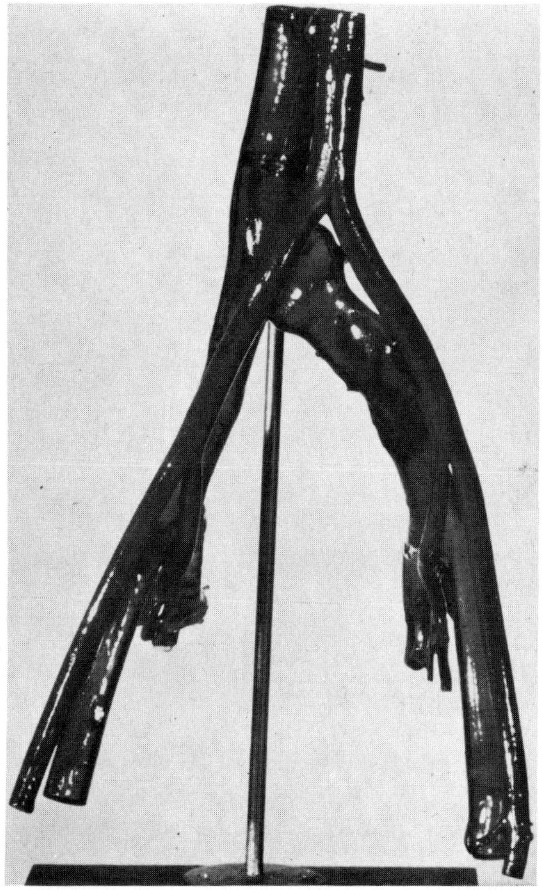

Fig. 3.34 Cadaver corrosion cast showing compression of the left common iliac vein where it is crossed by the right common iliac artery.

right common iliac artery. This combination results in varying degrees of anterior-posterior (or fore and aft) compression of the termination of the left common iliac vein (Fig. 3.34) (cast). It is sufficient to cause a radiological filling defect in about 50 per cent of patients with otherwise normal iliac phlebograms (Fig. 3.35) (Negus, Edwards and Kinmonth, 1968). This compression is compensated by an increase in lateral diameter, so that although the vein is flattened there may be little change in its cross-sectional area.

In a smaller number of otherwise normal subjects, the degree of compression is more marked and is accompanied by 'adhesion' or 'band' formation at the mouth of the left common iliac vein (Figs 3.36 and 3.37). These bands have been found in about 20 per cent of nearly 1,000 dissections (Table 3.1). In the

Table 3.1

Date	Author	Dissections	% Incidence of bands
1906	McMurrich	31	32·3
1943	Ehrich & Krumbhaar	399	23·8
1957	May & Thurner	430	18·6
	Present series	100	14·0
	Total	960	Mean: 22·2

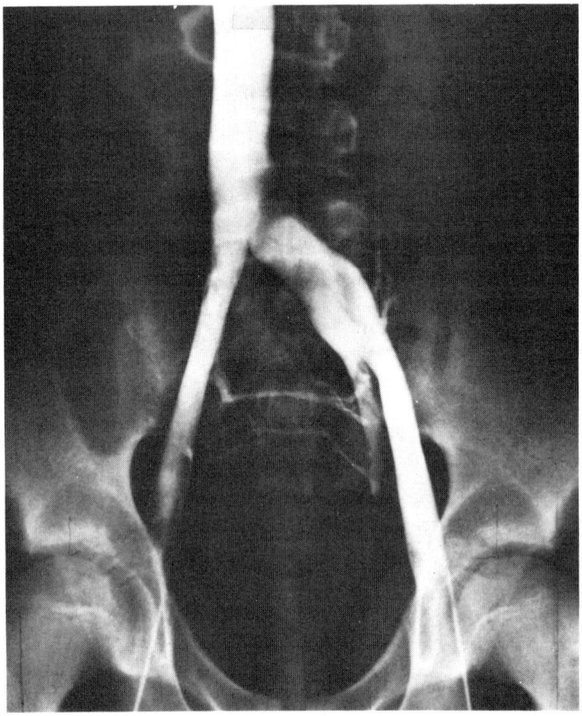

Fig. 3.35 Phlebogram showing left iliac vein compression in a 32 year old male with normal iliac veins and inferior vena cava.

author's series 'band formation' was always associated with marked compression of the vein and a decrease in cross-sectional area (Negus et al., 1968). (Fig. 3.38.).

Compression and band formation at the mouth of the left common iliac vein appear to be normal anatomical anomalies which usually cause no symptoms or physical signs in healthy, ambulant subjects. However, in the presence of a restricted venous flow and hypercoagulability which are associated with severe illness, operation or trauma, acute thrombosis of the left common iliac vein may be precipitated. It has long been recognised that iliac vein thrombosis or 'white leg' affects the left side more commonly than the right (Table

Table 3.2 Incidence of iliofemoral venous thrombosis

Date	Author	Total cases	% Incidence Left	Right	Bilateral
1902	Clarke	41	61	27	12
1940	Barker et al.	210	72	28	
1943	Ehrich & Krumbhaar	16	50	18·7	31·3
1951	Veal et al.	11	54·5	46·5	
1957	Gibbs	10	50	50	
1960	Sevitt & Gallagher	173	59·5	40·5	
1967	S.T.H. Series	88	53·5	27	19·5

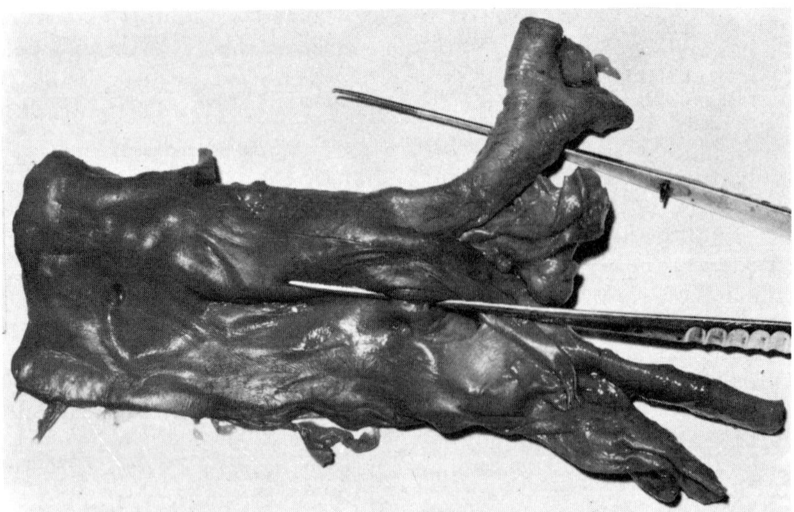

Fig. 3.36 Dissection of the inferior vena cava (opened along its right lateral side) which shows a 'band' crossing the mouth of the left common iliac vein. There was no evidence of recent or post-venous thrombosis in this patient.

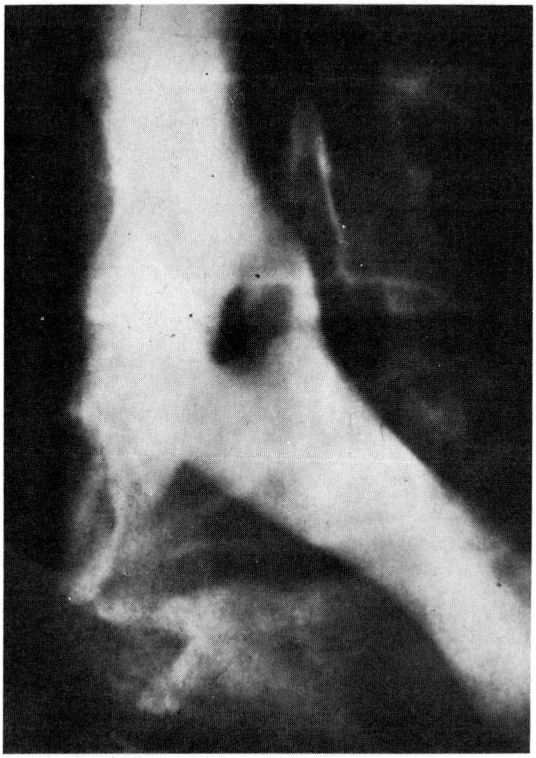

Fig. 3.37a Phlebogram showing a central band at the mouth of the left common iliac vein.

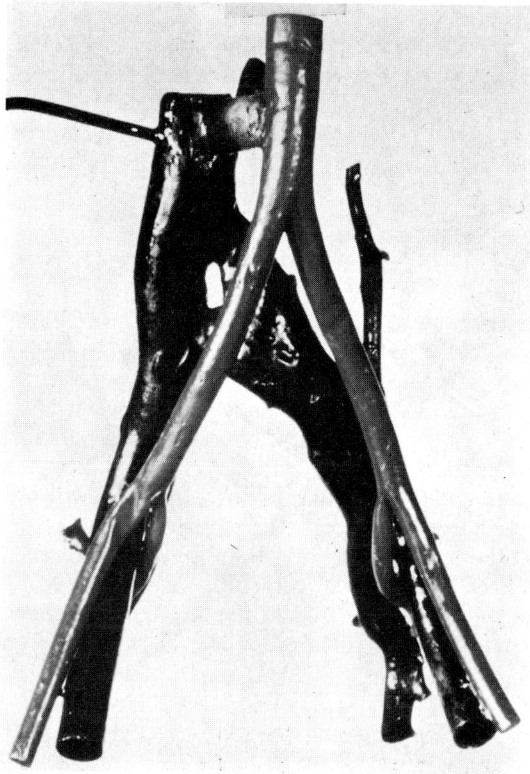

Fig. 3.37b Corrosion cast of the pelvic vessels of a 45 year old woman showing a large central filling defect, representing a band, at the mouth of the left common iliac vein.

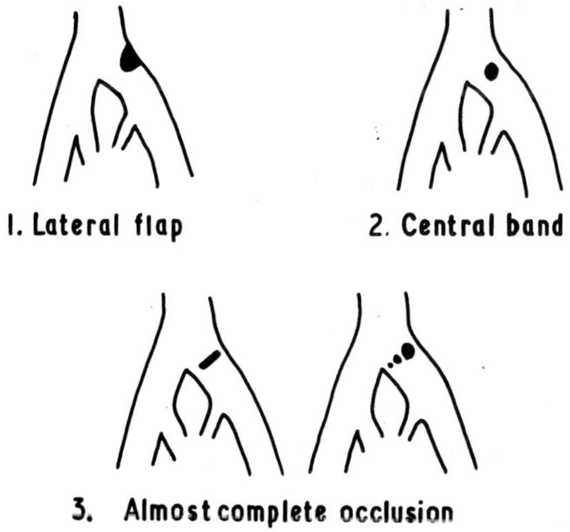

Fig. 3.37c To show the variety of bands found at the mouth of the left common iliac vein.

3.2), but the reason was obscure until the recent recognition of the predisposing anatomical factors.

Acute venous thrombosis in the left common iliac vein is often followed by failure of recanalisation and the permanent venous stenosis which is described in Chapter 16.

Tributaries

The iliolumbar vein is the only tributary of the common iliac vein. The right vein is usually smaller than the left. It is formed by the union of an iliac branch and the ascending lumbar vein. The former provides an important collateral pathway in obstruction of the external iliac vein by virtue of its communication with the left circumflex iliac vein, while the ascending lumbar vein is a valuable bypass in left common iliac vein obstruction, through its numerous communications with the vertebral venous plexus and later with the inferior hemiazygos vein (Fig. 3.38—Phlebogram).

THE INFERIOR VENA CAVA

This wide, thin walled trunk ascends from the level of the 5th lumbar vertebra to the right atrium, lying to the right of the vertebral bodies. Formed by the junction of the common iliac veins, it receives two pairs of short, wide lumbar veins, which connect with the vertebral venous plexus. In its upper half it is joined successively by the renal, right ovarian or testicular vein, adrenal, phrenic veins and the hepatic veins. It leaves the abdomen through the diaphragm at the level of the 8th thoracic vertebra, being somewhat fixed by its adrenal and hepatic tributaries.

In view of its complicated embryology, it is not surprising that there is some congenital abnormality in about 1 per cent of otherwise normal subjects. These include paired cavae, a left sided cava, or occasionally complete absence with compensatory enlargement of the azygos and hemiazygos systems.

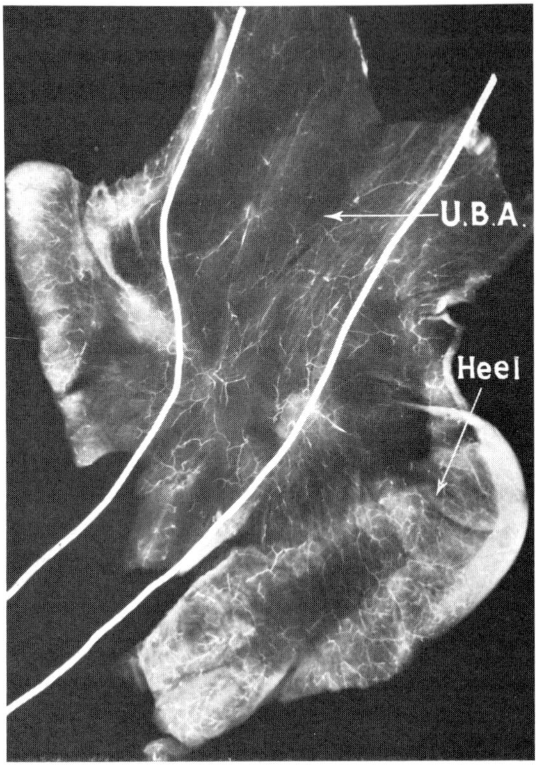

Fig. 3.39 The arterial supply of the ulcer bearing area (U.B.A). This is the X-ray of the skin, subcutaneous tissue and deep fascia of the lower third of the leg, which was dissected off in one piece and laid flat. The vessels had been injected with bismuth suspension. The two heavy lines enclose the 'ulcer-bearing area' (U.B.A). The relative avascularity of this area and the small size of the vessels compared with those of the heel and foot is noticeable.

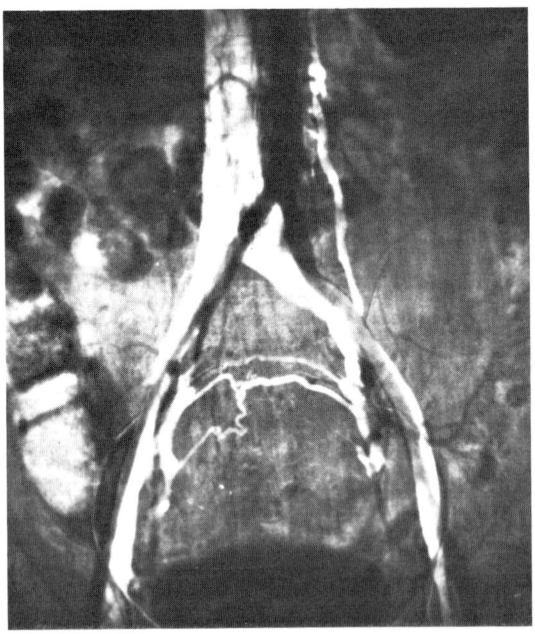

Fig. 3.38 Subtraction film (combined arteriogram and phlebogram) showing ascending lumbar vein enlargement in left common iliac vein obstruction.

Valves in the iliac veins and inferior vena cava

Valves are occasionally found in the external iliac veins (see Fig. 3.17). The tributaries of the internal iliac vein possess valves and valves are occasionally found in the main trunk. No valves have been seen in the common iliac vein. The inferior vena cava is valveless.

THE ARTERIAL SUPPLY OF THE SKIN AND SUBCUTANEOUS TISSUES OF THE LEG AND FOOT

Figure 3.39 shows an X-ray of the skin and subcutaneous tissues of the lower half of the leg, ankle region and heel which was removed from an amputated limb after the arterial system had been injected with a bismuth suspension (D. A. W. Edwards). It will be seen that the skin supply down as far as the ankle arises from small perforating arteries, which rapidly break up into a tree-like distribution of arterioles. Each perforating artery is more or less directly responsible for a small area of skin but at the periphery of this area the arterioles anastomose freely with those of the neighbouring veins.

Many of these small perforating arteries accompany the perforating veins, and in Figure 3.25 quite a large perforating artery can be seen accompanying the middle perforating vein although it is not closely applied to it.

The arterial supply of the skin of the foot, however, differs in being more profuse and coming from larger vessels. The heel particularly is seen to have a good arterial supply of many larger vessels arising more directly from the posterior tibial artery. Figure 3.39 brings out the difference between the profuse arterial supply of the foot and the sole in contrast to the sparse and poor blood supply of the skin of the ankle region (i.e. the ulcer-bearing area = U.B.A. in Fig. 3.39).

A study of these pictures is of interest in understanding the problems of venous ulceration. The small size and paucity of arteries supplying the skin of the lower third of the leg, particularly in the area where ulceration occurs, is striking. It is obvious that if there were a local rise in venous pressure (such as might occur in the vicinity of a large incompetent perforating vein) the effect on the local circulation would be worse than in a region with a larger arterial supply. The circulation to the heel and foot is so copious and carried by such large vessels that it is more difficult to imagine that ulceration would happen here. Clinical experience bears this out.

One further important practical point emerges. It is apparent that when operating on the lower third of the leg and undercutting a large area of skin in the subcutaneous plane, many of these perforating arteries would be divided and an area of skin easily made ischaemic. The only collateral arterial circulation would be by the anastomosis of small arterioles from neighbouring areas of skin whose perforating arteries had remained intact. Thus to minimise skin necrosis undercutting must be avoided.

REFERENCES

Barcroft, J. & Rothschild, P. (1932) *J. Physiol.*, **76**, 447.

Barrow, D. W. (1949) *Clinical Management of Varicose Veins.* London: Hamilton.

Basmajian, J. V. (1952) *Surg. Gynec. Obstet.*, **95**, 537.

Bauer, G. (1946) *J. Amer. med. Ass.*, **131**, 196.

Beesley, L. & Johnston, T. B. (1939) *Manual of Surgical Anatomy,* 5th edn. Oxford University Press.

Boyd, A. M., Catchpole, B. N., Jepson, R. P. & Rose, S. S. (1953) *Ann. Surg.*, **138**, 726.

Cockett, F. B. (1953) *Pathology and Treatment of Venous Ulcers of the Leg.* M.S. Thesis, London.

Cotton, L. T. (1967) *Cardio-Vasc. Research,* **1**, 249.

Eger, S. A. & Casper, S. L. (1943) *J. Amer. med. Ass.,* **123**, 148.

Fegan, G. W. & Pegum, P. G. (1968) *Brit. J. Surg.,* **61**, 124.

Gay, J. (1868) *On Varicose Disease of the Lower Extremities and its Allied Disorders: Skin Discoloration, Induration, and Ulcer.* London: Churchill.

Gray, H. (1954) *Anatomy,* 31st edn., p. 853. Edited by T. B. Johnston and J. Whillis. London: Longmans.

Kosinski, C. (1926) *J. Anat., London,* **60**, 131.

Le Dentu, A. (1867) *Recherches anatomiques et considerations physiologiques sur la circulation vein use du pied et de la jambe.* Thesis, Paris.

Negus, D., Fletcher, E. W. L., Cockett, F. B. & Lea Thomas, M. (1968). *Brit. J. Surg,* **55**, 369.

Negus, D., Edwards, J. M. & Kinmonth, J. B. (1969) *Brit. J. Surg.*, **56**, 481.

Powell, T. & Lynn, R. B. (1951) *Surg. gynec. Obstet.*, **92**, 453.

Quain, J. (1892) Ed. E. A. Schafer & G. D. Thane. *Elements of Anatomy.* Vol. II, pt. 2, p. 536.

Tompsett, D. M. (1956) *Anatomical Techniques.* London, Edinburgh: Livingstone.

Warwick, W. T. (1931) *The Rational Treatment of Varicose Veins and Varicocele.* London: Faber and Faber.

4. Applied Physiology of the Veins

JOHN LUDBROOK

The physiology of the veins in general, and particularly the fascinating problem of venous return from the muscles and subcutaneous tissues of the lower limb, are subjects which receive curiously little attention in the standard textbooks. Two outstanding facets of venous physiology have only been recently appreciated. These are:

1. The fact that the superficial veins have smooth muscle in their walls and the deep veins do not. Thus the deep veins are a more or less passive reservoir of blood capable of expanding and contracting only in response to circumstances such as internal venous pressure, external pressure on the veins (e.g. by muscles) and of course posture.

The superficial veins, however, react strongly by contracting in response to direct stimuli, cold and such drugs as ergotamine. They dilate in response to heat and smooth muscle relaxants (such as oestrin for example).

Any surgeon who has operated on the superficial veins and observed them contract on the stimulus of manipulating them, must be impressed at the contrast when he handles the big, deep veins, with their lack of reaction and willingness to bleed profusely. The very fact that the superficial veins can be 'stripped' without the patient losing torrents of blood is eloquent testimony to the contractile powers of the superficial veins.

2. The second outstanding fact is that the physiology of venous return from the leg is quite different when lying prone, and when standing up. In the prone position with the legs on the same level as the heart, blood flows evenly along all vessels superficial and deep towards the heart—propelled by the relatively small vis-a-tergo coming through the capillaries.

When we stand up, however, the beautifully intricate and efficient calf pump is the main mechanism. It has been aptly termed the 'peripheral heart' because not only does it propel the contained venous blood up to the heart on systole but in diastole it sucks in the venous blood from the subcutaneous tissue of the ankle region via the ankle perforating veins (see Fig. 4.5). So the flow from the whole of the skin and subcutaneous area of the ankle region is *inwards and up the deep veins*.

It is really impossible to begin to understand the abnormal physiology of the valve failures associated with varicose veins and the post-thrombotic syndrome, unless this important piece of normal physiology is appreciated.

Not only do the veins of the human lower limbs possess all the general properties of the venous system, but they also exhibit a number of anatomic and functional adaptations which are specific to man's assumption of the upright posture. Many of the disorders of the veins of the lower limb seem to result from failure of these adaptory mechanisms.

In the description which follows, most of the known properties of veins will be considered, though with particular respect to the veins of the lower limbs, and with greatest emphasis on those which are most immediately relevant to the venous disorders which form the main subject of this book. There have been several more or less comprehensive reviews of this general subject (Arnoldi, 1964; Ludbrook, 1966; Wood, 1965), and original articles will be cited only when they are of outstanding importance, or if they have not been considered within these reviews.

CONDUIT FUNCTION

The most obvious function of veins is to carry blood back to the heart. The total cross-sectional area of these effluent venous pathways is considerably greater than that of the arteries which carry the inflowing blood, and this is especially true in the lower limbs. A consequence of this is that the resistance to venous outflow is low. This is reflected in the very small pressure differential between the small veins of the foot and the femoral vein, and between femoral vein and right atrium, when the body is at rest in the horizontal posture (Fig. 4.1).

These pressure differences are part of an *hydraulic* pressure gradient, which comes about because of the resistance of the veins to blood flow. However, assumption of the upright posture creates an additional *hydrostatic* pressure gradient, the hydrostatic pressure being the pressure-equivalent of a column of blood extending to the right atrium. Thus the actual pressure within a vein at any point in the lower limb is the sum of these two components (Fig. 4.2). The level of zero venous pressure is sometimes called the

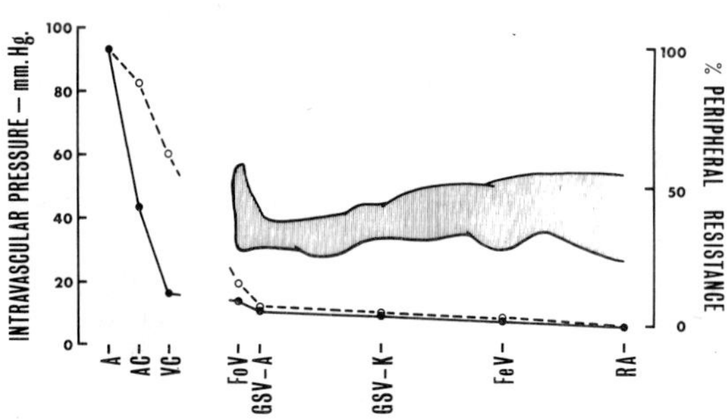

Fig. 4.1 The intravascular pressure gradient in the lower limb in the supine posture with *normal resting blood flow* (continuous line) and with *maximal blood flow* (broken line). A, artery; AC, arteriolar capillary; VC, venular capillary; FoV, foot vein; GSV-A or -K, great saphenous vein at ankle or knee; FeV, femoral vein; RA, right atrium.

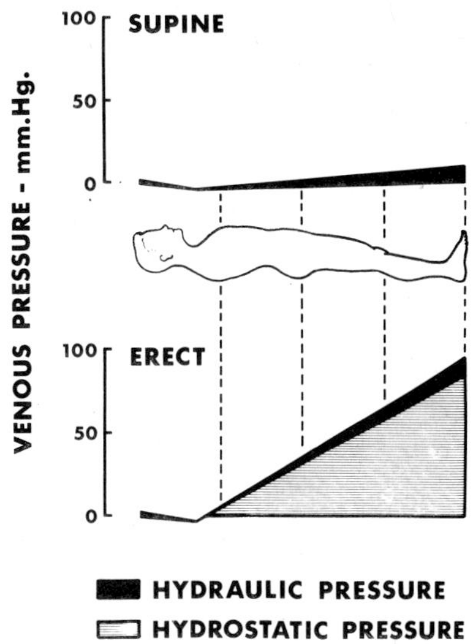

Fig. 4.2 The *hydraulic* and *hydrostatic* venous pressure gradients in the supine and erect postures.

phlebostatic axis (Winsor and Burch, 1945), and corresponds to the intersection of the mid-axillary plane, and a plane at right angles to this which passes through the fourth chondrosternal junction.

The shallow slope of the hydraulic venous gradient (Figs 4.1 and 4.2) is able to be maintained even when there is a great increase in total blood flow, such as occurs after exercise. However, whereas under resting conditions about nine-tenths of the total resistance to blood flow through the limb is accounted for by pre-capillary vessels, when blood flow is greatly increased nearly half the resistance may be provided by post-capillary vessels (Fig. 4.1). This relatively fixed resistance of the venules acts as a kind of governor which prevents an uncontrollable increase in cardiac output, or an uncontrollable fall of arterial blood pressure, in the face of violent muscular exercise.

During exercise such as walking or running the situation is further complicated. The venous valves intermittently interrupt the column of blood which extends to the right heart, and thus intermittently cut off the hydrostatic component of the venous pressure.

The physiologic significance of this will be considered in detail later.

Not only are the venous conduits of the lower limb multiple, and collectively of great cross-sectional area, but in face of physical blockage of the main veins the lesser veins have a remarkable capacity to dilate and act as collateral channels. The result is that complete occlusion of a major vein may cause little obstruction to blood-flow. Thus the immediate effect of ligation of the inferior vena cava is to produce only a small and transient rise in venous pressure distally (Gazzaniga et al., 1967) *under resting conditions*. In order for there to be a significant disturbance of the conduit function of the veins of the lower limb there must be either widespread obliteration of the major venous pathways (e.g. massive venous thrombosis), obliteration of a major vein at one of the critical points where there is limited potential for collateral development (e.g. the common iliac vein) (Mavor and Galloway, 1967), or a great increase in blood flow through the patent venous pathways must be provoked (e.g. by exercise). So while an anatomic obstruction to a major lower limb vein may be able to be demonstrated phlebographically, proof of impaired venous conduit function is more difficult to obtain. The presently favoured techniques are the demonstration of a rise in distal venous pressure during exercise (Negus and Cockett, 1967), or of a reduced rate of venous outflow from the limb when it is suddenly elevated (Ludbrook and Westcott, 1968).

CAPACITY FUNCTION

It is estimated that some 70 per cent of the blood volume is at any moment contained within post-capillary vessels: that is, veins of varying sizes. For this reason, the post-capillary vessels are known collectively as *capacity vessels,* in contrast to the pre-capillary *resistance vessels.* The main property of a capacity vessel is that the volume of blood contained within it can vary within wide limits with minimal change in pressure (Fig. 4.3).

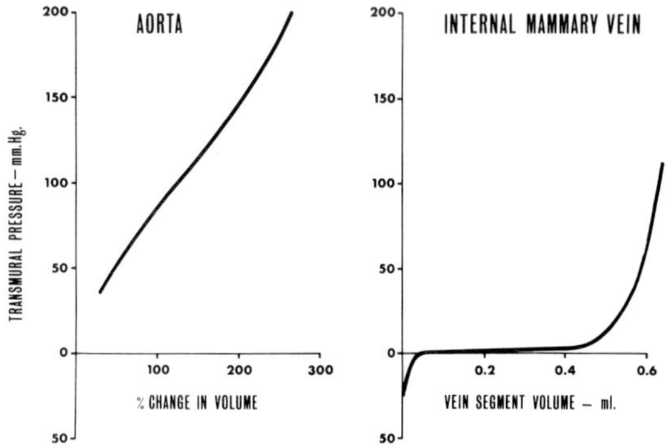

Fig. 4.3 The pressure-volume characteristics of an isolated human *artery* (after Hallock and Benson, 1937) and an isolated human *vein* after Ryder et al., 1944).

In contrast, as the volume of blood an artery contains is increased, the pressure rises in an almost proportional fashion because of the elastic properties of its walls. This is merely another way of saying that veins are collapsible, at any rate when they are isolated from the tissues which surround then.

With change in posture from horizontal to erect, each normal lower limb will accept about 350 ml of additional blood. Man is constantly changing his posture from horizontal to erect, but the geometry of his capacity vessels ensures that this efflux of about 10 per cent of the blood volume from the thorax into the lower limbs produces virtually no change in the filling pressure of the heart. However, if the geometry of the low pressure circulation is disturbed, as it may be in a patient with gross varicose veins, so is this nice balance. In such a patient, if the blood volume were to increase by an amount equal to the increased capacity of the lower limb veins, there would be an excessive rise in central venous pressure when he lay down. On the other hand, if the blood volume were unchanged there would be an excessive fall in central venous pressure when he stood up. The usual response to gross varicose veins is a compromise. There is a moderate increase in blood volume, but such patients often have an excessive tachycardia on standing up, and an excessive rise in central venous pressure on lying down.

The venous system does not merely act as a passive bag, but is able to some extent to alter its capacity (Wood, 1965; Browse, 1968; Mark and Eckstein, 1968; Webb-Peploe and Shepherd, 1968). Those veins which contain smooth muscle in their walls are enabled, by way of their sympathetic nerve supply or by circulating catecholamines, to contract actively. Generally speaking, the same stimuli produce this change as produce constriction of resistance vessels, and vice versa. These phenomena have been studied chiefly in human subcutaneous veins. They are clearly important in the matter of temperature regulation, where veins act as adaptable heat exchangers. They may be important in the fine control of the cardiovascular response to change of posture and muscular exercise. *However, the deep veins of the body, and of the lower limb in particular, are almost devoid of smooth muscle* (Horton, 1966), and such evidence as there is suggests that increase in venous tone can effect only a modest reduction in size of the vascular compartment as a whole.

Direct local stimuli are also able to cause profound—but localised—alterations in venous tone: thus the spasm which may accompany venepuncture or operative manipulation, and the dilatation which results from tapping the skin which overlies a vein.

Apart from the passive translocation of blood resulting from postural change, and active alterations in compliance of the vein wall, there is a third mechanism by which the volume of blood in the capacity vessels of the lower limb can alter. While some 350 ml of extra blood is accommodated in each lower limb when a person stands still, this reservoir is subject to the action of the musculovenous pumps of the limb during ambulation. Two effects derive from this. In the first few seconds of exercise a bolus of blood is ejected towards the heart, and is made available for the sudden increase in cardiac output: indeed, it may be one of the major stimuli to this increase. During continuing exercise, the blood which has been expelled from the lower limb veins is available for redistribution to the pulmonary vascular bed, and to opened-up capillary vessels in exercising muscle throughout the body.

While this chapter is primarily concerned with venous function under normal conditions, it would not be complete without mentioning briefly the place of the venous (capacity vessel) system in relation to haemorrhage. When blood is lost, it is the volume contained in the capacity vessel component of the vascular system which diminishes. The illogicality of estimating blood loss and blood replacement by measuring arterial pressure is now well-recognised. Instead, central venous (right atrial) pressure is used as an index of capacity vessel filling, or blood volume is measured directly. Many believe that on a whole-body basis an increase in venous tone can reduce the volume of the container (the capacity vessels), as a reflex response to loss of the contents (blood). However, the importance of this possible means of maintaining central venous pressure has not yet been clearly defined.

MUSCULO-VENOUS PUMP

The valved deep veins of the lower limb, enclosed within or between the muscles, comprise a series-parallel arrangement of reciprocating pumps (Fig. 4.4). The chambers of the pumps consist of the various intra- and inter-muscular veins in the calf and thigh. The lumina of intramuscular veins of the calf have been shown to be virtually obliterated during muscle contraction, while most of the intermuscular veins are greatly narrowed (Almén and Nylander, 1962; Arnoldi et al., 1966). The approximate volume of those in the calf is 100 ml, and of those in the thigh 200 ml. The arrangement of the valves has already been described (Chap. 3). The energising mechanism of the pumps is the contraction of the surrounding muscles, which develop pressures as great as 250 mmHg in the leg, and 115 mmHg in the thigh. Input of blood to the chambers of the pump comes by way of the distal deep veins, and from the superficial veins by way of communicating veins of

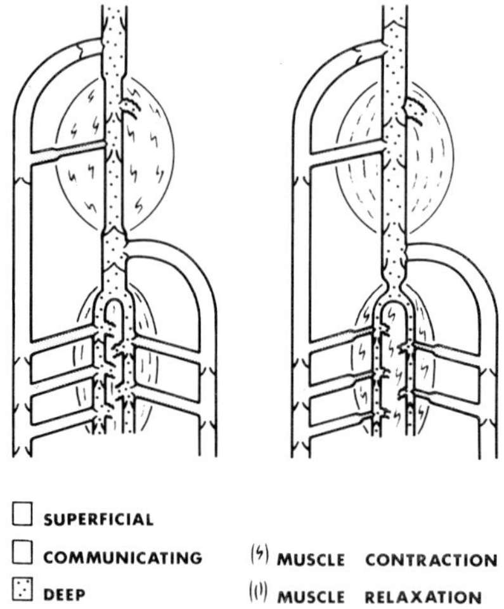

Fig. 4.4 The musculovenous pumps of the leg and thigh, showing the series-parallel arrangement, and the behaviour of the veins and their valves during reciprocal calf-thigh muscle activity as in walking.

the ankle region. However, the greatest contribution is made by the blood which has passed through the capillaries of the surrounding muscles. The output of the calf pump is delivered into the thigh pump, and from the latter into the great veins of the abdomen. However, the calf pump is much the more efficient mechanism of the two.

It is meaningless to describe the musculovenous pumps in terms of their volume-output of blood, for clearly this cannot exceed the volume-input (that is, arterial inflow). However, the power generated by the pumps can be calculated from the rate of blood flow through them, and from the lowering of hydrostatic pressure in deep and superficial veins which they achieve. The estimates vary (Ludbrook, 1966; Stegall, 1966), but it is clear that during ambulation the power developed by the lower limb muscles in driving the calf pump is but a small proportion of that devoted to propelling the body forward, or of that generated by the heart under the same circumstances.

The musculo-venous pumps appear to accomplish two things. First, they reduce the volume of blood which is contained in the capacity vessels of the lower limb during exercise, and permit this blood to be redistributed for other functions. Second, they lower the mean venous hydrostatic pressure in the lower limb, especially below the knee. Thus, during walking exercise, the mean posterior tibial venous pressure in the lower calf is reduced from about 80 mmHg to about 40, and that in the great saphenous vein by rather more (Højensgard and Stürup, 1952; Arnoldi, 1965; 1966; Ludbrook, 1966; Hjelmstedt, 1968; Fig. 4.5). This in turn has the effect of increasing the arteriovenous pressure gradient in the appropriate tissues by nearly 50 per cent (Fig. 4.6), and increases the potential for arterial through-flow by the same amount at any given level of resistance-vessel tone. This impressive gain in terms of lower limb blood flow is accomplished by a very modest energy input (*vide supra*). It may be, therefore, that the term 'peripheral heart' which has sometimes been applied to the musculovenous pump is not inappropriate, in that it permits a great increase in blood flow through the muscles of the lower limb during ambulation by a much more economic method than the alternative of a great increase in cardiac output. This appears to be yet another adaptation to man's assumption of the erect posture.

The function of the musculo-venous pump has a particular significance in venous disease.

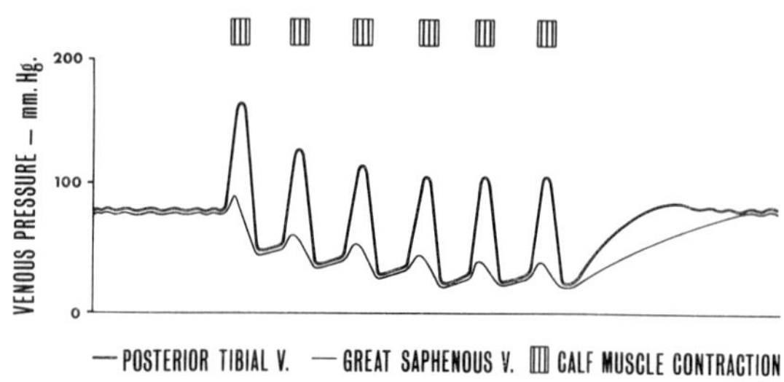

Fig. 4.5 Schematic representation of the behaviour of deep and superficial venous pressure at mid-calf level before, during, and after walking. During diastole of the calf pump, the superficial venous pressure also falls, and it is during this phase that the venous blood from the sub-cutaneous tissues of the ankle is flowing into the bottom of the calf pump, via the ankle perforating veins.

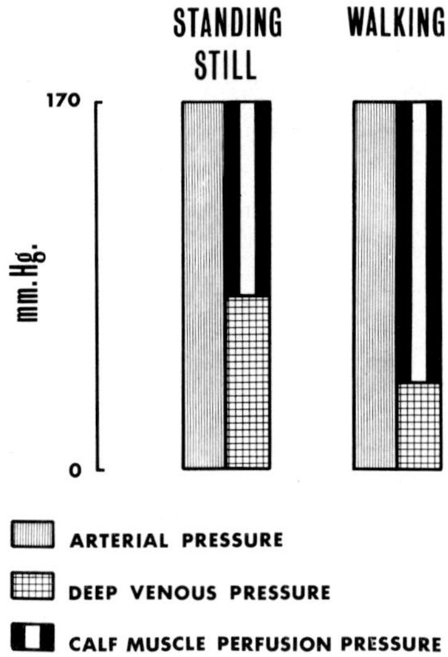

Fig. 4.6 The perfusion pressure (mean arteriovenous pressure difference) in the calf muscles at rest and during walking.

As will become clear later in this book, changes in the skin, ranging from eczema to frank ulceration, are a feature of legs in which the communicating veins have become incompetent. In many instances, the skin changes and the venous incompetence are able to be reversed by surgical or other means. By implication, therefore, an efficient musculovenous pump is necessary to the good health of the skin of the lower leg. The function of the pump which seems most closely related to this is its capacity to lower venous pressure in the superficial veins of the ankle during ambulatory exercise. It seems, therefore, that the skin of the lower limbs cannot withstand continuous exposure to a high venous pressure, and in normal everyday life is protected from this by the activity of the musculo-venous pumps, and the arrangement of the valves in the ankle perforating veins which prevent outward flow.

REFERENCES

Almén, T. & Nylander, G. (1962) Serial phlebography of the normal lower limb during muscular contraction and relaxation. *Acta radiol. (Stockh.)*, **57**, 264.

Arnoldi, C. C. (1964) The venous return from the lower leg in health and in chronic venous insufficiency. *Acta orthop. scand.*, Suppl. 64.

Arnoldi, C. C. (1965) Venous pressure in the leg of healthy human subjects at rest and during muscular exercise in the nearly erect position. *Acta chir. scand.*, **130**, 570.

Arnoldi, C. C. (1966) The influence of posture upon the pressure of the veins of the normal human leg at rest and during rhythmic muscular exercise. *Acta chir. scand.*, **131**, 423.

Arnoldi, C. C., Greitz, T. & Linderholm, H. (1966) Variations in cross sectional area and pressure in the veins of the normal human leg during rhythmic muscular exercise. *Acta chir. scand.*, **132**, 507.

Browse, N. L. (1968) The veins and cardiovascular reflexes. *Ann. roy. Coll. Surg. Engl.*, **42**, 307.

Gazzaniga, A. B., Cahill, J. L., Replogle, R. L. & Tilney, N. L. (1967) Changes in blood volume and renal function following ligation of the inferior vena cava. *Surgery*, **62**, 417.

Hallock, P. & Benson, I. C. (1937) Studies on elastic properties of human isolated aorta. *J. clin. Invest.*, **16**, 595.

Hjelmstedt, A. (1968) The pressure in the veins of the dorsum of the foot in quiet standing and during exercise in limbs without signs of venous disorder. *Acta chir. scand.*, **134**, 235.

Høјensgard, I. C. & Stürup, H. (1952) Static and dynamic pressures in superficial and deep veins of the lower extremity in man. *Acta physiol. scand.*, **27**, 49.

Horton, D. A'C. (1966) The veins of the human calf. *Proc. Univ. Otago med. Sch.*, **44**, 45.

Ludbrook, J. (1966) Aspects of venous function in the lower limbs. Springfield: Thomas.

Ludbrook, J. & Westcott, E. J. (1968) Venous outflow obstruction of the lower limb following plication of the inferior vena cava. *Surg. Gynec. Obstet.*, **127**, 1017.

Mark, A. L. & Eckstein, J. W. (1968) Venomotor tone and central venous pressure. *Med. Clin. N. Amer.*, **52**, 1077.

Mavor, G. E. & Galloway, J. M. (1967) Collaterals of the deep venous circulation of the lower limb. *Surg. Gynec. Obstet.*, **125**, 561.

Negus, D. & Cockett, F. B. (1967) Femoral vein pressures in post-phlebitic iliac vein obstruction. *Brit. J. Surg.*, **54**, 522.

Ryder, H. W., Molle, W. E. & Ferris, E. B. Jr. (1944) The influence of collapsibility of veins on venous pressure, including a new procedure for measuring tissue pressure. *J. clin. Invest.*, **23**, 333.

Stegall, H. F. (1966) Muscle pumping in the dependent leg. *Circulat. Res.*, **19**, 180.

Webb-Peploe, M. M. & Shepherd, J. T. (1968) Veins and their control. *N. Engl. J. Med.*, **278**, 317.

Winsor, T. & Burch, G. E. (1945) Phlebostatic axis and phlebostatic level, reference levels for venous pressure measurements in man. *Proc. Soc. exp. Biol. (N.Y.)*, **58**, 165.

Wood, J. E. (1965) The Veins: Normal and Abnormal Function. London: Churchill.

Part II
Pathology and Surgery of the Superficial Veins

5. Introduction

There are many causes and many types of varicose veins. Nearly all of them are progressive and get steadily worse throughout life—some types faster than others.

In spite of this wide diversity of types, and variation in the stage at which the condition is seen, it is universally referred to as just 'varicose veins'. One hears the question 'How do you treat varicose veins, by operation or injection?' One might just as sensibly ask the question: 'How do you treat chest disease?'

The first necessity when asked to see a case of 'varicose veins' is, as always, diagnosis. Below is set out a classification of the venous conditions of the leg which frequently masquerade under the all embracing term of varicose veins.

CLASSIFICATION OF VARICOSE VEINS

1. *Primary familial varicose veins*

A. Of the long saphenous system (the commonest type).

B. Of the short saphenous system (less common).

C. Primary ankle perforator incompetence (very uncommon).

2. *Secondary varicose veins*

These are the aftermath of a deep vein thrombosis and may be of three general types:

A. Those due to the generalised venous hypertension in the limb following the permanent blockage of a major iliac vein after an iliofemoral thrombosis (see Chap. 16). This general venous hypertension causes a steady gradual dilatation of all the small venules particularly in the distal part of the leg, ankle and even foot. All small veins and venules below the knee may partake in this, no one particular system being involved and without notable dilatation of the main saphenous veins.

B. Those due to destruction of the valves in the ankle perforating veins which is common after a deep vein thrombosis. Destruction of the valve at the mouth of the short saphenous vein, or even the long saphenous vein may also occur, and a secondary short or long saphenous incompetence will then follow a deep vein thrombosis.

C. Varicose veins round the lower pubis and abdomen. These are always the aftermath of an iliofemoral thrombosis (Chap. 16) and start life as collateral veins.

3. *Pudendal varicose veins*

These are peculiar to women and are a post-pregnancy phenomenon. They arise from the breakdown of the valves in the terminal part of the internal iliac vein just below the entry of the uterine veins. The enormous pressure and flow in the uterine veins during pregnancy may then leak into the leg via the obturator vein, and more particularly the internal pudenal vein (see Chap. 10). These veins appear in the labia and also spread from the vagina down the inner side of the leg and back of the thigh. They are usually small surface veins and are painful particularly just before the periods.

4. *Varicose veins secondary to arteriovenous fistulae* (either traumatic or of the generalised or local congenital type) (see Chapter 11).

5. *Varicose veins associated with various degrees of the congenital lateral venous anomaly known as the 'Klippel Trenaunay syndrome'*

These occur on the lateral aspect of the leg and are the remnants of the primitive sciatic venous system which normally disappears at about the third month of embryonic life.

6. *Capillary veins* (also known as venous stars, telangiectases, burst veins, etc.)

These little clusters of dilated capillaries appear on women's legs and thighs often during pregnancy, or sometimes in later life, for no obvious reason at all. Their main importance is their appearance as they are very visible and disfiguring. They may be unassociated with any other venous abnormality in the leg, and very little is known about their aetiology, except that their appearance has some connection with the level of oestrin or other sex hormones in the blood.

7. *Athletes hypertrophied veins*

Young athletic patients occasionally come with the complaint of prominent and sometimes tortuous veins in muscular legs with very little subcutaneous tissue. Often there is no demonstrable valvular incompetence, and the main complaint is of their appearance and sometimes of aching.

All these various types of varicose veins will be considered in this book. But it must already be clear that there is no one treatment which is applicable to all the types listed above, and which are commonly included under the name 'varicose veins'.

At one end of the scale are veins which are often better not treated at all! While at the other end there are certain secondary types of veins (notably the post-thrombotic group) which require early, energetic and understanding treatment to prevent the crippling sequelae of pain and ulceration.

The reason for treatment, the urgency of treatment and the type of treatment varies widely in the various types. The only key to successful management and treatment is a thorough understanding of the aetiology, pathology and progress of them all.

As always, the way to successful treatment is careful and complete diagnosis.

Finally, the type of leg in which the venous pathology is found has a great bearing on the symptoms and on the urgency of treatment. As a generalisation the thin, hairy male leg with a minimum of subcutaneous tissue stands up to venous incompetence and hypertension much better than the fat, hairless, cold female one. In this latter type of limb (commonly called the erythrocyanoid limb) the early symptoms of aching, burning and pain, may be very tiresome and genuine; later, venous incompetence of all sorts may precipitate the very painful and disabling lesion of 'fat necrosis', which once established leads on to a hard, fibrous plaque in the ankle with an ever present tendency to ulceration at the slightest trauma or infection. Hence venous incompetence in fat legs specially needs early and radical treatment (Fig. 5.1).

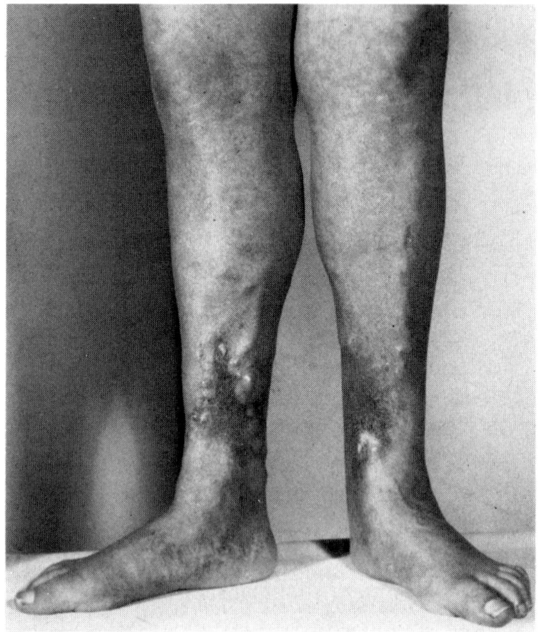

Fig. 5.1 The hard pigmented areas in the lower third of the leg resulting from fat necrosis.

Secondary venous disorders due to deep thrombosis are considered in detail in Part III of this book. The rest, with particular emphasis on the primary familial group (the commonest ones) are considered in this section.

6. Primary Familial Varicose Veins

AETIOLOGY

The fact that the human race gets varicose veins at all is probably due to our evolutionary adoption of the erect position. The superficial veins of the legs being between three and four feet below the heart, and unsupported except by connective tissue, are in a poor position to withstand continuous venous hypertension, The main long and short saphenous veins are strong and muscular and they can withstand sustained venous hypertension without becoming enlarged or varicose. However, their branches which run more superficially in the connective tissue just under the skin are thin walled and are unable to resist prolonged venous hypertension, so they become enlarged and tortuous (i.e. varicose).

The human leg has evolved a complicated and highly efficient method of protecting these veins from the effects of prolonged hypertension—which depends on the presence and efficient function of a large number of strategically placed valves.

Varicosity of the superficial veins occurs when certain of these valves, particularly those guarding the mouths of the long saphenous, the short saphenous and the perforating veins, are destroyed by thrombosis or appear to be absent or inefficient due to some other reason.

The prevalence and aetiology of the common primary varicose veins has been the subject of a very extensive literature which is well summarised in Anning's monograph (1954) and in Borschberg's recent monograph (1971). Such factors as heredity, race, obesity, intercurrent disease, chest disease, age and even constipation have all been the subject of prolonged investigation and discussion.

However, from amongst this welter of data, two factors are really outstanding and beyond doubt. These are the influence of heredity and race. Nearly all are agreed upon these two.

HEREDITY

In patients with primary varicose veins a family history is present even on casual direct questioning in about 70 per cent.

In a recent series of 200 consecutive cases of primary varicose veins seen by one of the authors 70 per cent had a close blood relative affected, and this was known without further research or prompting of the patient.

Virchow and Gay (1868) earlier recognised this.

In a more careful and detailed study Anning (1954) found that out of 102 patients with 'varicose ulcer' whose family history was known, 91 had a positive family history (i.e. 89.2 per cent). He also noted the hereditary factor in deep vein thrombosis.

When we consider what the heredity factor is, however, there is little exact information. The likelihood is that absence of one or more strategic valves is the defect which is inherited. Certainly there is evidence from the work of Cockett (1953) and Cotton (1951) that there is great variation in the number and siting of valves both in the iliac veins and in the great saphenous vein. Surgeons who are used to passing the stripper retrogradely are impressed by the fact that in many familial cases of long saphenous varicose veins, the stripper will pass from groin to ankle with no more than an occasional half-hearted hold up on a valve. Passage retrogradely down a normal vein, however, is made almost impossible by the number and efficiency of the valves.

RACE

One of the most remarkable things about varicose veins is the racial distribution. This extends not only to varicose veins but also to deep vein thrombosis.

Varicose veins are essentially a disease of the white European races, and of the peoples of the Mediterranean Basin. East of Suez, and South in the African Continent, the incidence of this disease falls so sharply that it is a rarity. Thus in the *pure black African,* in the *Arabic races,* the *Indians* and the *Asiatics,* varicose veins as we know them in the West, do not exist as a problem. Odd examples of varicose veins and deep thrombosis are occasionally seen in all these peoples, but it is exceptional.

By contrast, in France, Germany, Scandinavia, the British Isles, and the North Americas, including the coloured, varicose veins are so common that it has been variously calculated that between 10 and 20 per cent of the population are affected in some degree. In these countries also deep thrombosis and its sequelae are frequent.

Other aetiological factors

Thus, in general, it is probably heredity and race which determine basically whether one is going to acquire varicose veins. The rate at which they develop and get bigger and worse in any given individual is, however, influenced by some other aetiological factors, first amongst which are *pregnancy* and occupations involving *prolonged standing work, particularly in hot surroundings* (causing venous dilatation).

These are undoubtedly the two most important contributors to the progress of varicose veins. Most patients and many doctors have their pet theories on this subject—but such factors as trauma, shock, constipation, age, overweight, chest disease, diet play a minor part only (see Borschberg, 1971).

We have good evidence also that this prevalence of varicose veins is not a modern phenomenon, for John Gay, writing in 1861, reported that in that year 7,993 recruits for the army under the age of 25 were examined; of these 326 (just under 5 per cent) were rejected for varicosity. Moreover, it is interesting to note that in England the ratio was 27 per 1,000, in Scotland 54 per 1,000 and in Ireland 67 per 1,000.

SYMPTOMS

First, the symptoms associated with uncomplicated varicose veins will be considered, then those associated with their four great complications, which are: (1) haemorrhage; (2) thrombosis (or phlebitis); (3) eczema; (4) ulceration.

Uncomplicationed varicose veins

The symptoms of this condition and the reasons why patients present themselves for advice or treatment are diverse and defy classification. The patient's complaint varies according to the sex and psychological makeup, and with the type and degree of development of the veins. Some people seek help not because they have any symptoms related to the veins, but because they are worried about the future and by lurid tales that other vein-sufferers have told them. Others may seek treatment to make them fit for military service, or for emigration. One man presented himself because his large varicosities were a worry to his wife!

However, the most common symptoms may be grouped under three headings as follows: (1) disfigurement; (2) aching and pain; (3) swelling.

DISFIGUREMENT

The modern tendency to more and more exposure of the female leg (and even of the male) has made this one of the most frequent reasons for seeking treatment. It has been said that the voluminous Victorian skirt hid a multitude of evils: rickets, arthritis and almost certainly a lot of rather advanced varicose veins!

In the opinion of the authors the presence of an incompetent varicose saphenous system (long or short, with or without perforators) in a young and comely female leg is an adequate indication for curative operative treatment in the early stage.

Such veins progress steadily throughout life, and radical surgery has a better chance of cure when done early.

Beware however the patient who presents herself with minor surface veins, or thread veins—but without a demonstrable saphenous incompetence. Such persons are often pathologically 'leg and vein conscious', and any treatment by injection or other means often multiplies their symptoms and focuses their attention on their legs until a neurotic state is reached.

It is worth mentioning that nowadays when bathing on Mediterranean beaches is within reach of the many, more and more men present themselves for treatment for cosmetic reasons.

ACHING AND PAIN

By far the most common complaint in all types of varicose veins is of a leg which aches on standing. The typical story is that on standing still for any length of time (specially in hot climates, or in hot surroundings, e.g. at a cocktail party) the leg becomes increasingly uncomfortable and aches. Sometimes the main ache is specifically over a particular dilated group of veins. This symptom is rapidly relieved by *moving* the legs, or walking, or by lying down with the feet up. Nearly all varicose vein sufferers say that their legs are comfortable when moving or walking, but ache on standing.

There are four important points in relation to this symptom in varicose vein cases. These are:

1. In patients who complain primarily of pain in legs with varicose veins—always look for some other cause of the pain, besides the veins. Osteoarthritis of knee, or hip, and disc lesions, are common sources of discomfort in the leg, which often co-exist with varicose veins.

2. Patients with progressive primary varicose veins often complain of more static aching pain in the early stage when the veins are *small*, than in the late stage when the veins are large. *It may be said of varicose veins that the early stage is the stage of symptoms, while the late stage is the stage of signs and complications.*

3. There is one type of varicose vein that is notable in that excessive pain and aching is usually the presenting symptom. This is the post-pregnancy *pudendal* vein syndrome, where the pudendal veins and the small veins arising from them down the back of the thigh, become acutely distended and painful *during the two or three days just prior to the period* (see Chap. 10).

4. Varicose veins occurring in the erythrocyanoid limb in the female always give rise to more severe symptoms than in a normal leg. The erythrocyanoid limb with its rather avascular subcutaneous fat and general vascular instability, reacts very badly to even early mild varicose veins. Often these patients are categorised as 'neurotic' and 'unsatisfactory personalities' because their complaints about their legs seem to be out of proportion to the physical signs. However they are perfectly genuine, and they merit early radical treatment.

SWELLING

This is a variable symptom. As a rule swelling of the calf and ankle is absent in primary varicose veins. As shown in Figure 6.1 there may be large varicose veins in thigh and calf—but when the ankle perforating veins are competent the ankle region may be normal. When ankle perforators are incompetent, however, there is a different story—the rapid development of dilated veins and venules in this region, an ankle flare (Fig. 6.8) and slight swelling of the ankle occurs.

However, in women with the fat erythrocyanoid limb, swelling may be a complaint—although it is seldom marked. Such women may complain that the ankle *feels* swollen—(Fig. 6.2) although on inspection oedema may be minimal. Swelling of the ankle in the ery-

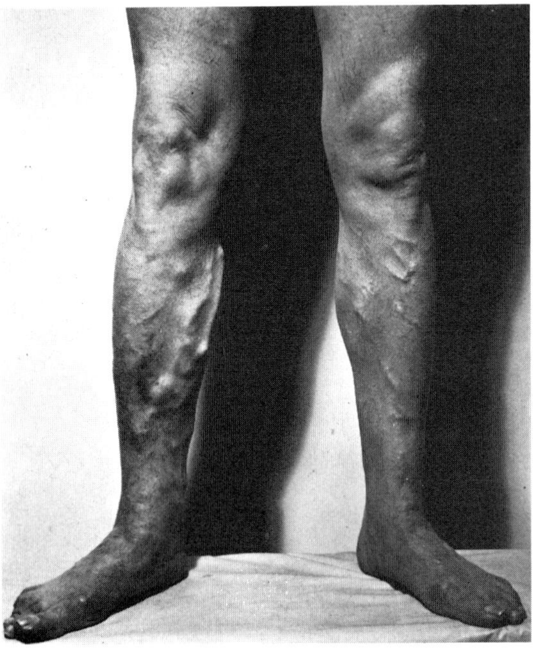

Fig. 6.1 Incompetence of the internal saphenous vein with good ankle skin and no swelling.

throcyanoid limb moreover may occur before the periods, in hot weather, or after alcohol even in the absence of varicose veins.

When gross swelling of the ankle is prominent some other more deep seated cause should be sought. This may be either:

1. An obstruction of the deep veins anywhether from the calf to the vena cava (Chaps 14 to 17).

2. A deep vein thrombosis (Chap. 14).

3. One of the more general causes of oedema such as heart failure, hypoproteinaemia or anaemia.

4. A lymphoedema (Fig. 6.3). The lymphatics are the main channel for clearance of tissue fluid and obstruction of the lymphatics is reflected quickly in swelling of the ankle, foot and toes. The commonest form of lymphoedema is the so-called 'lymphoedema praecox' of young girls, but it may be seen at any age (see Chap. 16). Secondary obstruction of lymphatics due to wounds on the inner side of the limb (surgically inflicted or otherwise), and various types of malignancy in the pelvis may also cause swelling of ankle.

RARER SYMPTOMS

Rarer symptoms are:

1. Various types of discoloration ranging from a mild brown staining over the varices or in the ankle region, to frank purpura in the lower half of the leg (see Chap. 19).

2. Cramp. Nocturnal cramps of the calf are seen particularly associated with short saphenous varices and mid-calf perforator incompetence.

3. Venous colic is a rare symptom sometimes complained of after taking excess of ergotamine tartrate by migraine sufferers.

4. Pain over the veins in bed at night is a rare complaint.

THE COMPLICATIONS OF VARICOSE VEINS

Haemorrhage

It is not generally realised that there is a steady mortality rate every year, mostly in the elderly, by haemorrhage from varicose veins. At St Thomas' Hospital there are between 6 and 10 emergency admissions per year, due to severe spontaneous bleeding from varicose veins.

Bleeding is of three types: spontaneous, traumatic, and subcutaneous.

SPONTANEOUS BLEEDING

This is the most dangerous. It occurs in the elderly patient with long-standing varicose veins, with numerous small dilated veins round the ankle covered by paper-thin skin. Usually the patient has an incompetent ankle perforating vein and thus the venous pressure in these cuticular venules is exceptionally high in the erect position (nearly 100 mmHg).

A common story is that a patient notices her foot or shoe is 'wet' and she looks down and sees to her horror, that she is standing in a small pool of blood. She may sit down, feel faint, and actually faint sitting with the leg dependent—in which case she has a good chance of rapidly bleeding to death! If she

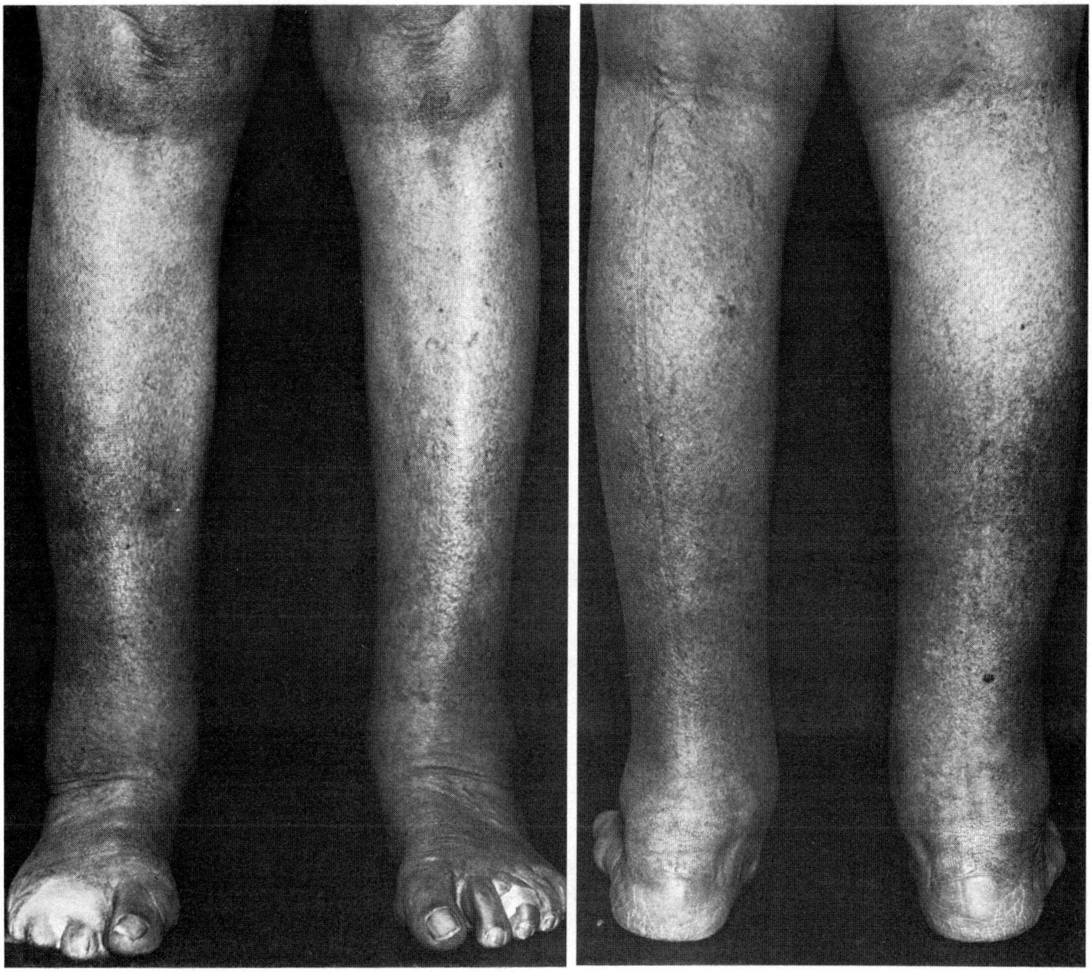

Fig. 6.2 The erythrocyanoid limbs showing the slight swelling.

faints flat on the floor, or lies down with the feet up, this lowers the pressure and the haemorrhage may cease, and the patient recovers sufficiently to call for help.

Such cases of severe and often repeated haemorrhage may occur with little or no obvious trauma, or merely a scratch with the finger.

TRAUMATIC BLEEDING

Severe and obvious trauma, usually around the ankle, may occasionally rupture a large varicose vein and cause profuse haemorrhage. On the whole this is a relatively rare occurrence—although much feared by those with large varicose veins who may come for treatment because of this particular worry.

Occasionally after some more major accident (like being knocked over by a car, or a fall) widespread and spectacular bruising may develop after subcutaneous rupture of varicose veins. A large haematoma may need evacuating.

SUBCUTANEOUS BLEEDING

Bleeding into the tissues is fairly common.

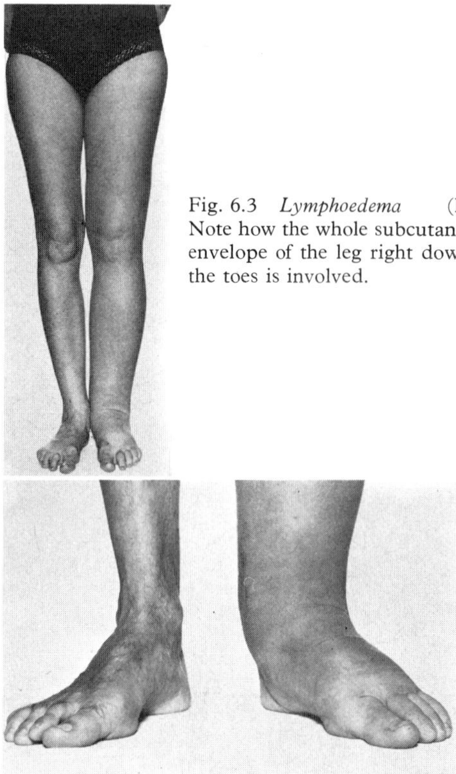

Fig. 6.3 *Lymphoedema* (left). Note how the whole subcutaneous envelope of the leg right down to the toes is involved.

Many young women with varicose veins, and particularly those with the erythrocyanoid leg tend to develop spontaneous, small haemorrhages, or 'ecchymoses', and are inclined to bruise easily after trauma.

THROMBOPHLEBITIS

This is a common and serious complication. Any patient who has varicose veins of any size may get it, but it is more common in the elderly with *big tortuous* varicose veins. It may start after an obvious trauma. More often it appears spontaneously in a group of varices, and a favourite group is the varices of the posterior arch veins just below and inside the knee (see Fig. 7.30).

Often it is a complication of enforced rest in bed during an operation or illness. There is no doubt that all patients with varicose veins who are immobilised in bed should wear elastic stockings or an efficient compression bandage on both legs, while they are in bed and for the whole time that they are immobilised.

SYMPTOMS AND SIGNS

The most obvious thing is that the group of varices concerned suddenly become *tender, hot, inflamed and hard or solid.* In a fat leg there may also be quite a lot of local oedema round the veins affected.

This is of course the picture of inflammatory reaction of the vein wall to the contained thrombus. The inflammatory reaction is more severe the younger the patient and the smaller the varicose vein. In old patients, with large fibrous tortuous varicose veins the inflammatory reaction may be so damped down that pain and redness round the vein may be minimal, although it is always painful to the touch.

When the inflammatory reaction is severe, there is often a high temperature, giving the impression of a bacterial infection. Patients are often put on antibiotics for this reason, but it is nearly always a sterile inflammatory reaction and there is no need for them.

PROGRESS

Superficial thrombosis in varicose veins has traditionally been regarded as a benign process without risk of pulmonary embolism. *Nothing could be further from the truth!* A glance at the causes of thromboembolism (Chap. 14) shows that a significant number of the cases of pulmonary embolism originate in the first instance in an attack of superficial thrombophlebitis, which has spread into the deep veins.

The danger lies in the fact that this deep spread may take place silently without patient or physician being aware that it is happening. A group of varices below the knee may show obvious thrombophlebitis (with pain and tenderness etc.) and it may appear to be settling, while a silent soft thrombus is spreading up to the saphenous orifice, or down towards a large perforator. Such a development in a main saphenous vein may remain fairly symptomless for two or three days before the vein becomes obviously tender. It may spread into the deep veins in three ways:

1. Into the femoral vein via the saphenofemoral junction at the groin in ascending long saphenous thrombophlebitis.

2. Into the popliteal at the junction of the *short* saphenous vein in the popliteal fossa—in ascending short saphenous thrombophlebitis.

3. Into the deep calf veins (posterior tibial) via one of the ankle perforators.

Once thrombus has entered the deep veins it has all the serious complications of a deep vein thrombosis, including fatal embolism.

TREATMENT

In our opinion superficial thrombophlebitis in varicose veins is a serious condition and merits urgent radical treatment. The best remedy undoubtedly is to treat the patient as a semi-emergency and operate on the affected system within a day or so of onset, doing a routine radical operation (flush ligation at groin *or* popliteal fossa with stripping, removal of thrombosed masses and closure of the perforating veins).

Sometimes it is not possible or feasible to do this for various reasons, in which case the second best method of treatment is *ambulation and bandaging*.

Thus the treatment of choice is:

1. *Emergency operation.* Saphenofemoral ligation (or saphenopopliteal in the case of the short saphenous) closes the upper escape for thrombus into the deep veins. Ankle perforator exploration and ligation then closes the lower escape route. Stripping of the system concerned with 'winkling out' of the thrombosed vessels through a small incision, completes the operation. This should be done within two or three days *of the onset* of the condition if it is to be safe and effective in limiting the spread and cutting out the danger of thromboembolic complications. It also has the merits of relieving the pain and curing the original cause of the condition (namely the varicose veins) so that there shall be no recurrence. An untreated long saphenous thrombophlebitis does not (as is the popular story) cure the varicose veins. The long saphenous thrombosis gradually recanalises and within a year the patient's varicose veins are back again, usually with increased symptoms of aching and pain, and also with an increased chance of recurrent phlebitis!

2. *Conservative treatment.* Where skilled emergency operative treatment is unavailable or not possible, the second best method of treatment is by *pressure bandaging* and *ambulation.* A soft gauze pad is placed over the actual area of thrombophlebitis and then the webbing elastic bandage is applied, as usual, from toes to just above the knee—giving firm even pressure over the whole ankle and lower leg. The patient is then instructed to walk and keep as active as possible during the day, and to raise the foot of the bed at night. The pressure bandage is worn during the day only, and is put on *before* the patient puts his leg down in the morning. This pressure bandaging is continued uninterrupted until the area of phlebitis has contracted to a small, *painless,* solid fibrous string—a process which normally occupies about four weeks.

Treatment may then be discontinued, and the patient should be warned to have an early elective operation on his varicose veins. Sometimes in the acute stage the mass of superficial thrombosed varices may be very painful, so much so as to make the wearing of a tight bandage impossible. This can usually be overcome by careful placing of soft gauze padding under the bandage. The pain can be eased in the early stage by giving aspirin or codis. It has become common practice to prescribe Butazolidine for thrombosis, but we are not convinced of its usefulness.

3. *How not to treat acute superficial thrombophlebitis.* The worst way of treating the condition is to put the patient to bed (often without elevation of the feet)—immobilise him, and perhaps give him an inadequate course of oral anticoagulant. This method (which unfortunately is often seen) practically ensures further spread of the thrombosis, often into the deep veins—and may convert what should be a short benign illness, into a prolonged serious one!

Doctors are often talked into this by the patient's complaint of pain over the phlebitis.

A NOTE ON THROMBOSIS IN NORMAL SUPERFICIAL VEINS

When thrombosis occurs in a *normal* superficial vein (*not* connected with a varicose vein system) in any part of the body, then a careful search for a cause should be instituted.

Patchy recurrent thrombosis in normal superficial veins occurs in patients with a hidden primary *carcinoma*. The authors have seen this as the presenting symptom in cases of carcinoma of lung (which is the commonest), carcinoma of pancreas, stomach and carcinoma of ovary. These are all sites where a primary tumour may grow to a considerable size without early symptoms, and a patchy unexplained thrombophlebitis may be the presenting symptom of the disease.

Blood diseases such as polycythaemia, thrombocythaemia, and leukaemia, may also present in this way.

Recurrent superficial thrombophlebitis in the legs of a young male patient should prompt a thought about Buerger's disease and all the foot pulses should be examined carefully.

'Mondor's disease' is a thrombophlebitis of the lateral thoracic vein, on the lateral aspect of the chest wall—and its occurrence should always prompt a search for a carcinoma somewhere.

DRIP THROMBOSIS

An important and common form of thrombosis is that caused by an intravenous drip in a superficial vein, either during an operation or in the course of illness, or pre- or post-operative care.

It usually comes on after a drip has been in the same vein for 48 to 72 hours. It is characterised by a high temperature (100° to 101°F) and *considerable pain* and swelling and redness over the vein. It pursues a long and painful course and the affected vein is often still tender 4 to 6 weeks after the onset.

The main factors responsible for a drip thrombosis are:

1. *Length of time that a drip is in a vein.* After 72 hours in the same vein the incidence of drip thrombosis rises sharply.

2. *Type of solution.* Normal saline and blood are the least thrombogenic. The more complicated intravenous solutions such as amino acids, and intravenous lipid solutions and glucose in stronger than isotonic solution are very thrombogenic.

3. *Local trauma to vein wall.* The modern plastic indwelling catheter is less traumatic than the old sharp steel ones.

SEPTIC DRIP THROMBOSIS

Occasionally a *septic* drip thrombosis occurs —this is signalled by the occurrence of *rigors*. Septic thrombophlebitis, even in these days of antibiotics and heparin, is always an extremely serious complication, owing to the accompanying septicaemia and pyaemia. It should be treated by *heparinisation* and *high dose antibiotic therapy*, after identifying the organism by blood culture. If possible ligation of the vein between the septic point and the heart should be considered.

Eczema

True, uncomplicated varicose eczema is the slightly pigmented scaly patch which is often seen over an enlarged group of varices in the leg (see Fig. 6.4). It is seldom of annoyance or significance in the early stage—causing a mild irritation or itching. If the varicose veins remain untreated it becomes chronic and sooner or later leads to trouble especially if the patient treats it with 'skin preparations'.

Another form of uncomplicated 'venous' eczema is the dry pigmented scaly patch seen over the internal malleolar area, as a precursor of venous ulceration. This is often the first reaction to the localised venous hypertension due to valve failure in the perforating veins.

At this early stage both types of eczema are easily and completely curable by radical operation, eliminating the varicose veins or the faulty perforating veins. Thus, if the local venous hypertension can be cured or ameliorated by operation at this early stage—this is the treatment of choice, and the time to do it.

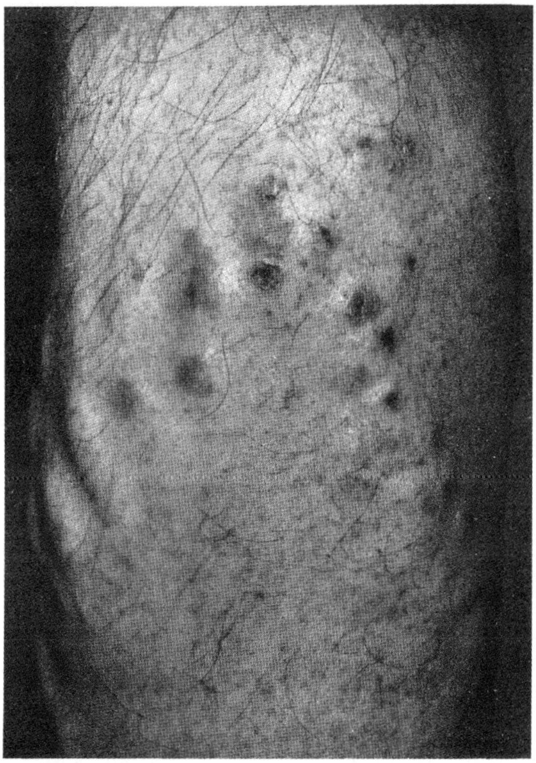

Fig. 6.4 Scaliness of the skin over varicose veins.

THE ROLE OF DRUG SENSITIVITY

Unfortunately many patients with either type of early eczema apply lotions and ointments to ameliorate the irritation or itching. Various preparations may be tried in succession either by the patient, or sometimes on a doctor's advice (*see* Fig. 6.5, *and* frontispiece).

This is a sure way of converting *a mild curable eczema* into a *major lifelong trouble.* The truth is that most of the severe so called 'varicose eczemas' that we see are drug induced. It is not generally realised that any mild eczema or irritation of the skin is 'sensitive' and the application of any apparently harmless preparation (to normal skin) can induce a serious and widespread sensitivity reaction.

The *first* thing is that most ointments have wool alcohol (Lanoline) as a base, and many medicated bandages and dressings and Zinc ointment also contain it. Skin sensitivity to this substance is common and easily induced by repeated application. The *second* frequent component of many 'medicated' dressings is 'balsam of Peru'. This substance adds a sort of 'medicinal aura' beloved by drug companies and advertisers, to dressings and applications —and is one of the most powerful eczema and sensitivity producing substances. It is contained in 'Tulle Gras' dressings and in many rectal suppositories, and ointments. The *third* enemy is skin preparations containing sulphonamide preparations, or antibiotics, they quickly produce eczema. Some of our worst and most persistent eczemas have been induced by penicillin cream which was originally applied to a venous ulcer. Neomycin cream also has an ugly reputation.

Other common skin applications which produce eczema are eusol, acriflavine and iodine.

Finally many patients are sensitive to *rubber* and as this is an essential constituent of many compression bandages, the difficulties are immense for the eczema patient—who may find it difficult to wear any form of support on the legs.

The subject of eczema belongs properly to the dermatologist—and specialist help should always be called in before an eczema becomes chronic—and a lifetime of misery begins if it is not quickly controlled. The present universal and long term application of *cortisone containing ointments* to skin lesions should be particularly condemned. Cortisone is a useful *short term control* for an acute eczema. If used over a long period sensitivity to the cortisone ointment itself may develop, as well as depression of the healing power of the skin locally by the cortisone and the production of a chronic ulcer (see Chap. 19).

In summary, when an early venous eczema appears, this should prompt an effort to get rid of the varicose veins and venous hypertension by early and effective surgery. Thus eczema should be a 'priority' indication for operation in all cases where this is required. If surgery is not appropriate (some generalised post-thrombotic cases) great care is taken not

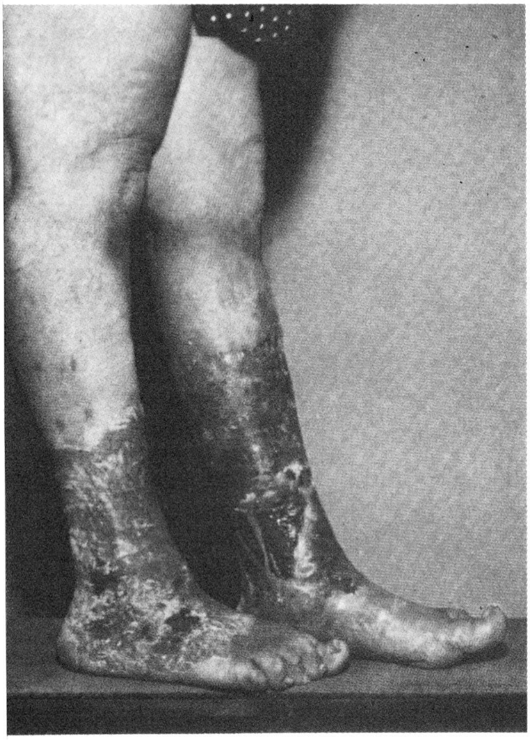

Fig. 6.5 Plaster dermatitis. (*See frontispiece*).

to put sensitivity producing applications on the skin.

Early uncomplicated varicose or venous eczema should not be treated by prolonged and varied skin applications aimed at relieving local irritation. In particular, 'medicated' ointments, 'medicated' bandages and 'medicated' dressings are avoided.

In the authors' experience pure olive oil, vaseline and Nivea cream, are permissible safe applications for cleaning flaky eczematous areas. Alcohol in the form of surgical spirit (60 per cent alcohol) is the safest application for surgical cleansing of the skin, without producing sensitivity, or normal saline.

Infected eczema

Nearly all severe eczemas teem with bacteria, and in particular the staphylococci and streptococci. They are always, therefore, a potent source of cross-infection in surgical wards. Such patients should be isolated, and on no account allowed near surgical patients.

When the skin is breached in an infected eczema, the staphylococci may then cause widespread skin destruction—giving rise to the widespread shallow ulcers—often mistakenly called 'varicose ulcers'.

The chain of events may be summarised as follows:

Venous hypertension
↓
Mild eczema (flaking)
↓
Sensitisation by skin applications
↓
Severe widespread eczema
↓
Infection with staphylococci, or streptococci
↓
Spreading shallow ulceration.

In such cases culture and vigorous high *parenteral* dosage with the right antibiotic, combined with rest in elevation and complete *cessation* of all local dressings, will often work wonders!

Lastly, in any patient who has an eczema from any other cause, it is always worse on the area affected by varicose veins, and made better by radical operation on the veins at fault.

Ulceration

This is the last, most feared, and best known of the four great complications. These lesions should be termed 'venous ulcers'. The old distinction between so-called varicose ulcers, stasis ulcers, gravitational and post-thrombotic ulcers is misleading and confusing because the basic pathology in all of them is venous hypertension in the subcutaneous tissues of the ankle.

The cause of the venous hypertension may be primary varicose veins, incompetent ankle perforating veins (post-thrombotic or otherwise), or perhaps a blocked iliac vein or sometimes all three together (see Chap. 17).

The clinical characteristics of these ulcers and their differential diagnosis is described in Chapter 19 and their treatment in Chapter 18. However certain basic facts are emphasised here.

Nearly all venous ulcers occur in that area of the leg termed the 'gaiter area' (being the area of the ankle covered by a 'Bishop's Gaiter') i.e. the lower third of the leg and dorsum of foot (Fig. 6.6).

This is the ankle skin whose main venous drainage is by the ankle perforating veins (see Chap. 3). All the severe venous ulcers in this territory are associated with valve incompetence in one or more of these perforating veins. The ulcer is due to a slow tissue necrosis caused by the high venous pressure in the capillary loops of the skin and subcutaneous tissues (Chap. 17), causing cellular oedema and then necrosis. The lesions are usually

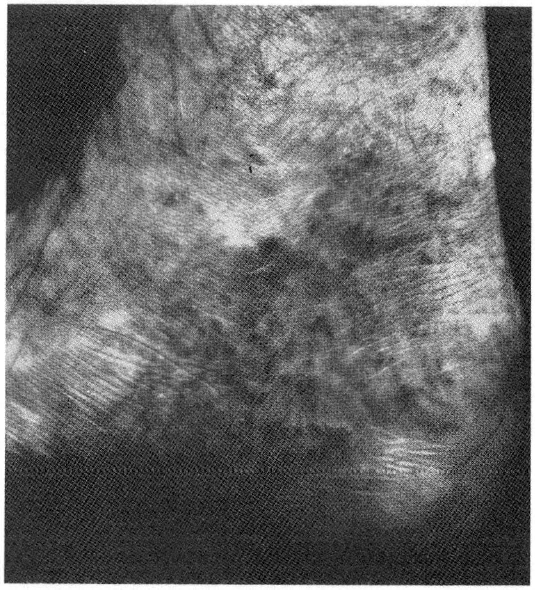

Fig. 6.7 Pre-ulcerous venular dilatation around the ankle.

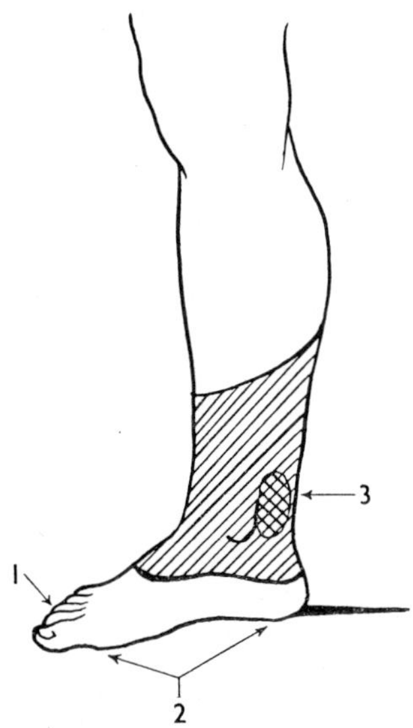

Fig. 6.6 Diagram of the main causes of ulcer of the toes, foot and ankle. 1. Chronic sores or ulcers of toes are due to: (a) Peripheral arterial disease (arteriosclerosis, diabetes, Buerger's Disease; (b) Chilblains; (c) Chronic fungus infection; (d) Trauma and bone infection. 2. Ulcers of sole of foot are due to: (a) Nerve lesions; tabes dorsalis, peripheral neuritis (diabetes), sciatic nerve lesion; (b) Peripheral arterial disease. 3. Gaiter area, over which venous ulcers occur.

on the inner aspect of the ankle just above and behind the internal malleolus.

Clinically there are two important precursor signs to show that an ulcer is imminent. In the *thin* leg (often male) there is an area of increasing venous congestion at the ankle (ankle flare, see Fig. 6.7) with a little pigmentation and a little scaling or flaking of the skin—often referred to as eczema.

In the fat leg, in addition to the above there may appear in the fat subcutaneous tissue a hard indurated area, often erroneously diagnosed as 'phlebitis'. This is actually a patch of 'fat necrosis' and is the typical reaction of subcutaneous fat cells to prolonged venous hypertension (Fig. 6.8). At first the fat necrosis is tender and red with surrounding inflammatory reaction, but gradually settles down and contracts to form a hard, fibrous plaque. Ulceration when it occurs on one of these pigmented areas of fat necrosis is one of the most difficult to heal.

It is at the stage of the early signs, *before the skin has broken down,* that radical treatment (either radical surgery or efficient support or both where appropriate) should be undertaken.

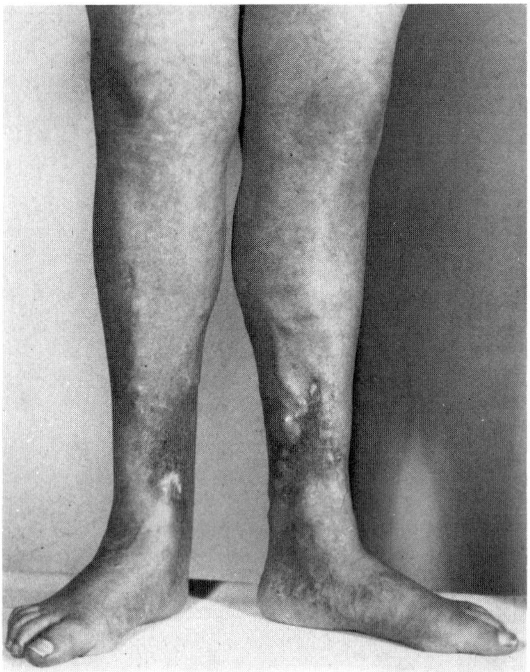

Fig. 6.8 Shows the early pigmentation of early fat necrosis and indurated plaque formation, over the ankle perforator area, which is the herald of ulceration to come. Note also the marked 'ankle flare'.

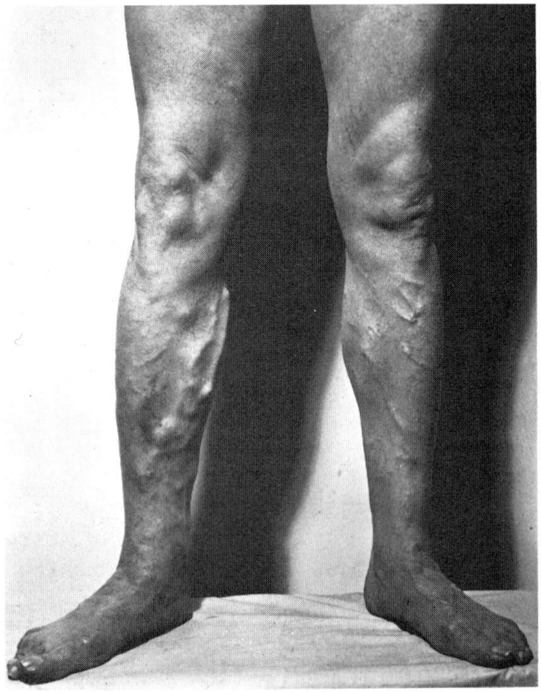

Fig. 6.9

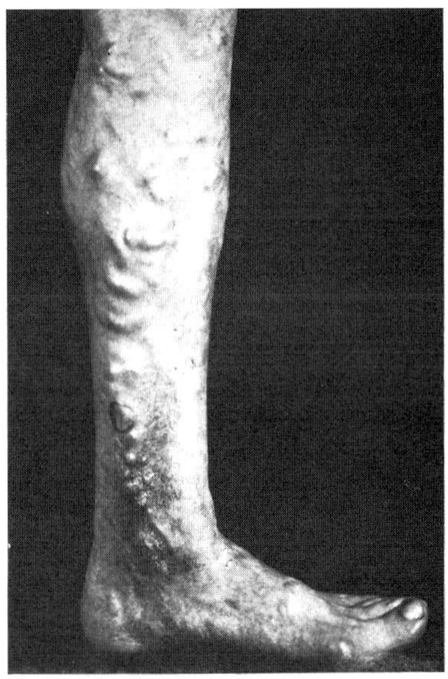

Figs 6.9, 6.10 These two figures show the contrast in the ankle skin between long saphenous incompetence, with normal perforating veins (Fig. 6.9) and long saphenous incompetence with, in addition, incompetent perforators (Fig. 6.10)

Particularly before the skin breaks down does operation give good results.

Once the skin is breached an important new factor makes its appearance—this is *infection*. Pain in the ulcer and rapid increase in size usually follows, and it is the two old offenders—the Staphylococcus and the Streptococcus which always do the damage. After an ulcer has enlarged and perhaps had some of the applications already deplored, put on it, secondary commensals appear and overgrow the original organisms *which, however, may still be there,* although difficult to culture.

The rules for the treatment of these ulcers are to be found in Chapter 18.

Serious ulceration very seldom occurs in uncomplicated long or short saphenous incompetence, provided that the ankle perforator valves are still competent. One often sees cases with enormous varicose veins, but perfectly clear ankle skin.

As soon as one of the ankle perforators becomes incompetent in such a case (as they often do) then engorgement round the ankle appears and eczema and ulceration follow rapidly (Figs 6.9 and 6.10). Exactly why the ankle perforator valve should suddenly become incompetent after many years in these cases is not clear. Possibly it is through sheer increase in size of the perforator, after years of handling increased flow and pressure, or possibly due to a minor subclinical thrombosis. Certainly it is in this type of case where one occasionally does see really enormous perforators, up to half the size of ones little finger!

REFERENCES

Anning, S. T. (1954) *Leg Ulcers*. London: Churchill.
Borschberg, E. (1967) *Prevalence of Varicose Veins in Lower Extremities*. Basel & N. York: S. Karger.
Cockett, F. B. (1953) *Pathology and Treatment of Venous Ulcers of the Leg*. M.S. Thesis, London Univ.
Cotton, L. T. (1951) *Br. Jnl. Surg.*, **48**, 589.
Gay, J. (1868) *Lettsomian Lectures, 1867*. London: Churchill.
Virchow, R. (1846) Die Verstopfung der Lungenarterie und ihre Folgen. *Beitr. exp. Path. Physiol. Traube*, **2**, 1. Berlin.

7. Diagnosis of Varicose Veins

Varicose vein disease is sometimes diagnosed with ease,
But oft the best attempts will meet with sad and sorrowful defeat.
So let us give you good advice.
Examine once, Examine twice:
Examine from the head to toes,
Before you dare to diagnose.
More harm is done because you do not *look*
Than from not knowing what is in the book.
Above all do not try to spot
Because you think you know a lot.
Spot diagnosis you should hate
Until you are a surgeon great!
By then of course you will have learnt
Some lessons bitter, and you darn't.

With apologies to Sir Zachary Cope.

The first thing to ask when a patient presents with varicose veins and symptoms in the legs is 'Are the varicose veins actually the cause of, or relevant to, the patient's complaint?'

So often patients are sent to see a surgeon or vascular specialist because they complain of aching or pain in the legs and are noticed to have varicose veins, and without more ado they are advised to seek treatment for them. The fact that they have osteoarthritis of the knee, or hip, or a disc lesion, which is the real cause of the pain and discomfort in the leg of which the patient complains, may have been overlooked in the first hasty examination.

This mistake is of everyday occurrence, and it is important not to subject any patient to an unnecessary operation or treatment for often quite minor varicose veins, when their symptoms are due to something else!

Differential diagnosis is also particularly important when a patient presents with an ulcer of the ankle. Again the first question should be 'Is this ulcer due to venous disease or to one of the numerous other causes of ulcer?' (The differential diagnosis of venous ulcers is dealt with in Chapter 19.)

If the condition of the patient's leg and his symptoms are judged to be due to some form of pathology in the venous system, then a detailed differential diagnosis of the exact type is required.

CLASSIFICATION OF MAIN TYPES OF VARICOSE VEINS

The main diagnostic subdivisions have been indicated in Chapter 5, but they are set out briefly here.

1. Primary familial varicose veins.
   (a) Long saphenous
   (b) Short saphenous
   (c) Ankle perforators.
2. Secondary varicose veins due to old deep vein thrombosis, either iliofemoral type or peripheral type or both (Chaps 15, 16, 17).
3. Pregnancy veins (Chap. 10).
4. Rarer types of veins (Hunter's canal perforator, pudendal, lateral venous anomaly, and secondary to arteriovenous fistula, etc.) (Chap. 11).

These four groups are borne in mind as one looks at a case of vein pathology with a view to further exact diagnosis (Fig. 7.1).

A description of the important steps in history taking and examination of a patient is now given.

HISTORY

1. The main complaint of the patient: is it pain, swelling, eczema, ulceration or just the appearance of the veins and the fear they might get worse? If the main complaint

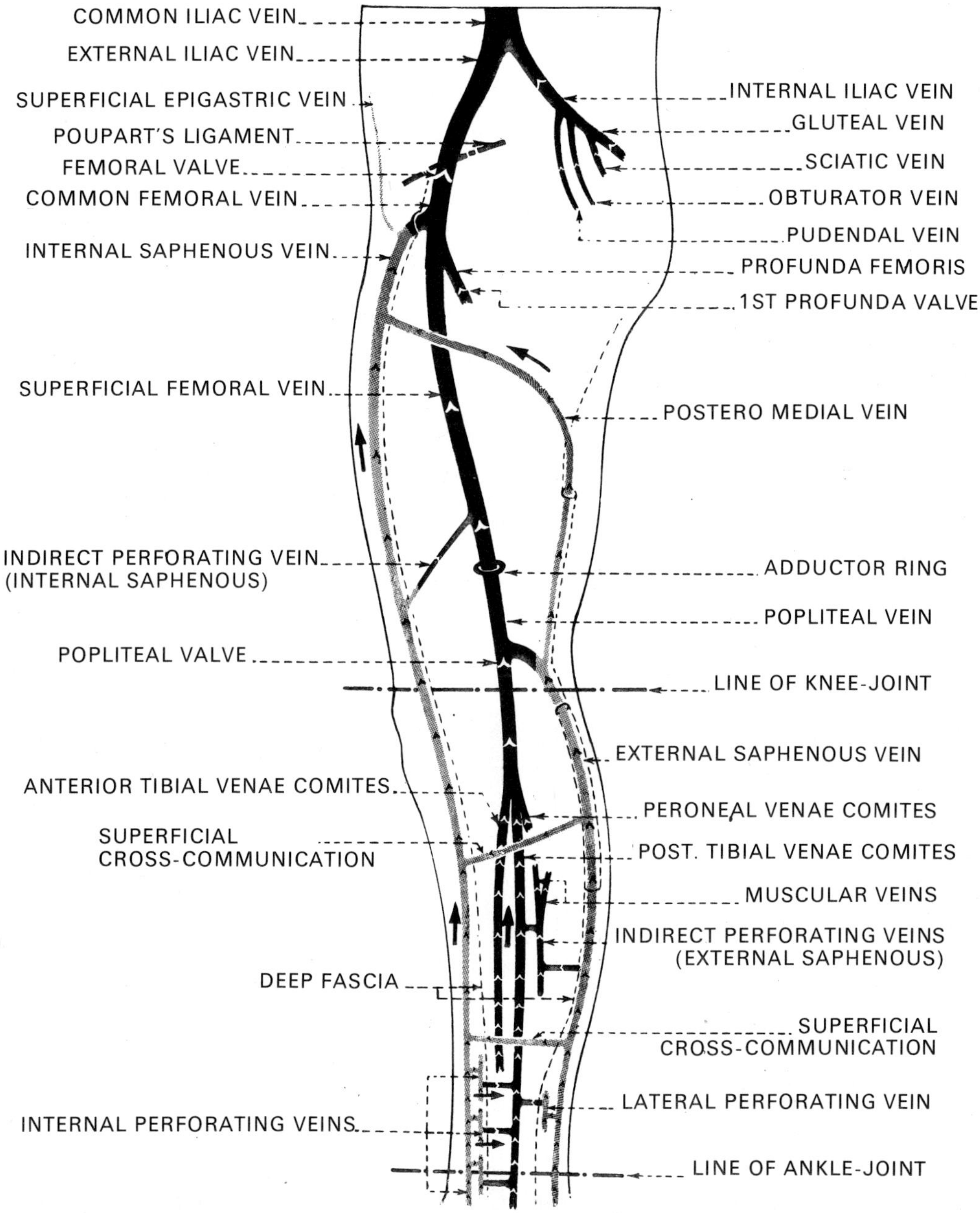

Fig. 7.1 A diagrammatic rendering of the veins of the lower limb.

is pain or swelling, then other causes of pain in the leg or swelling must be thought of and excluded.

2. Family history: Patients with primary varicose veins have a family history of the same condition occurring in a close relative in about 70 per cent of cases. Oddly enough there is also a significant number of cases of deep vein thrombosis who also give a positive family history (Fig. 7.2) (see Chap. 16).

3. If the patient is female, ask if periods are regular and has she missed a period recently—suggesting an early pregnancy.

4. In all cases enquire if there has been any previous history suggestive of deep vein thrombosis. Patients often forget about minor episodes of leg swelling, calf pain, or even quite major incidents—until their memory is stimulated by persistent direct questioning.

5. Ask the patient for details of any previous illness, accident, fracture, or operations. Information may emerge of great relevance to the diagnosis and treatment of the varicose veins. One patient admitted that he had had a testicle removed—this led to careful examination of the abdomen, and the discovery of a mass of secondary glands obstructing the vena cava!

EXAMINATION

The important part of the examination is *inspection in a good light in the erect position*, the patient standing on a stool. This is followed by palpation and certain special tests.

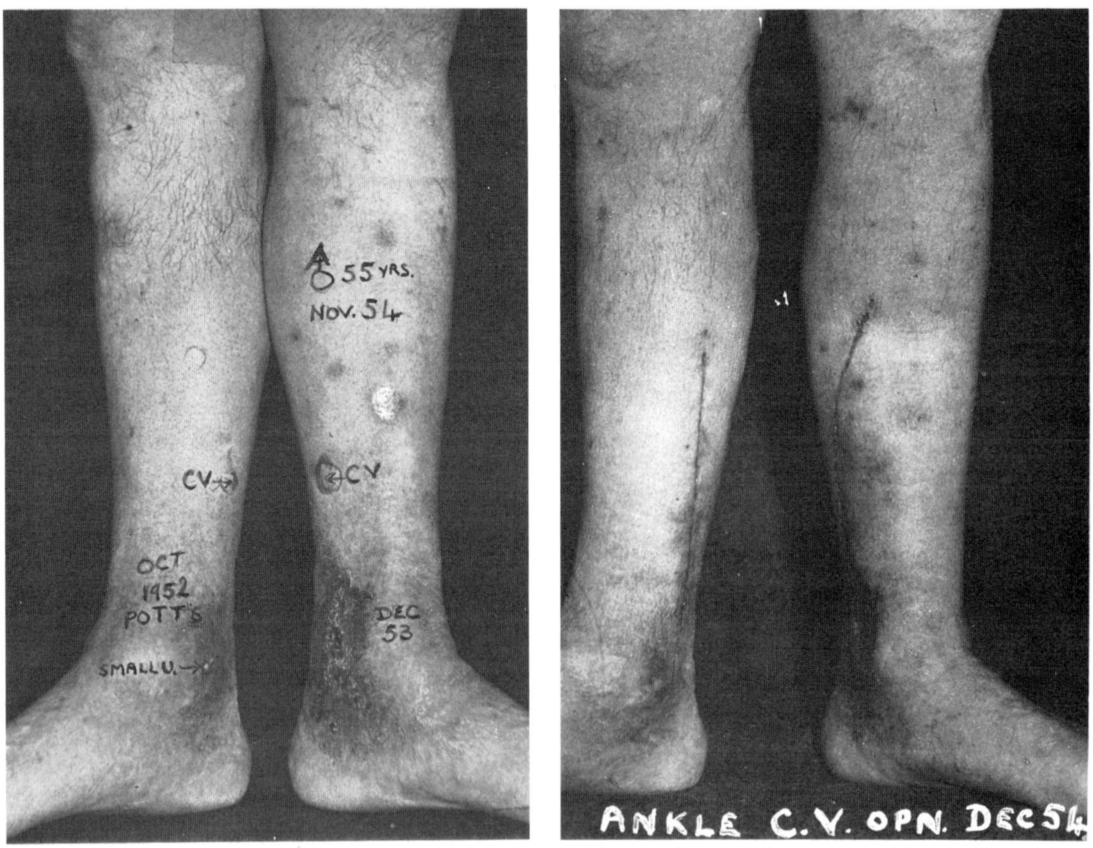

Fig. 7.2 Bilateral deep thrombophlebitis after a Pott's fracture, before and after ligation of the ankle perforating veins.

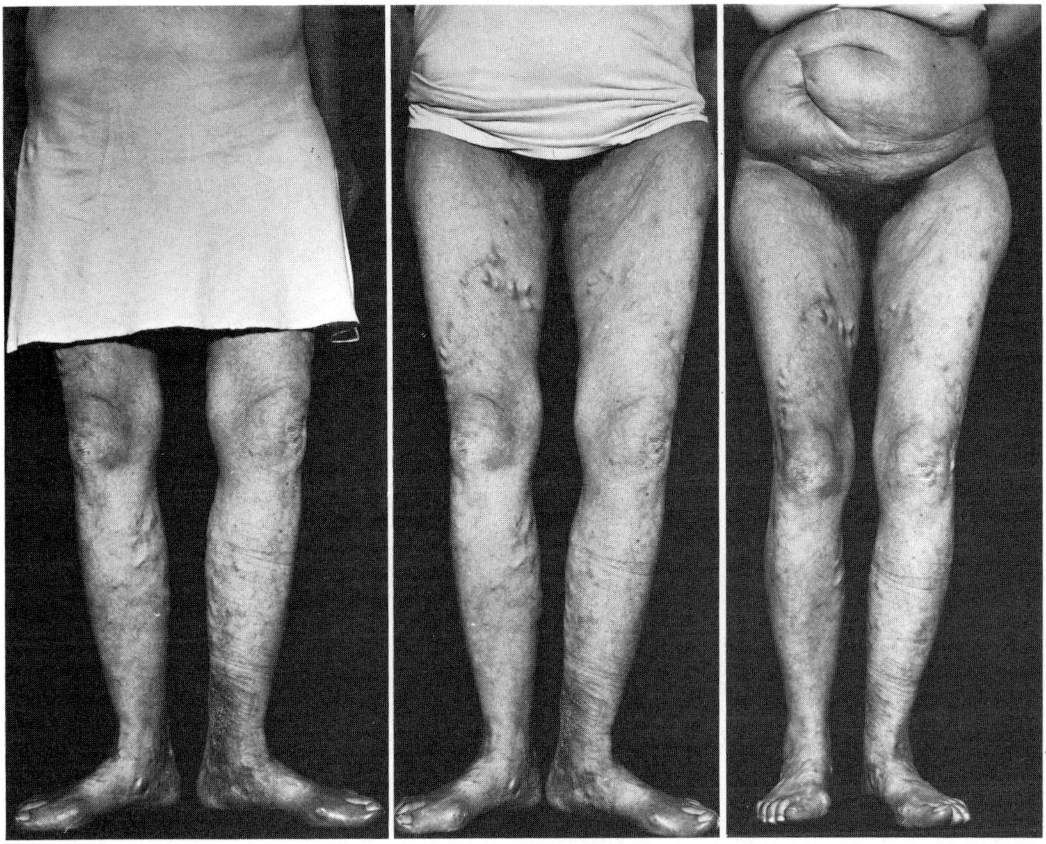

Fig. 7.3 Examination of patient, to illustrate the undressing required. Note the eczema of the left ankle of which the patient complained, the varicose veins, the swelling of the limb and the abdominal operation which was complicated by deep thrombophlebitis 12 years previously.

Inspection

Inspection should always follow a planned routine.

First the patient is *asked to stand* and is examined from the front.

It is important to look at the *abdomen* first.

The appearance of veins on the abdominal wall or running across the pubis is the 'give-away' sign of an old iliofemoral thrombosis. Scars of old operations are also noted, and may prompt further questions. An unduly protuberant abdomen may raise the question of pregnancy, or ovarian cyst or fibroid, (Figs 7.3, 7.4, 7.5).

Next, the eye runs down the legs and the general distribution of the veins is noted—

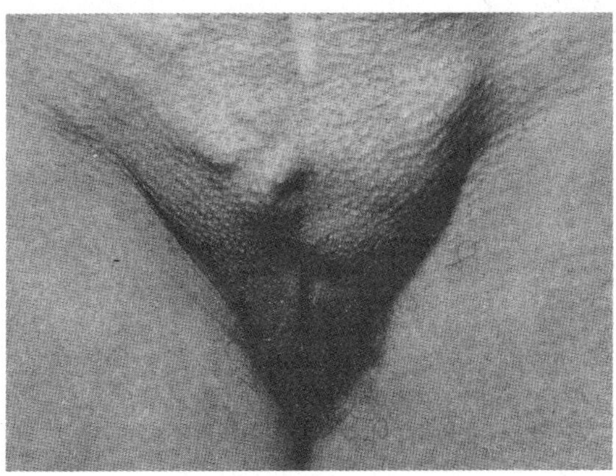

Fig. 7.4 Pubic varices usually indicate old iliofemoral thrombosis, with some residual obstruction of the iliac veins.

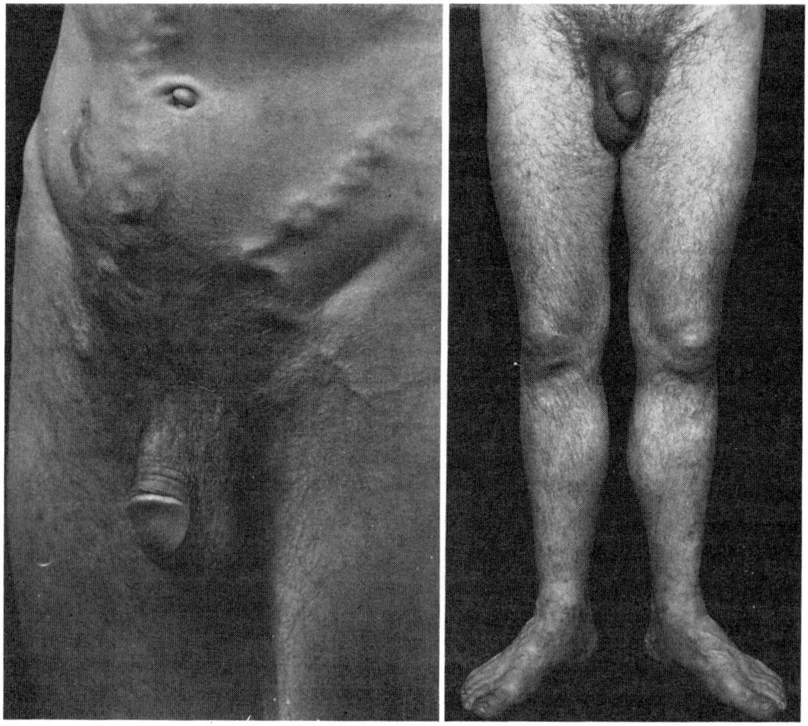

Fig. 7.5 Extensive abdominal collateral veins, following old iliofemoral thrombosis—with residual iliac vein obstruction.

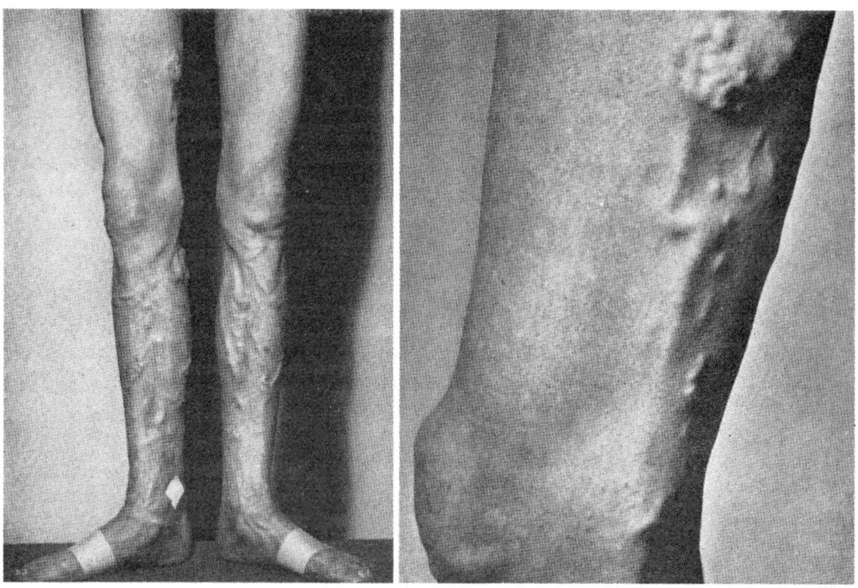

Fig. 7.6 Varices apparently arising from an incompetent communicating vein in Hunter's canal. The tests disproved this possibility; they are due to an incompetent internal saphenous vein.

whether they appear to be mainly in the long saphenous area, or on the lateral side, or mainly in the leg. If long saphenous incompetence appears to be present, it is worth making a quick diagram for record purposes of just which set of branches is affected (e.g. anterolateral branch of thigh or posterior arch of leg etc.).

Next, the ankle region is inspected carefully. Congestion of the ankle region, or prominent veins here and the presence of an ankle flare (see Figs 19.3 and 19.4) all suggest the presence of one or more incompetent perforators. Pigmentation, eczema, or actual ulceration in the ankle region makes this virtually certain. The sites of the main perforating veins are inspected carefully. Sometimes the incompetent perforator is obvious from the suggestive bulge as in Figure 7.12 but often it cannot be seen, and its presence is inferred from the congested veins and skin lesions in the 'gaiter area' of the ankle (see Chaps 17 and 18).

The patient is then asked to turn round, and the leg is inspected from behind. (A common omission!) (Fig. 7.7). The territory of the short saphenous vein is examined. In the same way as before, the ankle is looked at for signs of eczema, and the site of the lateral perforating vein is inspected.

Palpation and special tests

It is useful to feel the veins with the pulp of the fingers. They may be tender or fibrous or even thrombosed. Sometimes in a fat leg, a large, tense vein can be felt when it cannot be seen. This is important in cases of short saphenous incompetence, as the upper half of this vein lies beneath the deep fascia of the leg and even when enlarged, often cannot be seen. Yet if the knee is flexed slightly to relax the popliteal fascia, the vein can be felt easily if it is dilated.

SPECIAL TESTS

The cough impulse test

In this test, the finger is placed over the line of the enlarged internal saphenous vein below the foramen ovale (Fig. 7.8). Upon coughing, it is usual to feel an expansile impulse in a grossly varicose long saphenous trunk. This impulse is communicated to the varicose tributaries down the leg, and occasionally is so marked that it gives a thrill. The 'cough impulse' test is less delicate than the tourniquet test, but it is rapidly performed.

Technique. The pulps of the fingers are placed on the prominent enlarged veins in the leg or thigh; the patient is asked to turn the face to the ceiling and cough vigorously. The result varies from no impulse being felt to an expansile impulse and to a coarse thrill with the grosser valvular defects. The impulse is best felt 1 to 2 inches below the termination of the internal saphenous vein; the landmark for the latter is a point 1·25 inches outside and below the pubic spine. Sometimes a varix is visible or palpable here, or, in an average varicose internal saphenous vein, the enlarged vessel can be seen or palpated and rolled under the fingertips as an elastic cylinder. Enlarged saphenous glands may conceal it. Many healthy people are unable to cough, and the husky clearing of the throat, which they produce, might be mistaken for lack of cooperation.

Evaluation of the 'cough impulse' test. When a cough impulse is present it indicates not only incompetence of the terminal saphenous valve, but also that there is no competent valve between the saphenofemoral union, and the right auricle, i.e. that the valves in the common femoral and iliac veins are absent or ineffective. At operation on gross internal saphenous varicosity, the transmitted venous pulse and collapse with inspiration can sometimes be observed in it.

This test, to be truly positive, must give an impulse in varices in the thigh. At the foramen ovale the cough impulse can occur in the normal common femoral vein, due to the absence of valves in it and the external iliac vein (in 30 per cent of persons) although the terminal valve of the internal saphenous vein is sound.

A further error with the 'cough' sign is to regard the slight jerk of the muscular contraction that occurs in the lower limbs when some patients cough, as an expansile impulse.

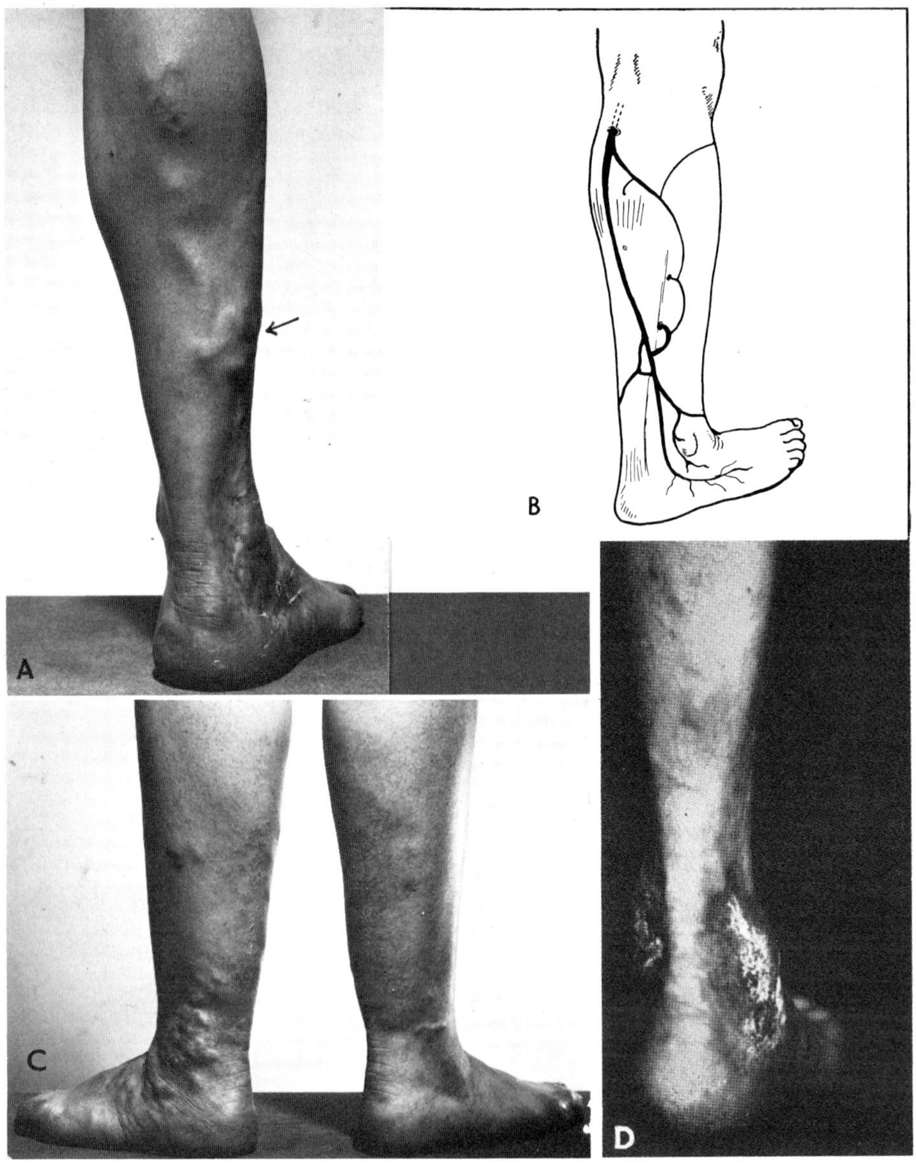

Fig. 7.7 Early and late cases of short saphenous with lateral perforator incompetence. A. Early case of short saphenous incompetence. Shows enlarged short saphenous, large lateral perforator (arrow), and early skin changes behind lateral malleolus. B. Diagram of the usual anatomy of the short saphenous vein and the lateral ankle perforator. C. Short saphenous incompetence in a fat leg. There is an eczematous skin reaction down the back of both ankles, and a bunch of dilated veins around the lateral malleolus. The short saphenous itself can neither be seen nor palpated through the fat. D. Advanced ulceration behind both malleoli, due to short, saphenous and lateral perforator incompetence.

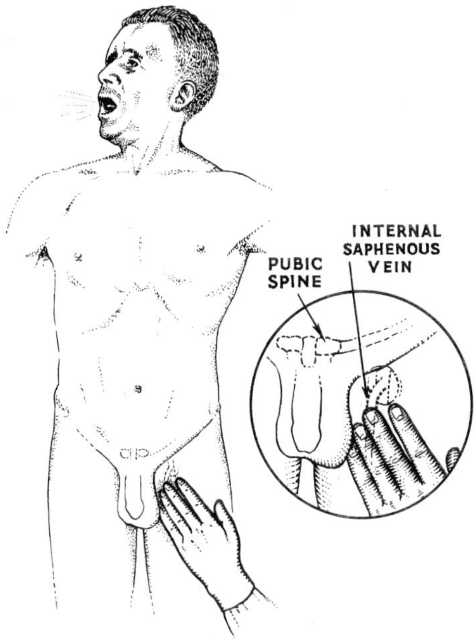

Fig. 7.8 The cough impulse test. The fingers must be below the foramen ovale for an impulse can occur here in the normal femoral vein and could be attributed erroneously to incompetence of the internal saphenous vein.

The percussion test (Schwartz's test)

This test described by Chevrier (1908) and associated with Schwartz's and Homan's name (1922) is carried out as follows:

With the patient standing, the examiner places two fingers lightly on the region of the foramen ovale whilst with the index finger of the other hand the varicosities below or above the knee are tapped smartly (Fig. 7.9). The test is also carried out in reverse. If the internal saphenous vein is enlarged an impulse is discernible by the lower or upper palpating fingers. It denotes an unbroken column of fluid extending from the saphenofemoral junction to the varicosities below. The test is used only in those with obvious varicose veins. In a person with an incompetent internal or external saphenous vein, an impulse can be made to pass up and down the defective vessels with the same rapidity that a vibration can be felt in a taut wire. It is especially of service for rapid approximate diagnosis in the gross varicosities. It is helpful in determining whether a group of varicosities are in direct connection with the long saphenous system or with the short saphenous system.

We regard the percussion test as more sensitive than the cough impulse test.

The Brodie Trendelenburg tourniquet test

This test is a good demonstration of valvular incompetence in the long saphenous system. It was described by Sir Benjamin Brodie in 1846. Later in 1891 Trendelenburg established its significance. Since that time the test has taken its place as one of the standard manoeuvres in demonstrating long saphenous incompetence.

Sir Benjamin Brodie's own original instructions were as follows:

(Fig. 7.10) 'If I put on a bandage and squeezed the blood out of the veins below and then put my thumb on the vena saphena magna above so as to stop the circulation through it, I found on taking off the bandage, the patient being in the erect posture, that the cluster of veins below filled very slowly and only from the capillary vessels; but if the patient being in the erect position I removed the pressure from the vein, the valves being of no use, the blood rushed downward by its own

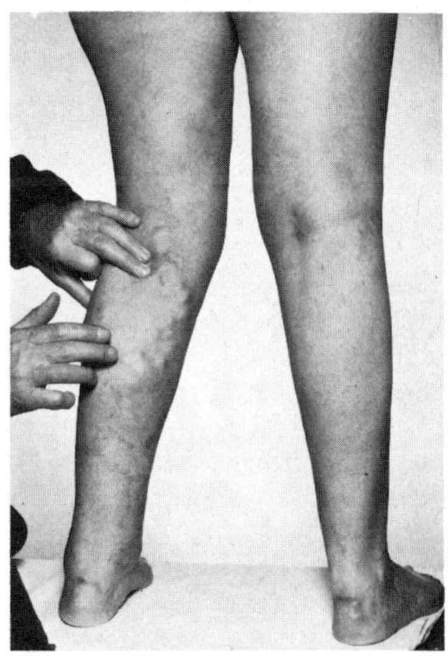

Fig. 7.9 The 'Schwartz Test' or Tapping Test, for an enlarged incompetent short saphenous vein.

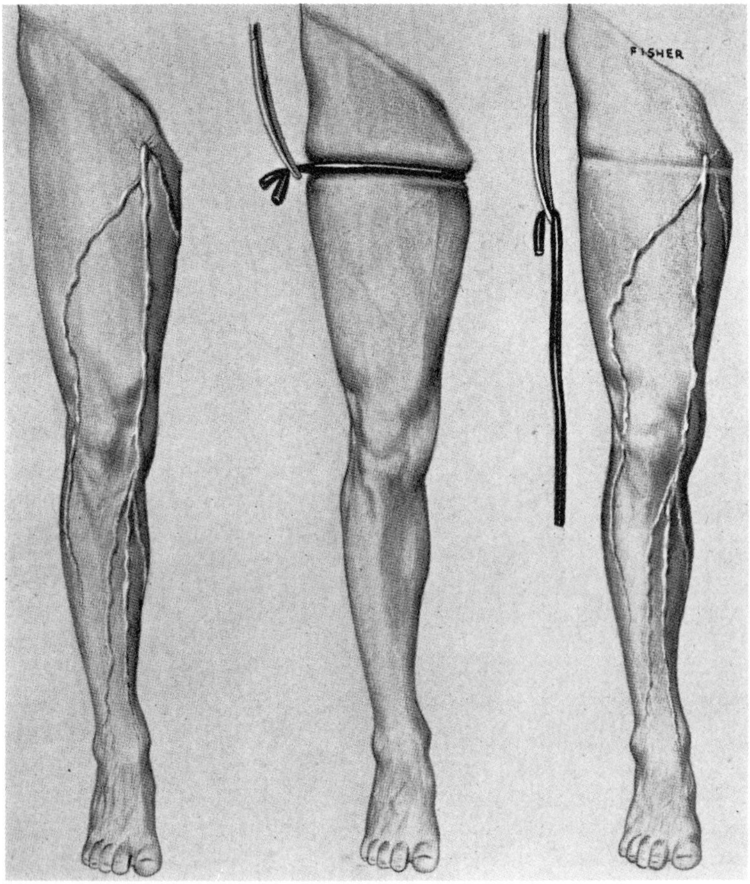

Fig. 7.10 The test for the incompetent internal saphenous vein.

weight contrary to the course of the circulation and filled the varicose clusters below almost instantly.'

In practice, in a patient with gross varices of the long saphenous system, he is asked to lie on a couch, the leg is raised, and the veins are emptied by stroking them firmly towards the groin. A light rubber band is then placed round the upper thigh, near but just below the saphenofemoral junction, and just tight enough to occlude the superficial veins efficiently. (This may require some practice, and several attempts on the same patient.)

The patient is then asked to stand up quickly, and stand still for about 15 seconds. The tourniquet is snapped off and if the long saphenous vein is incompetent, at once there is a cascade of blood down the veins, filling all the varices rapidly from above.

It is an impressive test.

Multiple tourniquet tests

Varicose veins are usually due to a leak of high venous pressure from the deep to the superficial veins. This leak is due to a faulty valve at: (1) the mouth of the long saphenous vein in the groin (the long saphenous leak); or (2) the short saphenous vein where it joins the popliteal vein in the popliteal fossa (the short saphenous leak); and (3) the ankle perforating veins—two on the inner side, one on the outer side, and one mid-calf—(the ankle perforator leak); (4) very rarely there is a perforator also in Hunter's canal (Chap. 11).

These escapes take place at different levels in the limb, and so it is theoretically possible to arrange a series of rubber tourniquets to cut off these leaks at various levels in the limb, and to diagnose at what level they are occurring.

These multiple tourniquet tests are time consuming, need experience to perform correctly, and can be difficult to interpret. Beautiful demonstrations can occasionally be obtained where veins are large and easily seen, and the diagnosis is obvious from inspection. Unfortunately in the more difficult cases (fat legs, legs with multiple leaks) the results of the tourniquet tests arc unrcliable, and possibly misleading. In some patients, the tourniquet tests are painful. Thus their routine use in diagnosis is *not* recommended.

However as they are occasionally helpful in demonstrations, one of the tests will be detailed here.

The double tourniquet test for short saphenous incompetence

This is useful when both the long saphenous leak and the short saphenous leak are present in the same limb.

The patient lies down and the leg is elevated to empty the veins, and two rubber tourniquets are applied, one at the groin and one immediately below the knee.

The patient then stands, the veins below the knee are observed (Fig. 7.11).

If they fill at once, there is a leak below the level of the tourniquets, i.e. in one or more ankle perforators. If they remain flat for about 10 to 15 seconds, the lower of the two tourniquets (which is controlling the short saphenous vein) is snapped off. If the veins below this immediately fill, this indicates a short saphenous incompetence, as the higher

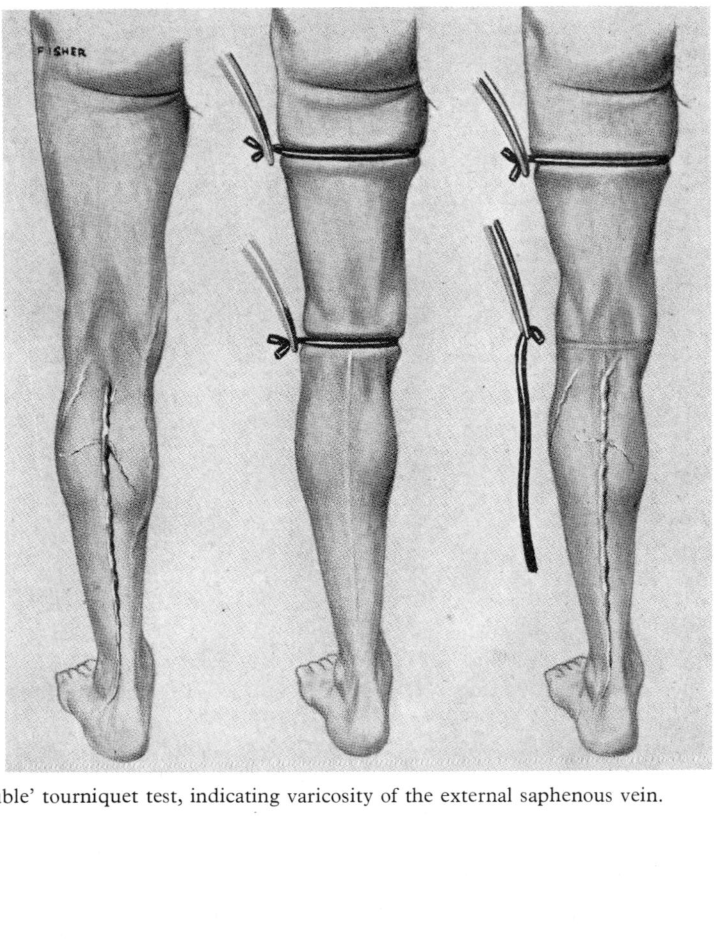

Fig. 7.11 The 'double' tourniquet test, indicating varicosity of the external saphenous vein.

tourniquet at the groin is controlling the long saphenous vein.

It is possible also to elaborate a triple tourniquet test as well, but the more complicated the test becomes, the more difficult it is to perform, and even then the diagnosis may be uncertain.

Tests for perforating veins

Probably the simplest test for a perforating vein is as follows: The suspected site of the perforator leak is firmly controlled by a thumb over it, the veins in the vicinity are stroked in a direction away from the perforator, to empty them, and the thumb is suddenly removed. Immediate and dramatic refilling of the veins from the spot compressed indicates the site of an incompetent perforator.

Unfortunately perforator leaks are seldom single, but are usually associated with a long or a short saphenous leak, or both—and clear cut results with a simple test like this is a rarity, as the veins around the perforator tend to fill rapidly from the other incompetent sources.

However there is one test which is occasionally helpful—this is the test known as Perthe's test.

Perthe's test (Fig. 7.12)

Where a patient has enlarged congested veins in the ankle area, this test will sometimes give a fair indication of the presence or not of incompetent ankle perforating veins.

The patient is observed while exercising the calf,

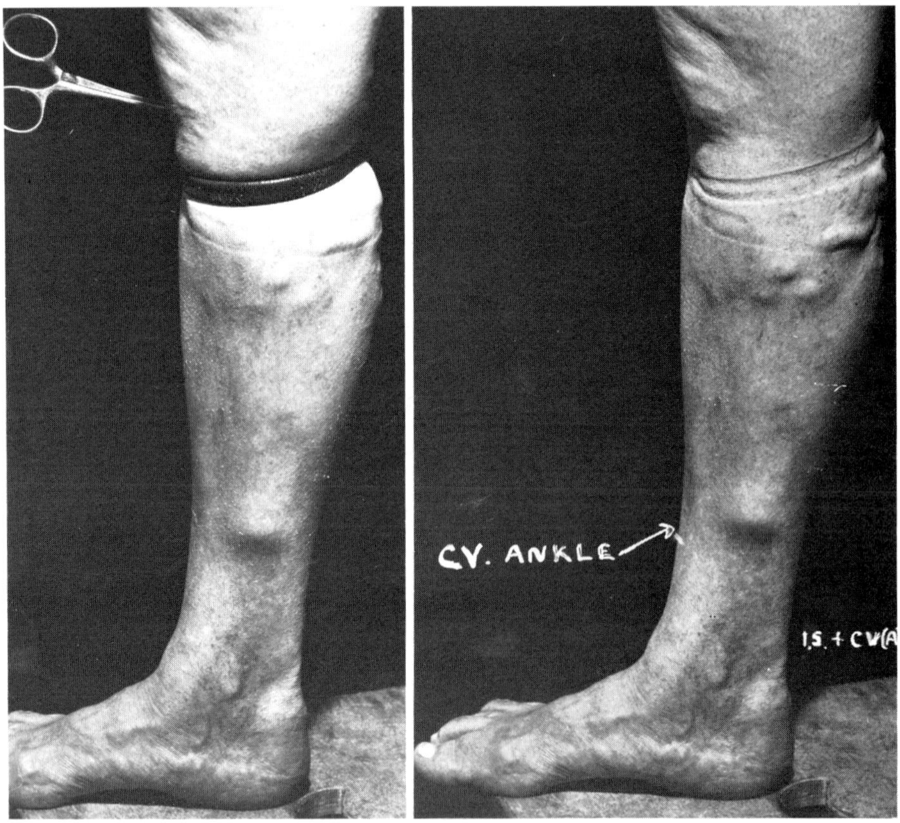

Fig. 7.12 '*Perthe's test.*' An incompetent upper ankle communicating vein with an overlying varix. The 'blow-out' fills after the veins have been emptied and a tourniquet applied. The varices in the upper leg are filled from this incompetent perforating vein. Tests for the long and short saphenous veins were negative. It will be noticed that this patient has as yet few skin changes at the ankle; only a little skin speckling and the beginning of filling of the retromalleolar groove.

by raising himself on his toes, and down again fairly rapidly. A tourniquet is applied to the upper third of the leg, tight enough to compress the superficial veins, and prevent filling from above (from an incompetent long or short saphenous system). The patient is again asked to exercise his calf and the veins in the ankle area are observed. (1) If they become *less prominent* and tense, this indicates that the muscular action has sucked blood from the superficial veins into the deep veins through the perforators whose valves must be sound. (2) If the veins remain the same or become *more* prominent during the exercise, it indicates that they are being filled via incompetent perforators below the tourniquet.

General assessment of tests for perforating veins

The above tests for perforating veins are often difficult, impossible to perform accurately, and difficult to assess clinically, without a great deal of practice.

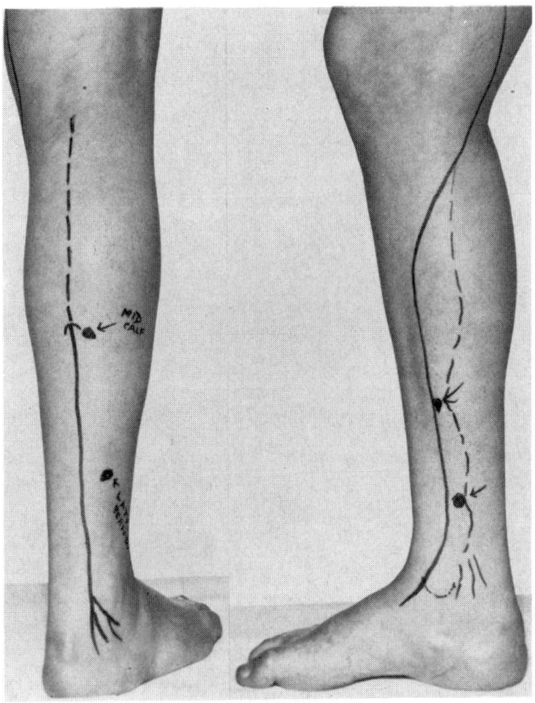

Fig. 7.13 The anatomical sites of the four main ankle perforators are shown. These sites are very constant. All four however may not be constantly present in the same patient, and their relative size and importance varies from case to case.

There is really no substitute for careful inspection. The presence of dilated veins or capillaries or skin lesions below the perforating veins in the ankle area, plus an exact knowledge of the anatomical location of the main perforators, are the requisites for the diagnosis. The four ankle perforators, which always have to be considered and looked for are shown in Figure 7.13.

Suggestive bulges or pits near enlarged incompetent perforators are often present—but they are by no means an infallible guide to the actual site of an incompetent perforator.

Thus the presence of incompetent perforators is often deduced by the signs they produce in the ankle area rather than by seeing or feeling the perforator itself. These early signs may be pigmentation, slight redness of the skin and the ankle flare.

THE MAIN CLINICAL PRESENTATIONS OF PRIMARY VARICOSE VEINS

Having reviewed the clinical diagnostic methods, the characteristics of the main common presentations of varicose veins must be illustrated.

The single incompetent long saphenous vein (see Figs 7.6, 7.14 and 7.23).

This is by far the most common presentation. In a reasonably thin person the enlarged vein may be seen over its course from groin to ankle, but this is relatively rare.

As the effect of venous hypertension in the vein builds up over the years the long saphenous trunk enlarges and thickens but it never gets grossly tortuous. It is much stronger than its tributaries. These are in the subcutaneous tissues just under the skin, and distend rapidly and become tortuous as the venous hypertension steadily stretches them over the years.

Thus the *tortuous varicose veins* on the surface are always the tributaries of the main saphenous trunk which is often not visible at all in a limb with the average amount of fat. The enlarged saphenous trunk remains relatively straight as it runs in its own slight

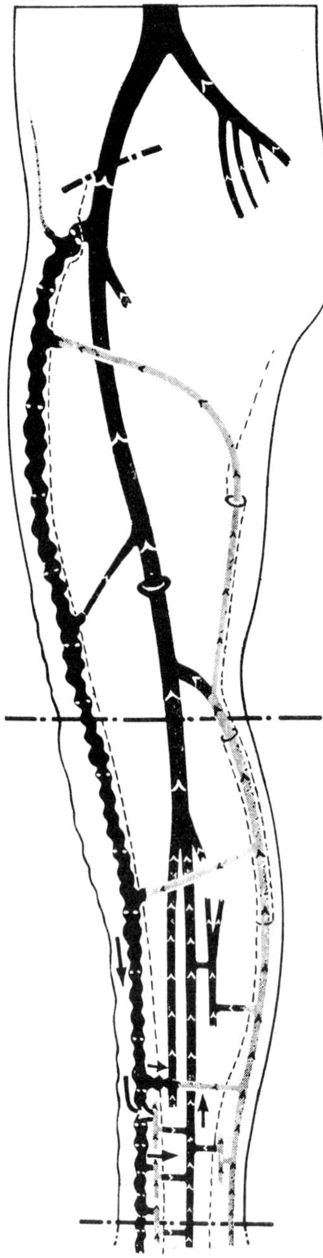

Fig. 7.14 The varicose internal saphenous vein (diagrammatic).

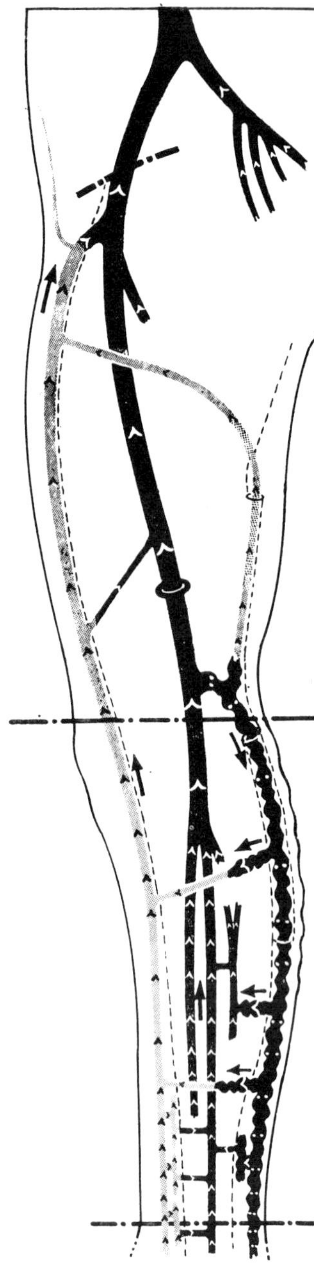

Fig. 7.15 The varicose external saphenous vein (diagrammatic).

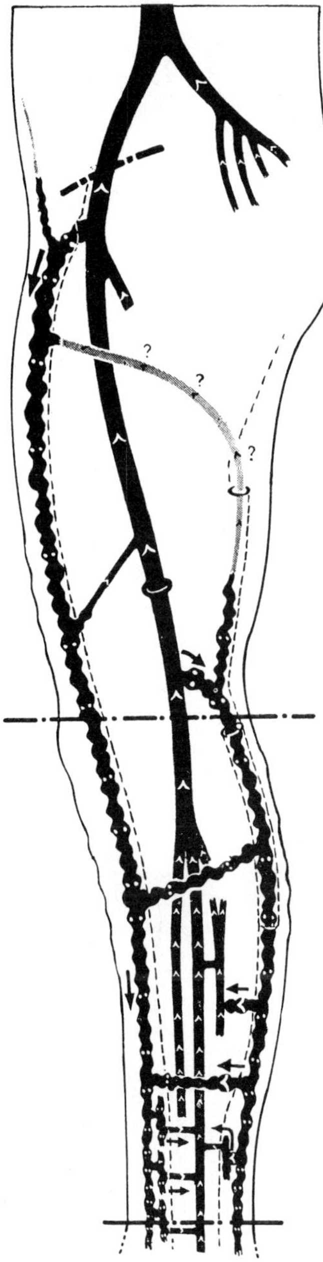

Fig. 7.16 The combined varicosity of the internal and external saphenous veins (diagrammatic).

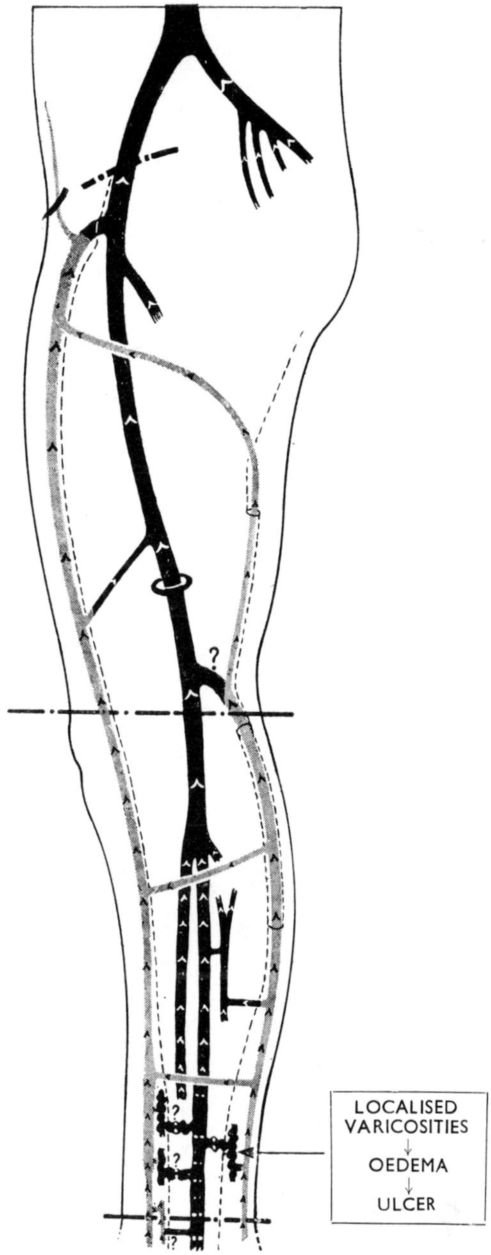

Fig. 7.17 The incompetent ankle communicating veins. The question marks indicate that not all those veins are necessarily incompetent at the same time (diagrammatic).

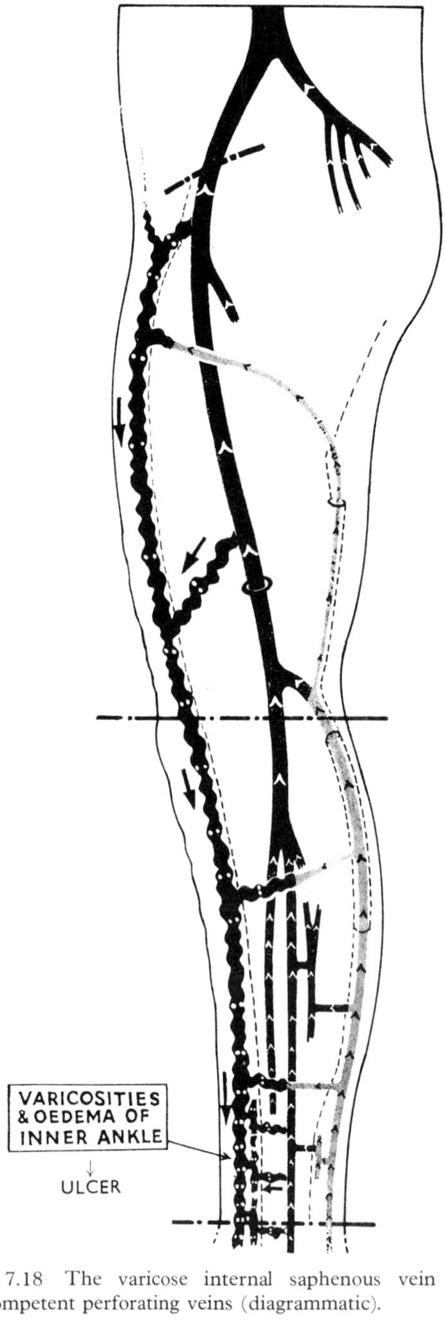

Fig. 7.18 The varicose internal saphenous vein and incompetent perforating veins (diagrammatic).

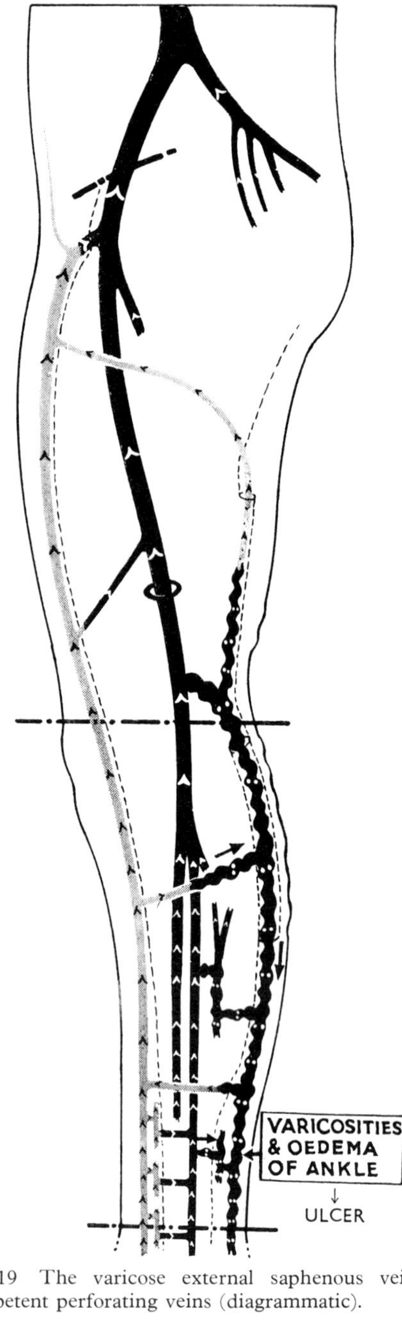

Fig. 7.19 The varicose external saphenous vein and incompetent perforating veins (diagrammatic).

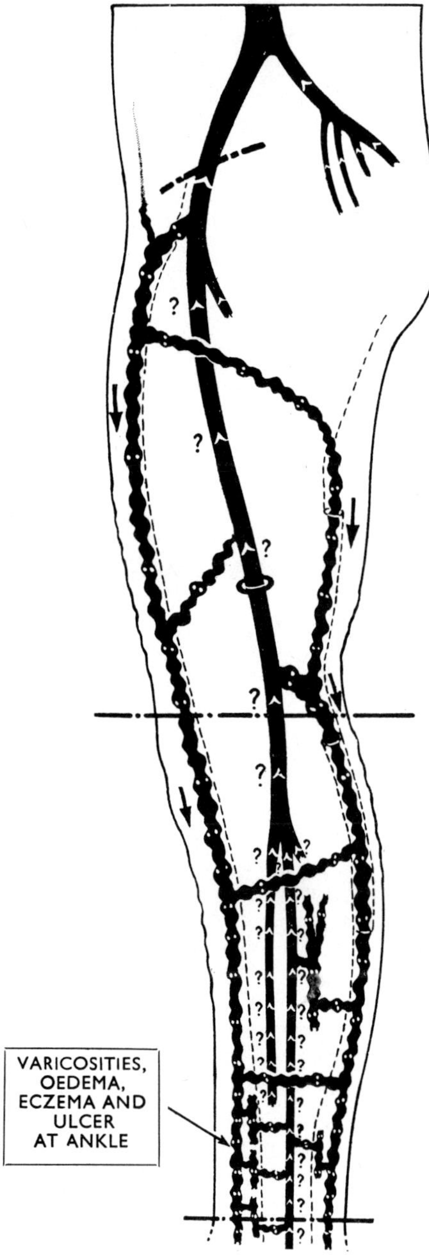

Fig. 7.20 The triple incompetence, i.e. varicosity of the internal and external saphenous veins and defective perforating veins. The question marks indicate the variable state of the valves of the deep veins (diagrammatic).

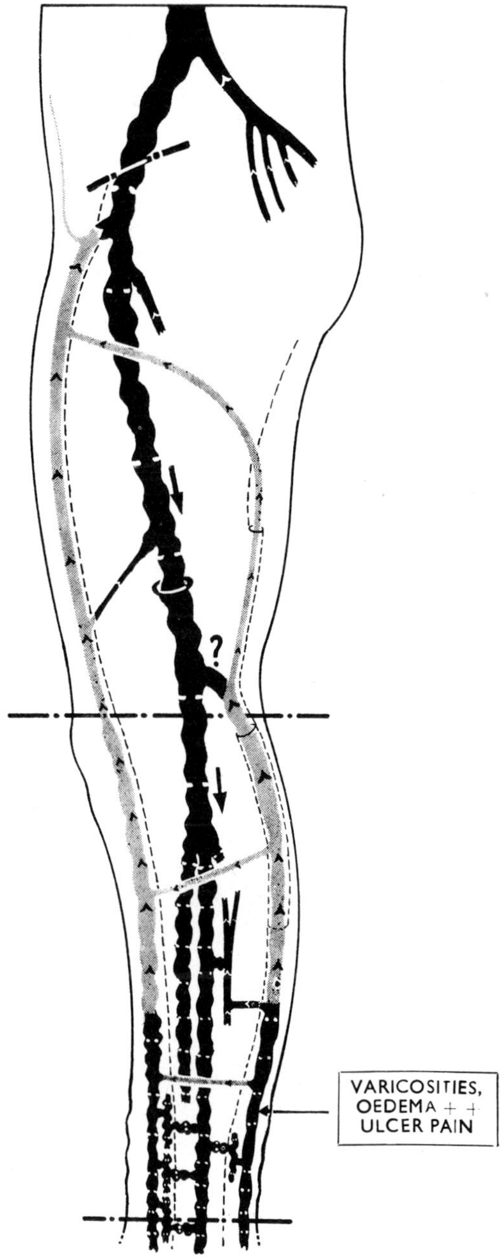

Fig. 7.21 Some later effects of deep thrombophlebitis (diagrammatic), incompetent deep and perforating veins.

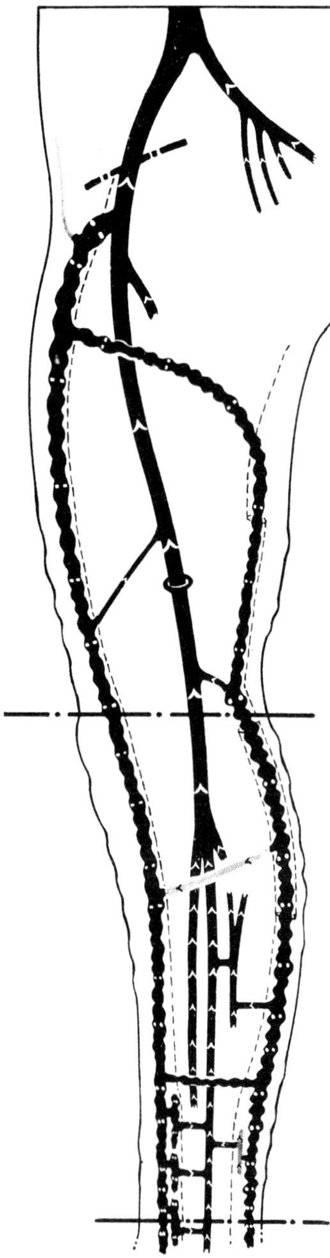

Fig. 7.22 Varicosity of the internal saphenous vein affecting the external saphenous vein.

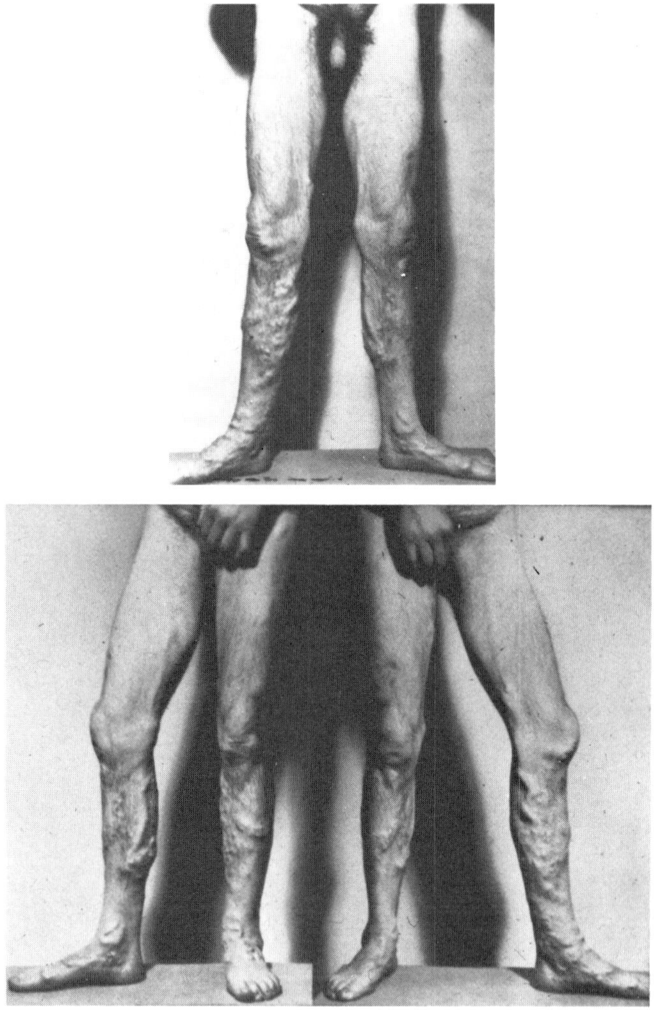

Fig. 7.23 A, B, C. Gross internal saphenous incompetence but with good ankle skin.

fascial compartment closely applied to the deep fascia. This is of course the reason why the 'stripping operation' is possible at all—as it is the enlarged and relatively straight main saphenous trunk down which the stripper is passed.

At the foramen ovale or near it in the groin a 'saphena varix' may be seen and felt. This varix is not usually on the main saphenous itself, but on the rather thinner walled antero-lateral branch. It is occasionally mistaken for a femoral hernia—but its pathognomonic physical sign—a thrill palpated by the finger over it on coughing—should differentiate the two, as well as the easy compressibility of the saphena varix (Fig. 9.2, p. 145).

There may be other globular dilatations or blow outs along the course of the main trunk. One just above the knee is frequent.

The distribution of varices on the limb depends on which combination of the main branches of the saphenous are involved, and this varies widely from case to case (Fig. 3.3, p. 20).

In the upper third of the thigh and usually arising very close to the saphenous orifice itself, are the two constant branches: (1) the *anterolateral* (Fig. 7.25) (or anteroexternal), running obliquely across the front of the thigh, often involved as a prominent tortuous vein;

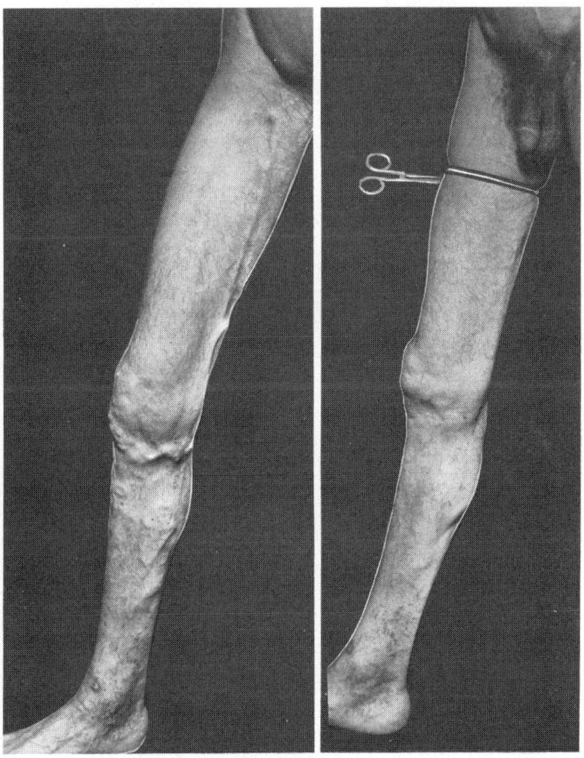

Fig. 7.24 A case of apparent simple varicosity of the internal saphenous vein, but the external saphenous is also incompetent.

(2) the *posteromedial vein* (or posterointernal) running down the inner side of the thigh to the popliteal space, often anastomosing with the short saphenous.

Note that the posteromedial vein may arise low, halfway down the thigh, when it gives the appearance of, and is often mistaken for, a mid-thigh perforating vein. Occasionally also the posterior arch about knee level, may arise half way up the thigh.

In the leg there are two important branches which arise about knee level (rather variable, sometimes just above the knee, or may be just below). These are: (1) the anteromedial again —sometimes known as the 'stocking vein' (Fig. 7.29) as it runs down the front of the shin and shows badly through women's stockings; (2) the important posterior arch vein, which runs down the inner side of the calf to anastomose with the inner ankle perforators (see Chap. 3). This branch is more often varicose than any other (see Figs 7.23 and 7.30).

In primary long saphenous incompetence the ankle skin is *usually remarkably healthy* (unless a faulty ankle perforating vein is present).

Particularly when walking, the normally functioning ankle perforators 'aspirate off' most of the superficial venous hypertension into the calf pump (see Chap. 4) thus protecting the ankle skin and lowering the pressure in the veins. So there may be large varicosities present with healthy ankle skin (see Fig. 7.23). This explains why nearly all patients with this type of varicose vein find that their *symptoms* (heavy, aching leg) are immediately relieved by movement and walking.

The double incompetence of long saphenous vein, and ankle perforator (see Fig. 7.18)

Many patients with gross long saphenous incompetence go for years without any lesions of the ankle skin, then suddenly, over six months or so, their symptoms change and the ankle skin becomes uncomfortable and congested—venules rapidly appear—and eczema and ulceration may follow in a year or two.

This change means that the valve in one of the ankle perforators has given way, and the

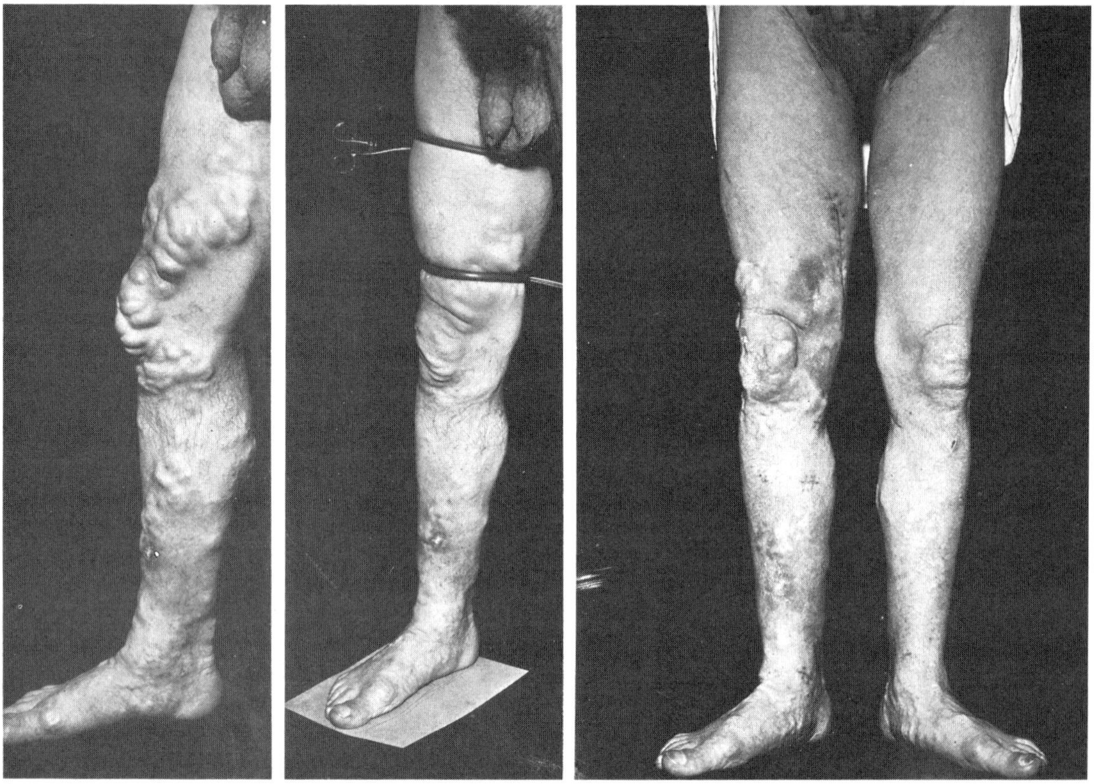

Fig. 7.25 A case of triple incompetence, i.e. varicosity of the internal and external saphenous veins and of a communicating vein in Hunter's canal.

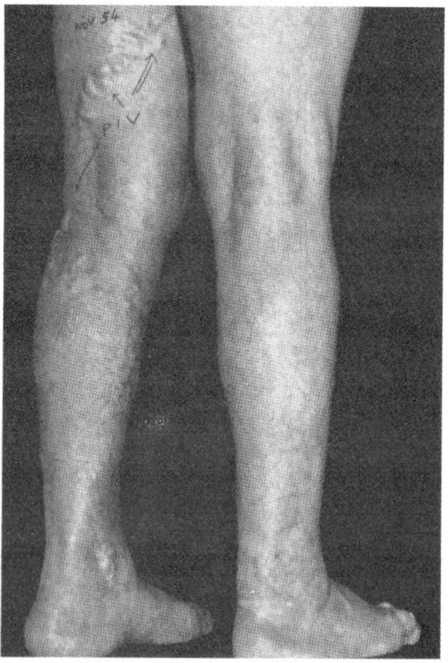

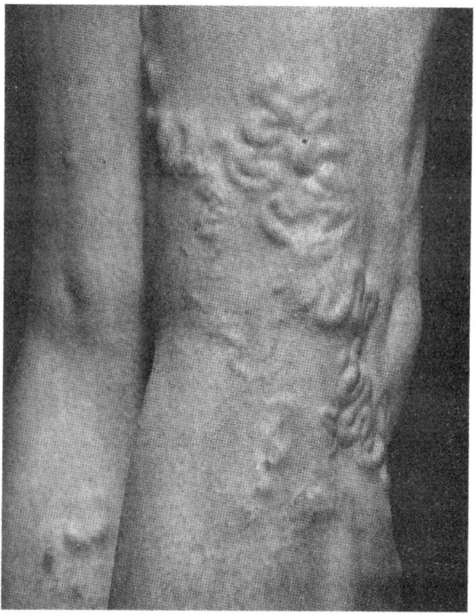

Figs 7.26, 7.27 Varicosity of the posterointernal tributary of internal saphenous vein.

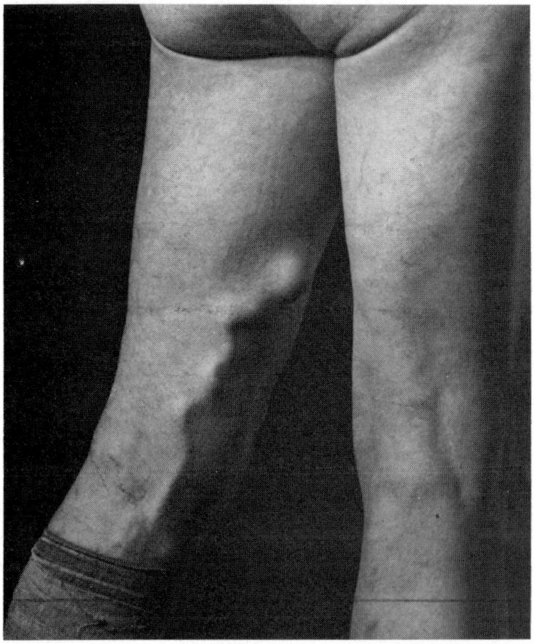

Fig. 7.28 High origin of posterior arch vein from long saphenous.

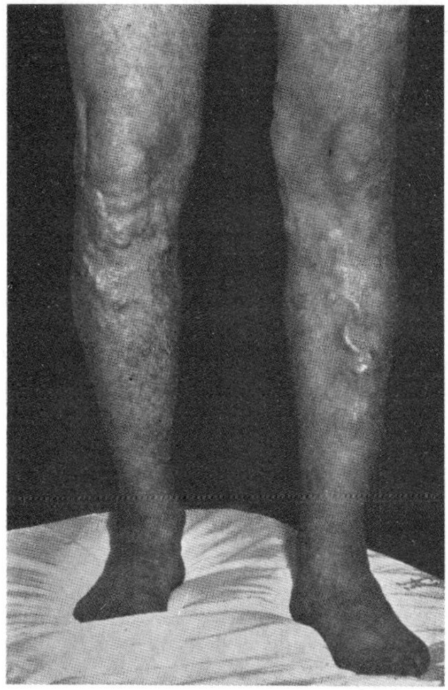

Fig. 7.29 Bilateral internal saphenous incompetence with marked varicosity of the anterior tributary in the left leg.

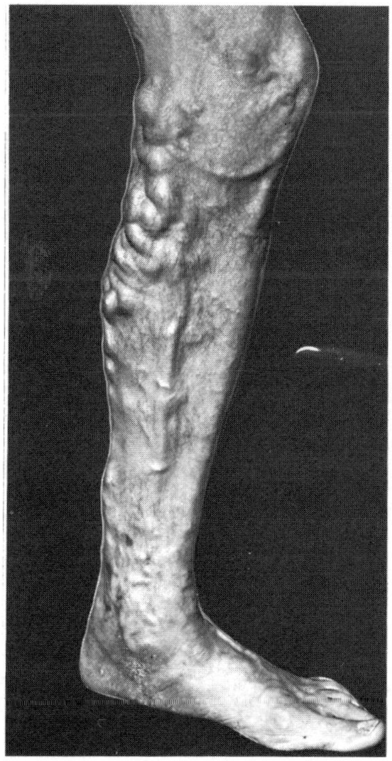

Fig. 7.30 Varicosity of posterior arch vein.

perforating vein is now *adding* to the venous hypertension round the ankle instead of *subtracting* from it.

This complication usually brings the patient to seek advice fairly rapidly, and it is a strong indication for radical surgery (stripping and perforator exploration) otherwise the patient will soon be crippled by an ulcer.

The photograph in Figure 7.23 shows the difference between uncomplicated long saphenous incompetence (right leg—normal skin) and long saphenous incompetence complicated by perforator incompetence (left leg—congested ankle skin). The later appearance is shown in Figure 7.34.

What causes the failure of the perforator valve after it has been functioning soundly for many years is not known precisely. In some a minor unnoticed episode of thrombosis or phlebitis may be the explanation.

The single incompetence of the short saphenous vein (see Figs 7.7, 7.15 and 7.31).

This is rarer (about 10 per cent of cases) and is strongly familial. The short saphenous vein runs deep to the deep fascia from the popliteal fascia to mid-calf, and it is only subcutaneous in its lower half. When it is enlarged it is seldom visible in the upper half of the leg, and its only obvious sign may be a group of enlarged veins round the external malleolus, possibly extending on to the dorsum of the foot.

It is often overlooked and misdiagnosed. The commonest reason for misdiagnosis is that it simply *is not looked for,* the necessity of *viewing the patient from behind* is omitted!

The most useful test is the percussion test. With a palpating finger over the short saphenous vein in the popliteal fossa, the varices lower down are tapped smartly—a transmitted thrill is then felt by the 'watching' finger (see Fig. 7.9).

The double incompetence of the short saphenous and the lateral or mid-calf perforators (see Fig. 7.19)

In the same way as the long saphenous leak and internal ankle perforator leak tend to occur together, so with the short saphenous vein, often this may be associated with a *lateral ankle perforator leak,* or a *mid-calf perforator leak* or occasionally both. The typical appearance of the combined leak is shown in Figure 7.7. This usually intensifies the lateral malleolar symptoms—causing eczema and patchy lateral malleolar ulceration, occasionally spreading round on to the dorsum of the foot.

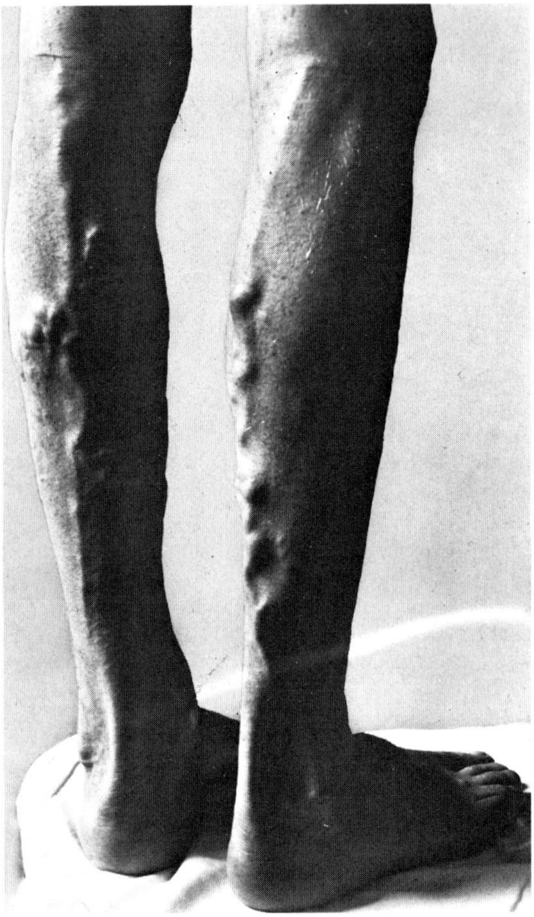

Fig. 7.31 Bilateral varicosity of the external saphenous vein.

Occasionally a short saphenous leak is combined with an internal ankle perforator leak—causing ulceration round both internal and external malleoli. Such a case is shown in Figure 7.7D, and 7.34.

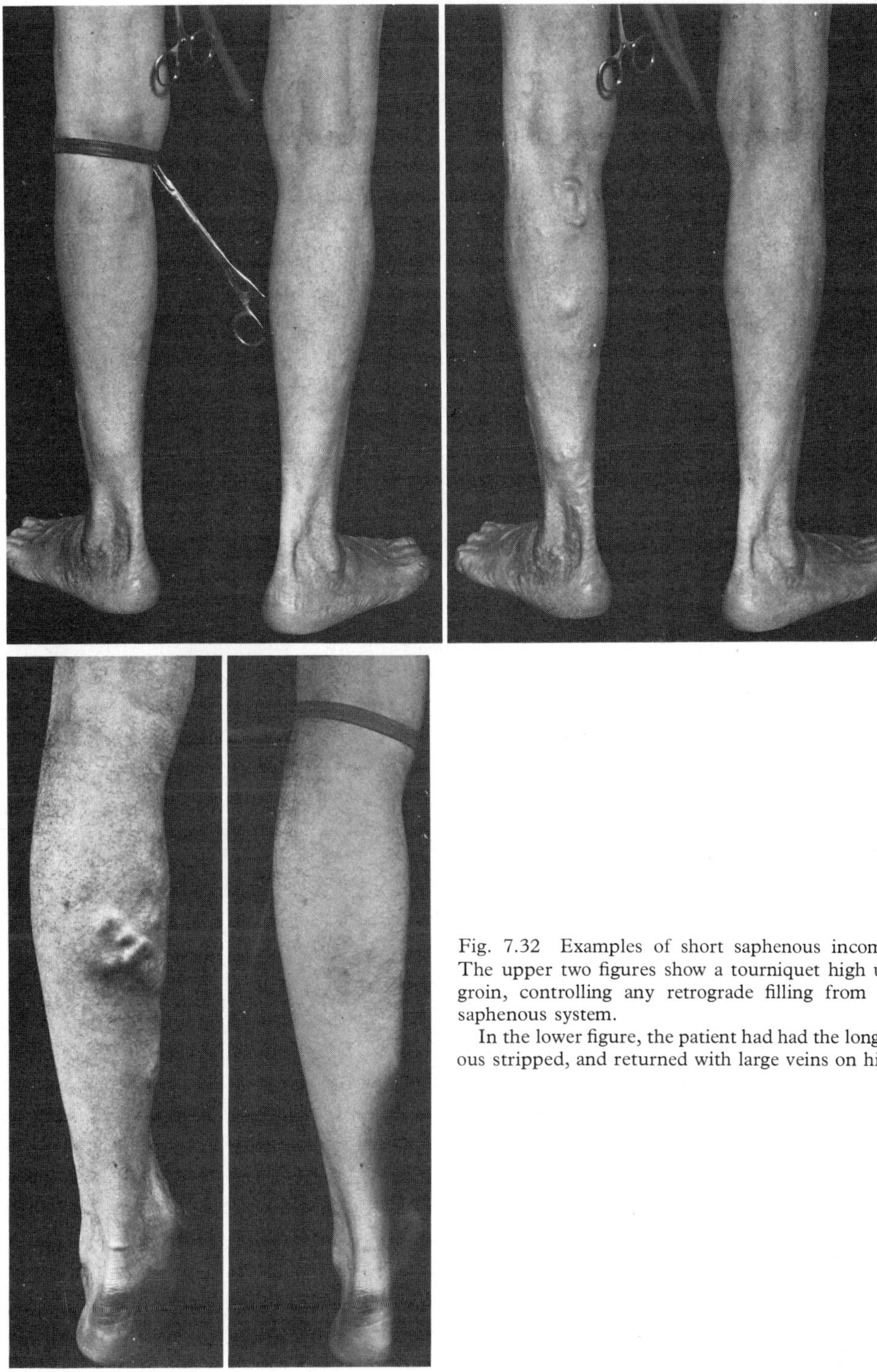

Fig. 7.32 Examples of short saphenous incompetence. The upper two figures show a tourniquet high up at the groin, controlling any retrograde filling from the long saphenous system.

In the lower figure, the patient had had the long saphenous stripped, and returned with large veins on his calf!

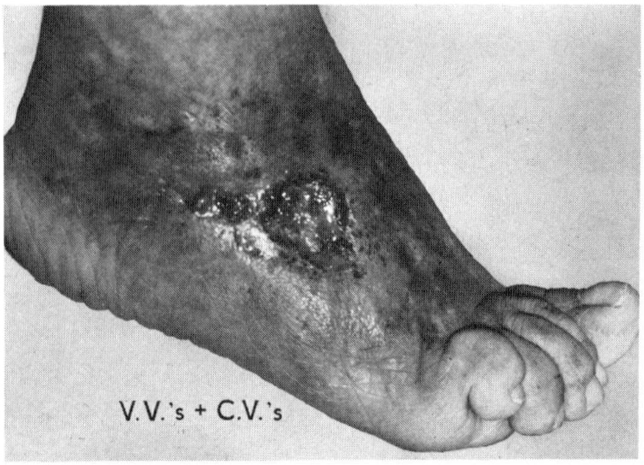

Fig. 7.33 Skin changes at the ankle and exceptional ulceration of the dorsum of the foot due to varicosity of the external saphenous veins and incompetent ankle communicating veins.

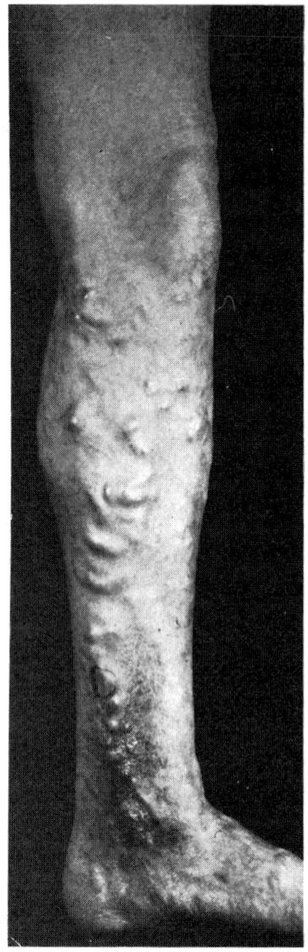

Fig. 7.34 Showing recurrent varicose veins due to an undiagnosed external saphenous vein. The internal saphenous vein has already been tied and stripped. Notice also the probable incompetent ankle perforating vein and pre-ulcerous skin changes.

Double incompetence of long and short saphenous veins (see Figs 7.16 and 7.24)

This combination is not rare and often comes to light because a patient has had an efficient stripping of the long saphenous system and returns with varicose veins in the calf. In fact the incompetent short saphenous system has been overlooked and not operated upon! The typical clinical appearance of such cases is seen in Figure 7.32.

Again, the essential in the diagnosis is to be aware of the possibility of this combination and to look for it. Such cases, having two high pressure leaks in the limb, usually have quite large veins, and always some veins round the lateral malleolus.

Primary incompetence of ankle perforating veins (see Fig. 7.17)

Nearly all cases of gross perforating vein incompetence (particularly those without co-existent long saphenous or short saphenous incompetence) are due to destruction of the perforating vein valves by old deep vein thrombosis (Fig. 7.21) and they are dealt with in Chapter 17.

However, very rarely a young patient may appear with a typical single ankle perforator

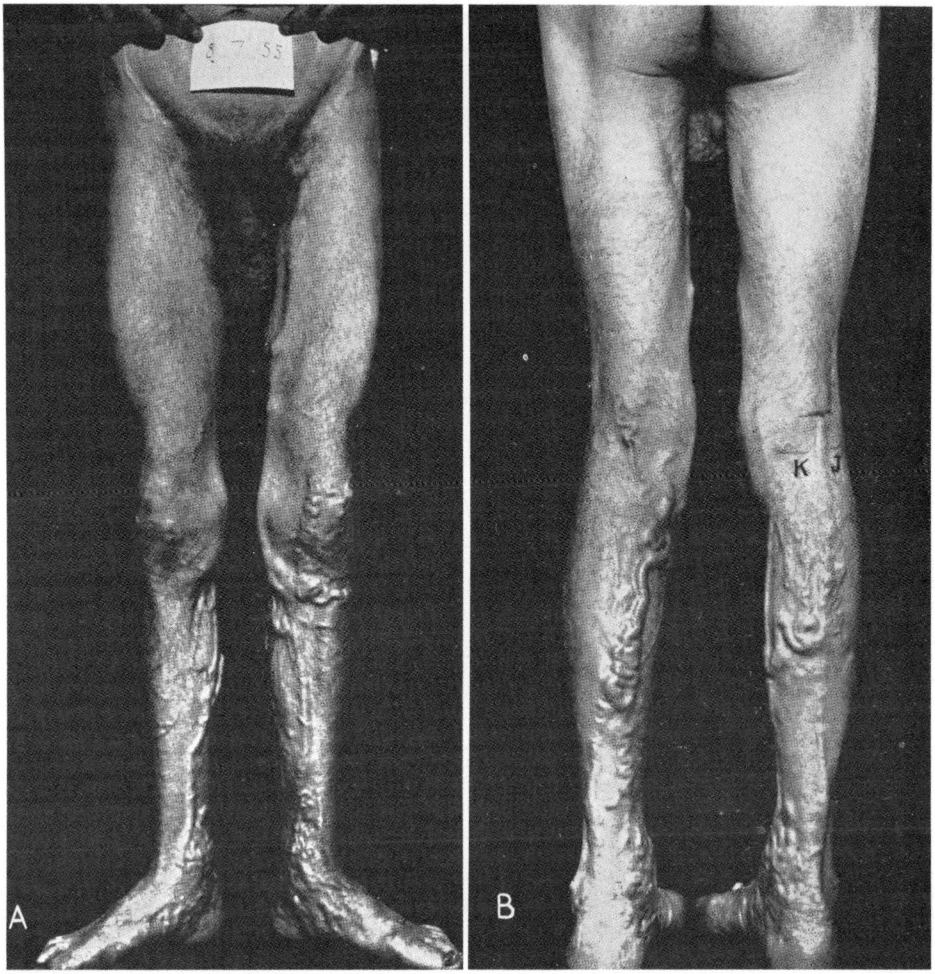

Fig. 7.35 A varicose right external saphenous and varicose left internal saphenous vein. Superficially these legs are alike and a 'spot' diagnosis would probably have been wrong. A. Front view; notice the left saphena varix and left varicocele. B. Rear view; note the level of the knee joint (K.J.) and the point where the external saphenous dips down into the popliteal space (right leg).

incompetence, ankle flare, and ankle skin changes—which appears to be primary—and not due to deep vein thrombosis. It must be emphasised that this is exceptional.

Rarer types of veins

If the presentation does not fit into any of the above categories one is probably seeing either:

1. Secondary veins due to old deep vein thrombosis (either below inguinal ligament type or iliofemoral) (Chaps 16 and 17), or

2. One of the rarer presentations of varicose veins, such as pudendal (internal iliac) veins, some form of the lateral venous anomaly (Klippel-Trenaunay syndrome) or venous stars (telangiectasia).

These are described in Chapter 11.

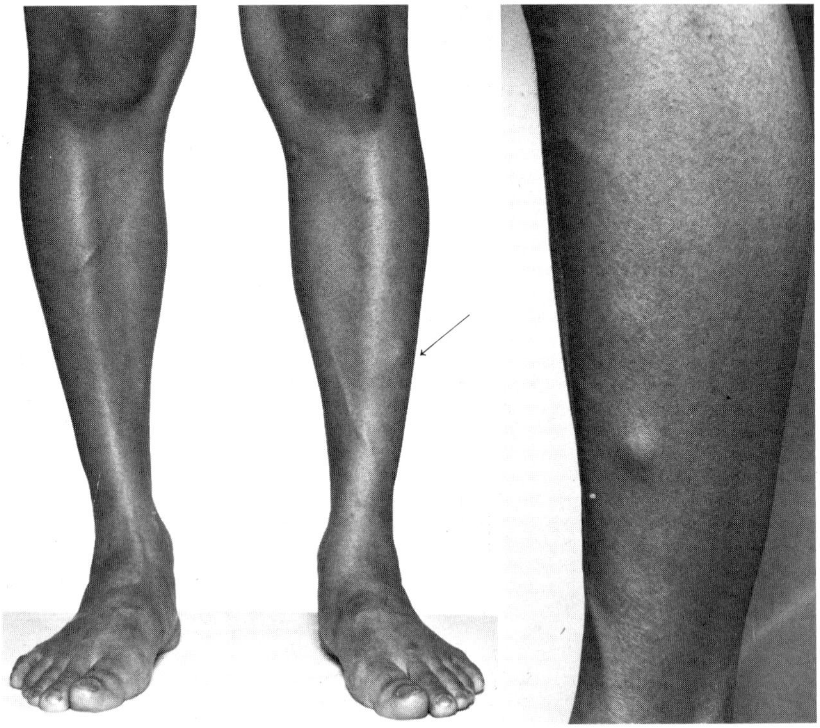

Fig. 7.36 A 'muscle hernia' over the anterior tibial compartment. This is often mistaken for a varicose vein, or perforating vein.

REFERENCES

Chevrier, L. (1908) De l'examin aux reflux veinaux dans les varices superficielles. *Arch. gen. Chir.*, **2**, 44–54.
Cope Zachary, alias Zeta. (1972) *The Diagnosis of the Acute Abdomen in Rhyme*. London: Lewis.
Homans, J. (1922) *Boston med. surg. J.*, **187**, 258.
Perthes, G. (1895) *Dtsch. med. Wschr.*, **21**, 253.
Ratschow, M. & Schwartz, E. (1930) *Arch. Clin. Chir.*, **150**, 720.

8. Management of Varicose Veins

1. Conservative Measures
2. Injection Treatment
3. Operative Treatment

'Varicose veins' on the whole is a very slowly progressive, non-lethal, increasingly disabling disease. It is this progression which must be kept in mind when planning management.

Varicosis takes its place with migraine, arthritis, rheumatism and back trouble as the happy hunting ground of quacks and 'fringe medicine practitioners of all sorts'. It is also the happy hunting ground of the drug companies, and one seldom opens a medical journal without spying some advertisement for either pills, complicated ointments or dressings, or the beloved 'medicated bandages' which are claimed to ameliorate varicose veins or ulcers.

The situation should now improve because exact knowledge about the pathology and behaviour of all forms of varicose veins is available—no longer largely shrouded in mystery and guesswork.

Three other things must be borne in mind when talking about the treatment of varicose veins. These are:

1. 'Varicose veins' is often used as an all embracing term covering all the venous disorders of the leg listed in Chapter 5, with their widely different basic pathology, but which manifest themselves by the appearance of dilated abnormal veins on the surface of the leg.

The management and treatment of all these venous disorders varies widely, because of their different pathology.

2. Whatever the basic pathology, nearly all types of varicose veins are improved temporarily by two simple measures, namely (a) rest, with the feet at or above heart level and (b) pressure bandaging.

Thus any treatment, however peculiar or esoteric, which incorporates one of these simple factors, will result in temporary improvement.

In the assessment of the effects of any form of treatment this always has to be taken into consideration.

3. *The time factor.* Venous disease is *slow.* It develops slowly and produces its damaging effects on the skin and subcutaneous tissues slowly over years. Treatment may cure or ameliorate rapidly, but if it has been ineffective in curing the *basic pathology* of the particular type of venous trouble, then the symptoms and signs either remain, or inexorably recur in one or two years. Thus when reporting the results of treatment for varicose veins or venous ulceration, *a long follow-up* assessment period is necessary. A follow up period of under two years is useless and at least five years are needed to claim that a type of venous pathology or ulcer has been cured or ameliorated by the chosen remedy.

This slow waxing and waning of venous disease over the years makes it a very special ailment to manage, and the real truth about many treatments only becomes apparent after the surgeon has been following and treating a group of patients for perhaps ten years or more.

The word 'management' of venous disorders is thus the operative word. Management may have to go on throughout the patient's and the surgeon's life. Operation, may be only an episode in the management. In primary varicose veins it may be a major and effective episode. In various forms of post-thrombotic syndrome it may be a less important episode.

CONSERVATIVE MEASURES

Not all cases of varicose veins need treatment. Some are better left alone and in others the more active remedies (injection or operation) should be avoided.

First, what types of varicose vein should *not* be treated?

Trivial capillary veins, and venous stars are often best not treated. The reason is twofold: (a) they are not progressive and never give rise to skin destruction or ulceration and (b) what treatment we have is unsatisfactory. Micro-injections into them occasionally give good results in big unsightly telangiectases, but injection into or around small ones often produces permanent brown marks which are more objectionable than the varicules. Skin cosmetics are available for covering such minor blemishes if the patient so desires.

Trivial veins, minor degrees of gravitational venous dilatation, and mild long saphenous incompetence in the elderly are usually best left alone. Such patients often come because they have been told there is a danger of 'phlebitis' or 'ulceration'. Reassurance is all that is needed. There are also certain groups of post-thrombotic syndrome patients who are managed by explanation and reassurance rather than anything active (Chap. 17).

Supportive treatment and treatment by posture

Elastic support by elastic stockings or elastic bandages is the main conservative measure in controlling the symptoms and effects of varicose veins.

From consideration of the Chapter on Physiology and Chapter 17, it will be apparent that the superficial venous hypertension generated by a leak into the long saphenous system at the groin is very much less than the enormous pressure transmitted outwards by a leaky perforating vein at the ankle.

Thus to control the symptoms of an early case of long saphenous incompetence, a light elastic stocking may be quite effective. But even a heavy elastic stocking may be ineffective in controlling the hypertension generated by an ankle perforator, and a heavy webbing elastic bandage is the only thing which will do the job.

So in general, the bigger the veins, and the lower down the limb the source of the venous hypertension, the stronger must be the elastic support to control the symptoms.

This then is the guide to the weight and strength of elastic support required. Figure 8.1 shows the various types of support available. Light elastic stockings are useful in trivial cases of minor varicose veins, whose legs ache when standing. They are very useful to relieve symptoms while patients are awaiting operation. (Hospital waiting lists may run to a year or more!) Heavier types of stocking may be worn during pregnancy.

The toughest and firmest grade must be prescribed however if the patient has ankle veins, early skin changes, or other evidence of ankle perforator leak.

Thick webbing elastic bandages are in our experience best to control actual venous ulceration (see Chap. 18).

Elastic stockings should be fitted professionally, should always have a full heel (see Fig. 8.1) and may be either of knee or thigh length. Where *heavy* stockings are necessary to control ankle varices, below knee stockings are adequate. Full length stockings, unless they are light, are uncomfortable and difficult to keep up, requiring complicated arrangements of suspender belts.

Nowadays quite effective light elastic tights are also made. All elastic stockings lose their elasticity after about two to three months wear, and must be renewed.

On the whole young and active patients dislike wearing elastic support, and prefer to have their veins cured by radical surgery if possible. In the elderly, however, there is not so much resistance to this form of palliative treatment. Many patients with eczema find it impossible to wear elastic stockings because of the skin irritation—many of them become allergic to rubber. In tropical climates, the wearing of elastic stockings may be unbearable. In some with the post-thrombotic syndrome, elastic support throughout life is necessary (Chap. 17).

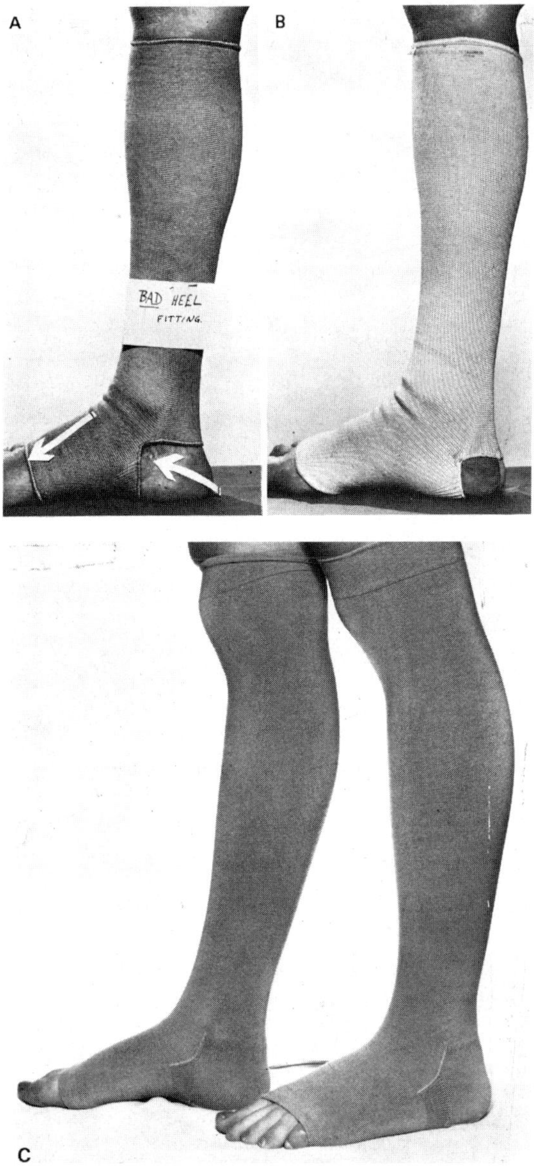

Fig. 8.1 Some examples of the defects in the fitting of elastic stockings. A. This is a bad fitting. The big gap over the heel means that there is no pressure just below the malleoli, where it is needed most. The stocking stops short of the root of the toes—oedema will develop in the skin between the end of the stocking and the root of the toes; this is a useless stocking. B. A slightly better stocking, it comes down to the root of the toes and the heel gap is less, but there are ridges over the instep; this will make it somewhat uncomfortable. C. The 'Suprema' knitted lastex yarn and nylon stocking. This fulfils the requisites for a good elastic stocking. It has an elastic heel which fits snugly and gives elastic pressure where required. It is free of ridges, and goes down to the root of the toes.

Treatment by posture—putting the patient to bed with the feet elevated just above heart level—is absolutely effective in all venous disorders, but it completely immobilises the person. If an ulcer is threatening to break down, or get out of hand—one week in bed with the feet up will start healing which may then continue under elastic support.

A week or so in bed every three months may become a valuable part of the routine management of patients with the more severe forms of post-thrombotic syndrome.

TREATMENT BY INJECTION

The purpose and effect of sclerosant injection

The purpose of injecting a sclerosant into a varicose vein is to destroy its endothelium in that area, and thus induce an aseptic thrombosis which organises and closes the vein.

History of sclerosant therapy

The injection of varicose veins developed shortly after the introduction of the hypodermic syringe. It arose out of the observation that an attack of spontaneous thrombophlebitis in varicose veins occasionally obliterated and cured them. Pravaz (1857) used sclerosant therapy in 1851, when he injected a solution of ferric chloride into an aneurysm in the hope of permanently thrombosing it. In 1853, Chassaignac (1855) introduced it into varicose veins hoping thereby to close them. Since then many substances have been tried.

In 1904, Tavel of Berne combined the ligation of varicose veins with injection of carbolic acid 5 per cent (a coagulant) and made a convincing case for his method. Schiassi (1908) injected 1 per cent iodine in aqueous potassium iodide. From 1912 onwards Linser (1916 and 1921) tried mercuric chloride, but its toxicity as shown by transient albuminuria and gross local damage stopped its use. Sicard (1922) introduced sodium salicylate injections, 2 ml of a 20 per cent solution being the first dose, and 2 to 3 ml of a 30 to 40 per cent solution after two to three days. He stated that it was effective, harmless and painless. He had tried salvarsan and sodium carbonate but had found them too caustic. K. Linser (1925) used a 15 to 20 per cent solution of sodium chloride. Sugar in various concentrations was also given (Kausch, 1917; Noble, 1926). Quinine was first used in 1913 (Hanschell 1928) and later urethane was added as a local anaesthetic (Genevrier, 1922). Subsequently, Maingot and Carlton (1928) and Harvey in 1936, used it synchronously with lithocaine (lithium salicylate 30 per cent and tutocaine 1 per cent) as a 'twin' injection.

In more recent years the introduction of less toxic substances such as Ethanolamine and sodium tetradecyl sulphate, has made injection treatment safer. Also, a much greater awareness of the care with which the injection has to be made and the importance of after-treatment has been emphasised by G. Fegan of Dublin (1967).

Principles of treatment by Compression Sclerotherapy

The term compression sclerotherapy was coined by Fegan to emphasise one of the important points in the practice of injection therapy, namely that the vein and the whole limb must be compressed efficiently after a sclerosant injection.

If a sclerosant is injected into a varicose vein which is still in contact with its filling source a bulky thrombus tends to be formed. This thrombus will in time, like all other thrombi in veins, recanalise and the varicose vein will reappear, rather thicker and more painful than before. This bulky thrombus can be prevented by accurate placing of compression pads over the injected vein, and then compressing the whole limb with an elastic bandage, especially including the compression pads. If this compression is efficient and maintained for a period of at least six weeks, then the walls of the vein are, as it were, 'stuck together' by the inflammatory reaction, granulation tissue and fibrosis, and a much less bulky obliterated vein is obtained which is more likely to remain permanently occluded.

The second principle of sclerotherapy is movement, which must be started within minutes of the injection. As long ago as 1949 Kinmonth and Robertson showed that an injection of radio-opaque sclerosant into the patient, supine and immobile, stayed in the veins for a minute or so, but with the least movement, it entered the deep veins of the leg where it stayed unless vigorous contractions of the calf was performed to move it onwards. These observations have recently been confirmed by one of the authors (H. Dodd).

It is essential that after the sclerosant has been injected and the leg bandaged that it should be vigorously moved, otherwise the sclerosant may 'hang around' in the deep veins and damage them and the perforating veins. This sequence of events has been observed by one of us several times—resulting in a post-injection perforating vein ulcer.

Moreover, while the thrombosis is taking place in the superficial injected vein, it is essential to maintain steady pressure and unremitting active movement to limit the superficial thrombosis to the treated vein and prevent *it* from spreading up and down and into the deep veins, possibly causing a deep thrombosis.

Thus the practical essentials of safe and efficient sclerotherapy are:

1. The accurate injection of a small dose (0·5ml) of one of the modern safer sclerosants into a short segment of vein, and its retention there for a minute or more to act on the vein wall.

2. The maintenance of steady pressure over the injected segment for at least six weeks—to compress the vein, stick its walls together, and prevent the formation of a bulky thrombus which will recanalise.

3. Elastic compression and active movement of the whole leg, starting within minutes of the injection.

These principles have been clearly enunciated by Fegan in his writings. Successful and safe sclerosant therapy in suitable cases can only be achieved if these principles are adhered to carefully.

Indications for sclerotherapy

One of the main troubles with sclerotherapy is that it is only a temporary palliative type of therapy, never curative, as it is never aimed at the basic pathology of venous disease, namely the main perforator leaks. Only surgery can do this. It can successfully close large unsightly branch veins to the temporary gratification of the patient, but if the basic leak from the perforating vein (saphenous or ankle) is still in operation, the result will be temporary and further veins will reappear in place of the one blocked off. These can then be sclerosed on subsequent occasions and so on.

Thus one of the best applications of sclerotherapy is to close off residual veins, which are annoying the patient *after* an accurate surgical closure of the saphenous orifice in the groin, or any other perforating vein has been done.

The other point which is of great relevance in sclerotherapy, is that the *greater the venous hypertension in the veins, the less successful, and the more positively harmful are the results of sclerotherapy.* The venous hypertension transmitted into the great saphenous system by a valvular incompetence in the groin is quite small, compared with the large venous pressure transmitted outwards by the ankle perforators and the short saphenous vein. So injections in branches of an incompetent long saphenous system, particularly higher in the thigh, are much more likely to be successful than those given to high pressure veins in the lower leg (which we consider dangerous, for reasons to be mentioned). Successful injections in long, single tortuous superficial branches of an early incompetent long saphenous system may thus give a good result for a number of years before recurrence takes place. Lower down the leg and especially in the ankle region, injection therapy *gives bad results, is unsafe and has no place.*

Injection therapy also has an occasional place in treating trivial, isolated, superficial varices and some larger venous stars and telangiectases.

Technique of injection

The technique of injection is important for a safe and effective injection therapy. The three solutions which we consider best and safest for sclerosant therapy are:

1. Ethanolamine oleate (monoethanolamine 5 per cent with benzyl alcohol 2 per cent)—trade names are Ethanolomin, Monethan, Neovaricaine. It is sterilised by autoclaving.
2. Sodium tetradecyl sulphate 3 per cent, in benzyl alcohol 2 per cent—trade names are Thrombovar and S.T.D. It is sterilised by autoclaving.
3. Phenol-glycerine fluid (phenol 2 per cent in glycerine 25 to 30 per cent)—it is sterilised by autoclaving.

There is very little to choose between these three solutions as sclerosants—all are safe and effective if used properly. As regards dosage, no more than 0·5 ml should be used at any one injection site, and no more than *four injections* should be given at any one sitting (2 ml total dose) (Fig. 8.2).

Injection is done with a fine, sharp needle, with the patient *reclining, not standing.* The vein can be filled, enough for the needle to enter it, by stroking it down towards the needle. In small veins it is sometimes necessary to put the limb down for a moment, allow the vein to fill, enter the needle, and then return to the horizontal. The 0·5 ml injection is made slowly into the vein (after first ensuring that the needle is safely in the vein lumen by withdrawing a little blood). The injection is retained in a short segment of vein by compressing it with the fingers just above and below the injection site for just under a minute. Sometimes the patient will complain of a slight stinging sensation during this manoeuvre. Any complaints of pain or real discomfort means that the injection is being made *outside* the vein, and it must be stopped at once.

A local compression pad, which may be a

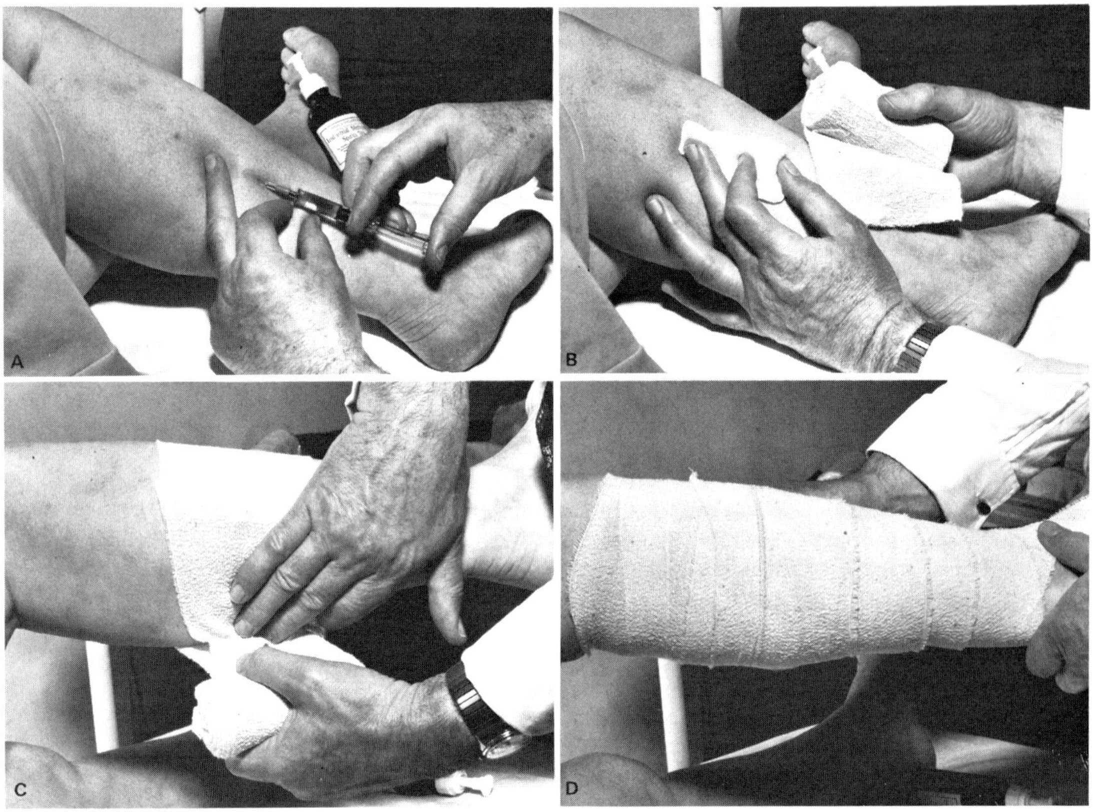

Fig. 8.2 Injection of a 'residual' varicose vein on the outer side of the leg. A. With the patient lying down, the segment of residual vein is isolated with the fingers of the left hand as shown, and 0·5 cc of ethanolamine is injected into it and allowed to remain for 1 minute. B. The vein is then accurately compressed with a pad of three or four layers of rolled-up gauze. C. & D. The compression pad and whole calf are firmly bandaged with a good crêpe, and the patient at once walks about. The crêpe bandage should remain untouched for about 10 days.

piece of gauze, rolled up like a cigar, or a piece of felt, is then placed over the vein, and a firm compression bandage (either crêpe or some other light extensible material—*not* heavy webbing elastic) is applied to the *whole limb* from ankle to just above the injection site in the thigh. The patient is instructed to walk round the room *immediately*. Further instructions are then given to do *as much active walking as possible* during the succeeding week or so.

The exact time that the bandage remains on (untouched) is subject to some variation—but for an average injection in small thigh veins, a period of about one week is adequate. However if bigger veins are being injected, and particularly the large, higher pressure ones below the knee—in the upper calf, then about six weeks (as recommended by Fegan) is desirable. In such cases, however, it becomes a little problematical as to which is doing the most good—the injection or the bandage (see p. 270)—as six weeks firm bandaging will cure many minor ulcers even without an injection!

Summary of main indications and contraindications for injection therapy

BEST INDICATIONS

1. Residual veins after operation (but *not* true recurrent veins—see Chapter 9).

2. Occasional small isolated vein dilatations and cosmetic veins.

3. Large venous telangiectases.

RELATIVE INDICATIONS

1. Dilated branch veins, mainly in thigh and round the knee of an early incompetent long saphenous system. Such veins can be safely ablated by good injection technique—but recurrence over a period of years is to be expected.

CONTRAINDICATIONS

1. Veins in the lower third of the leg and ankle, particularly those arising from incompetent ankle perforators or the short saphenous system.

2. Veins on the foot.

3. Veins in the elderly.

4. Veins in fat legs. These are often unsuitable for two reasons:

(a) The difficulty of bandaging such legs efficiently.

(b) The severe perivenous reaction in the fat sometimes amounting to a painful fat necrosis.

5. Any person who is for any reason immobile and incapable of active movement immediately after injection.

6. The post-thrombotic syndrome (Chap. 17).

7. Veins in limbs with extensive eczema, or a dirty ulcer.

Complications of sclerotherapy

1. Failure to sclerose the vein—usually due to poor technique.

2. Production of a painful thrombus. When this occurs the pain is very persistent and prolonged.

3. Extravenous injection may produce either a local inflammatory focus, or sometimes an injection ulcer, which may be extremely indolent and need surgical excision.

4. Permanent brown staining of the skin. This is one of the serious drawbacks to treatment of small veins for cosmetic purposes. The permanent brown mark left on the skin may be considered more disfiguring that the original vein, and a dissatisfied patient may result.

5. Sensitivity reactions to the injection material may occur. These are rare but very disturbing. They range from an erythematous rash, to severe anaphylactic reactions requiring treatment with adrenaline.

6. The authors have seen both deep thrombosis and pulmonary embolism as a result of injection, again mostly ill-advised excessive injection in the lower leg area.

7. *Post-injection gangrene.* The most severe complications, however, may occur when an injection near the ankle perforators is attempted. The authors have seen four cases of partial gangrene of the foot and one traumatic arteriovenous fistula as a result of ill-advised injection attempts in this area. Periarterial injection or intra-arterial is an ever present danger, because the posterior tibial artery becomes comparatively superficial in the lower third of the leg. Fegan and Pegum (1974) have recently reported a further series of eight injection injuries arising in this way and have also emphasised the danger of making injections in the region of the internal ankle perforating veins.

Medicosocial aspects

The concept that there are two treatments for 'varicose veins' namely injection or operation, is one which has severely damaged the image of vein treatment. This is not helped by the frequent and often foolish controversy indulged in by otherwise responsible medical men on this subject.

As this book has endeavoured to show, there are all sorts of venous disorders covered by the general title 'varicose veins' and each type needs first a diagnosis and then its specific treatment. There is a definite, though limited place for injection therapy as we have indicated.

Where skilled surgery is unavailable or unattainable for any reason, then injection therapy may be pushed a *little* further than our strict indications. This, however, brings with it the necessity for increasingly careful attention to the details of technique by an experienced staff, and careful after-treatment and supervision—otherwise the complication rate rises.

The worst aspects of injection therapy are seen when 'varicose vein' cases are herded into 'injection clinics', often seen by junior, or even temporary staff, or by part-time practitioners. Injections are given to all who attend, there is little attempt at real diagnosis, and minimal follow up, and the science of management of venous disorders falls to a low ebb in such circumstances. Patients may attend for years not even knowing that a simple operation may cure their misery. Even more seriously, early and remediable cases of severe venous disorder may be 'nursed along' until they become chronic and when a surgical opinion is asked, the chance for early, efficient and successful surgery has passed.

OPERATIVE TREATMENT

This chapter on the operative treatment of primary varicose veins is based mainly on our personal, large experience. We have had the opportunity for an exceptionally long follow up evaluation of the operative methods. Bad results of varicose vein surgery have a habit of 'coming home to roost'.

Operations for varicose veins and their associated complications are important and merit the attention of all members of a general surgical team. The practice of deputising diagnosis and treatment entirely to juniors is deprecated.

The procedures exact high standards of diagnosis, investigation and technical skill and are rewarding in their results. They are excellent training for other major operations which often occupy the senior surgeon, but which do not always contribute so much to the well-being of the patient and community.

The development of operations for varicose veins (1891–1974)

For over 2,000 years varicose veins have engaged surgeons, their remedy has been ligature, excision, or both.

The observation of Sir Benjeman Brodie in 1846, confirmed by Trendelenberg in 1890, that some varicose veins filled retrogradely from the groin, and that pressure here after emptying the veins kept them empty for a time was a landmark. Based on this, in 1891, Trendelenberg advised ligating the long saphenous trunk above the large varices in the thigh. He specified the junction of the middle and lower thirds of the thigh or a little lower. This step attracted wide attention. A shrewd assessment of it was made by W. Thelwall Thomas in April, 1896 which was supported by Robert (later Sir Robert) Jones, both of Liverpool. Because Thomas' article illustrates the essentials still necessary for success we detail it.

The conditions are:

1. Knowledge of the venous and arterial anatomy of the lower limb.
2. The location of leaks of hypertension from the deep veins into the superficial veins.
3. Exact division (not ligation) of these vessels at their source from the deep veins of the lower limbs.

Regarding Trendelenberg's operation, W. T. Thomas wrote that he 'followed Trendelenberg's operation in two cases but alas, new veins formed along the branches which entered the saphena above the site selected by Trendelenberg'. He continued, 'Since 1893 I resolved to tie and cut the internal saphena immediately below the saphenous opening and have operated on fifteen cases in this manner with perfect results . . . if the external saphenous is at fault it is dealt with at the lower end of the popliteal space and if a mass of varices is proved to have deep connections it is excised. The internal saphenous is ligated twice and the portion between the ligatures is either divided or a piece cut out to prevent subsequent recanalisation.'

He reported: four divisions of the internal saphenous at the saphenous opening; three divisions of the long and short saphena (one patient both sides); two divisions of the long and short saphena and excision of a group with deep connections; six divisions of the internal saphena and excision of a bunch of varices.

Thomas writes: 'Trendelenberg's operation has become a favourite on the Continent and is finding its way here but I venture to think that interference with the internal saphena at its highest available point is a better proceeding and I have no hesitation in commending it to your notice'. At this meeting Jones said that he had operated on nine cases, in three of which he had tied the external saphena as well. In tying the internal saphena he had tied it high up in the same position as that described by Thomas and he thought that there was great advantage in letting the ligature lie above the points of entrance of all the veins entering the saphena. Jones said that he 'thought much more of this operation than he did of excisions of varicosities'.

Readers will notice the familiarity of these persons with the problem of multiple leaks into the superficial veins, and their precise division of the termination of the internal saphena.

Another milestone was passed in 1921 when G. H. Cole of Aberdeen described high ligation of the internal saphena and saphenectomy by a Babcock's stripper from the groin to the knee and excision below it.

Cole's reason for the high saphena division was that of ensuring closure of its two main branches, the posteromedial and the anterolateral veins. He observed that the long saphenous trunk may be duplicated in part and further he was aware of injury to the saphenous nerve by writing: 'no injury done to the saphena nerve up to the time of discharge'. We stress this danger later! The need if necessary to strip or extract the short saphenous trunk is stated. So Cole established the value of stripping as described by Mayo (1906) and Babcock (1907).

In the 1920s injection of varicose veins became popular. In 1927 McPheeters, H. O. described his technique of their treatment by the use of sclerosing solutions. It had been reported by Tavel in 1904 when he ligated the saphenous vein and injected carbolic acid 5 per cent as a sclerosant.

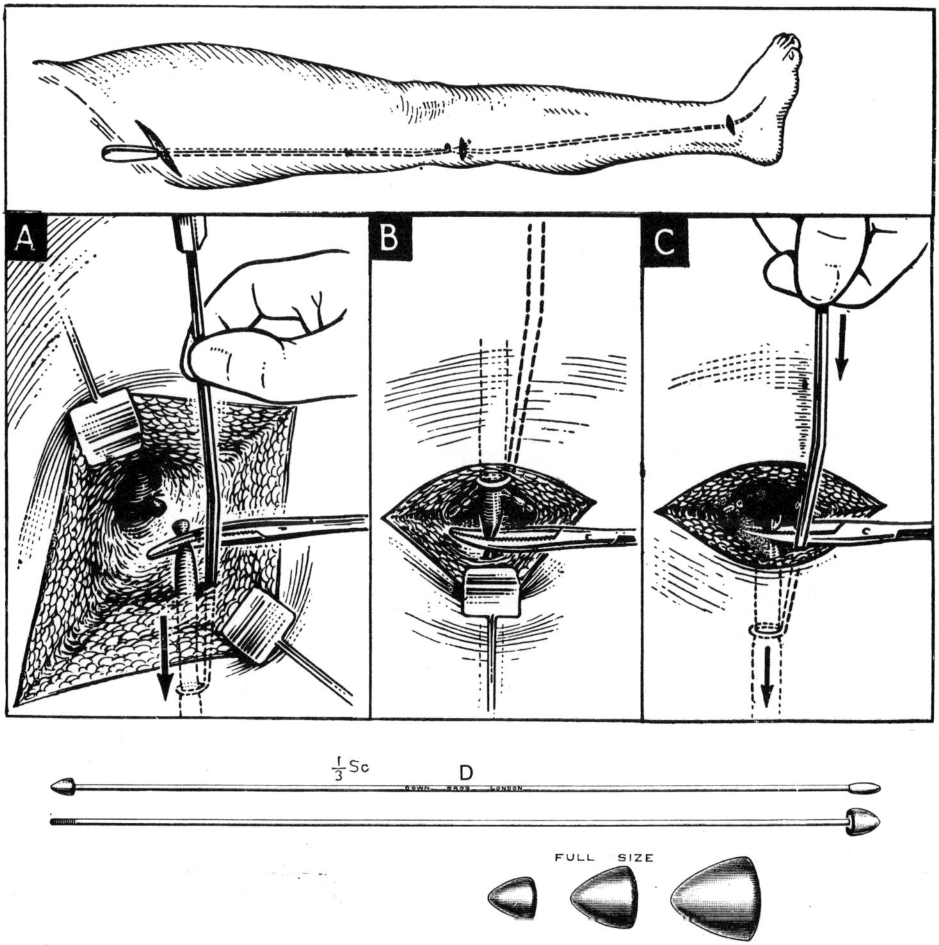

Fig. 8.3 A, B & C. External stripping by a Mayo's type of stripper. D. Babcock's stripper. (By courtesy of Down Bros.)

De Takats (1930) wrote on the injection treatment of varicose veins, recommending dextrose 50 per cent with sodium salicylate 15 per cent. Regarding the operation he said: 'The stump of the ligated saphenous vein should be as short as possible, i.e. as near to the common femoral vein as feasible. The long saphenous vein can be stripped above the knee but below the knee, the main object of the operation is to interrupt all perforating veins. This is far more important than the removal of an isolated dilated segment. . . . In close to 400 cases, operation was performed 16 times (4 per cent).'

Thus De Takats was aware of incompetent communicating veins other than the saphena, and the need for precise operation on the long saphenous vein. He was also impressed by the value of sclerosant therapy which was his chief theme.

Ligature and injection of a sclerosant was a convenient treatment for varicosities and stripping tended to fall into abeyance.

W. Turner Warwick (London) published his handbook on the *Rational Treatment of Varicose Veins and Varicocele* (1931). Although he detailed the following radical operation, he too favoured injections. His operation consisted of (1) ligation of the saphenous vein close to its termination proximal to all its tributaries; (2) removal by Babcock's probe of the internal saphenous between the knee and the saphenous opening; (3) 'Below the knee, the main trunk of the vein is exposed by an oblique incision in the upper half of the leg and a second one in the lower half. Through the incisions, the main trunk of the internal saphenous was removed, particular care being given to tracing and ligating the main perforating branches below the deep fascia.' 'The skin and subcutaneous fascia are dissected back from the deep fascia and the varicose veins removed from the deep aspect of the flap. By this procedure other undescribed perforating veins can be secured.'

'The external saphenous vein and its indirect perforating branches are treated in the same way.' 'This technique gave a higher proportion of successes . . . but for success repeated attacks are necessary.'

W. T. Warwick (1931) wrote: 'When I first turned to the injection method, if I found the Trendelenberg test positive, I performed a Trendelenberg operation before commencing injection, but for the past three years (i.e. since 1928) I have given up preliminary ligation. . . . In very few cases has any resort to operation been necessary and today (1931) surgery has a very small field in the treatment of uncomplicated varicose veins.'

One of us began operating on varicose veins in the 1930s by terminally dividing the saphenofemoral and saphenopopliteal unions and injecting a sclerosant distally into the saphenous trunks (Dodd and Oldham, 1940). A further refinement was to abrade the interior of the vein by a rough-ended long needle as well as the insertion of small doses of sclerosant along the vessel. This was an attempt at saphenectomy *in situ* and it gave good results.

The injection of sclerosants into varicose veins both at operation and for ambulant patients tended to get out of hand in the years 1930 to 1950. Larger

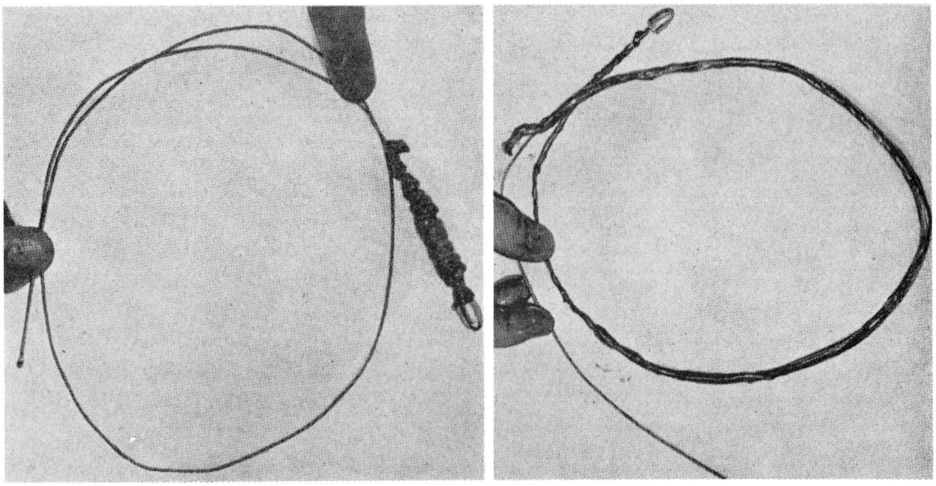

Fig. 8.4 Myers' stripper (without stripped vein telescoped and opened out) (By courtesy of Down Bros.)

doses of better and stronger sclerosants were the fashion and regrettable cases of deep thromboses and skin necrosis were seen frequently in well conducted surgical clinics to which they ultimately gravitated.

The dangers were sounded repeatedly by Professor Michael Boyd of Manchester and from his Department (1945–1955) instruction was published and heeded so that these, plus disillusionment with the results, restored sanity. The adoption of stripping also reduced their use.

Fegan's disciplined technique for ambulant sclerosant compression therapy is increasing the effectiveness and safety for the lesser forms of varicosities and post-operative remnants.

Stripping as a valuable method was resuscitated by R. R. Linton (1949). After terminal saphenous ligation he stripped the saphenous vein, and in the leg cut down to the deep fascia, dividing incompetent communicating veins subfascially. This was an arresting publication of a radical remedy and stripping was done increasingly.

T. Myers (1954) invented a flexible stripper and also confirmed Linton's good opinion of terminal ligation and stripping.

In the decade 1950 to 1960 surgeons were captivated by the facility of stripping and tended to revert to a ligature 'somewhere' in the groin or popliteal space putting their emphasis on stripping. The inevitable recurrences in 1 to 5 years brought the necessary correction, so that today the accepted canons are a flush saphenofemoral or sapheno-

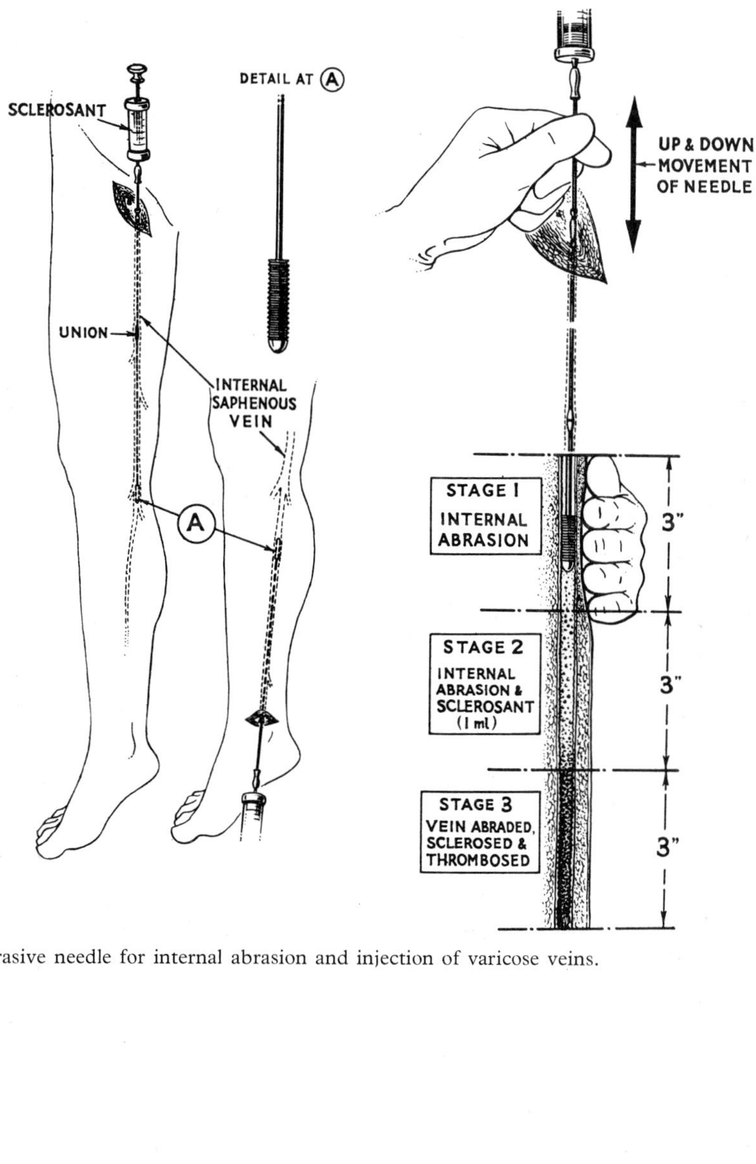

Fig. 8.5 The abrasive needle for internal abrasion and injection of varicose veins.

popliteal ligation and division of any faulty communicating veins, plus stripping, plus the 'worming' out of prominent subcuticular varices.

Leaks from deep connections spoken of by Thomas in 1896 and ligated by Warwick and Linton, earned surgeons' intellectual acceptance when in 1953 F. B. Cockett and D. E. E. Jones described the precise anatomy of the ankle perforating veins and also how they were made incompetent in deep thromboses. Their exact location ensured their certain division.

In the late 1960s a series of investigations by R. May of Innsbruck, and Cockett and Lea Thomas of London established the importance of pathology of the iliac veins and inferior vena cava. These play a great part in the clinical presentations of some problems in the lower limbs and must be considered as will be described in Chapters 13 to 17.

BASIC RATIONALE OF THE MODERN OPERATION

The modern operation of 'flush ligation' and stripping, for primary varicose veins, is designed to cure both the cause of the varicose veins and to remove the actual dilated varicose veins themselves—as completely as possible.

The '*flush ligation*' part of the operation cuts off accurately the source of the high pressure leak from the deep veins.

The *stripping* part of the procedure merely removes the 'dilated veins' themselves which are the result of the high pressure leak.

It follows, therefore, that the most important part of the procedure, if recurrence is to be avoided, is the accurate location of these points of leak from the deep veins, which may be either at the groin (long saphenous) or in the popliteal fossa (short saphenous) or in the lower leg (perforating veins) or any combination of all three.

Flush ligation. The superficial varicose system is ligated and divided precisely at its deep connection with the high pressure filling source, e.g. by a saphenofemoral or saphenopopliteal ligation. Less frequently the venous hypertension is conveyed by an inefficient communicating vein or veins between the superficial varices and the deep system in the thigh or leg, and these must be located, ligated and divided. This ligation procedure to eliminate the high pressure filling is fundamental; the other steps which aim to destroy the varicose saphenous trunk and its tributaries are subordinate and complementary to it. The division of one or more incompetent communicating veins above the ankle is usually necessary when swelling, ulceration or eczema are or have been, present or threatening.

Elimination of saphenous trunks and their branches by stripping. If this obliteration is omitted, these defective trunks and their tributaries fill with blood from other venous sources. They are an eyesore and a possible site of thrombophlebitis. Although they are disconnected from their proximal high pressure venous filling by the terminal saphenous ligation, they refill from normal branch veins as well as other points.

Operation according to diagnosis

The various common clinical presentations of primary varicose veins requiring operation are as follows:

1. The incompetent internal saphenous vein. This is ligated at the saphenofemoral union and ankle and the saphenous trunk between these two points is removed by stripping.
2. The incompetent external saphenous vein. This is ligated at the saphenopopliteal union and at the external malleolus, and the intervening vessel is excised by stripping.
3. The incompetent communicating vein or veins in the leg or in the thigh require location, ligation and division. The gross subcuticular varices adjacent to them are excised.
4. Simultaneous varicosis of the internal and external saphenous veins; these require treatment as in 1 and 2.
5. The faulty internal saphenous vein with a defective communicating vein in the thigh or ankle is treated by high ligation and ablation of the former and division of the latter.
6. The defective external saphenous and communicating veins are treated as in 2 and 3.
7. The triple combination of varicose

internal and external saphenous veins, together with defective communicating veins, is relieved by ligation and division of all three, with ablation of the saphenous trunks.

8. Recurrent varicose veins usually include one or more of the above and are treated accordingly.

Thus, the three operations advised for varicose veins are those of:

1. Ligation and division of the sapheno-femoral junction, with saphenectomy of the long saphenous vein from the groin to the ankle by stripping.

2. Ligation and division of the sapheno-popliteal union, saphenectomy of the varicose short saphenous vein from the popliteal space to the ankle by stripping.

3. The ligation and division of a faulty communicating vein or veins located usually in the lower third of the leg or thigh. **The act of stripping does not necessarily destroy incompetent perforating veins** (*see* p. 130).

Ligation and division of the great saphenous vein at the groin and its ablation to the ankle is the commonest operation; the external saphenous vein is incompetent in about 9 per cent of cases (Slevin, 1948). In a personal series, there were 1,303 patients with internal saphenous incompetence, 137 with external, and 46 with both internal and external varicosities. Failure to detect inefficiency in the short saphenous vein or the ankle perforating veins has been a cause of persistent varicose veins, eczema and recurrent ulceration, especially of that situated around the external malleolus. The following is an all too typical case history.

Mrs M. S., aged 50, was first seen in May, 1947, when she complained of varicose veins of the left leg with gross ulceration at the external malleolus. The tourniquet test revealed an incompetent internal saphenous vein, and on 6.6.47. the operation of ligation, abrasion and injection was carried out at the left groin and ankle. By 27.6.47. the ulcer was healed and the leg improved, although requiring a few further injections. The ulcer recurred at the end of August but with Lestreflex bandaging it was healed by October, 1947. In October, 1948, re-ulceration occurred following a knock, and incompetence of the external saphenous vein was diagnosed after a little difficulty as it was obscured by an enlarged semimembranous bursa. Injections were made into this vein on two occasions. The ulcer recurred in January, 1949, and a 'twin' injection was given into the external saphenous vein on 3.3.49. The ulcer, however, did not disappear completely and in April ligation, abrasion and injection of the external saphenous vein was carried out. By 7.7.49. the leg had recovered, and it remained well until in January, 1954, following a kick on the ankle, the ulceration re-appeared over the external malleolus, which healed with compressive bandaging. In May, 1954, the supramalleolar areas were explored for inefficient communicating veins, the middle internal perforating vein was found enlarged and defective; it was ligated. When seen in July, 1955, the result was perfect, but as she is over fifty years old, faithful care and protection by a robust elastic stocking was emphasised. This tedious story could have been avoided by a complete diagnosis and operation when she was first seen.

Selection of patients for operation

If the general health is good, the diagnosis of varicose veins is firm, and the patient's need is clear, the radical operation may be offered to all persons almost irrespective of age.

We have operated on patients from the age of *eight* to *eighty-two*. Many older patients who are gainfully employed may be treated satisfactorily, but there are two important points to check before operating on patients over the age of 60 to 65:

(a) They must be fully mobile.

(b) There must be no peripheral arterial disease or obstruction.

Incisions and stripping procedures in the periphery of a limb with artery obstruction may fail to heal and give rise to serious complications.

A FREQUENT QUESTION

Many patients when advised to undergo an operation for stripping of their varicose veins ask how the circulation is carried on without them, and whether this does not involve a 'strain' on the other veins. The reply that the main venous return is via the deep veins of which there are a large number usually satisfies the patient, together with the explanation that the blood in the varicose veins is either 'static' or 'going backward'.

The explanation that the saphenous vein is quite surplus to requirement, rather like the appendix, is also helpful.

One can get very deeply involved in trying to explain the basic physiology of venous return to a patient!

Pre-operative marking of the veins

As varicose veins of course disappear when the patient lies down on the operating table it is essential to mark out the course of the major superficial tortuous veins to be removed before operation (see Fig. 8.6).

This is best done with a felt-tip 'Pentel' pen. The marks made by this pen are indelible, and are not washed off by spirit or other liquids used for sterilising the skin at operation. The major saphenous vein itself does not need marking as its situation and course is very constant. The dilated branches which are tortuous and run close under the skin are very variable in situation and they must be carefully marked in every case. After stripping of the main saphenous vein at operation, these secondary prominent branches are stripped out by 'worming' through very small incisions placed directly over them (see Fig. 8.8–8.12). It is evident, therefore, that to get consistently good results, the marking of these secondary veins must be very accurate.

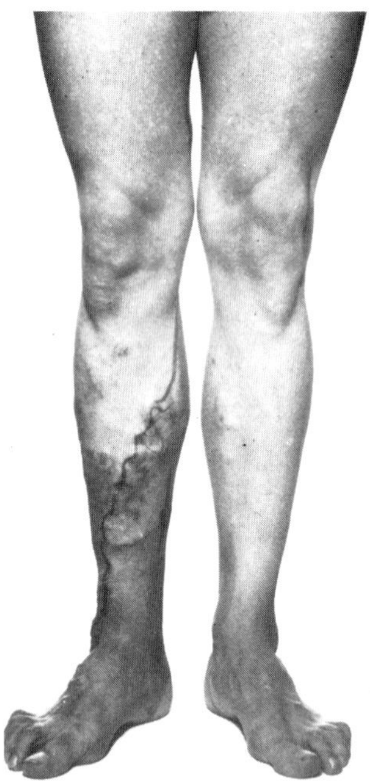

Fig. 8.6 Showing the prominent anterior branch of the long saphenous vein in the leg just below the knee, marked out pre-operatively with a 'Pentel' pen. It will be removed by the 'worming technique'.

The anaesthetic

With modern relaxants and light background anaesthesis there is seldom any reason for doing the operation for varicose veins under anything but general anaesthesia.

Local anaesthesia can of course be used but its indications are extremely few now. However a technique for local anaesthesia is included in this section.

Inhalation anaesthetics which cause vasodilatation should be avoided—especially *halothane*—as these may cause considerable haemorrhage during a stripping procedure.

TECHNIQUE OF LOCAL ANAESTHESIA

The incision at the groin. The incisions are marked out accurately (see later), and a considerable area around them is infiltrated generously (Fig. 8.7), the skin being raised in pig-skin wheals; then the subcutaneous tissue a little deeper is injected more widely,

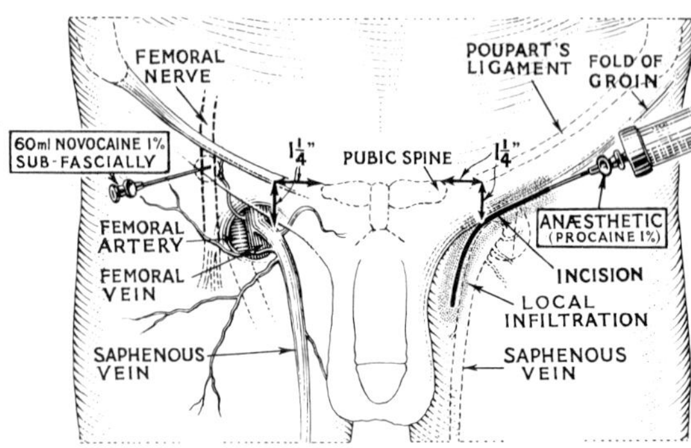

Fig. 8.7 Local analgesia. The infiltration of the groin for the saphenofemoral ligation. The right side shows the anterior femoral nerve being infiltrated; this is necessary for painless stripping.

and last, a layer close to the deep fascia is also infiltrated freely. Cutaneous sensation is lost in five minutes.

Stripping of the internal saphenous trunk. For 'stripping' of the internal saphenous trunk (and ankle communicating vein ligation) the femoral nerve must be injected in order to desensitise the anterointernal aspect of the limb from the groin to the ankle. This large nerve trunk lies immediately to the outer side of the femoral artery, underneath the deep fascia (Fig. 8.7). The pulsation of the artery midway between the symphysis pubis and the anterior superior iliac spine is located by direct palpation above the fold of the groin, the nerve lies immediately external to this point. The needle is passed vertically downwards here until the resistance of the deep fascia is felt, and overcome by further pressure. Aspiration is applied to the needle, to ensure that its point is not in the femoral artery, and if nothing is withdrawn, 20 ml of analgesic is injected to block the nerve, the needle being advanced a little whilst doing so. Confirmation of the accuracy of the injection is usually obtained by the patient feeling a sharp pain when the nerve is pricked by the needle.

By the time the saphenofemoral ligation has been done, the long saphenous vein exposed at the ankle, and the stripper threaded into the vein the limb will be anaesthetised sufficiently to permit a painless stripping from the groin to the ankle or vice versa.

Infiltration for the incision at the ankle. During the pause for the development of anaesthesia in the groin, the region about the internal malleolus where the ankle incision will be made is infiltrated superficially and deeply. The line of this incision is scratched on the skin because the swelling made by the local analgesic will have subsided when the time for this part of the operation arrives. An alternative marker is to leave the hypodermic needle in the skin after the injection. It is valuable to mark the long saphenous trunk at the internal malleolus pre-operatively, as this facilitates its exposure.

OPERATION FOR LONG SAPHENOUS VARICOSE VEINS

Operative procedure (See Fig. 8.8, 1–14)

Position of patient. This is very important. The whole table is tilted head down to an angle of about 10°, or if the patient is on a fixed table the leg is raised 10° on a padded board (Fig. 8.2).

This brings the legs just above heart level, causing the venous pressure in all the veins to fall to zero. This manoeuvre is in fact

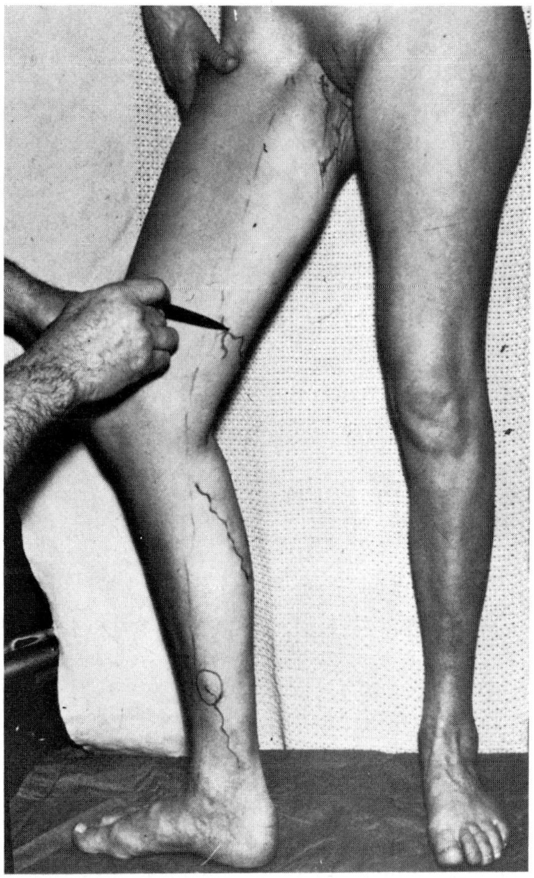

Fig. 8.8 1. Pre-operative marking of the varicose veins with 'Pentel' felt-tipped pen. Note that this patient has (a) a suspicious bulge and vein arising in the ankle perforator area (marked with a circle) and (b) some large pudendal varices, as well as two prominent varicose branches of the long saphenous. *(contd.)*

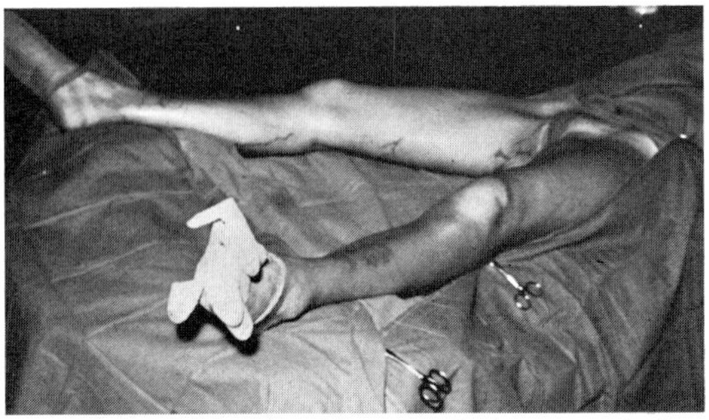

2. Position for operation. Note that the legs are *raised*, as the table is tilted head down. The leg not being operated on will be covered by another towel carefully excluding the groin and anal region.

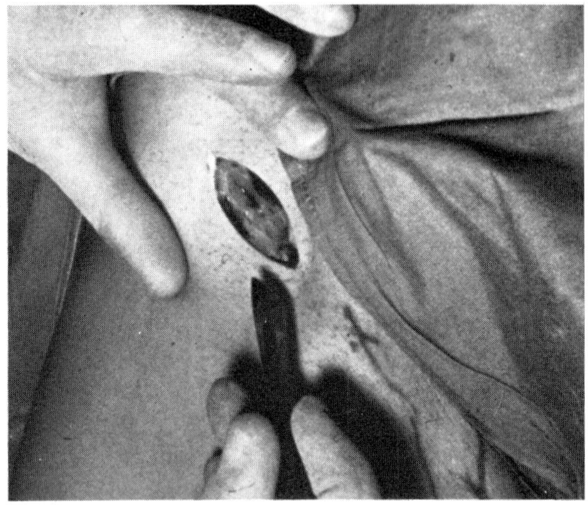

3. The incision in the groin. Note the operator's left middle finger is on the 'pubic tubercle' to give the correct siting of the incision.

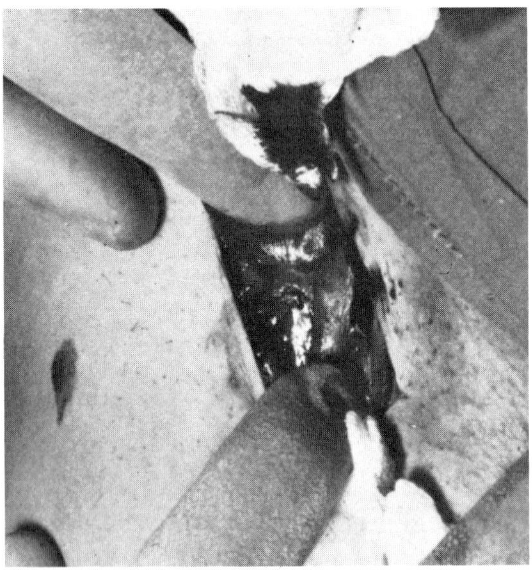

4. After division of the deep layer of fascia, the exposure of saphenofemoral junction is done by two swabs wiped firmly up and then down.

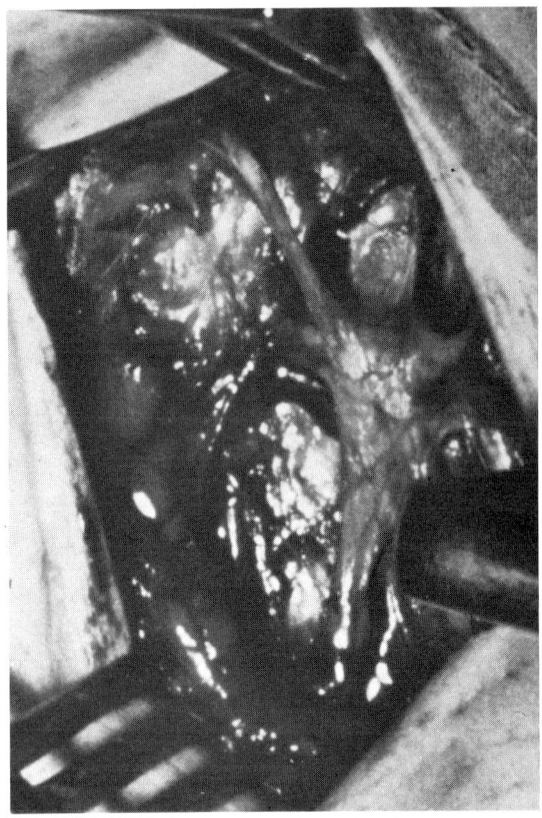

5. The saphenofemoral junction cleanly exposed by swab dissection.

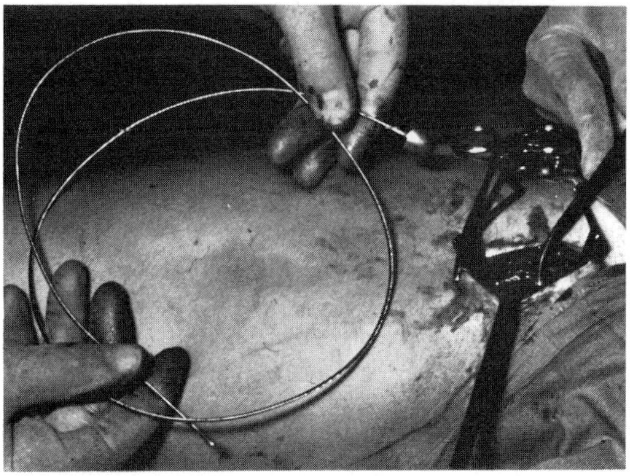

6. The flush saphenofemoral ligature has been done, and the stripper is about to be inserted in the distal end of the saphenous vein at the groin.

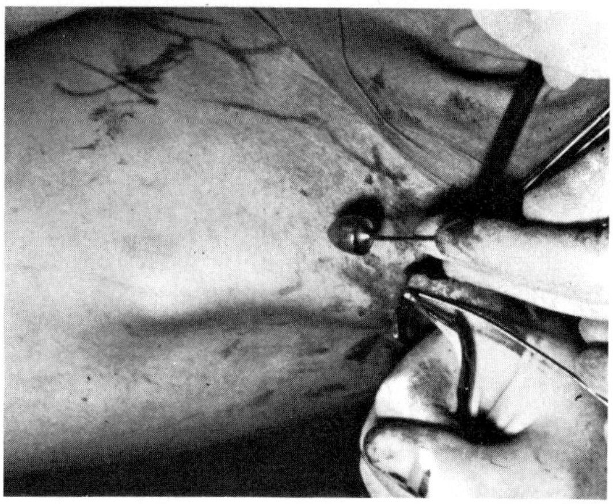

7. The stripper passed down the saphenous vein' being directed into the correct channel by the forefinger inserted down the wound.

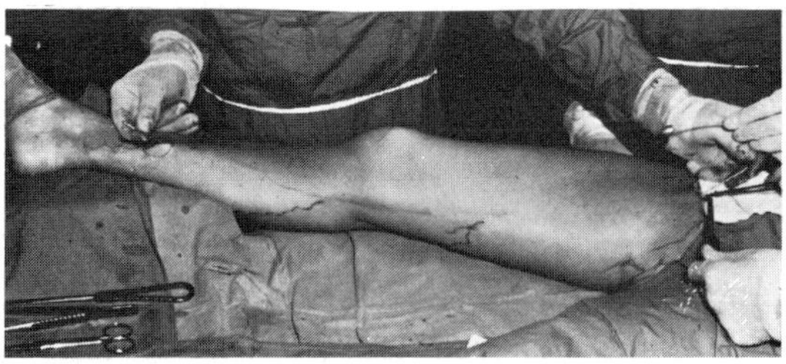

8. The stripper is passed down to the ankle region and is being extruded through a small vertical wound over the site of the enlarged middle ankle perforator. (The perforator was tied first.)

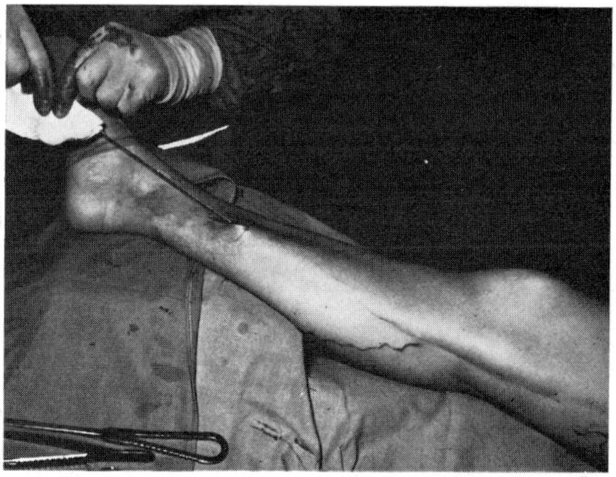

9. The stripper is slowly and steadily drawn down out of the lower wound. Note that the stripper is *not* bent or wrapped round the finger (which ruins it!) but is held firmly in a piece of gauze.

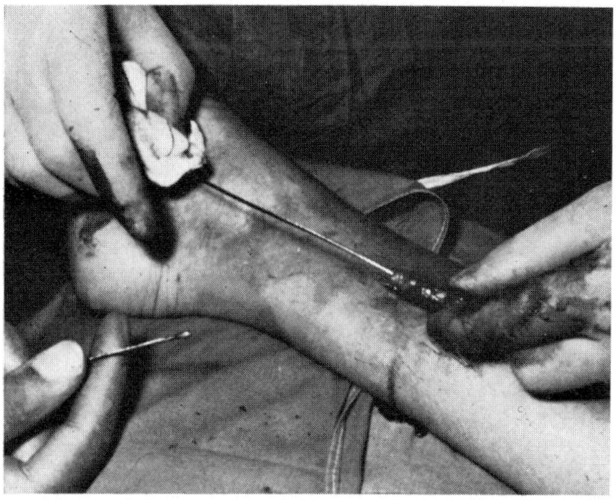

10. The 'vein bolus' is withdrawn slowly from the lower wound.

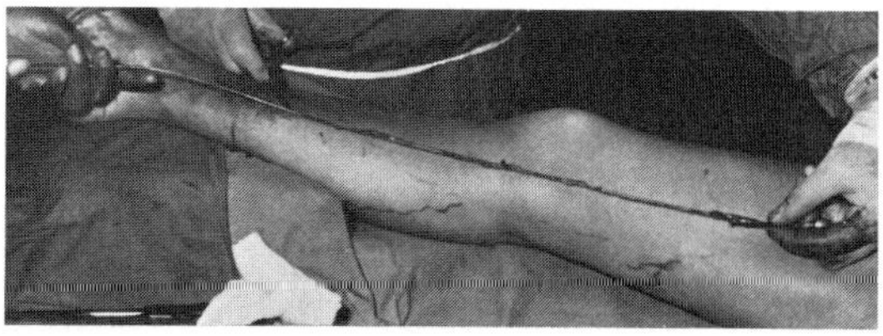

11. The complete saphenous vein on the stripper.

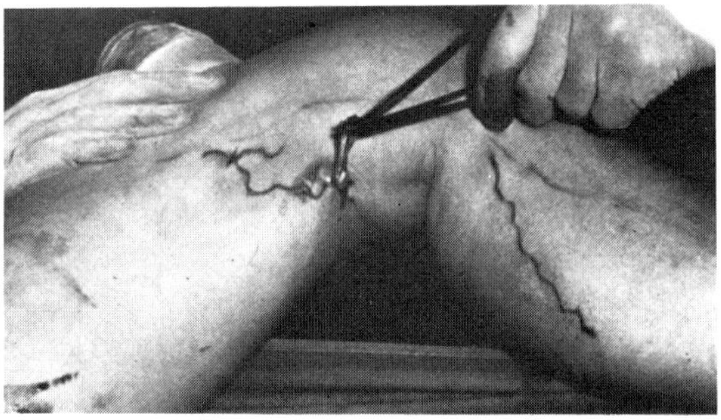

12. The secondary branches (carefully marked) are then removed by the 'worming technique', through separate very small incisions.

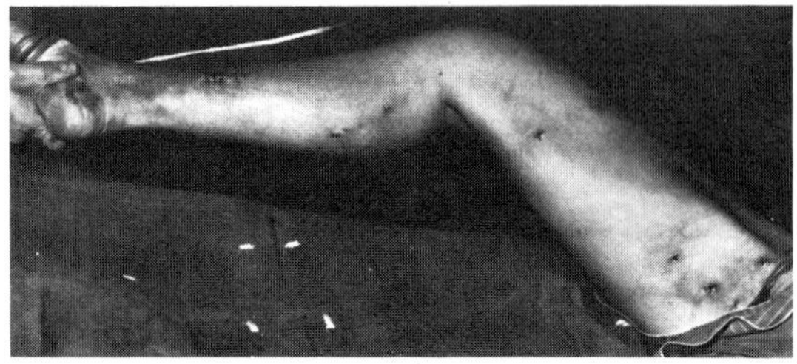

13. The completion of the operation. All incisions are closed with fine plastic silk. Note the small incisions over the prominent branch veins, where they have been wormed out.

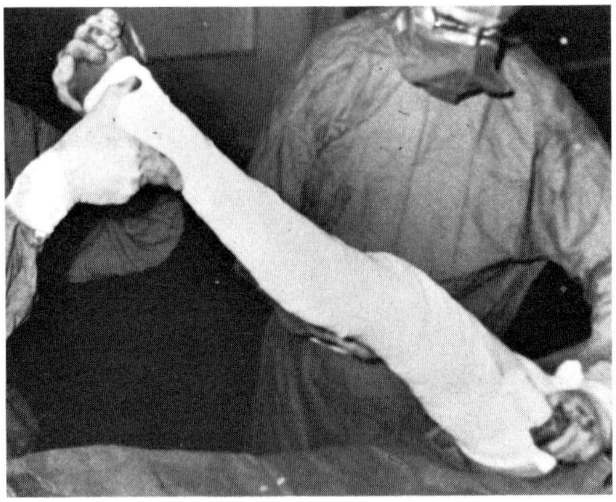

14. The last act of the operation; the application of a firm sterile crêpe bandage over dry gauze dressings, over the whole limb by the surgeon himself.

necessary for nearly all vascular operations on the legs, as it empties the veins and decongests the whole limb and is the *single most important factor controlling haemorrhage during vein stripping*.

It is equally important not to have the legs *too* high, otherwise if a large vein is opened accidentally air may be sucked in with the danger of air embolism.

The legs are abducted, the heels resting on a padded cross board (see Fig. 8.8).

TEMPERATURE OF THEATRE

The theatre should not be too hot, as this causes general vasodilatation and may contribute quite a lot to blood loss (see also avoidance of halothane, already mentioned).

EXPOSURE OF THE SAPHENOUS VEIN AT THE GROIN

A wide exposure of the saphenofemoral junction is absolutely necessary in order to achieve the essential flush ligature on the wall of the femoral vein above all the tributaries. Only by a generous exposure can the frequent variations of the venous anatomy and sometimes of arterial anatomy be recognised and dealt with.

Landmark of the saphenofemoral junction. The saphenofemoral junction is at a point 2·5 to 3·5 cm (1 to 1·25 inches) below and lateral to the pubic tubercle (Fig. 8.9). All the incisions have their centre at this point; we emphasise the importance of accurately determining pubic tubercle before making the incision.

The variable level of the fold of the groin in relation to Poupart's ligament is not generally realised; it depends on the obesity of the patient. In the stout the crease is 3 to 5 cm lower than the ligament. In thin subjects the skin crease and Poupart's ligament are almost superimposed and an approach here will be found too high for the saphenofemoral junction. We advise that the skin crease be ignored when planning the incision.

The incisions

Two incisions will be discussed: the curved or 'hockey-stick', for wide access, and the oblique.

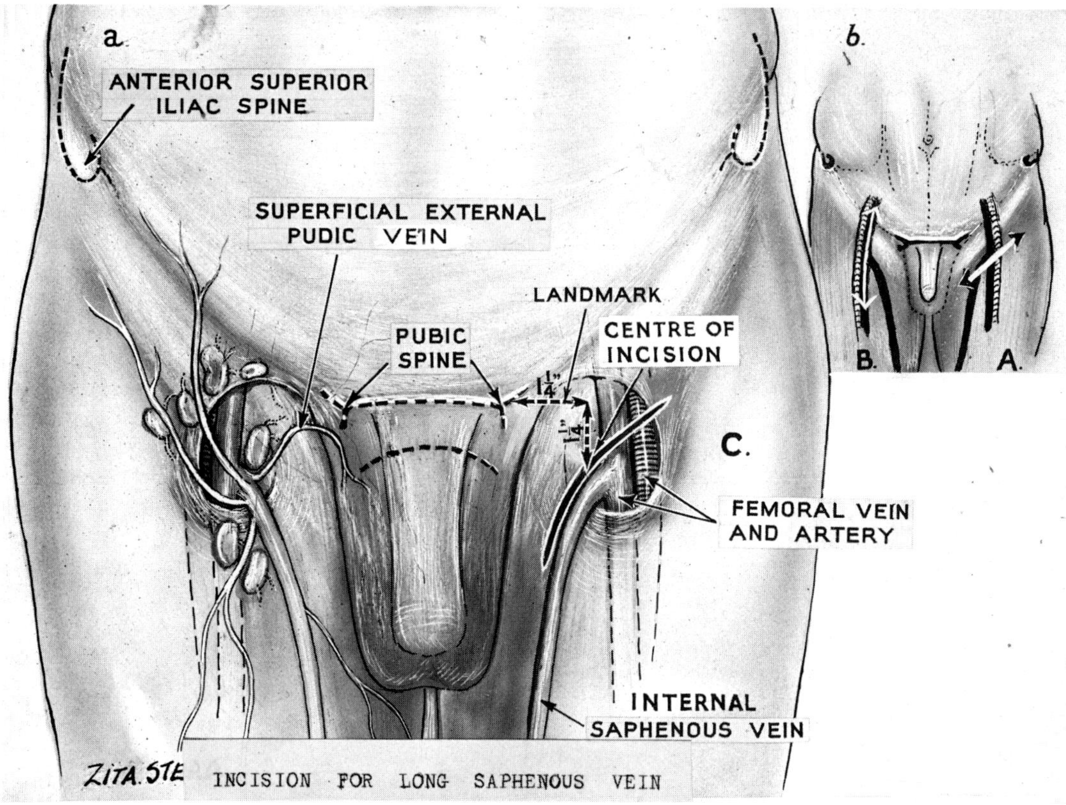

Fig. 8.9 The incisions for exposure of the termination of the internal saphenous vein.

The curved or 'hockey-stick' incision (Fig. 8.9). This was evolved from a combination of the oblique and vertical incisions, being 8 to 12 cm long. Its outer half lies in the gutter of the groin and the inner half curves downwards to the thigh. The incision, as its name implies, is shaped like a hockey-stick and lies over the terminal 5 to 7 cm of the internal saphenous vein. It is centred as above.

The outer portion of the incision exposes the saphenofemoral union, and the inner part, when strongly retracted downwards, will reveal up to 10 to 12 cm (4 to 5 inches) of the internal saphenous trunk. The incision is especially designed to give access to its posterointernal tributary, which often joins it at its upper third.

A good scar remains after it (Fig. 8.10).

The oblique incision (Fig. 8.9 inset). This must be centred accurately over the surface marking of the saphenofemoral junction. It is 7 to 10 cm long and adequate retraction of the wound edges by an assistant is necessary to gain a complete exposure. It heals with a fine scar. It is parallel to the fold of the groin.

The length of the incision. One of us began to ligate the internal saphenous vein with the idea that it should be done through a one-inch (2 to 3 cm) incision. This was an error; with an opening so small it was easy to miss the saphenous vessel entirely, to mistake one of its large tributaries for it, to overlook feeding veins, or, surprising as it may seem, even to ligate the femoral vein. A generous incision has avoided such pitfalls. 'The surgeon should operate by sight, and not by faith' (Maingot, 1953). No additional incapacity follows a wide

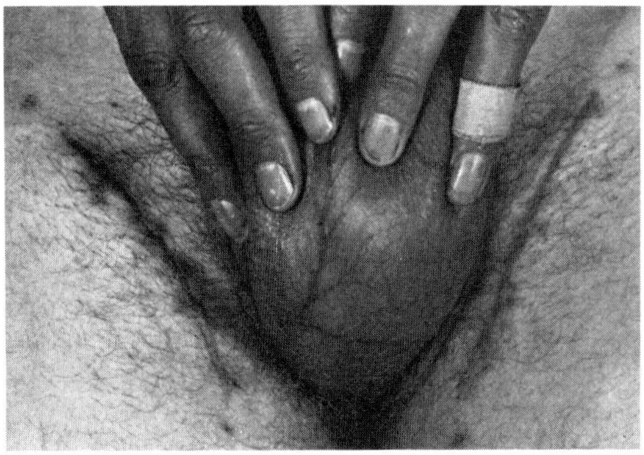

Fig. 8.10 The scars after bilateral ligation of the sapheno-femoral junction.

exposure, and the dependable results confirm its suitability. Many of the recurrences after operation have resulted from working through an inadequate and wrongly-placed approach.

THE EXPOSURE OF THE INTERNAL SAPHENOUS VEIN

After the incision through the skin has been made, the lips of the wound are elevated (Fig. 8.11) and the incision carried straight down through the fat until the layer of the superficial fascia is encountered. This is opened by a stroke of the knife. The saphenous vein lies deep to this layer of fascia (Camper's fascia).

When this layer has been opened, a small gauze swab is taken and quite firmly wiped upwards and then downwards in the wound. This simple manoeuvre exposes the whole saphenofemoral junction rapidly and safely, and avoids cutting lymphatics and small arteries (see Figs 8.12 and 8.8—No. 4).

In patients with an ulcer or eczema of the leg, there is often adenitis and periadenitis of the vertical and horizontal groups of saphenous lymph nodes; these are avoided by retracting

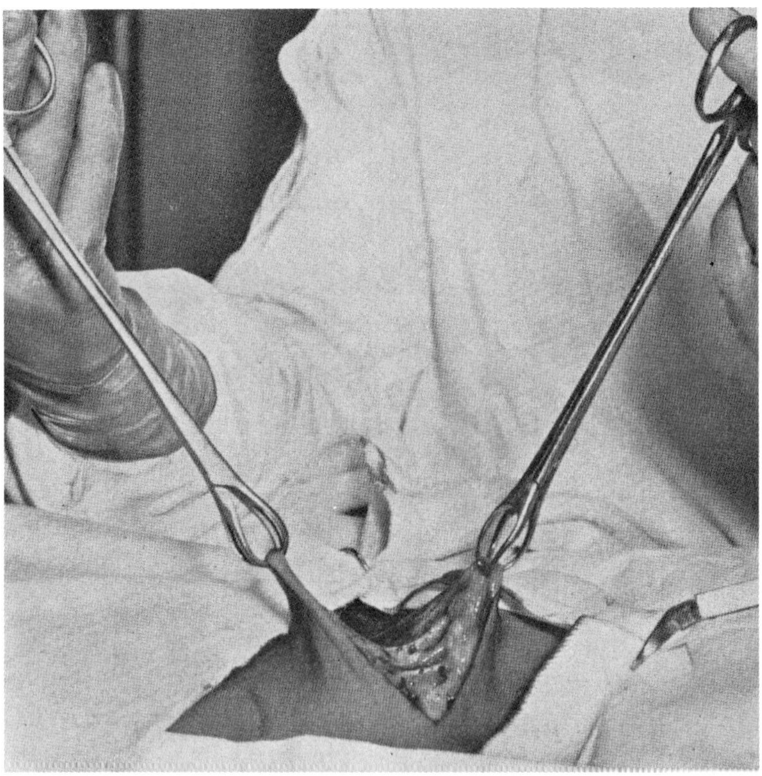

Fig. 8.11 Forcible elevation of the skin edges after making the skin incision.

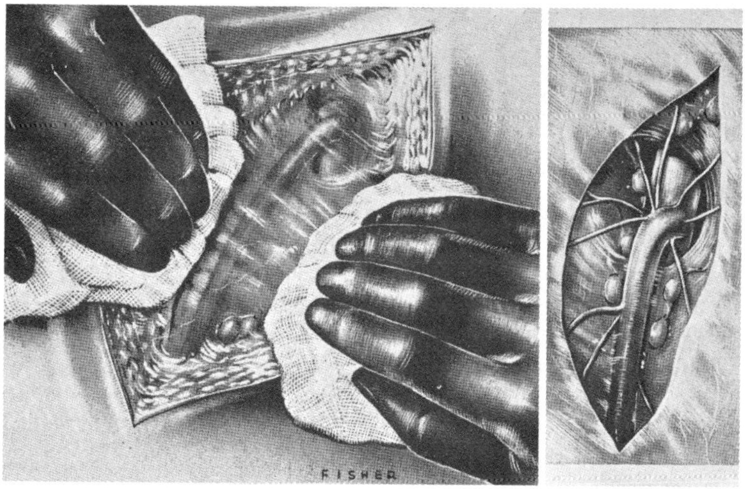

Fig. 8.12 Location of the internal saphenous vein by stretching of skin and fat. Inset—the average finding of the internal saphenous vein.

them downwards and outwards. Distended lymphatics can occasionally be seen passing into the femoral canal. By siting the incision correctly and deepening it vertically, the embarrassing bleeding which follows the division of matted lymphatic nodes is avoided. If the glands are unduly enlarged, one should be removed and sectioned; in this way one patient with an ulcer of the ankle was found to have lymphatic leukaemia.

LOCATING THE INTERNAL SAPHENOUS VEIN

Occasionally, on dividing the two layers of superficial fascia, especially if the incision is incorrectly placed, the long saphenous vein is not apparent, but fascia covering the pectineus muscle may be exposed instead. By inserting two swabs into the depths of the wound (Figs 8.8 and 8.12) and pressing its fatty sides gently and steadily apart, the saphena magna will be seen through the fat as it is retracted. If this fails, an alternative guide to it is that of tracing any presenting vein (almost invariably present in the wound). This leads to a larger tributary and thence to the long saphenous vein. Superficial veins encountered whilst making the incision are better not divided until the saphenofemoral junction itself is located.

A self-retaining retractor is inserted into the wound; Travers' is a suitable pattern (see Fig. 8.8).

THE TECHNIQUE OF DISSECTION OF THE VEIN (Fig. 8.13)

The vein strips best on its nude, shiny wall, and not outside the thin layer of adventitious fascia that ensheathes it and also obscures its tributaries. A rapid, clean dissection is possible by using Mayo's straight, round-

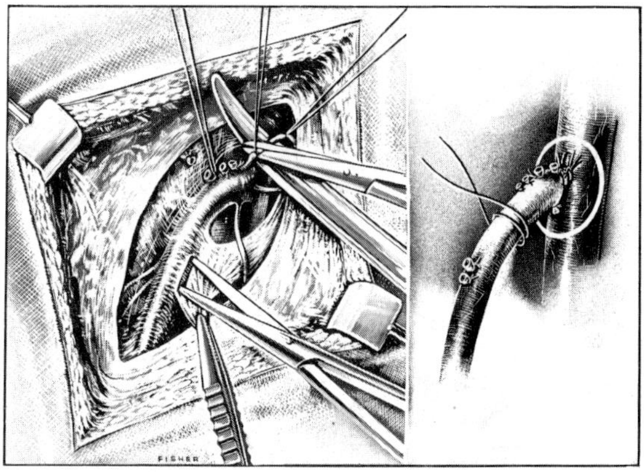

Fig. 8.13 The technique of the dissection of the internal saphenous vein and the ligation and division of the tributaries.

pointed scissors. Further, it is undesirable and unnecessary to grasp any vein wall with the dissecting forceps because varicosities are unpredictably and disconcertingly friable and bleed copiously if torn.

The fascia immediately outside the vein wall is held by the dissecting forceps, and the space between it and the vein is systematically displayed by gently opening the points of the scissors between them parallel to the vessel (Fig. 8.13). It is quick and effective and small tributaries are seen readily. The saphena magna and its radicals are dissected steadily until the faint white line indicating the union with the femoral vein is seen just inside the foramen ovale. The dissection includes opening the femoral sheath which has a thin continuation on to the internal saphenous vein (the cribiform fascia). The femoral vein is exposed for 0·5 to 1 cm above and below the foramen ovale and for half of its circumference. The saphenofemoral union and the terminal 0·5 cm of internal saphenous vein are closely invested by the femoral sheath and, as already mentioned, this is snicked by the scissors, opened and reflected from the junction of the long saphenous and femoral vein.

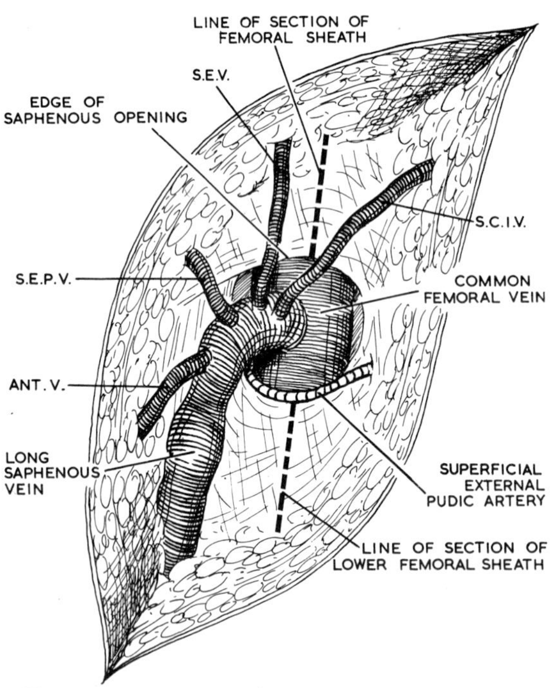

Fig. 8.14 Diagram showing the usual position of superficial external pudic artery.

Two observations during this procedure are of interest:

1. The enlarged varicose vein contracts down to normal proportions as a result of the dissection necessary to display it.

2. On watching some gross varicose veins, their distension and collapse synchronous with respiration and the heart beat are apparent.

THE SUPERFICIAL EXTERNAL PUDIC ARTERY (Figs 8.14 and 8.15)

This vessel is important and runs medially in various relationships to the end of the internal saphenous vein. Generally it runs underneath it in the lower edge of the foramen ovale but it may pass over the long saphenous vein (25 per cent of cases) and requires section, for in this superficial position it conceals the superficial epigastric vein and the saphenofemoral union. Less often it divides and both branches pass either superficially or deep to the saphenous vein, or one may pass over and the other under it on the deep fascia. They are divided as necessary, no attempt is made to preserve them.

THE TRIBUTARIES OF THE INTERNAL SAPHENOUS VEIN (see Figs 8.9 and 8.15 and also p. 20)

There are six significant veins joining the terminal 1 to 15 cm of the internal saphenous vein. It is seldom that one is absent, although they present in bizarre combinations (see Chap. 3). All but the posterointernal vein lie in the superficial fascia; the latter is on the deep fascia. They are as follows:

1. The superficial circumflex iliac vein, entering from above and laterally.

2. The superficial epigastric vein, passing vertically downwards from the fat of the lower abdominal wall.

3. The superficial external pudendal vein, from the external genitalia and perineum. These three vessels usually join the last centimetre of the internal saphenous vein.

4. The posterointernal (accessory saphenous) vein runs upwards on the deep fascia from the posterointernal aspect of the thigh to join the inner aspect of the internal saphenous vein. This vessel is always sought and divided, because it usually connects directly with the external (i.e. short) saphenous vein, which may, therefore, become secondarily dilated in a primary long saphenous incompetence, through this channel (see Fig. 7.22). Normally the posterointernal vein joins the last 5 to 10 cm of the internal saphenous vein, and is readily seen. When it is not apparent, here it may be even lower down, or inside the foramen ovale where it may be beside or joined by the deep external pudic vein (Fig. 8.16). Figure 8.16 indicates how the ligature must be placed.

5. The anteroexternal tributary runs subcutaneously diagonally across the thigh upwards and inwards from the anteroexternal aspect of the leg and knee, and joins the outer side of the last 2·5 cm of the long saphenous vein. This vessel (when varicose) is visible through the skin. When it is large and straight it may look like the internal saphenous vein, itself, particularly as it approaches the saphenofemoral junction. Its termination near the foramen ovale is frequently the site of the so called 'saphena varix'.

6. The deep external pudic vein (Fig. 8.16). In 30 to 40 per cent of cases this vein is present and joins the saphena magna on its posterointernal aspect precisely at its termination inside the foramen ovale. It is to expose this that half the circumference of the femoral vein is cleared, especially on its inner side, and gentle traction outwards is made on the internal saphenous vein. Not infrequently it is joined by the posterointernal vein (Fig. 8.16(4)).

Variations

The tributaries vary greatly in their pattern of union; it is unusual to find the same combination twice. Figure 8.15 tells the story.

We repeat that a full exposure of the femoral vein for at least 0·5 cm above and below the saphenofemoral junction is essential, as a superficial vein occasionally joins the parent vessel between these points. Much of the permanent success of the operation depends on the ligation and division of every tributary, because if one remains connected with the femoral vein and if the femoral or external iliac valve is incompetent, the high intravenous pressures would still be transferred to this subcutaneous vein and would keep the venous dilatation active, even after stripping of the saphenous trunk. From such an undivided vein over a period of years, a plexiform mass of thin-walled subcutaneous varices develop, ultimately connecting it with the saphenous trunk (if present) and its tributaries below (see Chapt. 9).

Unless all the subordinate vessels of the internal saphena are tied and cut, it is usually impossible to do a flush saphenofemoral ligation.

In spite of being alert, it is surprisingly easy to overlook the superficial epigastric and circumflex iliac veins. One of us recalls demonstrating the procedure for the varicose internal saphenous vein to some visiting surgeons and on completing it was asked to recapitulate the steps, naming the ligated vessels. During it the undivided superior epigastric vein was revealed; it had remained concealed by the superficial external pudic artery passing over it in the upper edge of the wound (Fig. 8.17).

LIGATION OF TRIBUTARIES

1. When all the tributaries are defined, they are divided between ligatures. The outer ligatures are cut short but those on the internal saphenous vein are held long, for traction on them elevates it to the surface and facilitates the operation.

2. The deep external pudic vein, when present, is divided and if it is possible to include it in the ligature of the saphenofemoral junction, it is an excellent step. This avoids submitting the ligated stump of a small thin-walled vessel to the high thoraco-abdominal pressures which may reach 200 mmHg during vomiting and coughing—a tie

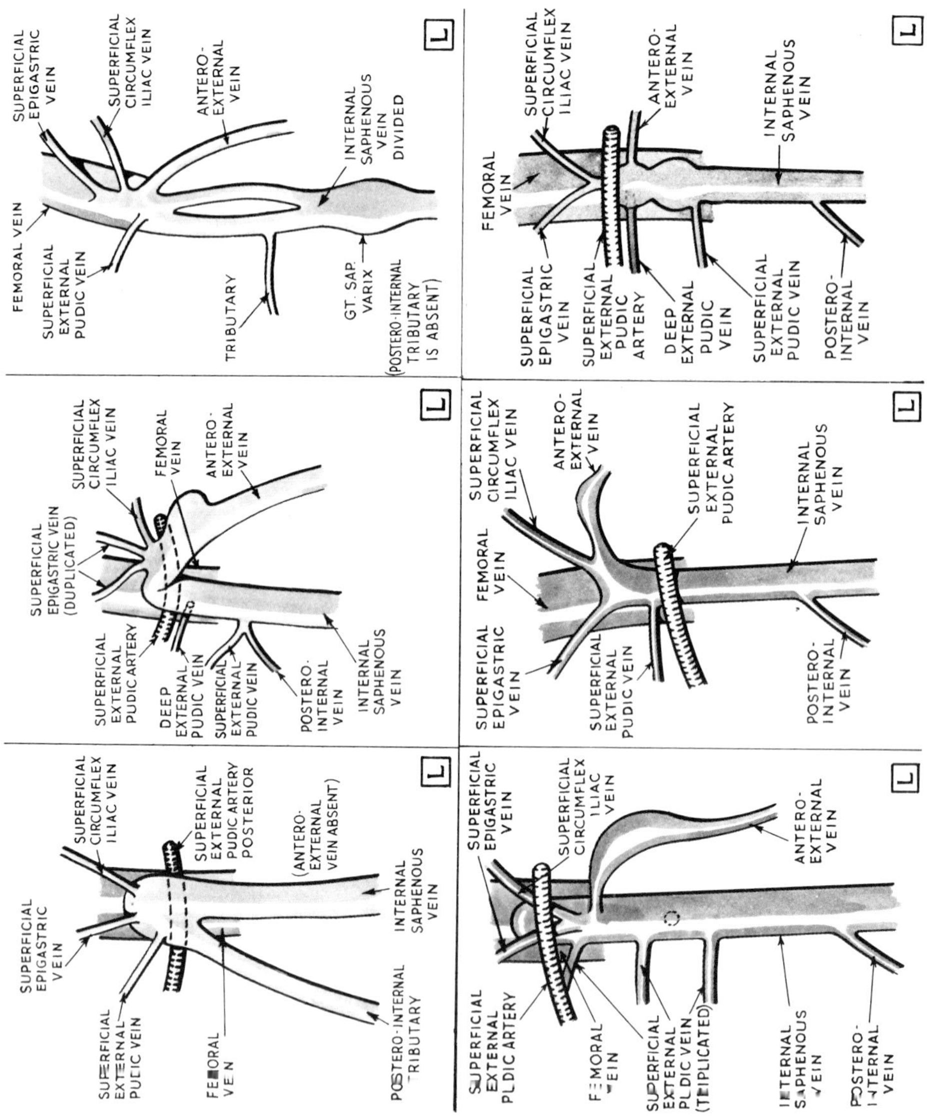
FEMORAL VEIN
SUPERFICIAL EPIGASTRIC VEIN
SUPERFICIAL CIRCUMFLEX ILIAC VEIN
ANTERO-EXTERNAL VEIN
INTERNAL SAPHENOUS VEIN DIVIDED
SUPERFICIAL EXTERNAL PUDIC VEIN
TRIBUTARY
GT. SAP. VARIX
(POSTERO-INTERNAL TRIBUTARY IS ABSENT)
L
SUPERFICIAL EPIGASTRIC VEIN (DUPLICATED)
SUPERFICIAL CIRCUMFLEX ILIAC VEIN
FEMORAL VEIN
ANTERO-EXTERNAL VEIN
SUPERFICIAL EXTERNAL PUDIC ARTERY
DEEP EXTERNAL PUDIC VEIN
SUPERFICIAL EXTERNAL PUDIC VEIN
POSTERO-INTERNAL VEIN
INTERNAL SAPHENOUS VEIN
L
SUPERFICIAL EPIGASTRIC VEIN
SUPERFICIAL CIRCUMFLEX ILIAC VEIN
SUPERFICIAL EXTERNAL PUDIC ARTERY POSTERIOR
(ANTERO-EXTERNAL VEIN ABSENT)
INTERNAL SAPHENOUS VEIN
POSTERO-INTERNAL TRIBUTARY
L
FEMORAL VEIN
SUPERFICIAL CIRCUMFLEX ILIAC VEIN
ANTERO-EXTERNAL VEIN
INTERNAL SAPHENOUS VEIN
SUPERFICIAL EPIGASTRIC VEIN
SUPERFICIAL EXTERNAL PUDIC ARTERY
DEEP EXTERNAL PUDIC VEIN
SUPERFICIAL EXTERNAL PUDIC VEIN
POSTERO-INTERNAL VEIN
L
SUPERFICIAL CIRCUMFLEX ILIAC VEIN
ANTERO-EXTERNAL VEIN
FEMORAL VEIN
SUPERFICIAL EXTERNAL PUDIC ARTERY
INTERNAL SAPHENOUS VEIN
SUPERFICIAL EPIGASTRIC VEIN
SUPERFICIAL EXTERNAL PUDIC VEIN
POSTERO-INTERNAL VEIN
L
SUPERFICIAL EPIGASTRIC VEIN
SUPERFICIAL CIRCUMFLEX ILIAC VEIN
ANTERO-EXTERNAL VEIN
SUPERFICIAL EXTERNAL PLDIC ARTERY
SUPERFICIAL EXTERNAL PLDIC VEIN
POSTERO-INTERNAL VEIN
L

contd.

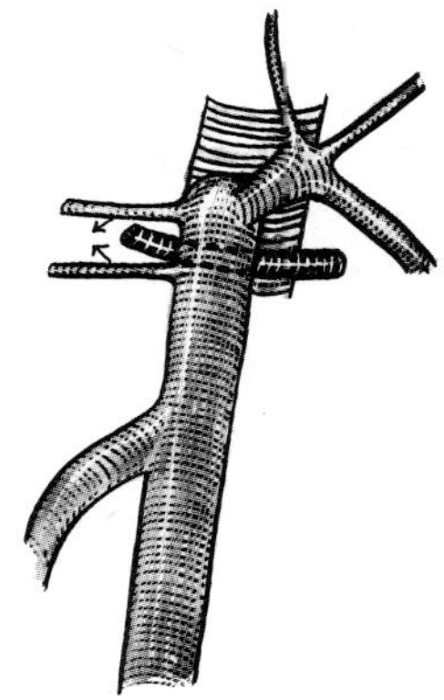

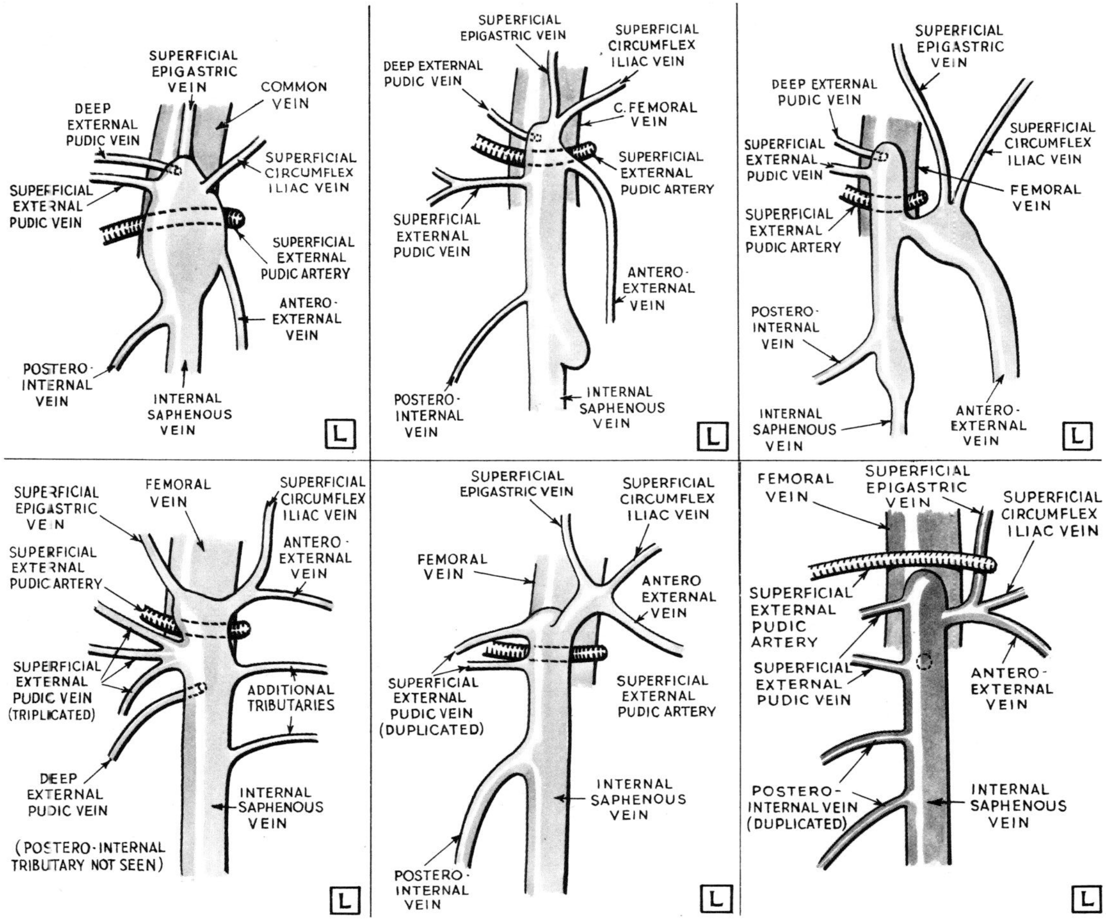

Fig. 8.15 Twelve consecutive dissections of the termination of the long saphenous vein. They are different although some are bilateral veins (the right have been transposed to the left to facilitate comparison).

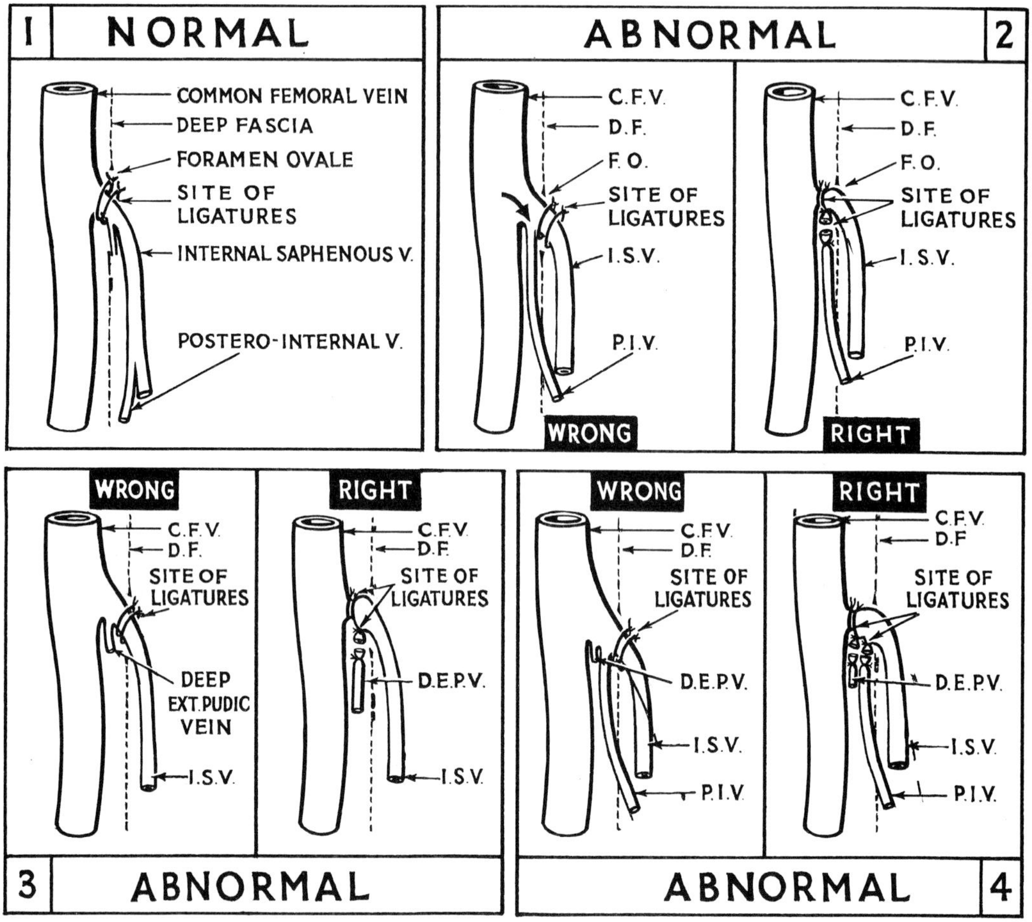

Fig. 8.16 Variations of the posterointernal and deep external pudic veins as they join the termination of the internal saphenous vein inside the foramen ovale. The right and wrong ways of placing the ligatures are indicated. The 'tie' must be flush on the femoral vein.

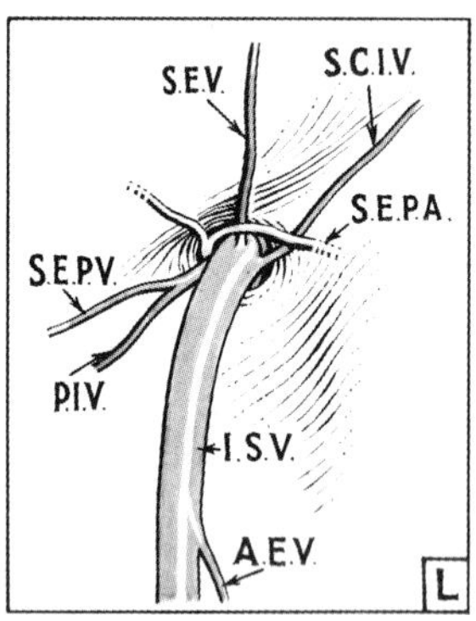

Fig. 8.17 The superficial epigastric vein concealed by the superficial external pudic artery which is also abnormal in this patient for it is emerging on the inner side of the internal saphenous vein instead of the usual outer side.

which could yield under such strain (see also Fig. 8.16).

Ligation of the internal saphenous vein. The end of the long saphenous vein is ligated with stout silk or linen thread. This material bites into the vessel wall and ties with a non-slipping knot. Catgut ligatures on the proximal end of the saphena magna have yielded occasionally, with fatal or critical haemorrhage. To make the saphenous stump safe, a second ligature is applied to it, or better still, it is transfixed with fine silk or thread, and tied as is a hernial sac (Fig. 8.18). The great surgical master, Halstead (1893), showed that transfixion is the certain way to secure an important vessel, and that an encircling liga-

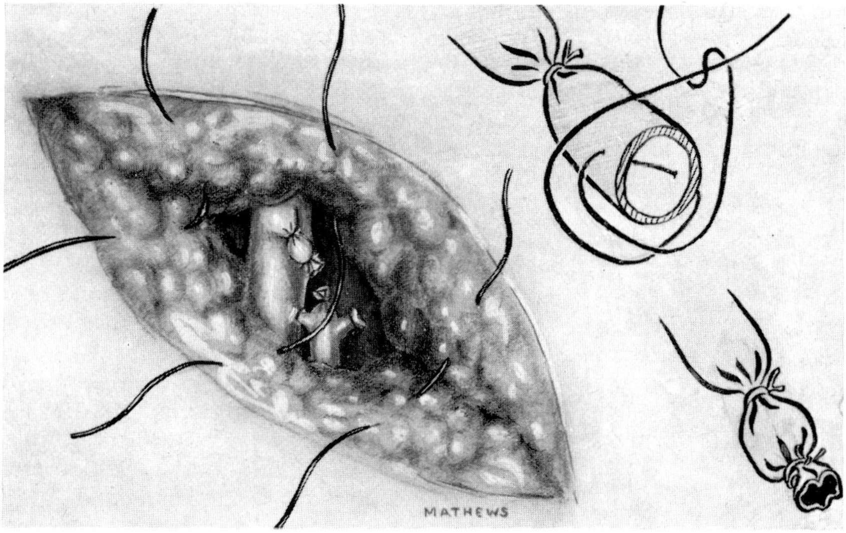

Fig. 8.18 Ligation and transfixion of the stump of the internal (or external) saphenous vein, also the closure of the dead space by interrupted sutures.

ture can be 'shot off' like a pea from a pea-shooter. As the pressures exerted on the stump of an incompetent internal saphenous vein may equal or exceed those in an artery, the need for security is obvious.

Inspection of the common femoral vein. Before tying the end of the saphenous vein, the femoral vein is inspected for a short distance above and below the junction. It is essential to see it, as it may be mistaken for the long saphenous especially in very thin patients.

AN ALTERNATIVE METHOD OF SAPHENOFEMORAL LIGATION

Another method of ligating the internal saphenous vein at the groin is mentioned. This consists of first exposing the sapheno-femoral junction by gauze dissection, and then having carefully identified the saphenous trunk, it is divided between haemostats a centimetre or so below the junction. The upper forceps is then used to elevate and put some traction on the stump of the saphenous vein. The tributaries are then easily defined by further gauze dissection and are divided until the saphenofemoral union is displayed. The flush ligature is then applied and tied. This technique should be used with caution, as the following episode illustrates:

In 1951 one of us after twenty years of varicose vein surgery exposed 3 to 4 cm of the femoral artery in an emaciated patient under the impression that it was the internal saphenous vein. The error was realised by the absence of tributaries, then the pulsation was noticed, and the necessary re-orientation

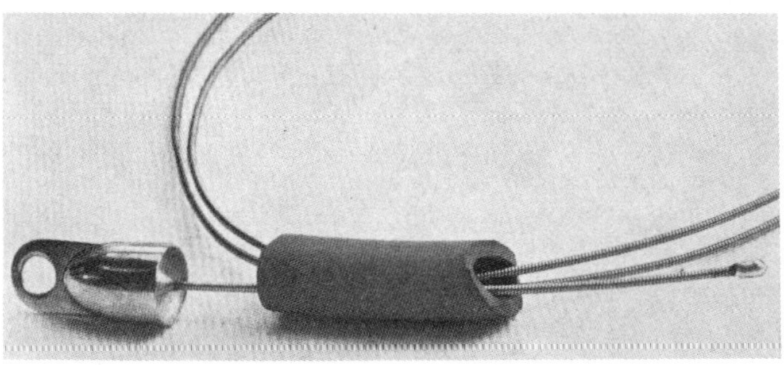

Fig. 8.19 Modified Myers' stripper.

followed. This incident served to show how serious the preliminary division of the vessel would have been. It occurred when operating with an excellent assistant and good conditions in every way.

It may be said that these are theoretical objections but our experience is that every error can occur in spite of care and we suspect that others find it so: 'The more care we take, the fewer mistakes we small make.' (Milligan, 1954).

STRIPPING OF THE INTERNAL SAPHENOUS VEIN

After the flush saphenofemoral ligation the saphenous trunk itself remains to be stripped.

Stripping is possible because even in gross varicose veins, when the branches are numerous, large and very tortuous on the surface of the limb, the saphenous trunk itself, although it enlarges, remains relatively straight on the deep fascia. A stripper can, therefore, be introduced and made to pass along the whole length of the vein either from below upwards or from above downwards.

Various modifications of the Myers flexible stripper are now in routine use. There are also strippers with interchangeable heads which are useful (except that loose heads can be lost with the passage of time!). Disposable plastic strippers are also available.

SURGICAL ANATOMY OF THE LOWER PART OF THE LONG SAPHENOUS VEIN AND THE SAPHENOUS NERVE

Figure 8.20 shows the important surgical relationship of the saphenous nerve to the internal saphenous vein in the lower third of the limb. It will be seen that the saphenous nerve is closely related to the vein and bifurcates over the vein about 2 or 3 inches above the ankle. It is in this situation that the passage of a bulky stripper head with vein telescoped on it, may damage the saphenous nerve. It will be readily appreciated that if the bulky stripper is pulled upwards, it may well get caught in the fork of the nerve, avulsing the whole or part of the saphenous nerve. This may cause a most annoying patch of anaesthesia and later hyperaesthesia over the internal malleolus. Sometimes in cases of actual nerve rupture (as opposed to mere bruising) a troublesome saphenous neuritis may persist for many months.

On the other hand, passage of the stripper downwards, although it may bruise the nerve carries much less risk of disrupting it.

Thus in order to minimise the risk of saphenous nerve injury it is either best to: (1) strip the vein from above downwards; or (2) avoid this area altogether with the stripper, and remove the vein either through a modified ankle perforator incision, 2 or 3 inches above the ankle or just below the knee.

If the saphenous vein is very large, however, and it is considered desirable to strip it right down to the ankle, it should be stripped from above downwards (Cox et al. 1974). Alternatively it can be stripped in two parts, through two incisions.

TECHNIQUE OF STRIPPING

Stripping downwards

For this a relatively stiff stripper of the cable type is required. The small tip is passed into the cut end of the saphenous vein at the groin, and the stripper is gently passed down the limb following the anatomical course of the long saphenous vein. It tends to wander into the branches, and it has to be gently kept 'on course' by frequent small withdrawals and advancements. Getting it past the remains of valves and varices in the wall of the vein occasionally causes difficulty, but they can usually be passed by gently 'shaking' the stripper up and down the vein a few times.

The end of the stripper is advanced either to the ankle perforator region (where it is cut down upon through a small vertical incision, through which often the perforators can be explored as well (see Fig. 8.8)) or to the ankle just *below* the internal malleolus (where it is cut down on and extruded by a small transverse incision).

When the stripper is extruded from the vein, the distal part of the vein going down towards the foot is divided and tied off. Then the acorn is firmly tied in the vein at the groin and the whole stripper is gently and firmly

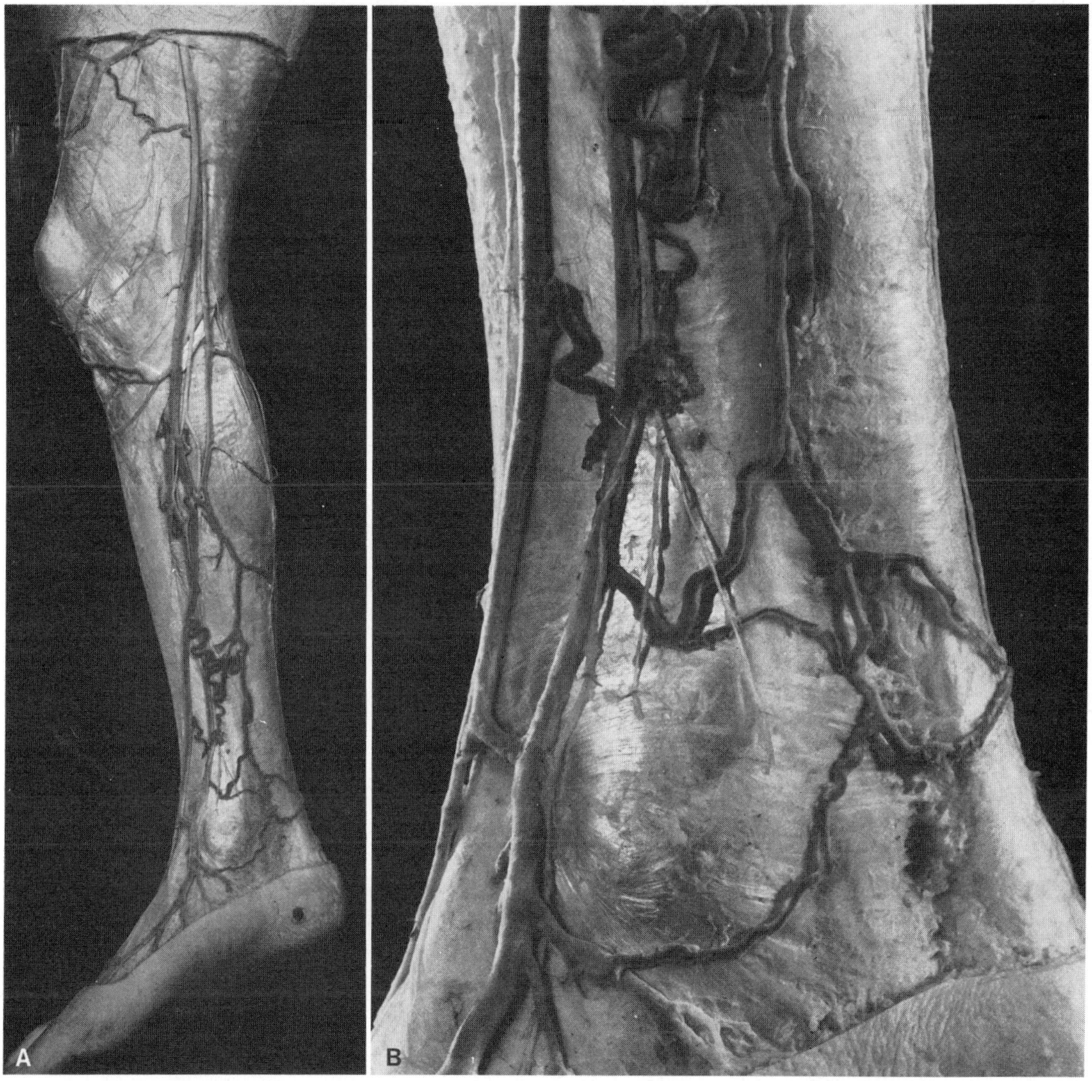

Fig. 8.20A, B These dissections show the close relationship of the saphenous nerve to the saphenous vein particularly in the lower part of the leg. 'B' in close up, shows the bifurcation of the nerve just above the ankle, in which a stripper head passing upwards may get caught, thus avulsing and permanently damaging the nerve.

withdrawn with the vein telescoped on it (see Fig. 8.8).

If the leg is well elevated and the theatre not too hot, there is very little bleeding into the stripper track.

If there are incompetent ankle perforators in the limb, however, they should be dealt with through the separate perforator incisions *before* the vein is stripped out, as otherwise they may cause considerable bleeding back into the stripper track, if they are large.

The stripper track is compressed gently with a big swab or rolled towel for about three minutes while coagulation occurs and the

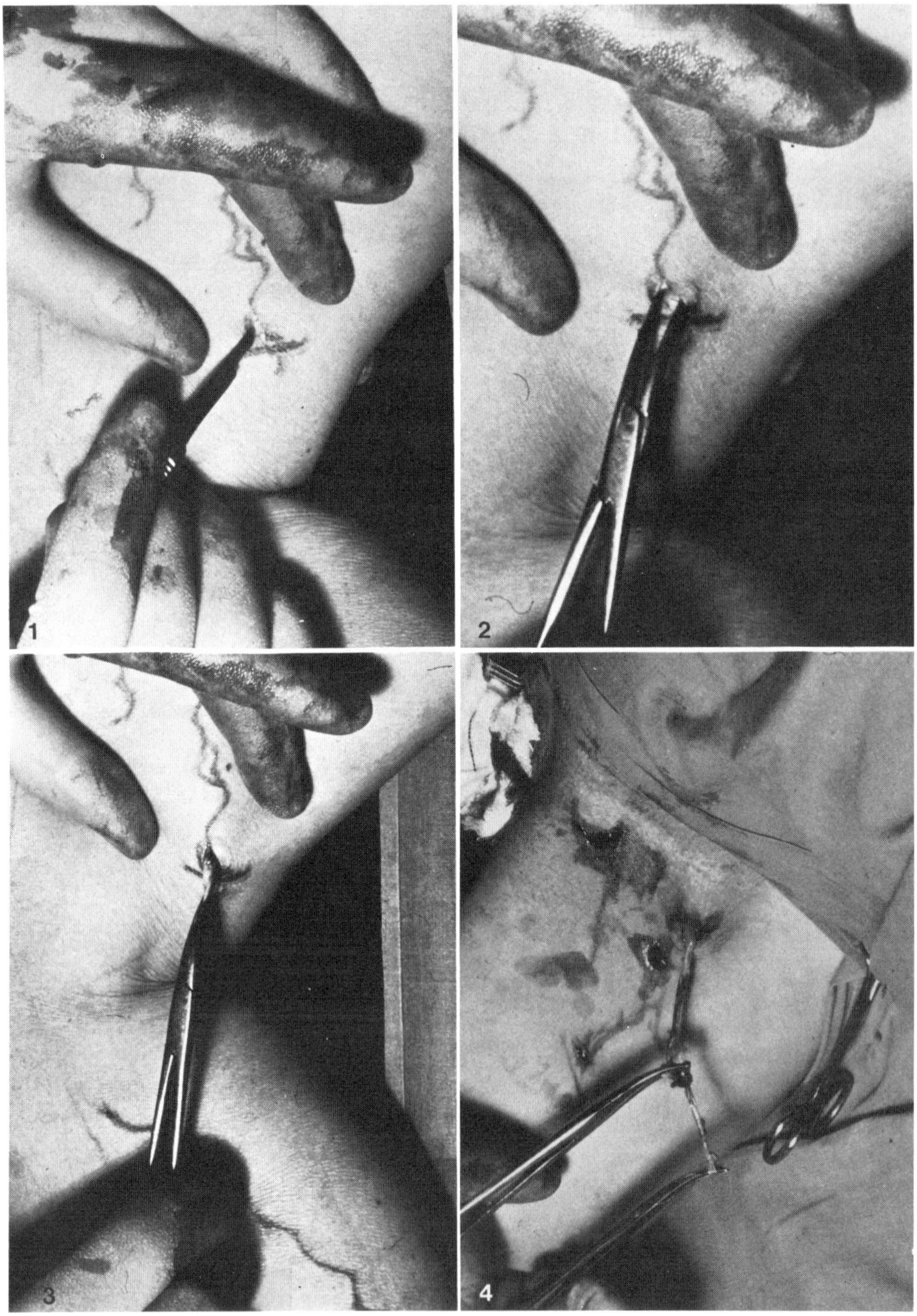

Fig. 8.21 'Worming technique' for removing small branch veins. 1. The vein is carefully marked on the skin and a 2 millimetre long incision is made over it. 2. A fine-ended forceps is thrust into the small wound and opened and closed several times to burrow into the subcutaneous tissues until the small vein is seen. 3. The small vein is seized in the forceps and by a gentle to and fro movement is eased out of the wound. 4. Long lengths of small tortuous veins can be 'wormed out' of these small wounds by this technique.

torn off branches contract and then the clot is massaged from out of the track first down, then upwards.

Stripping of the secondary branches

After the main saphenous trunk has been withdrawn, then the secondary stripping of the dilated branches which have been marked beforehand is carried out.

Particular branches which frequently have to be removed are the tortuous anterolateral vein of the thigh and the tortuous posterior arch vein on the calf (Fig. 8.8).

These vessels are removed by very small incisions placed along their course, by the technique known as 'worming' (see Fig. 8.21). This name has been applied because the technique is in every way similar to that employed by birds on the lawn in the early morning, who extract worms from the turf with their beaks!

A fine artery forceps is thrust into the tiny incision over the vein and opened once or twice, until the white vein wall is sighted. This is then grasped and with a side to side movement, quite long lengths of the tortuous vein can be withdrawn from each little incision in a very short space of time and with little bleeding.

Having completed these subsidiary vein removals all incisions are sewn up with fine 4° silk—after a final massage of the stripper track to force out the last of the clot.

The limb is then held up by the foot, by an assistant, a flat piece of gauze is put over each incision, and a 6 inch crêpe bandage is applied with moderate pressure from toes to groin.

Interrupted stripping

Sometimes the tip of the stripper impacts on its way down and no amount of manipulation will get it to move on. In such cases there are two alternatives:

1. One can cut down at the point of impaction—withdraw the stripper, reinsert it and continue the downward strip.

2. Make a fresh incision over the long saphenous vein in the lower leg (ankle perforator incision) or at the ankle reinsert the stripper, and pass it upwards.

Stripping upwards

Many surgeons prefer to insert the stripper in a fresh incision at lower leg or ankle, after doing the flush saphenofemoral ligation, and pass the stripper upwards. Theoretically this should be easier than passing it downwards, because the valves should not hold it up. However, in practice the stripper is quite often held up even in its upward passage, by branches, kinks and blowouts on the side of the vein.

As has been already indicated, stripping by pulling the large acorn head upwards from the internal malleolus gives an increased risk of saphenous nerve complications.

This, however, can be overcome by having a stripper with a detachable acorn head, which can be fitted on either end. If this instrument is available it can be passed upwards to the groin, the heads swapped from one end to the other, and the vein stripped out from above downwards.

Residual veins after stripping

Figure 8.22 shows the state of the internal saphenous vein drainage area after stripping. The branch veins shown, if they are large and varicose should be removed after the main strip by the 'worming technique' already described.

If they are not removed they tend to fill by gravity and spoil what would otherwise be an excellent cosmetic result.

Post-operative bandaging (see Fig. 8.8)

As soon as the wounds are closed and the skin cleaned from blood stains, the limb is held up by the foot by an assistant and the sterile firm crêpe pressure bandage is applied evenly from foot to thigh. This bandage is left untouched until the seventh day when the stitches are removed.

The application of the pressure bandage is the most important final step in the operation, and it should be applied by the surgeon himself, not left to an assistant or nurse, who may not appreciate its important functions, which are as follows:

1. It effectively controls all further venous bleeding and oozing over the operated areas, prevents the formation of large haematomas

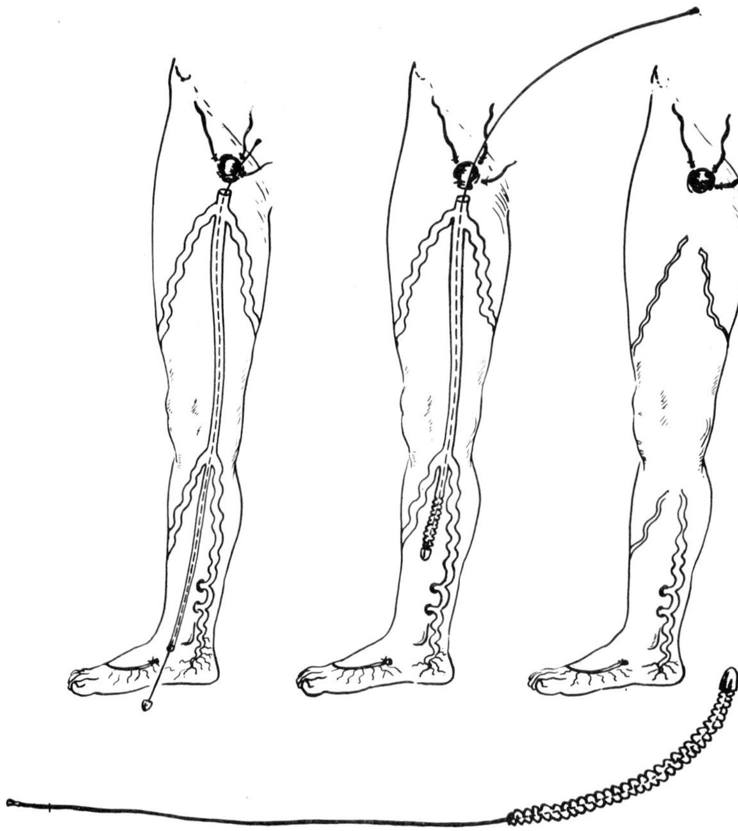

Fig. 8.22 The internal saphenous area after stripping. 1. Note that the tributaries are still interconnected and will fill up again if linked with a source of venous hypertension, or they will fill by gravity when the patient stands.
2. Note that stripping does not destroy the ankle perforating veins, therefore these must always be approached and tied as a separate manoeuvre through a special incision if this is necessary.

in the vicinity of the stripped veins, and generally contributes considerably to post-operative comfort and freedom from pain.

2. It compresses not only the superficial veins, but the deep veins as well and is therefore an important contribution to freedom from post-operative deep vein thrombosis.

The bandage should ideally be of the *light crêpe bandage,* or *linen elastic bandage* type. These bandages can be put on the unconscious patient at full stretch without exerting dangerously high pressure. *Webbing elastic bandages should never be used on the unconscious patient* as they exert so much pressure that they may occlude the arterial circulation, especially in elderly patients, or women with delicate limbs and skin.

Bloodless stripping (Fig. 8.23)

If the techniques as detailed above are carried out in a reasonably cool theatre, with elevation of the legs and with an anaesthetic agent which does not cause vasodilatation, then blood loss is not a serious problem and can always be easily controlled.

However, some surgeons like to pressure bandage the limb following the stripper head up as it is pulled up and out of the stripper track. The pressure bandaging is done by an

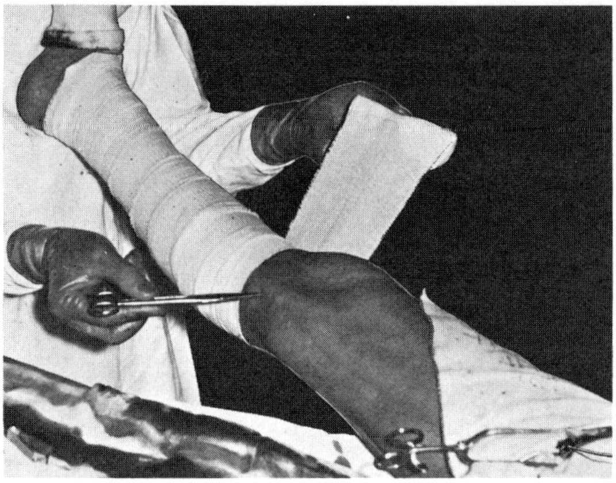

Fig. 8.23 Clean stripping of the internal saphenous vein. The wound at the ankle has been sutured and dressed. As the stripper is drawn from the ankle the limb is firmly bandaged with a sterile crêpe bandage. The haemostat tip is indicating the position of the stripping shoulder. (The staining on the towel is not blood but iodine.)

assistant as the stripper is slowly withdrawn from the track. It is claimed that this technique minimises haemorrhage and haematoma formation and discoloration in thigh and leg.

However it has the disadvantage that the numerous secondary avulsions of branch veins, which go to improve the final result so much, are not possible if this method is used. If multiple avulsions are attempted before the secondary veins are disconnected from their filling sources by stripping (and ankle perforator ligation) then copious haemorrhage may ensue. It is mainly for this reason that we do not recommend this stripping technique as routine practice.

OPERATIONS FOR THE SHORT SAPHENOUS VEIN

Surgical anatomy

The short saphenous vein begins half way between the *external* malleolus and the outer margin of the tendo achilles, by the coalescence of a series of veins draining the outer side of the dorsum of the foot, and the outer side of the heel. It runs straight up the middle of the calf to the centre of the popliteal space. In its lower third it lies *on* the deep fascia, but at the musculotendinous junction of the gastrocnemius at the middle of the calf, it penetrates the deep fascia and runs beneath it, to end in the popliteal vein, in the midline of the popliteal space. The exact level of the saphenopopliteal union is variable, but in most cases it is somewhere between the two horizontal skin grooves at the back of the knee.

The anatomical variations have been listed by Kosinski (Chap. 3) but in our experience they are rarer than his figures purport to show (Fig. 8.24).

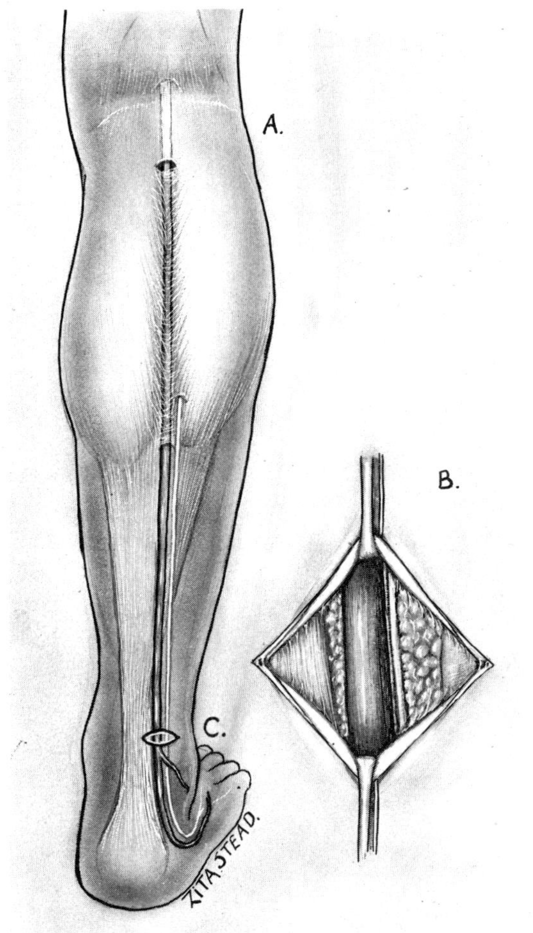

Fig. 8.24 The nerve-vein relationship at the ankle, i.e. the external saphenous vein and sural nerve.

However there are two important variations which are not uncommon and these are:

1. Just before its entry into the popliteal vein, the short saphenous is joined by a large branch coming from above: this is the postero-medial branch of the great saphenous vein (see Chap. 3) and is one of the important routes by which the great saphenous communicates with the short saphenous. Occasionally it is large, and almost replaces the normal junction with the popliteal vein. It always has to be sought at operation and ligatured and divided.

2. The two pairs of gastrocnemial venae comites normally pass up towards the middle of the popliteal fossa and join the popliteal vein just below the entry of the short saphenous.

However, frequently there is some communication between these gastrocnemial veins and the terminal inch or so of the short saphenous. Occasionally the short saphenous appears to end in one of these large gastrocnemial veins, and they present an irregular varicose appearance.

When this anomaly is found it is important not to tie the gastrocnemial veins thus interrupting their discharge into the popliteal vein. The short saphenous is then tied at its junction with the gastrocnemial vein, which is not interrupted.

The nerve vein relationship

The sural nerve is very closely applied to the short saphenous vein—especially in its lower third (Fig. 8.24). It is quite a large nerve and can easily be mistaken for a vein in a dissection round the external malleolus. Injury or division of this nerve may result in anaesthesia of the lateral half of the foot. It is not so vulnerable to bruising by the stripper as is the saphenous nerve in stripping of the long saphenous vein. It is more often injured during the dissection at the ankle where it may be beside one or more of the branches.

The operation

The standard operation for an incompetent short saphenous vein is 'flush ligation' at the point where it enters the popliteal vein, combined with removal of the vein to the external malleolus or just below it by stripping.

The patient must be face down and the knee is flexed a little by placing a sandbag under the ankle. The foot of the table is tilted up a little, so that legs are above the heart. The same remarks about anaesthesia and theatre temperature apply here as in operations on the great saphenous vein.

Exposure in popliteal fossa

If the short saphenous vein can be felt preoperatively with the patient standing up, it is wise to mark it on the skin as a guide. The vein is approached by a generous incision, at least 2 inches long, *transversely* across the popliteal fossa. It can usually be made in one of the transverse lines of skin about level with the knee joint.

The incision is deepened until the deep fascia is seen and the short saphenous vein lies *deep* to this. The fascia is then divided transversely in the line of the incision. The short saphenous vein is then seen or sought for between the two heads of gastrocnemius. This manoeuvre is best carried out by opening and closing the blunt tips of a short straight Mayo scissors.

As soon as it is identified, it is lifted up in a pair of artery forceps and the *knee is flexed still further by an assistant.* This *latter* manoeuvre is extremely important as with the

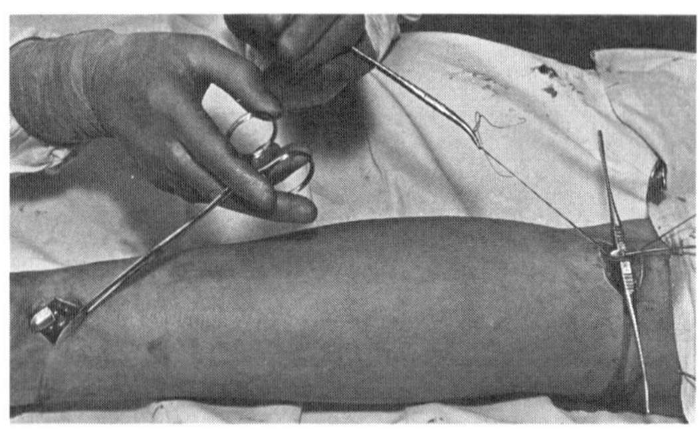

Fig. 8.25 The stripper passed through the external saphenous vein from the ankle to the wound at the popliteal space.

knee straight the structures in the popliteal fossa are 'on the stretch' and it is a difficult dissection. As soon as the knee is *flexed* all tension in the popliteal fossa is released and dissection of the short saphenous vein down to the popliteal vein is made easier. This dissection (the following of the short saphenous vein down into the popliteal fossa) is done with a small gauze swab ('Lahey Dab') or with the Mayo scissor blunt technique. A pair of small retractors in the popliteal fossa will be necessary to part the structures and allow the popliteal vein to be visualised. The short saphenous vein is now cut across and the proximal end lifted so that it can be more easily followed down into the fossa.

As in a great saphenous ligation at the groin, it is extremely important to ligate all side branches of the short saphenous right up to its junction with the popliteal vein. The large branch going upwards in the fat of the popliteal fossa (the posteromedial branch of the great saphenous—Chap. 3) is the most constant branch which has to be ligatured.

The short saphenous itself is then ligatured as close as possible to the popliteal vein. We usually use one piece of medium linen thread for this or a transfixion stitch.

Where the short saphenous seems to enter a large gastrocnemial vein (see above, surgical anatomy) the short saphenous is best ligatured flush against it and it is better not to divide the gastrocnemial vein.

The stripper is then made ready to pass down distally. Its small end usually runs down the vein to the point below the external malleolus where the vein originates. It is cut down upon here through a small transverse incision. The vein is dissected out cleanly by blunt dissection—the indwelling stripper being a useful guide. The sural nerve is carefully avoided. When the vein is cleanly dissected it is opened and the stripper passed out of it. The popliteal end is already secured and is now divided. The stripper is withdrawn downwards with a *steady slow* pull, with the short saphenous vein telescoped upon it.

The stripper is often held up at the mid-calf where the short saphenous vein emerges from the deep fascia, through a little curved foramen. A large branch often originates at this point which may need removal through a separate incision. It is also near here that the important mid-calf perforating vein emerges. For both these reasons it is advisable to cut down on and explore the mid-calf point, if the stripper impacts there, or if there is a large bunch of veins arising there (which may be winkled out). These explorations at mid-calf are done through a 1 inch *vertical* incision.

Cases with large bunches of veins round the external malleolus, with or without external malleolar eczema

In these cases (see Chap. 7) it is best to dissect out the large wormlike bunches of veins round the external malleolus by one or more transverse incisions. This thorough removal, *in addition* to stripping the short saphenous, immeasurably improves the result. In these cases the sites of the lateral and mid-calf perforating veins must be carefully inspected and if there is any doubt a separate exploration of these should be made (Fig. 7.12 perforating vein sites).

Incisions for exploration of the short saphenous vein

In general the rule that incisions should be *transverse* when over or near a joint, and *longitudinal* in the limb between joints, should be adhered to. These incisions give by far the best scars.

For exploration of the termination of the short saphenous vein in the popliteal fossa, a generous transverse incision is nearly always adequate. If, however, it is found to be wrongly sited in a particular case, either too high or too low, then a further small transverse incision can be used (the so-called 'step-ladder incision').

Curved and S-shaped incisions which have been recommended in the past should be avoided.

If a really wide exploration of the popliteal fossa has to be made for any reasons (e.g. extensive exploration of the artery or deep vein) then a straight vertical midline incision in the popliteal fossa is the best. Such incisions sometimes give rise to fibrous and keloid scars and this is their main disadvantage. However, if the deep fascia is sewn up carefully with fine plain catgut, and the skin is closed accurately with fine silk sutures, the chance of this 'spreading of the scar' is much reduced.

IMMEDIATE POST-OPERATIVE CARE

A full stripping operation for varicose veins should not be regarded as a 'minor' operation. It requires the same careful post-operative regime that would be accorded to a case of haemorrhoids or hernia or breast removal.

There has been a tendency to regard these cases as so minor that they can be discharged home after two days or so. Our experience has always been that this brings with it a train of annoying complications ranging from wound rupture and sepsis to swollen painful legs.

A careful standard post-operative regime should be insisted on to avoid all these irritations, some being major ones!

The three factors in the first week after operation are:

1. The maintenance of firm elastic pressure over the whole limb.
2. Insistence on regular movement and exercise of the legs.
3. The elevation of the foot of the bed 6 to 9 inches so that the legs are just above the heart level when the patient is in bed.

If the patient is allowed to have the legs down, without movement, and without support soon after operation, the venous pressure in them rises rapidly (see Chap. on Physiology), and may cause reactionary haemorrhage into the stripper track, and congestion and intense pain in all the areas from which the veins have been removed.

This high venous pressure must therefore be avoided particularly in the first post-operative week, so patients must stick firmly to the following regime:

Position. The foot of the bed is raised 6 to 9 inches and the patient is not allowed more than two pillows. Sitting up a little more for meals is permissible but the major part of the time is spent with the legs at or above heart level, so ensuring a low venous pressure for the greater part of the day. The legs and feet are moved about as much as possible, even when lying in bed.

Bandaging. The original firm crêpe bandage put on at the operation should remain untouched for seven days, unless it slips, when it is carefully re-applied.

Getting up. The patient gets up for short periods of active walking, starting 24 hours (or in the case of extensive perforating vein surgery 48 hours) after the operation. Before putting his legs to the ground the ankle and calf and knee are wrapped in an *extra* firm webbing elastic bandage put on fairly tight over the original crêpe bandage to counteract the high venous pressure. When this is on, the patient is told to walk actively, without standing still, for five minutes. During succeeding days the patient is allowed up two, three and then four times a day, for increasing periods of active walking in pressure bandages. After walking he gets into bed with the feet up.

After seven days the wounds and stripper track are healed enough to withstand a certain amount of high venous pressure.

On the seventh day, therefore, the stitches are removed and the patient leaves hospital. A firm webbing elastic bandage from ankle to knee is worn throughout the day for a whole fortnight. He is told to be as active as possible and do numerous short walks and move his legs about, especially if a prolonged period of standing has to be endured.

The bandaging routine and the insistence on movement adds greatly to the patient's comfort and freedom from pain during the post-operative period.

In most average cases the leg should be completely out of bandages three weeks after leaving hospital. In cases of extensive ankle perforator exploration, a further two weeks' support may be necessary as the post-operative ankle swelling is more and takes longer to settle. The elderly need longer support.

Stitches. Closure of all these small wounds

on the groin, leg and ankle, should be done with special care. Rough, coarse suturing may precipitate wound breakdowns and infection. These incisions should all be regarded as cosmetic problems, and the finest suture materials used, and meticulous skin apposition aimed at. Any fine non-reactive material such as fine silk, or braided nylon can be used. Some surgeons prefer subcuticular monofilament nylon, although in the authors' experience, this gives coarser scars than conventional apposition with very fine silk.

Stitches in general need to be left in about seven days, although the stitches in the small transverse groin wound (where there is no tension) may be removed earlier, about the fourth day.

The venous 'trophy'. When the telescoped vein on the Myers' stripper is extended a varying length is revealed which has the stumps of several avulsed tributaries 2 to 4 cm long attached to it (the entire saphenous trunk may measure 24 to 28 inches (60 to 70 cm). On examining the vein it may be found to be complete. Sometimes a portion of its wall, especially about the knee level, for several centimetres is torn away, presumably where a tributary has proved to be stronger than the parent stem. The vein may be in two pieces where a subordinate vessel has retained an entire piece of the saphenous trunk. Many varicose veins have been injected with sclerosing agents so that they are perhaps anchored by scar tissue. Occasionally the vein is found to be turned inside out, the stripping shoulder having been pulled inside a very dilated trunk; gentle traction on the inverted vessel usually extracts it entire.

The interior and valves of stripped veins. The removed vein is opened and its lumen and valves are inspected. The lumen may be clear and patent but it is easy to recognise a vessel which has recanalised after thrombophlebitis for in it are numerous interlacing white fibres passing in all directions from the wall, especially about the valves (honeycombing describes it well); it demonstrates how a deep vein reopened after thrombosis must always be incompetent. There may be one or more complete longitudinal septa for several centimetres across part of the vessel making two or occasionally three passages (Fig. 8.26). A thrombus completely or partially occluding the lumen may be present; it is usually firmly adherent to the vein (Fig. 8.26). Only a few have been seen and they were distal to a valve. The valves after thrombophlebitis are disorganised with irregular clumps of slightly pink fibrous tissue and the cusps have disappeared.

Varices. Eccentric dilatations are frequent on the saphenous trunk situated at a valve. They stimulate thought as to their formation. They are sometimes immediately distal to the valves, occasionally they are proximal, and in several specimens there has been an eccentric dilation above and below a valve cusp.

A varix forming above a valve is understandable as arising from excessive thoracoabdominal pressures exercised on the vein wall just above the closed valve and the vein wall yielding.

A varix below the valve is more difficult to explain (Fig. 8.27). The yielding may occur at the valve ring itself between the attachment of the cusps, and the site of the varix, above or below, is then fortuitous.

The valves. The valves found in the removed saphenous trunks are mostly bicuspid and of three types:

1. *Major valves.* There are one or occasionally two strongly developed valves in the terminal 1 to 2 inches of the internal and external saphenous trunks (2·5 to 5 cm). Occasionally another such valve occurs below the entry of the large tributaries at the knee. There is a well-marked dilatation of the vein above them.

2. *Ordinary valves.* There are a varying number of more delicate but apparently complete valves ranging from 1 to 8 from the groin to the ankle. Their cusps are delicate, there is no apparent valve ring as in the major valves, nor is the vein dilated above them.

3. *Ghost valves.* These are barely visible. There may be a suggestion of cusps but as a rule there is but a faint V mark on the endothelium, suggesting either an imperfectly formed valve or one which has disappeared leaving only the line of attachment of the cusps to the wall.

The valves are demonstrated by trickling a fine stream of water on the opened vessel opposite to the direction of blood flow. This floats the cusps outwards and causes the water to eddy or bounce back as it impinges on them.

On a few occasions, a tricuspid instead of a bicuspid valve has been observed.

The number of valves (types 1 and 2) found in the varicose internal saphenous trunks varies from 2 to 8.

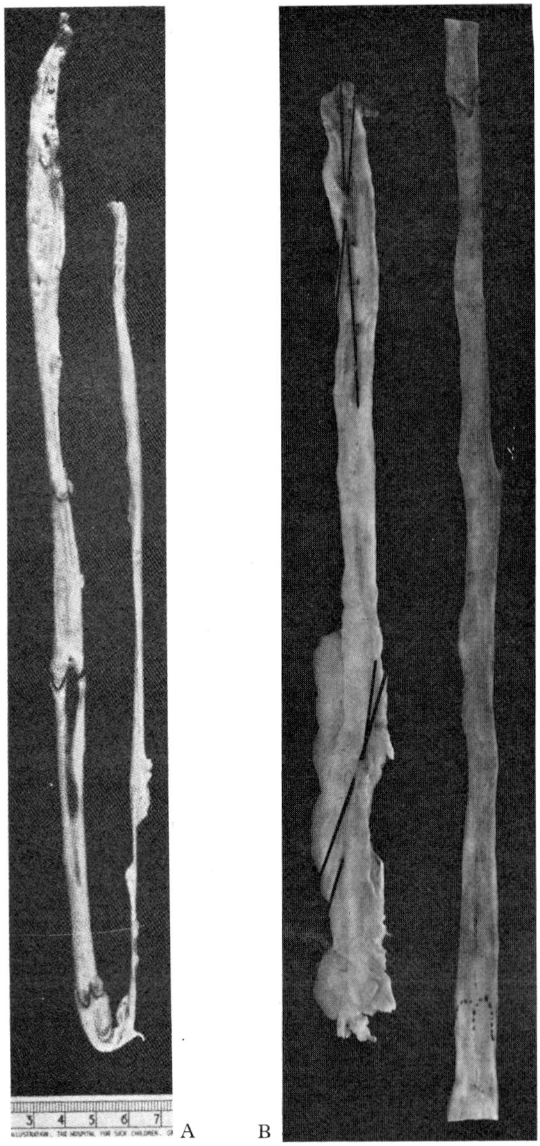

Fig. 8.26 A. A stripped long internal saphenous vein; it has been opened. It shows loss of part of it in the region of the knee and also a firmly adherent thrombus. The edge of the valve cusp has been marked with ink. B. Illustrating two stripped veins (laid open). That on the left is a recanalised thrombosed vein and the other an average varicose vein. Note that the left is lighter in colour (i.e. it is more fibrous), it has several channels as illustrated by the bristles inserted into them. It is thickened and fat is adherent to it from perivenitis. The other vein is a large thin-walled vessel with two valves showing faintly.

In 28 complete specimens of the internal saphenous trunks examined from 17 women and 11 men the average number of valves was 5. The highest number was 13, 1 had 10, 2 had 8, 3 had 7, 4 had 6, 2 had 4, 3 had 3, and the remaining 8 had 2. The average number of valves was 5·5 in the men and 4·5 in the women. The valves are more frequent in the leg portion than the thigh.

The varicose external saphenous trunk has proportionately more valves, although it is but half the length of the internal saphenous trunk. The average of 10 stripped specimens being 4·3, the highest number being 7 and the lowest 2.

Injection of stripped trunks. Some of the stripped saphenous veins have been injected retrogradely after ligating the snapped tributaries. Two findings have been noted. First, that of undoubted varicosity of the entire trunk to the ankle and, second, in some specimens the incompetence has been partial. Thus, in one internal saphenous trunk the fluid would not pass beyond the union of the anterior and posterior leg tributaries; below the knee it was sound. In one external saphenous vein it was found to be sound below the centre of the calf. This partial incompetence of the trunk of a varicose system will explain some variation in the physical signs and symptoms.

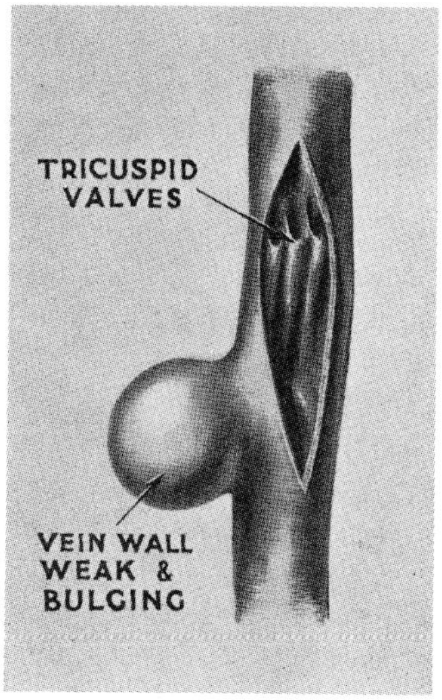

Fig. 8.27 An artist's drawing from a specimen showing a tricuspid valve and a varix distal to it; both are somewhat unusual.

DIFFICULTIES AND DANGERS OF THE OPERATIONS

Dangers

Most of the operative troubles arise from two causes: (a) failure to obtain an adequate exposure; (b) failure to appreciate the variations of venous and arterial anatomy to be found during both saphenofemoral and saphenopopliteal ligation.

The 'saphena' varix. A saphena varix, varying in size from a marble to a walnut, is fairly frequent on the terminal 2 or 4 inches of the internal saphenous vein and also, but less often, of the short saphenous vein. It is usually a saccular dilatation, but can be fusiform; it seldom affects the last centimetre of the vein. Even more frequently it is found on the terminal centimetre of the antero-external vein of the thigh. We have never seen one *precisely* at the saphenofemoral point, which is fortunate for surgeons.

Bleeding from a torn varix. Varices are disconcertingly friable and the copious bleeding that occurs when they are torn compels gentleness and alertness. In spite of care, a varix or large vessel may be torn by a slight touch and the bleeding may be profuse. The remedy is to press a pad firmly into the wound for two minutes (by the clock) and to tilt the operating table a little more, with the legs higher. The venous pressure and haemorrhage are thereby much reduced. The swab in the wound is rolled aside slowly, and the bleeding point or points, as they are revealed, are either under-run by a fine stitch or grasped with the special venous forceps (see Chap. 9) and tied. If the varix is grasped by even lightweight haemostats, they often tear away, and the dilation is injured further. Trying to clip the bleeding point in a pool of blood is dangerous; it may lacerate the femoral vein, and less often the artery is inadvertently damaged.

Another help is that of an efficient sucker which will remove the blood as rapidly as it issues and thereby reveal the exact site of the tear, allowing it to be dealt with.

Patience, gentleness and a wide dissection ensure freedom from accidents in this operation.

Division of the common femoral vein. This vein has been mistaken for the internal saphenous vein, and ligated, especially in thin subjects. On three occasions one of us was on the point of ligating it before realising the error, whilst on a fourth it was tied and injected retrogradely with sclerosing fluid. Because the vein continued to be distended and did not collapse, as does the varicose internal saphenous vein after ligation, the mistake was retrieved. The situation was treated by temporarily occluding the femoral vein superiorly, opening it distally between stay sutures, and allowing it to bleed for 5 to 10 seconds, thereby discharging the sclerosant; no clots were seen to emerge. The volume and power of its circulation was impressive. The vessel was sutured and no complication, either immediate or remote, followed.

Injury to the common femoral vein. This usually occurs from flurried attempts to stem bleeding from a torn saphena varix. The torrential bleeding which occurs from a side hole in the femoral vein can be stopped immediately by the tip of the gloved finger placed directly on the spot. While the assistant's finger is continuously so held, the table is tilted so that the legs are elevated, and the wound is enlarged. The femoral vein above and below the foramen ovale is steadily exposed. The fingertip pressure is transferred to directly above and below the site of the tear, which will then usually reduce the leak to a trickle, which it is easy to see and deal with by a lateral suture of fine thread or silk on a vascular suture round bodied needle. This procedure takes time and gentleness. Remember to use the sucker.

INJURY TO THE FEMORAL ARTERY

Injury. Accidental injury of the femoral artery is handled by the same technique as the injured femoral vein. Indeed in the older patient the restoration of the arterial flow is essential if gangrene is to be avoided. In younger patients, the vitality of the limb may remain after ligation of the femoral artery but its repair is better.

Ligation. Another accident (personal communications from various surgeons) is that of accidental ligation of the femoral artery, which has necessitated amputation of the leg in some patients. At first sight it is hard to visualise the perpetration of this mistake but, as already mentioned, in 1951, in a very thin man one of us almost committed this error.

A large, accurate incision, a good light and deliberate operating will avoid this catastrophe. It is noteworthy that the femoral and popliteal vein and artery are surprisingly superficial in thin persons.

High bifurcation of the femoral artery. As mentioned in Chapter 3, the femoral artery occasionally divides into its superficial and profunda branches immediately below Poupart's ligament. The profunda artery passes downwards and inwards over the femoral vein, and above or under the saphenofemoral junction, the internal saphenous vein being separated from it only by the anterior layer of the femoral sheath. It is an impressive presentation and the profunda artery could readily be injured if the saphenofemoral junction were approached roughly and through a small incision (see Chap. 3); Figure 8.28 shows a recent finding of this condition.

Difficulties of stripping

The bulk of the stripped vein. Occasionally *the bulk of* the telescoped vein as it is pulled down towards the ankle is so large that considerable difficulty may be experienced in drawing it past the knee, or over the lower third of the tibia. If there is difficulty on this

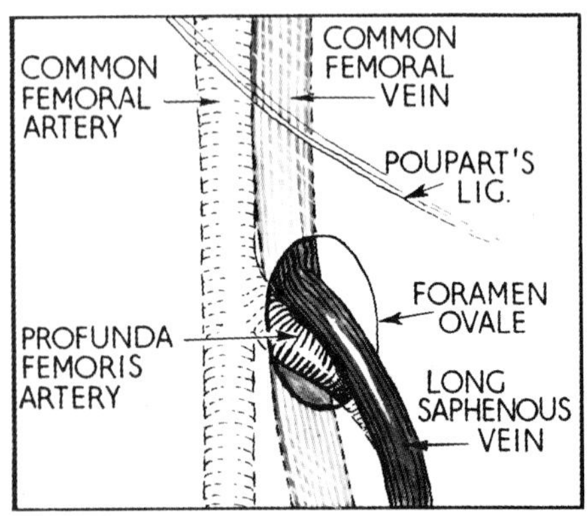

Fig. 8.28 High bifurcation of the femoral artery, with the profunda passing immediately under the saphenous junction. 'Beware of this anatomical variation.'

account, it is advisable to cut down on the mass at the hold-up and take it out with the stripper. If necessary the next stretch of vein can be removed separately.

It is inadvisable to pull large bulky masses of telescoped vein down through a small ankle incision, as this may cause an unnecessary amount of trauma to the saphenous nerve and ankle skin.

Inversion of the vein. With a stripper with a small shoulder, or a very large varicose trunk, the shoulder of the stripper may pass into the vessel's lumen and turn it inside out, but even so, with careful, gentle traction on it, the trunk will strip out completely. Usually this accident is not recognised until the venous trophy is drawn from the wound.

Pulling the stripper through the vein. When a varicose vein is very large, and the ligature round the vein and stripper has been omitted, the stripper may be pulled through the vessel splitting it, without removing it. The modified Myer's stripper with a larger shoulder and a concave face has prevented this.

Passage of the stripper into the femoral or popliteal veins. One must be always aware of this possibility. Interesting and significant variations were when the stripper ran by way of a large direct communicating vein into the popliteal (once) and femoral vein (twice). In one case the stripper passed from the ankle to its full length but it did not appear in the saphenous vein at the groin. It was ultimately felt in the femoral vein, having passed inwards by a large direct perforating vein at the middle of the thigh. Communicating veins are usually linked to tributaries of the internal saphenous veins rather than directly to its main trunk as in this patient, although the perforating vein passing into Hunter's canal is one of the few that can pass directly.

In the second person the stripper entered a large direct perforating vein in the lower third of the leg. In the third case the stripper passed into the popliteal vein by a direct communicating vein from the middle of the calf.

Copious haemorrhage. Occasionally alarming haemorrhage may occur into the stripper track.

The usual causes of this are:

1. The foot of the table has not been tilted up enough. This position with the legs above the level of the heart is *essential* in all operations on the peripheral veins (and arteries).

2. The external temperature is too high causing vasodilatation. In a hot theatre under powerful lights the leg may be warmed up appreciably causing full vasodilatation particularly in the foot.

3. The use of a vasodilator anaesthetic agent such as halothane. This should be avoided.

4. The avulsion by the stripper of an incompetent perforating vein. This may cause copious bleeding from the deep veins into the stripper track. Normally, such incompetent perforators should be diagnosed, exposed and tied *before* stripping the saphenous vein. However if copious bleeding into the stripper track from the perforating vein area does seem to be occurring, then a full ankle perforator incision should be made (see Chap. 18) and the perforators sought and tied.

Bad haemorrhage can always be controlled at once by raising the foot high, and pressing with a folded towel along the course of the track for three minutes. Copious haemorrhage occurs particularly with big veins in old people. In young people the retraction and contraction of the branches which have been avulsed is much more active and immediate in stopping haemorrhage.

A thrombosed saphenous trunk. Occasionally an unsuspected thrombosed saphenous vein may be found at operation. If the stripper can be made to pass retrogradely down the vein, such veins can be stripped out in safety (see Chap. 6). However, the bulk of these stripped veins is usually considerable and it may be necessary to use two or three incisions down the leg, the final one being in the perforating vein area of the ankle, finishing by tying the ankle perforators. Occasionally also one finds an unsuspected recanalised old thrombosis. The same remarks about stripping apply to this.

Large tributaries of the internal saphenous vein. Occasionally the stripper as it passes down the trunk will wander into a large tributary. It may be into the posterointernal tributary, and the instrument appears in the popliteal space. If this is detected, attempts are made to rectify it by withdrawing and re-directing the stripper. The apparent duplication of the internal saphenous vein below the knee has been mentioned and the instrument may pass down by the posterior arch vein or across the front of the leg towards the external malleolus by way of the anterior vein of the leg; all these large varicose veins may be stripped with advantage, but the removal of the greater part of the saphenous trunk is also advisable.

The use of sclerosants at varicose vein operations. Sclerosants should never be used in a patient who cannot be immediately active and moving. This is a rule which automatically prohibits the use of sclerosants on unconscious patients during vein operations.

The danger of causing widespread skin necrosis and deep vein thrombosis is considerable, and it should never be done.

Boyd and Robertson (1949) and Kinmonth (1947) showed that if in the supine patient enough radio-opaque sclerosant fluid is injected retrogradely into the internal saphenous vein, some of it passes quickly into the femoral and popliteal veins and tends to be held up at their valve cusps. Obviously this would cause a real risk of damage to deep veins and deep vein thrombosis.

Operations for bilateral varicosities. Provided the patient is fit and the veins not too extensive or large, both legs may be operated on at the same session. However, it is important that each leg should be done as a separate operation. If two operators attempt to 'do a leg each' at the same time, the result is usually a certain amount of confusion and breaches of sterile technique.

It is significant that nearly all the cases of 'swabs left behind' in the wound have been when two operators have been working synchronously. In one such case the *stripper itself* was left in the leg and was not removed until many months afterwards, after insistent complaints from the patient! (Records of Medical Defence Union, 1966.)

There is no reason why the short and the long saphenous vein and/or the perforators should not be done at the same operation. This will involve turning the patient over under the anaesthetic. Great care must be exercised in turning these patients as many are old and osteoarthritic. Post-operative 'lumbago' or 'stiff neck' may be caused by rough and inept turning of the unconscious patient.

If the veins on both legs are unusually large and widespread it is best to do one per session, with at least a week between each operation.

Long, trying, bilateral varicose vein operations lasting one and a half to two hours or more should be avoided as they fatigue the surgical team, and their concentration and performance may deteriorate.

POST-OPERATIVE COMPLICATIONS

At the outset it should be said that a well conducted operation for varices, correctly diagnosed with proper pre- and post-operative care, is one of the most successful and trouble free operations of surgery.

The complications listed below are, and should be rare.

Haematoma and bruising

Some discoloration and bruising along the stripper track is normal of course, and at about one week after stripping, the patient's leg looks 'black and blue'. It is important to warn the patient about this, to avoid alarm. Normally the bruising is absorbed within three to four weeks.

Occasionally there is some reactionary haemorrhage in the groin wound which raises a small haematoma. This is usually best left to absorb, unless it is large (size of a lemon or more) when it should be evacuated under anaesthesia and full sterile conditions.

Lymphatoma

Occasionally a small collection of lymph occurs in the groin wound causing a painless egg-sized swelling. This tends to occur rather later than a haematoma, about the fifth to sixth post-operative day and is due to severance of some of the groin lymphatics. If left it usually absorbs completely after a week or two or sometimes longer. It is best not to interfere with it or drain it, as this may cause a troublesome *lymphatic fistula* which may go on for weeks before it closes.

These lymphatomas tend to occur specially when an extensive dissection of the groin has been necessary, such as in re-explorations of the groin for recurrent varicose veins.

Wound sepsis

This occasionally occurs, but should be rare if these operations are accorded the meticulous aseptic technique that is given to any major operation of surgery.

In this connection it should be specially mentioned that careful towelling off of the groin and anal regions is necessary. With the table tipped feet up, instruments and strippers tend to slip off the tilted surface of the table towards the anal region.

Inadequate towelling of the groin and incomplete shaving are two frequent errors.

If the patient has an ulcer or eczema, it is highly likely that the skin will harbour some staphylococci. Open ulcers should always be in a 'healing phase' before any operation on the leg is contemplated. Moreover, if operation is undertaken near an ulcer or any eczematous skin (which is often necessary) it is wise to have the patient on a *systematic course* of wide spectrum antibiotic which is effective against staphylococci before, during and after operation. *Pre-operative culture* of eczemas and open ulcers is necessary and the appropriate antibiotic can be chosen according to the result of the bacterial culture. We have found Erythromycin or the combination of Ampicillin and Cloxacillin to be the most effective drugs. Erythromycin particularly has the great advantage that sensitivity reactions are rare.

Post-operative saphenous neuritis

Turning to Figure 8.20 it will be seen that in the distal third of the leg, the saphenous nerve has a very close relation to the saphenous vein.

If the distal third of the saphenous vein is stripped by a relatively bulky stripper head (whether the stripper is passed up or down) some temporary nerve damage often ensues.

This amounts to an area of anaesthesia often no bigger than a 50p piece, but sometimes a little bigger. The patient does not notice this immediately after the operation, but two to three weeks later when nerve recovery is taking place, a troublesome feeling of 'pins and needles' appears in the area, and hypertensitivity to touch. This phase usually lasts two to three weeks and then dies away as normal sensation returns.

However, in some cases there may be actual nerve rupture or division. This tends to occur when a large stripper head is dragged upward towards the groin, its shoulder impacting in the bifurcation of the saphenous nerve, 3 to 4 inches above the ankle. A permanent fairly wide area of anaesthesia may result and around its edge an uncomfortable zone of hypersensitivity may persist which the patient may complain of bitterly. This is usually loosely called 'saphenous neuritis'. It is fortunately becoming less common as surgeons become aware of the danger of rough upward stripping in this area (Cox et al., 1974).

Lymphoedema of leg

Considering that nearly all the lymphatic trunks from the lower leg are grouped around the long saphenous vein, it is surprising that this complication is so rare after stripping.

A chronic minor lymphoedema of the leg and ankle is seen quite frequently after the ex tensive dissection of the long saphenous vein when it is removed to use as an arterial replacement (vein bypass). However, this complication has been seen only twice as a compli cation of stripping as such by one of the authors. In each case there was unusually severe haemorrhage and fibrosis of the stripper track.

Induration of the stripper track

After the third week when the haematoma in the stripper track has absorbed, it is infiltrated by fibrous tissue and the stripper track becomes an uncomfortable indurated cord down the inside of the leg. The patient often complains that there is a 'stiff' feeling down the inside of the thigh which may persist for a month or so, before the fibrous reaction dies down and is completely absorbed.

Occasionally, when there has been a larger haematoma than usual in the stripper track, this induration may be excessive and last for several months. However, in our experience, even in these more severe cases it does absorb and disappear in time—occasionally leaving a little skin puckering.

Deep thrombosis and embolism

Deep thrombosis and embolism should be no more frequent after these operations than it is in the generality of cold surgical cases. Indeed if all the post-operative precautions (bandaging, movement, activity) are adhered to it should be less frequent.

Certainly clinically evident thrombo-embolism should not be seen in more than *0·1 to 0·2 per cent* of the cases.

We are indebted to Professor J. B. Kinmonth for the figures in Table 8.1 showing the incidence of non-fatal pulmonary embolism in several large series.

Table 8.1

	Cases	Embolism
St Thomas's Hospital, London (1949–1954)	204	1 (0·5%)
St Bartholomew's Hospital, London (1950–1954)	157	1 (0·6%)
University College Hospital, London (1954, Bolton Carter)	237	1 (0·4%)
Mayo Clinic, Rochester, U.S.A. (1947–1951, Myers)	711	3 (0·4%)

RESULTS OF SURGERY

'The good results of surgery are the results of good surgery.'

This aphorism applies nowhere more strongly than in the results of varicose vein operations. The long-term follow up of patients who have had radical surgery, of the type described in this chapter, for primary hereditary varicose veins has been excellent.

Most of the poor results and recurrences are due to: inaccurate diagnosis and inaccurate surgery.

The main causes of recurrence of varicose veins after operation are dealt with in the next chapter.

Any assessment of the results of varicose vein surgery must take in a follow up period of at least five years. Series have been reported by Bolton Carter (1954) and by Myers (1954 and 1955) reporting good results.

It is peculiarly difficult to get a good base-line for assessing the results of varicose vein surgery in a proper scientific manner, as in unending ways the results defy scientific assessment.. Many patients who have had what the surgeon deems an excellent result are dissatisfied because small veins are still showing here and there. Other patients are extremely grateful for and satisfied with the results of surgery, even though many residual veins still show. Other patients have been prevented from having an ulcer. Yet others are mainly grateful for relief from aching and pain.

As far as the authors' are aware, no good long-term follow up studies have been published taking adequate account of all these different factors. However, what we can say is that technically accurate and painstaking surgery, on a basis of accurate diagnosis, for primary hereditary varicose veins produces good long-term results. About 1 in every 10 patients return after five years or more with some minor residual veins or occasionally a true recurrence due to valve breakdown in a perforating vein. These may need minor local re-operation.

More recently a painstaking long-term follow-up (10 years) of primary vein surgery has been reported from the Mayo Clinic (Larson et al., 1974). Taking account of all the difficulties mentioned above, they found that 85 per cent of the patients maintained a 'good' to 'excellent' result over ten years' follow up. Even in the fifteen per cent not classified as good, they were mostly small and un-important recurrences. This paper gives an excellent unbiased account of what may be expected in the way of good long-term results, from accurate and meticulous vein surgery.

REFERENCES

Bolton Carter, J. F. (1954) *Lancet*, **1**, 743.
Boyd, A. M. (1947–1953) with Robertson, D. J. (1947) *Brit. Med. J.*, **2**, 452.
Boyd, A. M. with Robertson, D. J. (1948) *Proc. R. Soc. Med.*, **41**, 631, 633.
Boyd, A. M. with Catchpole, A. N., Jepson, R. P. & Rose, S. S. (1953) *Ann. Surg.*, **138**, 726.
Brodie, B. (1846) *Lectures Illustrative of Various Subjects in Pathology and Surgery*. London: Longmans.
Babcock, W. W. (1907) *N.W. Med. Jnl.*, **86**, 153.
Chaissaignac, E. (1855) *Nouvelle Méthode Pour le Traitement des Tumeurs Haemorrhoidalis*. Paris: Baillière.
Cockett, F. B. & Jones, D. E. E. (1953) *Lancet*, **1**, 17.
Cockett, F. B. & Lea Thomas, M. (1965) *Br. J. Surg.*, **52**, 816.
Colt, G. B. (1921) *Br. J. Surg.*, **8**, 486.
Cox, J. J. et al. (1974) *Br. Med. J.*, **1**, 415.
De Takats, G. (1930) *Surg. Gynae. & Obstr.*, **1**, 545.
Fegan, W. G. (1967) *Varicose Veins, Compression Sclerotherapy*. London: Heinemann.
Fegan, W. G. & Pegum, J. M. (1974) *Br. J. Surg.*, **61**, 124.
Génévrier, M. (1921) *Soc. Med. mil. franc.*, **15**, 169.
Halstead, W. S. (1893) *Bull. Johns Hopk. Hosp.*, **4**, 17.
Hanschell, H. M. (1928) *Br. Med. J.*, **1**, 542.
Harvey, R. S. (1936) In Maingot's *Post-graduate Surgery*, Vol. 2, p. 3281. London: Butterworth.
Jones, Robert (1896) *L'pool Med. Chir. Jnl.*, **278.**
Kausch, W. (1917) *Dtsch. med. Wschr.*, **43**, 712.
Larson, R. H. et al. (1974) *Mayo Clin. Proc.*, **49**, 2, 114.
Lensen, P. (1916) *Med. Klin.*, **12**, 897.
Lensen, P. (1925) *Derm. Wschr.*, **81**, 1345.
Linton, R. R. (1949) *Minn. Med.*, **32**, 38.
MacPheeters, H. O. (1927) *Surg. Gynae. & Obstr.*, **45**, 541.
Maingot, R. & Carlton, C. H. (1928) *Lancet*, **1**, 806.
Maingot, R. & Carlton, C. H. (1954) Personal communication.
May, R. & Thurner, T. (1957) *Angiology*, **8**, 419.
Mayo, C. H. (1906) *Surg. Gynae. & Obstr.*, **2**, 385.
Milligan, E. T. C. (1954) Personal communication.
Myers, T. T. & Cooley, J. C. (1954) *Surg. Gynae. & Obstr.*, **99**, 733.
Myers, T. T. & Janes, J. M. (1955) *Surgery*, **37**, 2, 184.
Nobl, G. (1926) *Wien Klin. Wschr.*, **39**, 1217.
Pravaz, J. quoted from Pravaz, J. C. T. (1857) *Sur le Traitment des Aneurismes par les Injections de Perchlorure de Fer Méthode Pravaz*. Paris thesis.
Schiassi, B. (1908) *Sem. med.*, **28**, 601.
Slevin, J. G. (1948) *Amer. J. Surg.*, **75**, 469.
Sicard, J. A. & Gaugier, L. (1926) *Pr. med.*, **34**, 689.
Tavel, E. (1904) *CorrespBl. schweiz. Arz.*, **34**, 617.
Thelwall Thomas, W. (1896) *L'pool Med. Chir. Jnl.*, **278.**
Turner Warwick, W. (1931) *The Rational Treatment of Varicose Veins and Varicocele*, pp. 117–120. London: Faber & Faber.

9. Recurrent Varicose Veins

Nothing gives the operation for varicose veins such a bad name as a gross recurrence after surgery, possibly producing a leg which appears to be worse than it was before.

Such tragedies are unfortunately still seen and the plain fact is that the great majority are due to inept and inaccurate surgery, often coupled with a wrong diagnosis.

It is still fairly common for a patient to present with gross varicose veins after a high ligation of the saphenous vein. The patient has a scar, roughly in the right place in the groin, yet under the incision the saphenous vein can be felt and tapped out (Schwartz test) and is still present. It had obviously never been found at operation! One can only presume that in such cases an inexperienced surgeon had been 'having a go' without adequate teaching or supervision!

This is only one fairly common example of what may be found in a case of so called recurrent varicose veins!

Classification. It is important to differentiate between three groups of veins which persist after operation.

1. Residual veins.
2. True recurrent veins.
3. Persistent venous dilatation due to deep vein obstruction.

RESIDUAL VEINS

When an incompetent saphenous vein is ligatured accurately flush against the femoral vein in the groin, and the trunk is stripped completely to the ankle, there may still be left one or two dilated tortuous tributaries. The commonest are: (a) the anterolateral vein ascending across the thigh; (b) the posterior arch vein, giving a cluster on the posteromedial aspect of the calf and thigh and (c) the anterior branch just below the knee—coursing diagonally up from the outer ankle. There may be other variants on this pattern.

Unfortunately even if the long saphenous vein is tied and stripped accurately these tributaries, if of any size, do not atrophy or thrombose. They remain patent and when the patient exercises after operation they fill by gravity through the venous network.

They are not distended by the pathological high pressure of an incompetent communicator and therefore they are not pro-

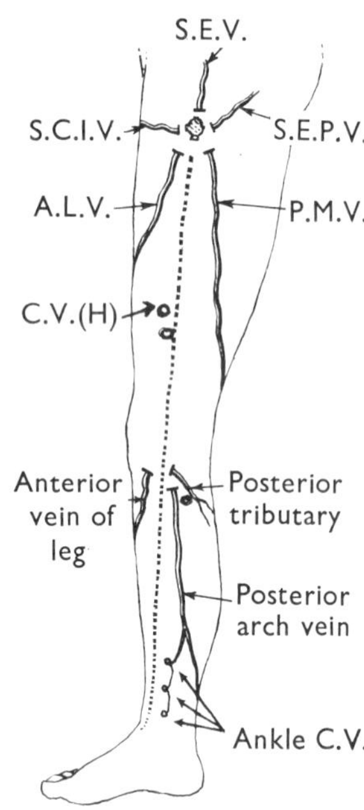

Fig. 9.1 This figure shows the main 'residual' veins left after clean stripping of the main saphenous trunk only.

gressive and only enlarge very slowly. Yet they mar the good result of the operation from a cosmetic and symptomatic point of view, although they are not true recurrent veins.

These prominent varices should be marked carefully before operation and removed through small subsidiary incisions by the technique of 'worming' as described in the previous chapter. If some of these are missed and the patient comes back with one or more of these residual veins there are three courses open:

1. Re-admission for a night or so and complete the operation by avulsing the offending vein through one or more small incisions. In some cases this can be done adequately under local analgesia as an out-patient, without admission. Local excision gives the best results.

2. One can treat the residual veins by the injection compression technique (Chap. 8).

3. One can do nothing. Many patients with small residual veins return full of woe because they think that their 'varicose veins are coming back', all they need is reassurance or in some cases a pair of light support stockings.

TRUE RECURRENT VEINS

True recurrent veins occur when an incompetent communication between the deep and superficial veins has been left undivided or has become so since the operation. This means that the veins remaining are subject to an abnormal venous hypertension or leaking outwards from the deep veins. They progressively enlarge, become more tortuous and prominent, and alarm the patient by growing and spreading perhaps more rapidly than before the operation. This is the main and important difference between residual veins and true recurrent veins.

True recurrent veins are a common problem, and are often a severe diagnostic and operative challenge to the surgeon.

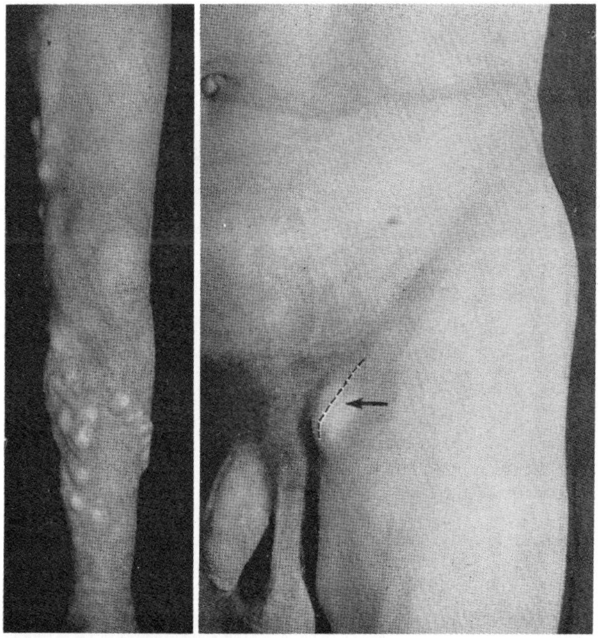

Fig. 9.2 Recurrent internal saphenous veins with a saphena varix due to failure to ligate the internal saphenous vein. The first incision is inked-in; a considerable varix underlies it.

The main causes of true recurrent varicose veins

These may be summed up as: (1) inadequate technical performance of the operation; (2) incomplete or incorrect diagnosis and therefore often failure to operate on the veins at fault.

Inadequate operative technique

FAILURE OF FLUSH HIGH SAPHENOUS LIGATION

Strange as it may seem this simple operation is often badly performed. The two common faults are: (a) failure to find and ligate the main saphenous trunk. A large tributary is treated instead; (b) a non-terminal or non-flush saphenous ligation.

If, at the original operation, the long or short saphenous veins were *not* ligated at their ending close on the femoral or popliteal veins so that one or more of their tributaries remained undivided between this tie and the saphenofemoral or saphenopopliteal junction respectively, then the high intravenous pressure in the femoral or popliteal veins continues to pass into these uninterrupted tributaries. Such vessels progressively dilate and by diverse anastomotic channels ultimately connect up with the trunk of the internal or the short saphenous vein and their radicals distal to the ligature and fill them with blood under high pressure. Some of these vessels would be already varicose or in due course would become so from the sustained hypertension to which they are subject. This re-appearance of varices with symptoms demanding attention usually takes one to three years. The omission to ligate all the saphenous tributaries is almost inevitable when the internal or external saphenous vein is divided at varying distances below the actual junction with the parent vein, and the more distal it is the more tributaries will remain, so bypassing the point of section with restoration of the back-pressure into the saphenous trunk and its area of drainage. *The fault lies in the surgeon's failure to expose clearly the saphenofemoral or saphenopopliteal junction* and to see a portion of the deep vein (i.e. femoral or popliteal) above and below the union before placing the critical ligatures. From personal experience we can vouch that this requires: (a) familiarity with the basic venous anatomy; (b) a correctly placed and large incision; (c) a display and identification of the venous tree before divisions are made.

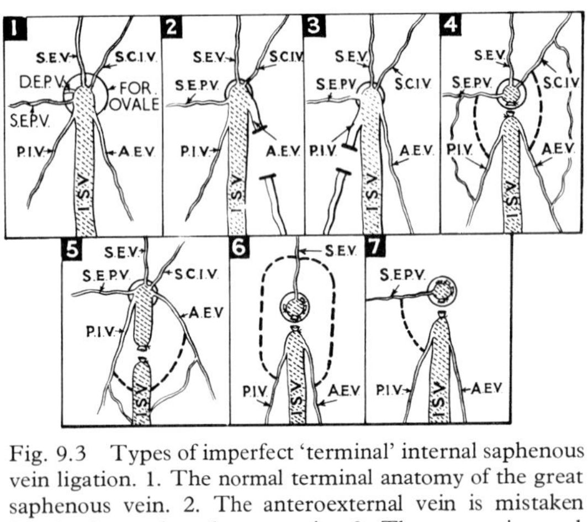

Fig. 9.3 Types of imperfect 'terminal' internal saphenous vein ligation. 1. The normal terminal anatomy of the great saphenous vein. 2. The anteroexternal vein is mistaken for the internal saphenous vein. 3. The posterointernal vein is tied instead of the long saphenous vein. 4. The internal saphenous vein is almost terminally ligated, but not all its tributaries. 5. A 'low' division of the internal saphenous vein; all the tributaries are intact. 6. Another type of so-called 'flush' tie, with the superficial epigastric vein untied. 7. A 'top' tie, except that the superficial (or deep) external pudic vein remains undivided.

UNLIGATED TRIBUTARIES

The omission to divide all the tributaries at the termination of the long saphena or short saphena merits emphasis as contributing to the re-appearance of varices.

The deep external pudic and posterointernal veins

In connection with overlooked tributaries, the surgeon must be aware of the occasional presence inside of the foramen ovale of the deep external pudic veins (40 per cent), and of the posterointernal tributary. They occasionally join, but may be separate. As these veins unite at the inner and slightly inferior aspect of the saphenofemoral union, they are easily missed, and the main ligature will be placed distal to their ending and varices will

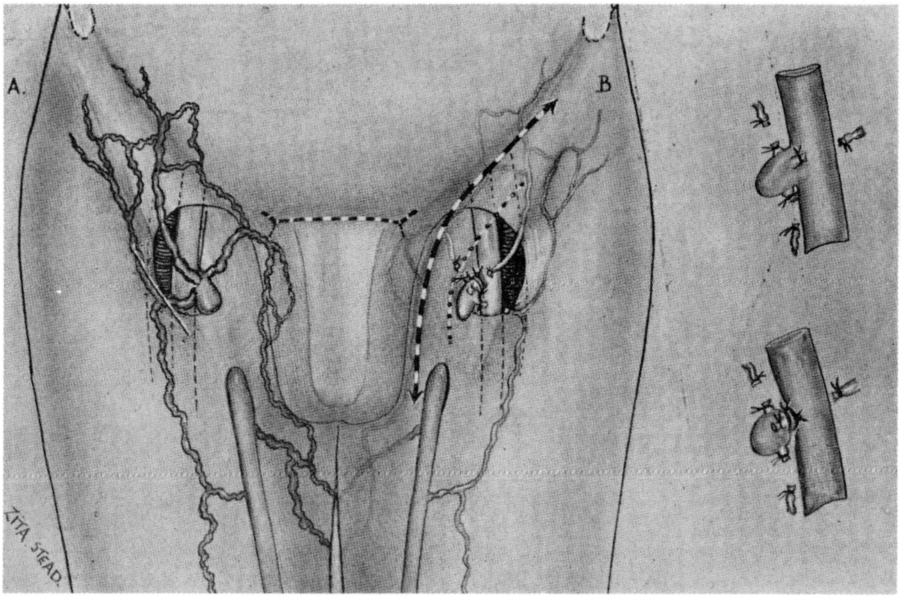

Fig. 9.4 The right side (A) shows the average finding in a case of recurrent veins after a low internal saphenous ligation; note the short incision placed too low. The left side (B) shows (1) the large high incision for recurrent long saphenous varices in contrast to the usual incision for saphenofemoral ligation (dotted-in) and (2) the ligation of tributaries and the double tie at the saphenofemoral level.

persist in the inner and posterior thigh and perhaps in the calf (Fig. 9.5). Less often in 1 to 2 per cent the posterointernal vein joins the femoral vein directly half an inch to one inch below the saphenous confluence, where again it can be overlooked unless the lower edge of the foramen ovale is divided (Fig. 9.6).

Other internal saphenous tributaries. The other four terminal saphenous tributaries must be found and divided to the satisfaction of a critical assistant, just as in biliary tract operations the cystic, common bile and hepatic ducts are displayed before cholecystectomy is performed.

Since the practice of naming each tributary individually has been adopted, it is rare to find one absent, although their combinations are bizarre. At our numerous procedures for recurrent internal saphenous varices, all the radicals have been found undivided at one time or another. The insistence on the ligation of the internal saphenous vein precisely at its union with the femoral vein is because this ensures that all the tributaries are divided and disconnected from the high pressure of the deep veins.

In rare instances, one of the tributaries of the internal saphenous vein from the lower abdominal wall may join the femoral vein direct, above the saphenofemoral union. If the valve immediately above (external iliac) or below Poupart's ligament is sound, this abnormal arrangement would not be surgically significant, but as this valve is absent in over 36 per cent of patients (Eger and Casper) then the high and varying thoracoabdominal pressures can pass into these superficial veins and the varices ultimately re-distend and extend. Thus it is advisable to see the common femoral vein for an inch above and below the saphenofemoral union.

RECURRENCE AFTER STRIPPING

It must be stressed that stripping is just as liable to recurrence as any other method. Stripping only removes the main saphenous trunk and leaves its tributaries available for dilatation by any source of venous hyper-

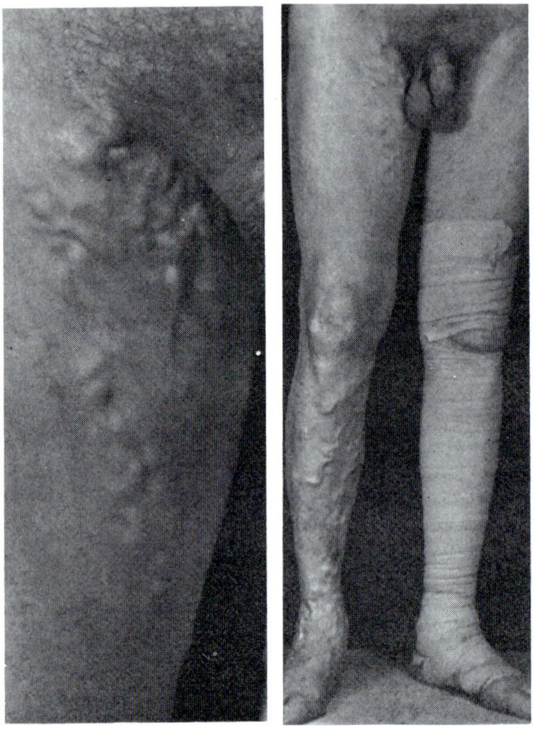

Fig. 9.5 Recurrent right internal saphenous varices, and recurrent left external saphenous varices causing eczema of the popliteal space and ankle (for which the limb is pressure bandaged). Both were due to non-terminal ligations of the internal and external saphenous veins. Sclerosant injections of phenol glycerine had been given, but without effect.

tension remaining connected with them from the groin to the ankle.

One of the worst, most painful and quickest types of recurrence occurs when a surgeon has stripped the main long saphenous trunk, but failed to do a flush saphenofemoral ligation. The venous hypertension then rapidly finds its way into the smaller, thinner-walled tributaries of the long saphenous system, which enlarge and dilate all over the leg. Patients understandably are very distressed at this sort of result!

We have met surgeons who had the impression that when they stripped the long saphenous trunk, they also tore it from the ends of the ankle communicating veins which then sealed off by thrombosis, thereby making

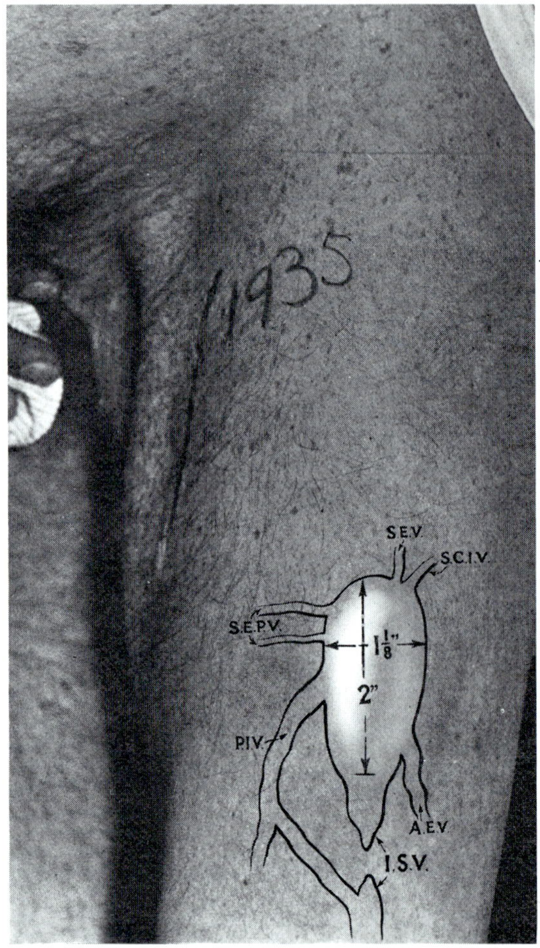

Fig. 9.6 A recurrent internal saphenous varicosity due to an inaccurately placed longitudinal incision (shown by the line). The internal saphenous was tied too low. The curious longitudinal fold to the inner side of the incision is a huge saphena varix 1 inch diameter by 2 inches long; the largest that one of us had seen. The inset shows the findings at the second operation. I.S.V. = internal saphenous vein; P.I.V. = posterointernal vein; S.E.P.V. = superficial external pudic vein (duplicated); S.E.V. = superficial epigastric vein; S.C.I.V. = superficial circumflex iliac vein; A.E.V. = anteroexternal vein.

the need to diagnose and tie them unnecessary. *Nothing could be further from the truth.* It must be emphasised that stripping of the long saphenous vein does not affect the incompetent perforating veins either at the ankle or thigh. These, if incompetent, must be diag-

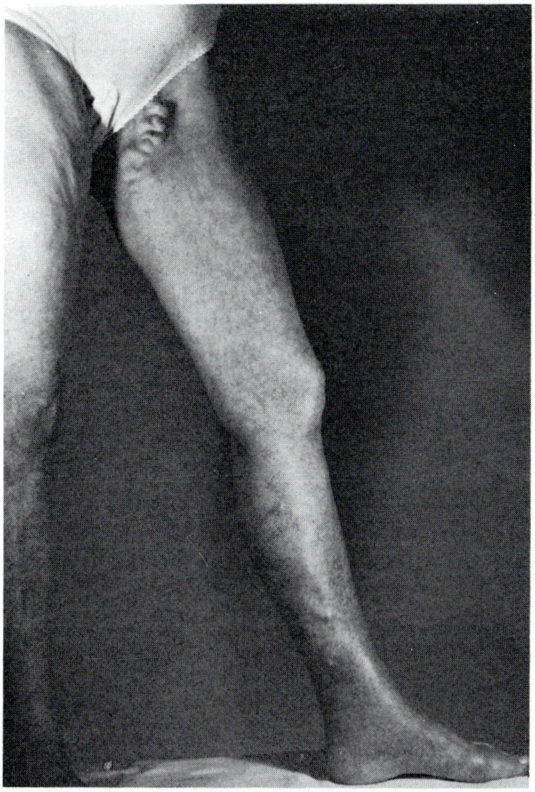

Fig. 9.7 Recurrent varicose veins due to low (non-flush) ligature of the saphenous. The large collateral in the groin appeared just one year after the faulty operation. She was also found to have an incompetent ankle perforator as one might suspect from the appearance of the ankle in the photograph; this was a second cause for her recurrence.

nosed and sought for specifically through another incision and tied as a separate manoeuvre (see Figs 8.22 and 9.1).

The incision at the groin

In many cases, a glance at the incision in the groin makes it clear that a flush ligation could not have been performed. It is either too short, or misplaced—often being inches from the right spot.

The incision must be centred over the saphenofemoral junction, which is 2·5 to 3 cm (1 to 1·5 inches) below and lateral to the pubic tubercle. In fat subjects it is essential to have the pubic tubercle marked by one's own left forefinger which should rest upon it as the incision is made (Fig. 8.8/3), otherwise it may be anything up to 2 or 3 inches too low.

It is difficult for an experienced surgeon to do an adequate exposure of the saphenofemoral junction through an incision an inch or two in length, it must be at least 2 to 3 inches long.

One year one of us operated on 33 patients with recurrent internal saphenous varicosities. Table 9.1 shows the causes.

Table 9.1

1. Internal saphenous vein unligated (Figs 9.2 and 9.6)	7
2. 'Low' ligation of internal saphenous vein, with bypassing through the tributaries and a mass of varices (Figs 9.3, 9.4 to 9.7)	24
3. Undiagnosed communicating vein in the thigh (Fig. 11.14)	1
4. Multiple ligation	1
5. Associated with incompetent ankle communicating veins	10
The symptoms the recurrences caused were:	
Swelling of the ankle	2
Eczema	5
Ulceration	7
Varicose veins	19

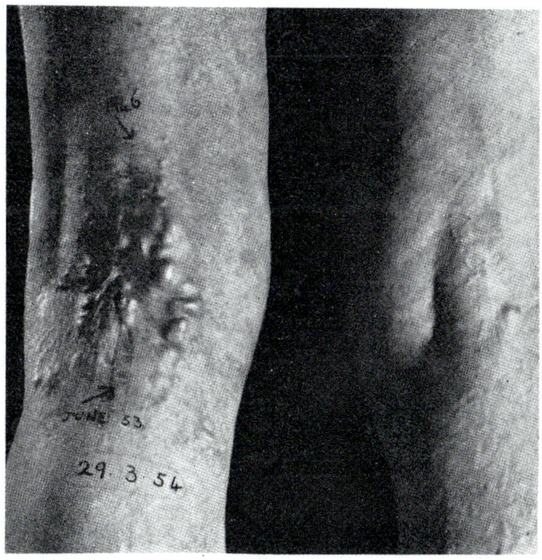

Fig. 9.8 Twice recurrent varicosity of the external saphenous vein (due to non-terminal ligation) before and after operation. She also had recurrent internal saphenous incompetence that has also been re-treated.

The recurrent short saphenous

From a perusal of the previous chapter it will be evident that the operation for flush ligation of the short saphenous vein is more difficult than the high ligation of the long saphenous vein, for it is subject to more anatomical variation.

The main sources of error have been:

1. An inadequate or wrongly placed incision (see Chap. 8).

2. A 'low-level' tie. It is just as necessary here, as in the groin, to achieve a flush ligation on the popliteal vein proximal to any branches. If this is not done, a large spray of recurrent small veins may appear in the popliteal fossa, which has been likened to a 'Medusa's head'. This recurrence may take place within two years and occasions the patient pain and aching (see Fig. 9.8).

Re-operation to find the stump of the short saphenous and to ligature it in the right place is a severe test of surgical skill. It should be done through an extended transverse incision.

3. Failure to find and tie the short saphenous vein. This again is a not uncommon fault. The short saphenous vein in the popliteal fossa lies *deep to the deep fascia*, and we have seen several operations where the deep fascia has never been divided! The higher up the popliteal space the sapheno popliteal union is the more deeply does it lie and it needs painstaking exposure and retraction to display it.

Inadequate diagnosis

This is the second great cause of so called recurrent or persistent varicose veins.

These cases stem from the fact that there is often *more than one* incompetent communication between the superficial and deep veins.

Recalling the Chapter on Diagnosis these are the 'points of high pressure leak' from the deep veins.

1. The long saphenous junction in the groin.

2. The short saphenous junction in the popliteal fossa.

3. The direct ankle perforating veins which may be either (see Fig. 7.12). (a) upper internal; (b) middle internal; (c) lateral; (d) mid-calf; (e) adductor (Hunter's) canal perforator.

'These five main direct perforating veins which are relatively constant in their anatomical situation account for 95 per cent of the perforator leaks. For the rarer and unusual ones see Chapter 11.

There may be any combination of these perforator leaks in a limb—although certain combinations are more common (Chap. 7).

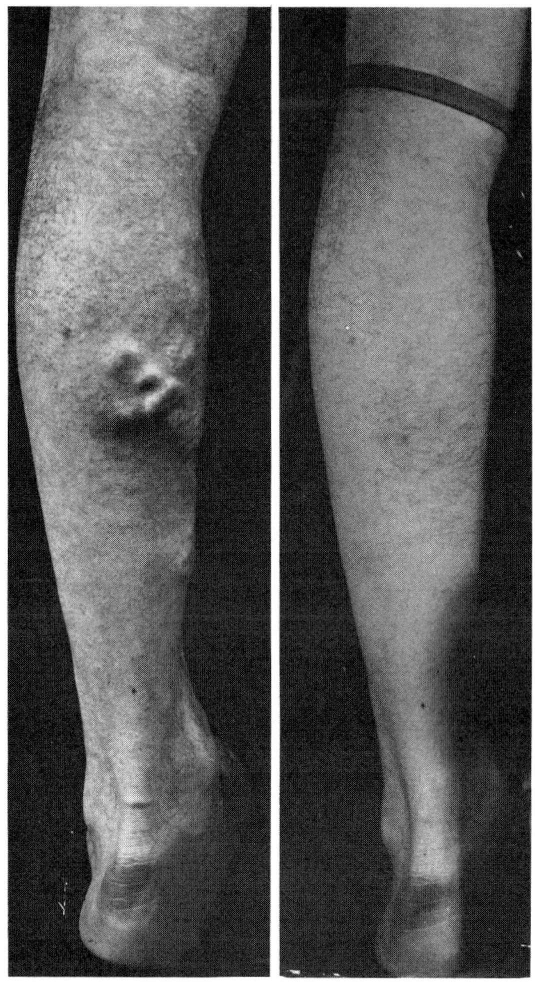

Fig. 9.9 Persistent varices after stripping of the internal saphenous vein, due to overlooked varicosity of the external saphenous vein.

One cause of recurrence is where one system (i.e. long saphenous or short saphenous) has been correctly and adequately operated upon, but the operator has overlooked an incompetent perforator.

Figure 9.9 is a good example of this where severe varicose veins persisted after a good long saphenous ligation and strip but the concomitant short saphenous incompetence had been overlooked.

Figure 9.10 shows another severe recurrence where a long saphenous had been stripped correctly but a large incompetent ankle perforator had been left. The deterioration of the ankle skin and veins continues unchecked until the ankle perforator is exposed and divided flush from the posterior tibial veins.

Thus where there is a recurrence after what appears to have been a proper operation on the long or short saphenous system—all the perforator sites must be looked at carefully and checked, particularly for large veins round the lower leg and ankle.

Another cause of recurrence particularly in women are incompetent pudendal veins (see Chap. 10).

The exact diagnosis of recurrent varicose veins can often be difficult and needs a good deal of clinical experience. It is certainly no job for the beginner! A venogram may be required.

PERSISTENT VENOUS DILATATION DUE TO DEEP VEIN OBSTRUCTION

In operations on the perforating veins and on the saphenous veins in cases of deep vein thrombosis and particularly in cases of iliac compression syndrome (Chap. 16) some recurrence or persistence of dilated veins is expected. In these the object of the operations is to deal with the main *local* causes of venous hypertension (i.e. the incompetent perforating veins) for in many there is still a generalised deep venous hypertension of the limb, which can never be completely cured by surgery (particularly in iliac vein obstruction from iliac thrombosis). Here the object of the surgery is carefully explained to the patient who is given to understand that some progressive venous dilatation even after operation is to be expected. Elastic stockings and regular periods of exercise and of rest with the legs elevated may also be necessary to make life bearable in the severer cases (Chaps 16 and 17).

Occasionally one sees this persistent superficial vein dilatation after either traumatic division of the deep femoral vein (i.e. after wounds, some fractures) and mistakes at operation by ligation of the common femoral vein as a rare accident during a saphenofemoral exposure.

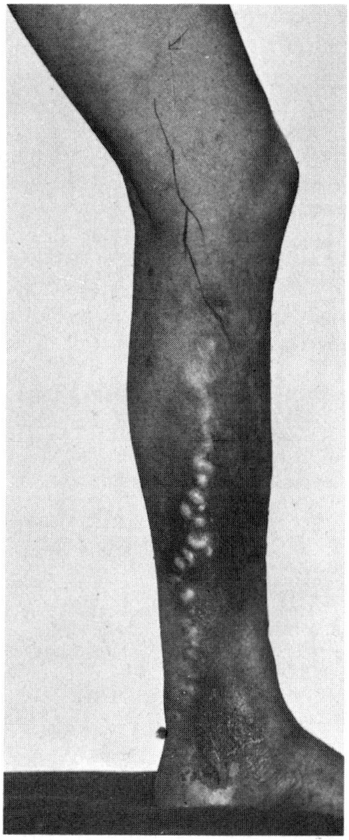

Fig. 9.10 Recurrence of lower leg veins after a high ligation and strip. A large internal ankle perforator has obviously been untouched in this case and is the cause of the persistent veins and skin changes in the lower leg.

In all these cases the dilated veins on the surface need careful assessment—in many instances they may be valuable collaterals in whom operation would be a disservice (Fig. 9.11).

DIAGNOSIS AND TREATMENT

Patients with recurrent or persistent varicose veins need care and skill with diagnosis. The apparent persistence or recurrence may have some previously overlooked deep-seated cause—such as a pelvic tumour or old iliofemoral thrombosis or one or more undiagnosed perforating veins.

Thus a careful history is taken, involving previous operations and especially anything suggestive of deep vein thrombosis. An awareness of pelvic abnormalities is essential.

Case history. A man of 55 came complaining that the veins in his right leg were coming back after an operation two years ago. On examinion his right thigh was somewhat swollen and its veins were slightly distended and there were traces of vein distension suprapubically. On close questioning he admitted to increasing frequency and difficulty with the urinary stream. Rectal examination showed a fairly advanced carcinoma of the prostate—causing a right iliac vein thrombosis!

The patient must stand in a good light and the whole of the lower abdomen and legs must be inspected (Fig. 7.3).

The distribution of the recurrent veins is noted. The typical spray of dilated small tortuous veins arising from the region of the previous groin incision is an unmistakable sign of low and inadequate ligation here (see Figs 9.6 and 9.7). However, the presence of a scar here without obvious varices should not lull one into thinking that the saphenous has been tied. The Schwartz (percussion) test, and the presence of a cough impulse in the veins below it may reveal that the saphenous is still incompetent and has not been touched or bypassed (see Fig. 9.2).

Then the short saphenous vein is inspected and palpated carefully and its competence assessed (Chap. 7).

Finally all the common perforator sites—adductor canal, mid-calf, internal and external ankle perforators (see Fig. 7.13) are individually considered. The pudendal area is inspected (especially in females).

If the recurrence does not fit into one of these patterns, unusual, rarer causes are thought of such as arteriovenous fistula and the lateral perforator anomalies (Chap. 11).

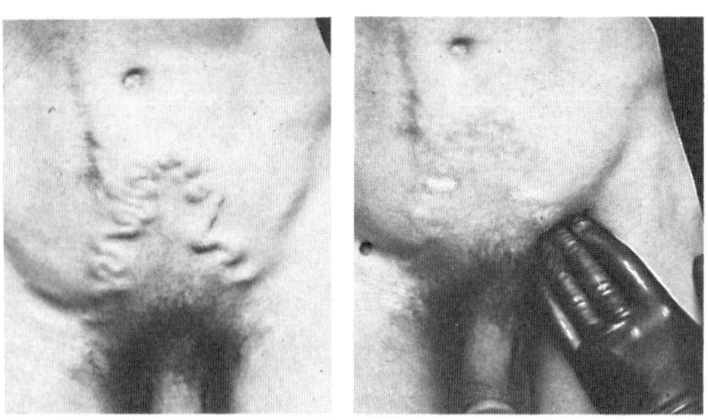

Fig. 9.11 Abdominal varices mainly of the superficial epigastric veins, following acute appendicitis with general peritonitis and deep thrombophlebitis.

Operations for recurrent veins

Re-exploration of the groin in a case of low or inadequate ligation here may be one of the most testing operations of surgery, and requires a good deal of experience and operative skill. It is not for a beginner!

The same may be said of opening of the popliteal fossa for recurrent short saphenous varices.

But apart from these two operations, exploring and tying the various perforating veins, and removing the masses of tortuous superficial veins which often occur are in no way different from operations on these veins described in Chapters 8 and 18. In the filleting out of the numerous long tortuous veins the technique of 'worming' them through a number of small incisions described in Chapter 8 is very useful.

Re-operation at the groin

A few guidelines as regards this operation may be useful.

Where the previous operation scar has obviously been an inch or so too low—a correctly placed incision over the saphenous orifice often reveals an untouched saphenous junction, and there are no serious difficulties in achieving a flush tie. The same applies where there has been a 'complete miss'.

The really difficult operations are those where the original incision has been about right and a mass of tortuous veins are coming from the saphenofemoral area but matted by scar tissue—indicating a 'near miss'.

The best plan is to dissect out and expose the common femoral vein on its medial aspect, keeping away from the matted hard fibrous tissue interlaced with varices on the anterior aspect of the vein. A long incision of the curved or 'hockey-stick' variety just below the inguinal ligament is used, going down on the inner side of the thigh for an inch or two (Chap. 8). It passes through the two layers of superficial fascia to the deep fascia. The position of the pubic tubercle is checked and the pulsation of the femoral artery is felt for. This gives the operator the position of the femoral vein which lies just medial and slightly posterior to the artery. The femoral vein is uncovered by incising its sheath on the *medial* aspect (away from the artery) and the femoral vein is uncovered and traced upwards. As the vessel is dissected upwards the stump of the internal saphenous vein will be seen protruding from its anterior surface adherent to the femoral sheath although sometimes it is normal and untouched in these cases and the femoral vein strips smoothly away from its surroundings. Working very delicately with the blunt tips of a pair of curved Mayo scissors is a good way to do this. Once the saphenofemoral junction is seen by working up towards it, a ligature of thread can be slipped round it with a curved artery forceps or an aneurysm needle.

The other end of the cut saphenous vein (if present) is best located by passing a stripper up from the ankle to the groin where it can be felt and stripped out without too much haemorrhage from the mass of small friable veins. (These have been cut off from their main filling source, by the flush ligature of the stump of the saphenous vein as it joins the common femoral vein.)

Re-operation on the short saphenous

Some authorities (including one of us) advocate a longitudinal incision for this, as it gives a wider exposure. However the poor healing qualities and liability to keloid and contracture makes this unattractive. An adequate wide exploration of the popliteal fossa can often be achieved by a large transverse incision. Apart from the trouble with bleeding from superficial varices, the operation proceeds on the same lines as detailed in Chapter 8. It is essential to see the popliteal vein and the saphenopopliteal union before placing the ligatures.

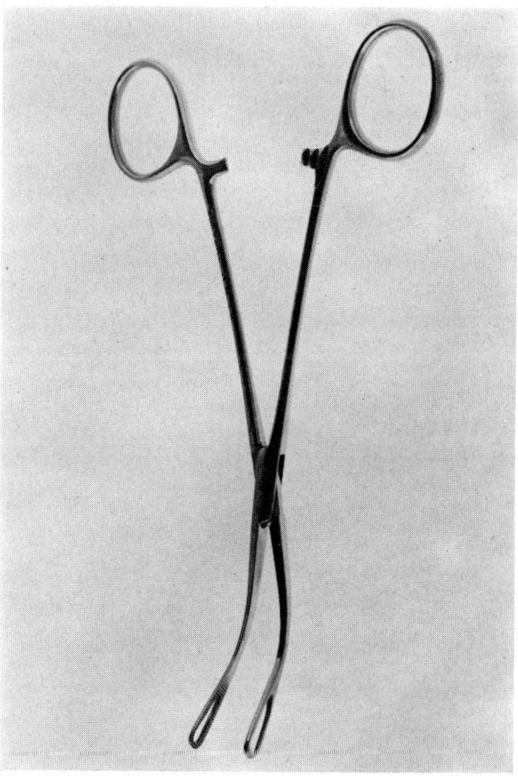

Fig. 9.12 Venous forceps.

CONCLUSION

Recurrent superficial varicose veins can be cured or greatly relieved if time is given to make a diagnosis, to plan and execute a radical treatment. The re-operation may take two hours or more. The bypassing recurrent veins are always thin-walled, tortuous, numerous and fragile. The occasional gross haemorrhage and dissection in scar tissue calls for patience and skill. Only those trained in venous procedures, and surgeons of considerable experience, should undertake them. They should always operate with adequate assistance, a good light, and have a sucker handy! A sucker may be life-saving to locate a copious bleeding point. We have been amazed at the torrential haemorrhage that can emerge from a tiny tear in a thin-walled varix. A double stitch by an ophthalmic or arterial needle is an effective and non-traumatising form of control. Haemostats may 'chaw' the friable venous wall and aggravate the bleeding.

One of us has found the venous forceps (Fig. 9.12) valuable for a laceration in a large varicose vein; its grip is secure and gentle.

REFERENCES

Eger, S. A. & Casper, S. L. (1943) *J. Amer. Med. Assoc.*, **123**, 148.

10. Varicose Veins in Pregnancy

Varicose veins which appear and seem to increase alarmingly during pregnancy are a common problem. All the three types of pregnancy varicose veins (classified below) enlarge more rapidly and give more trouble in the first three or four months. Oddly enough they often give less trouble and may even recede slightly during the later months, after the uterus has risen out of the pelvis.

Three distinct varieties of varicose vein are seen in pregnancy.

1. *The ordinary primary hereditary varicose veins* (long saphenous or short saphenous incompetence with occasionally perforator incompetence).

Patients who already have such valvular incompetence of this type usually find that there is an alarming and rapid increase in size and number of these veins during the early months of pregnancy. In fact this phenomenon is of use sometimes in diagnosing pregnancy in the early months.

2. *Vulval and pudendal veins.* These are a special type of varicose vein *only* associated with pregnancy.

3. *Multiple capillary naevi* (*or spider naevi*). These are capillary dilatations in the skin and are not strictly speaking varicose veins—although they are commonly and universally referred to as such. They are also sometimes called 'telangiectases' or 'venous stars' or 'skin staining'.

THE CAUSES OF PREGNANCY VARICOSE VEINS

The causes of the alarming increase in number and size of varicose veins in the early months of pregnancy may be grouped under two headings: (1) mechanical and (2) hormonal.

Mechanical causes. There are two factors here which together cause a gradual rise in resting venous pressure in the legs in pregnancy. These are first, the enormously increased flow through the pelvic veins, and secondly the increasing bulk of the gravid uterus in the pelvis which gradually exerts an obstructive effect until it rises out of the pelvis just after the third month.

Hormonal causes. Oestrin has a definite relaxant effect on smooth muscle and particularly on that of the vein wall. As the hormonal concentration in the blood rises this relaxant effect on smooth muscle of the vessel walls becomes very marked. It is not confined to the veins—patients with severe Raynaud's disease, due to digital artery spasm, usually find this symptom disappears or gets much better during pregnancy!

The rise in sex hormone concentration in the blood has a much more specific effect on the production of the 'spider naevi' in the skin. The degree of sensitivity of different patients to developing these 'spiders' differs widely. They usually regress to an amazing degree after delivery has occurred, although sometimes the venous capillary dilatation remains and is considered disfiguring.

The natural history and treatment of these three types of varicose veins seen in pregnancy will now be considered.

PRIMARY HEREDITARY VARICOSE VEINS

The patient who has a very slight primary long or short saphenous incompetence will find that this vein will increase in size, will become conspicuous and sometimes quite painful, particularly in the early months.

After delivery the vein may almost disappear. Repeated pregnancy however, has a steadily damaging effect, and after two or three babies complete resolution of the veins does not occur. The patient may then be left with a progressive long or short saphenous incompetence at a relatively young age.

Treatment during pregnancy

Treatment during pregnancy is by elastic stockings or elastic bandages. Occasionally it may be necessary to advise the patient to lie down with the legs up just above heart level, for one or two short periods during the day.

It is not advisable to treat such veins actively either by operation or injection during pregnancy. Operation is particularly difficult and accompanied by a high blood loss as the veins are dilated and full. Moreover they seldom give rise to any more active symptoms than dismay on the part of the patient and regress considerably after delivery.

Treatment after pregnancy

Approximately three months after delivery is the time to assess the veins and to perform elective surgery if this is necessary.

If the veins are still large and giving concern, then radical operation should be advised forthwith, before further pregnancies.

However if the veins have regressed well, and are no more than very slight, it might be well to defer operation until after the next pregnancy or even until the family is complete. This needs careful individual judgment, as the degree of regression of veins after delivery varies from case to case.

VULVAL AND PUDENDAL VEINS

These veins, which are peculiar to pregnancy, appear in the vulva and labia and on the inner side and back of the thigh. These veins arise predominantly from the internal pudendal and obturator veins, which are tributaries of the *internal iliac* vein (see Lea Thomas et al., 1967). Sometimes there is also a contribution via the superficial external pudendal branch of the saphenous vein, at the saphenofemoral junction (Figs 10.1 and 10.2).

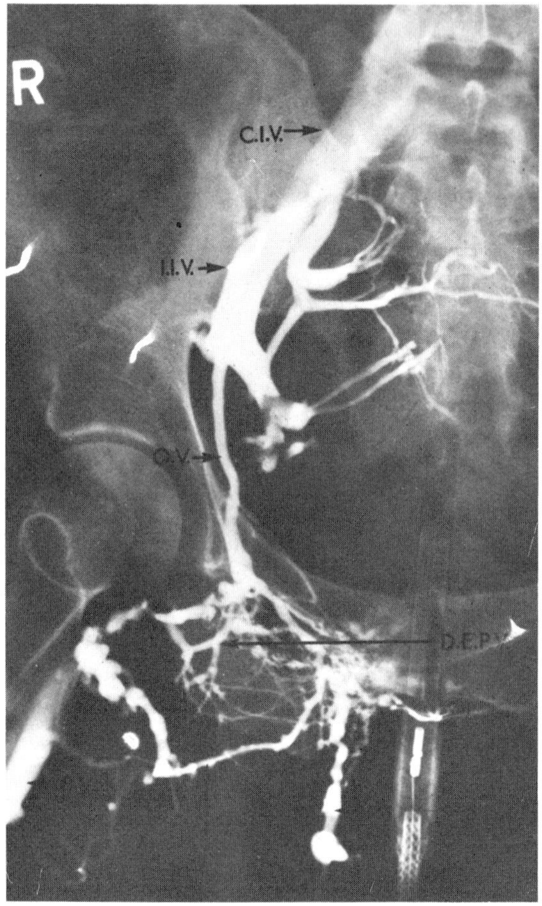

Fig. 10.1 Direct cannulation of a vein entering the right vulval varices. Superficial and deep external pudendal veins joining saphenofemoral junction. Obturator vein (O.V.) entering internal iliac vein. A radiation dosemeter has been inserted into the vagina.

As the internal iliac vein is the main drainage of the uterus, the increased venous pressure and flow from this organ (when gravid) leaks out along these two pathways to the relatively small thin-walled veins in the vulva and inner side of thigh. These dilate rapidly and occasionally present an alarming

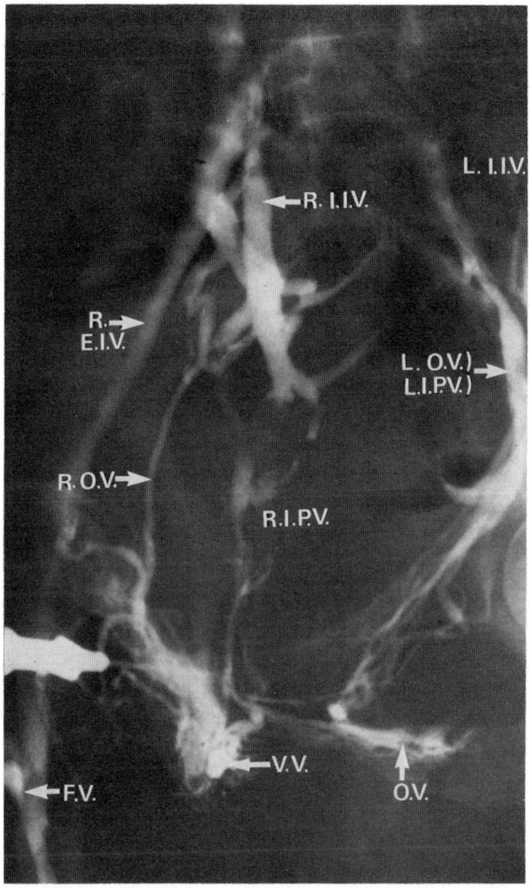

Fig. 10.2 Intraosseous phlebography into right os pubis. 40° oblique projection. Vulval varices (V.V.) Internal pudendal vein (I.P.V.) Obturator vein (O.V.) Femoral vein. Note cross-filling of opposite internal iliac venous system.

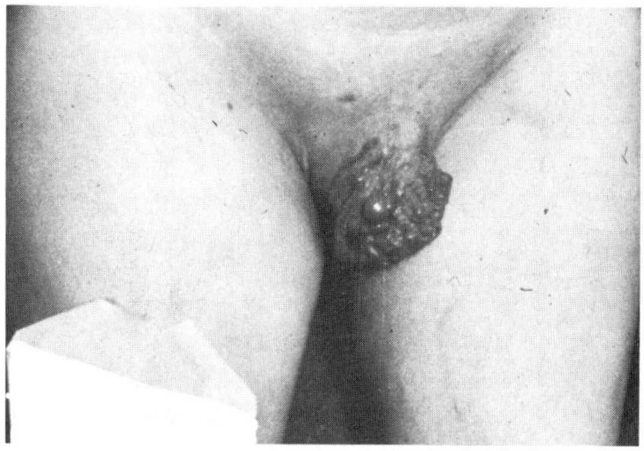

Fig. 10.3 Grape-like bunches of large vulval varices.

picture by the third or fourth month of pregnancy, rather like a 'small bunch of black grapes' in the vulva (Fig. 10.3).

However, in spite of their size they almost never give rise to any serious complication such as haemorrhage or thrombosis either before pregnancy, or during delivery. Afterwards and with the shrinking of the uterus, they diminish within hours and sometimes completely disappear.

Occasionally this 'leak' into the upper and posterior part of the thigh does not entirely disappear, but the incompetent channel remains, causing an annoying bunch of veins just lateral to the vulva. Usually just before the periods these swell and the whole of the back of thigh and outside of the leg may become congested and painful (Figs 10.4 and 10.5).

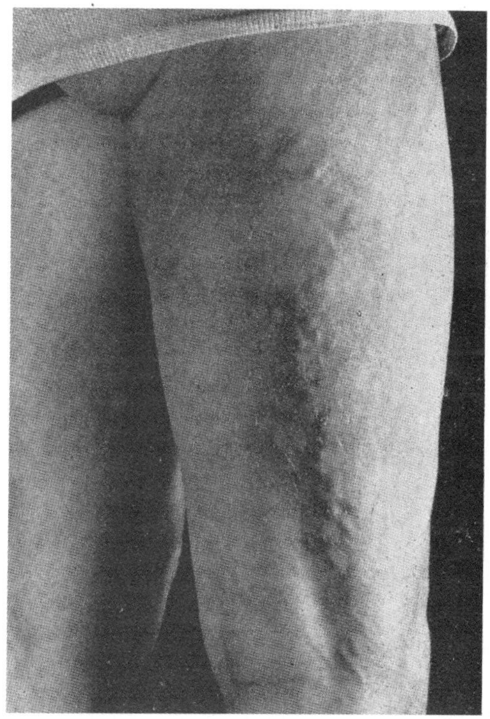

Fig. 10.4 Internal iliac incompetence. Varicose veins due to incompetence of a peripheral tributary of the internal iliac vein.

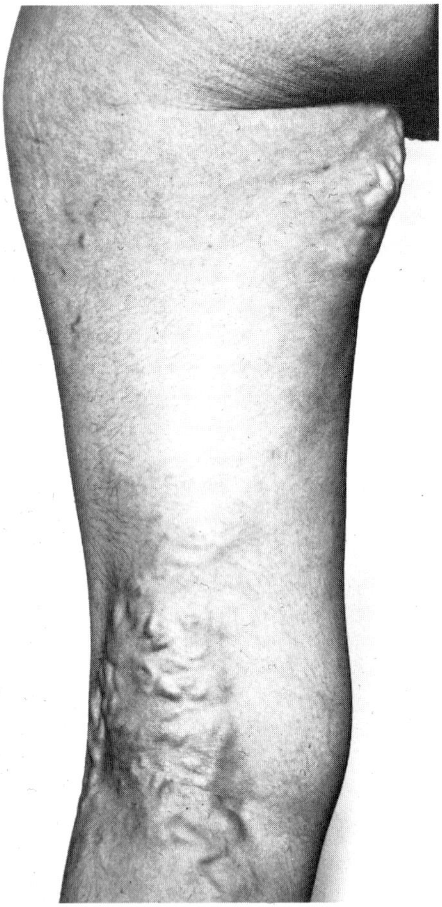

Fig. 10.5 Pudendal varicose veins. View of the back of the thigh, showing the bunch just lateral to the vulva—spreading down the back of the thigh and giving rise to large veins in the popliteal area.

Occasionally the pain may be so great that for a day or two before the period the patient is forced to lie down to gain relief.

Treatment

Once again no treatment is advisable during pregnancy.

If the pudendal veins persist and give rise to periodic symptoms then the only treatment that the authors have found effective is surgical.

The veins are carefully marked out with the patient standing. Then small incisions are made high up lateral to the vulva and the main visible veins descending from this region are freed and avulsed (by the worming technique described in Chapter 8). The main veins are then followed down across the back of the thigh and if necessary down the lateral side of the leg by a series of small 2 millimetre incisions and the veins wormed out and avulsed. Although this is a somewhat tedious and 'finicky' procedure it does produce great relief of symptoms from the patient's point of view, and of course a good cosmetic result.

Injections in this group of veins on the whole produces poor results, a painful pigmented area and no relief of pain.

MULTIPLE CAPILLARY NAEVI

These are often called 'spider naevi' or 'venous stars'. Their connection with a rise in hormone concentration in the blood has already been indicated. They also occur in other conditions in which a rise of blood oestrogen takes place—for instance in cases of cirrhosis of the liver, where oestrin breakdown by the liver fails, and the blood level rises.

In susceptible individuals on the contraceptive pill, these naevi may appear in crops.

Any young female who comes complaining of the appearance of spider veins on the legs should always be checked for early pregnancy or are they taking the 'pill',

But apart from this there appear to be certain susceptible individuals who break out in 'spider veins' on their legs for no very obvious reason, and the tendency is often familial.

Treatment

1. Treatment should if possible be directed towards the cause. If the patient is on the 'pill', this must be explained, and she must weigh up in her own mind the advantages (contraception) and disadvantages (spider veins).

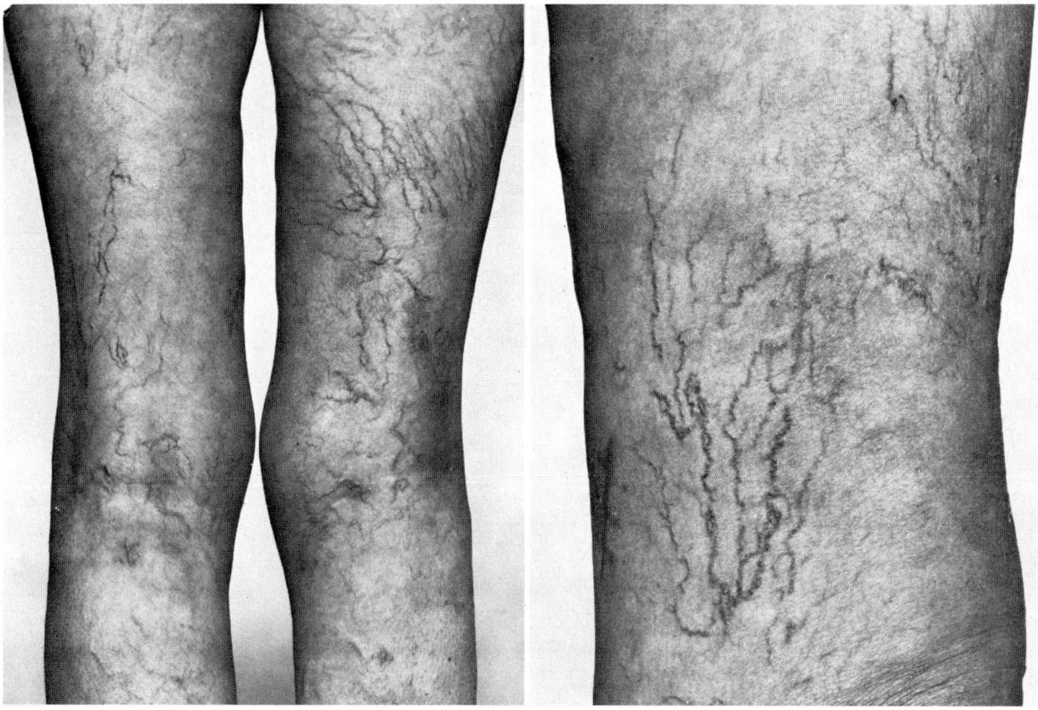

Fig. 10.6 Spider naevi (capillary veins or spider veins).

If an early pregnancy is present, an explanation is all that is required.

2. Local treatment to persistent spider veins is often requested by patients because of the cosmetic appearance. The greatest caution should be exercised here, as local treatment by diathermy, injection or electrolysis may well result in a worsening of the condition by unsightly brown scars, and the appearance of more capillaries, and a progressively dissatisfied patient.

Where many spider veins are also associated with a gross long or short saphenous or perforator incompetence, then appropriate radical surgery of the major veins may quite considerably alleviate the congestive appearance of the lesions and this is always worth doing.

Local injections should be reserved for reasonably localised and rather *gross* venous stars. Quite good results can be obtained by using a very fine needle and small syringe (a so-called serum needle). In a good light, with the patient lying with the legs down it is possible to enter one of the capillaries directly and on injecting about 0·2 ml of ethanolamine slowly the whole spider will suddenly 'blanch'. A pressure pad is rapidly applied over it and the leg pressure bandaged for about five days. Considerable improvement in the appearance may be obtained in localised cases by this method, although often a faint brown stain remains.

The smaller and finer venous stars, however, are best left alone, after an explanation of their aetiology to the patient.

REFERENCES

Lea Thomas, M., Fletcher, E. W. L., Andress, M. R. & Cockett, F. B. (1967) *Clin. Radiol.*, **18**, 3.

11. Rare and Congenital Forms of Venous Anomalies

1. The Klippel Trenaunay Syndrome
2. Arteriovenous Fistulae
    a. Congenital
    b. Acquired
3. Haemangiomas
4. The Mid Thigh Communicating Vein
5. Athletes Prominent Veins
6. Pure Stasis Veins and Ulcers in Old People

KLIPPEL-TRENAUNAY SYNDROMES
(or lateral venous anomaly)

In early intrauterine foetal life the limb has two main vascular systems: (1) a ventral—the primitive femoral artery and veins and (2) a dorsal—or sciatic system. During the second month, the latter atrophies almost completely, and the femoral system takes over.

Normally the only remnants of the old sciatic system are the internal iliac and inferior gluteal vessels and in the leg, the artery of the sciatic nerve.

In certain cases the old sciatic venous system may persist in various forms giving rise to a large group of venous anomalies in the limb, under the general title of 'Klippel-Trenaunay syndromes' or 'lateral venous anomalies'. In fact the original paper only described one type (Klippel and Trenaunay, 1900) (Malan and Puglionisi, 1964).

All forms of the syndrome have two things in common however: (1) they are congenital—the condition is *present* at birth, although it develops considerably with further growth; (2) it affects the *lateral* and *posterior* surface of the limb predominantly, often going up and affecting the buttock and general vascular territory of the internal iliac vein and artery.

There are three main clinical degrees or types of the anomaly. These are:

Type 1 (Figs 11.1 and 11.2)

The fully developed anomaly

In this type there is marked skin angioma over the whole of the lateral side of the leg, from foot right up to the buttock. Deep to the skin and spreading through subcutaneous tissues, muscle and sometimes affecting bone too, there is diffuse angiomatous abnormality consisting of many small and large venous and lymphatic spaces. Sometimes the venous spaces may have conglomerated into large venous sinuses, or actual large abnormal veins. These usually communicate at the top of the limb with the internal iliac vein, via a series of large abnormal veins of the inferior gluteal group.

There may also be a greater or lesser degree of precapillary arteriovenous fistulae in these patients, and these may result in greatly increased blood flow into the limb and an increase in the rate of bone growth—producing eventually a leg which may be 2 or 3 inches longer than the other side (see Fig. 11.2).

The vascular abnormality may rarely go right through all the tissues of the pelvis including the rectum and we have seen two cases in which troublesome recurrent haemorrhages from the rectum, with large very vascular haemorrhoids, was a feature.

Treatment. On the whole these cases are

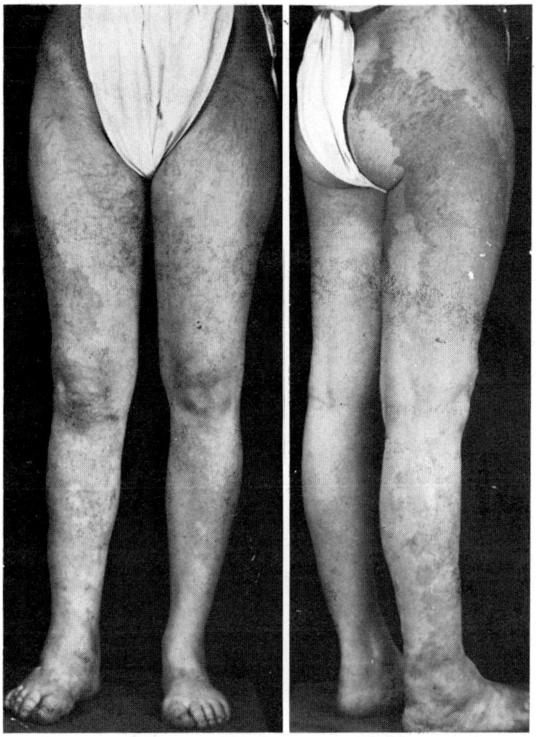

Fig. 11.1 Type 1, fully developed Klippel-Trenaunay syndrome. Congenital lateral venous anomaly with extensive skin staining, and increase in leg length and girth, showing the presence of numerous small arteriovenous fistulae.

best left alone. A light, full length elastic stocking helps the symptoms and disguises the appearance.

In particular, injudicious large incisions in or over the haemangiomatous areas of skin must be avoided. Such incisions may break down and ulcerate and lead to years of unhealed ulceration and misery.

Surgery may be indicated for two reasons only. These are: (a) if there is a big venous element with large sinuses, it helps if the big communicating veins feeding these sinuses from the internal iliac system, or deep veins, are divided. This must be carefully worked out with the aid of detailed phlebograms; (b) if the increase in rate of growth of the limb is excessive compared to the other normal limb, then fixation of the epiphysis round the

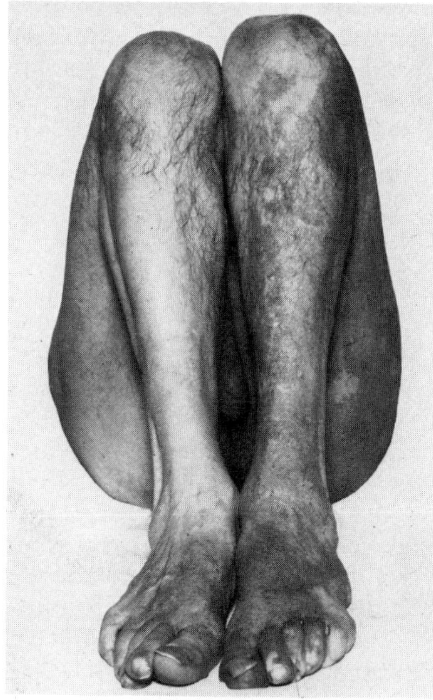

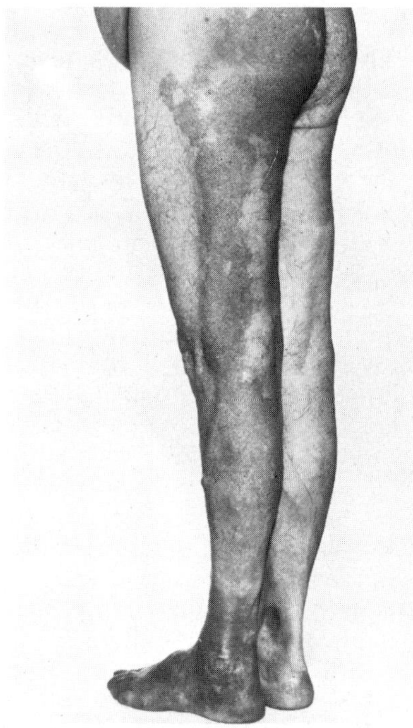

Fig. 11.2 Another case of Type 1—Klippel Trenaunay showing the typical skin staining and increase in leg length.

knee at the age of 13 or 14 years should be done. This can be done by the relatively simple orthopaedic procedure of stapling and is very worthwhile. In extreme cases, amputation may be necessary, for various reasons.

Type 2 (Fig. 11.3)

Pure venous anomaly

In this type there is no arteriovenous fistula element, and therefore no bony involvement and no increase in limb length. The main feature is a diffuse cavernous haemangioma entirely consisting of large and small venous spaces. Often these spaces are in fact well differentiated large veins, with a proper venous wall (Fig. 11.3). These large abnormal veins and venous spaces often communicate direct with the internal iliac vein above, or by large abnormal lateral communicating veins with the deep femoral or profunda system. There is usually a diffuse capillary haemangioma, often patchy (Figs 11.3 and 11.4) over the lateral and posterior surface of the leg and thigh.

Apart from the appearance, the main complaint of these patients is of heaviness and swelling of the leg. Phleboliths and small tough thrombi sometimes occur in the venous spaces, and where there are big communicating veins—these may give rise to minor recurrent pulmonary embolism and may lead to pulmonary hypertension in young adult life.

Treatment. Once again, support with a good, full length elastic stocking is the basic treatment. Surgery, however, has a place in the treatment of many of these patients. Where large communicating veins with the internal iliac system, or the deep veins, can be demonstrated by phlebogram, considerable benefit can be obtained by tying these surgically. This results in great relief in the symptoms of heaviness and aching and often reduces the size of the haemangioma materially. Radical excision of large, well organised veins can sometimes be done successfully—but only if the skin over them is normal. *Big incisions in purple haemangiomatous skin should be always*

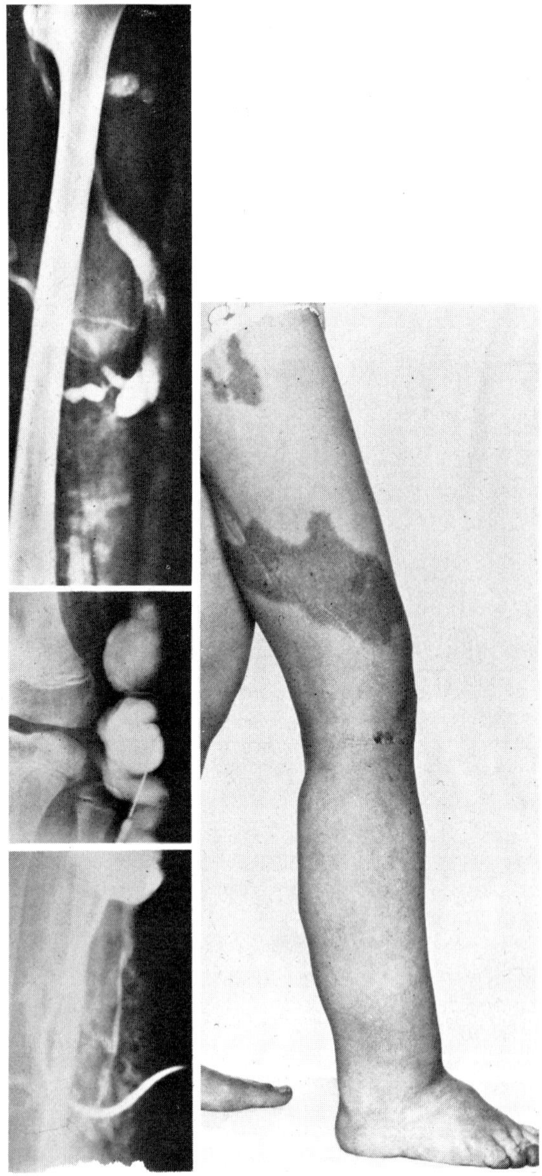

Fig. 11.3 Type 2—Klippel-Trenaunay (the pure venous anomaly). The phlebogram of this leg shows the large well organised venous spaces, and the big communicating veins with the profunda system.

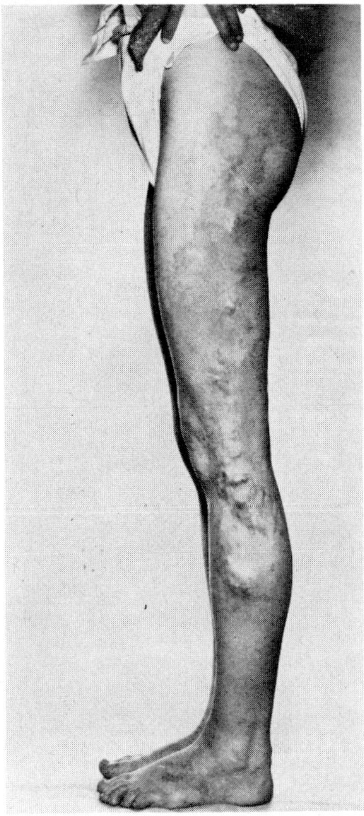

Fig. 11.4 Another Type 2 Klippel-Trenaunay (pure venous anomaly). Showing large venous sinuses and skin staining going right up over the buttock in the typical distribution.

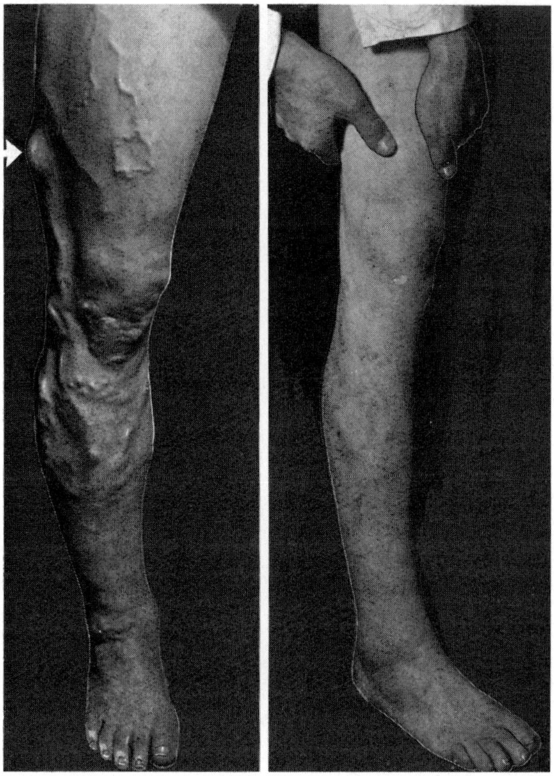

Fig. 11.5 A 'blow-out. from an abnormal lateral communicating vain passing through the tensor fasciae femoris.

avoided, as these may fail to heal—breaking down to form large chronic fibrous ulcers.

Type 3

Minor forms of the syndrome

Minor forms of the syndrome are not uncommon, presenting as diffuse varicose veins on the lateral side of the thigh and leg, arising from one or two lateral perforating veins usually in the thigh. Figures 11.5 and 11.6 show good examples of such cases. There is often no capillary haemangioma of skin in these cases, or one or two small patchy ones.

They present simply as small tortuous lateral varicose veins, usually without evidence of any long or short saphenous incompetence.

Treatment. These cases can be treated successfully by surgery. The abnormal perforating vein on the outer side of the thigh is found and tied. The site of this perforator is usually fairly obvious clinically (see Figs 11.5 and 11.6).

Then the veins arising from it are avulsed with forceps (worming technique) through a number of very small incisions placed along the length of the vein.

ARTERIOVENOUS FISTULAE

1. Congenital type

A. DIFFUSE TYPE

In these individuals small precapillary size arteriovenous fistulae persist throughout the limb. They are so small and diffuse that they

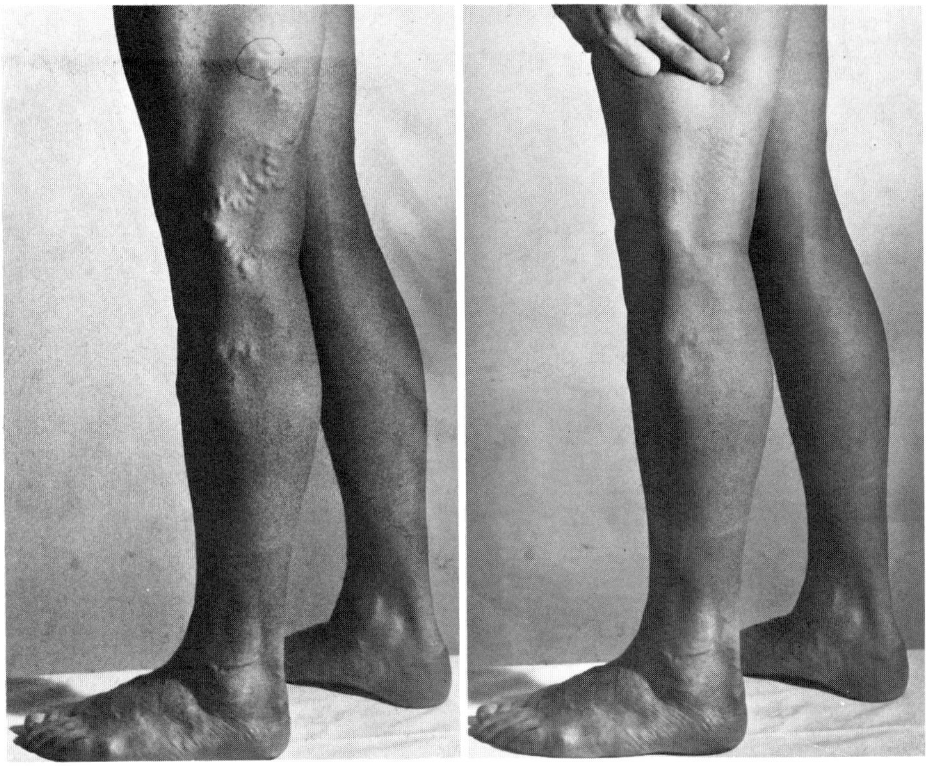

Fig. 11.6 Minor forms of the Klippel-Trenaunay anomaly—another abnormal lateral perforator.

cannot be demonstrated by the usual arteriographic techniques. The main symptom is a warm limb which *grows faster* than the other one. There may be obvious associated congenital haemangiomatous changes—as in the type 1 Klippel-Trenaunay syndrome, but often there may be no skin abnormality at all, and *no enlarged veins*. These cases are not amenable to surgical treatment. Surgical control of the excessive growth of the limb, by fixing the epiphyses round the knee, at age 12 to 14 may be required.

B. LOCALISED TYPE

In this type the fistulae are larger, but localised to a small area of the hand or foot. Figure 11.7 is a typical example occurring in the hand and Figure 11.8 shows one in the foot. In these cases all the signs of arteriovenous fistulae are present—a localised machinery murmur, large and often pulsating veins, increase in finger or toe length, and often chronic venous ulceration.

The treatment of these cases is surgical. Radical ablation of the whole length of artery involved in the fistula is usually necessary—often associated with amputation of a toe or a finger. Even such radical measures as these often fail to cure the localised condition completely—but it is possible to diminish considerably the total volume flowing through the fistulae and this ameliorates the local condition considerably.

2. Traumatic type (Fig. 11.9)

Traumatic arteriovenous fistulae are of course mainly seen during wartime, and in the limbs particularly. They are usually the result of *small* penetrating wounds by either a fine sharp instrument or a small flying piece of shrapnel.

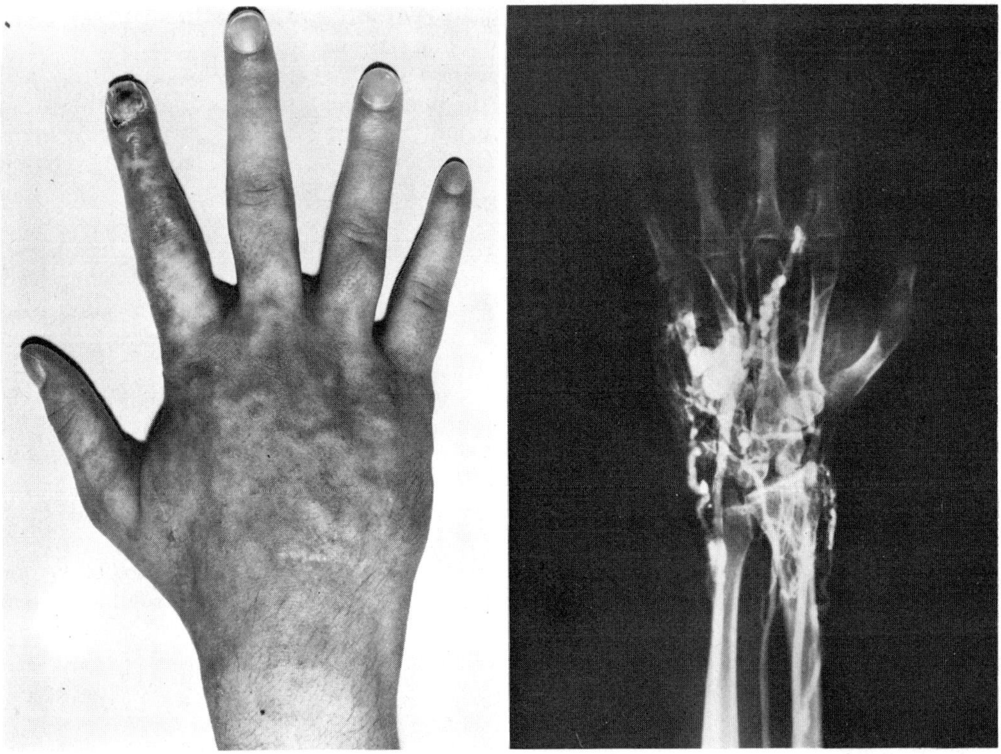

Fig. 11.7 Localised congenital arteriovenous fistula, affecting ulnar artery distribution in hand. Note the venous staining and ulceration and increase in length of the fore and middle fingers. Arteriogram shows enlarged ulnar artery and big venous dilatations near the site of the fistula. Note the large mass of dilated veins on the dorsum. There was a distinct local machinery murmur heard over the palm of the hand. Treated by ablation of the whole ulnar artery arch in the hand.

As the wound is often small and trivial and as the artery bleeds directly into a vein, no large haematoma develops, and for this reason the *diagnosis of arteriovenous fistula is often overlooked* at the time of wounding. In fact at this early date the only sure sign of the establishment of an arteriovenous communication is the typical continuous machinery murmur which is heard if a stethoscope is applied over the area.

If the diagnosis is missed, then the patient may be unaware of it for two to three months, when dilated veins gradually start appearing in the vicinity of the fistula. The patient may complain of these and it is at this stage that he may be sent to a surgeon with a diagnosis of varicose veins.

Thus any patient who has had an injury in the vicinity of varicose veins which have recently appeared and are enlarging, should be suspected of having an arteriovenous fistula. A stethoscope is the essential diagnostic instrument and careful auscultation over the course of the main artery should be done.

Arteriography will reveal the full site and extent of the fistula.

HAEMANGIOMAS

Haemangiomas are not true tumours or new growths, but are more or less localised congenital malformations (or hamartomas).

As the primitive vascular system in the embryo differentiates, the arteries, the veins, and the lymphatics become separated off as

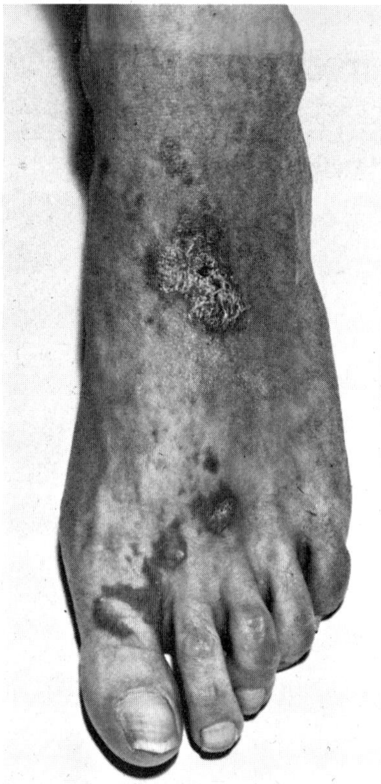

Fig. 11.8 Localised arteriovenous fistulae (congenital) in foot. Typical pigmented venous ulcerating lesions, engorged veins and a hot foot, bigger than the other side. But no murmurs heard in this case, as the fistulae were too small.

different systems. However, at a very early stage of development they are not so differentiated and so many of these malformations of the vascular system contain elements of all three systems.

We have already seen one excellent example of this in the type 1 Klippel-Trenaunay syndrome.

However there are a large number of vascular malformations in which the venous element predominates by far and these may be properly termed haemangiomas.

The two main types of haemangioma are the surface capillary haemangiomas and the deeper-seated cavernous haemangiomas.

Capillary haemangiomas

The flat ones are the lesions known as 'port wine stains' which may occur on any part of the body. These may be single lesions or more often they may be part of a more extensive, deep-seated cavernous haemangioma. (see Figs 11.1 and 11.2.)

Unless they can be completely excised and replaced by normal skin they are best not interfered with. Incisions and wounds over areas of capillary haemangioma tend to heal badly, ulcerate, and give rise to chronic distress.

Sometimes babies are born with single or multiple *raised* capillary haemangiomas which have received the very descriptive term of 'strawberry mark'. These are soft, raised lesions, crimson or dark blue and tend to occur on the chest wall, back and scalp particularly. They cause great distress to the parents. They should not usually be treated,

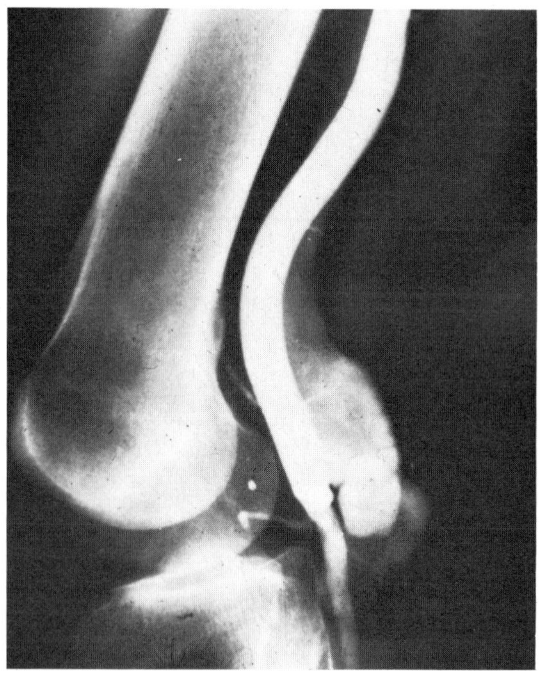

Fig. 11.9 Traumatic arteriovenous fistula of the popliteal artery (due to entry of a small spike of glass).

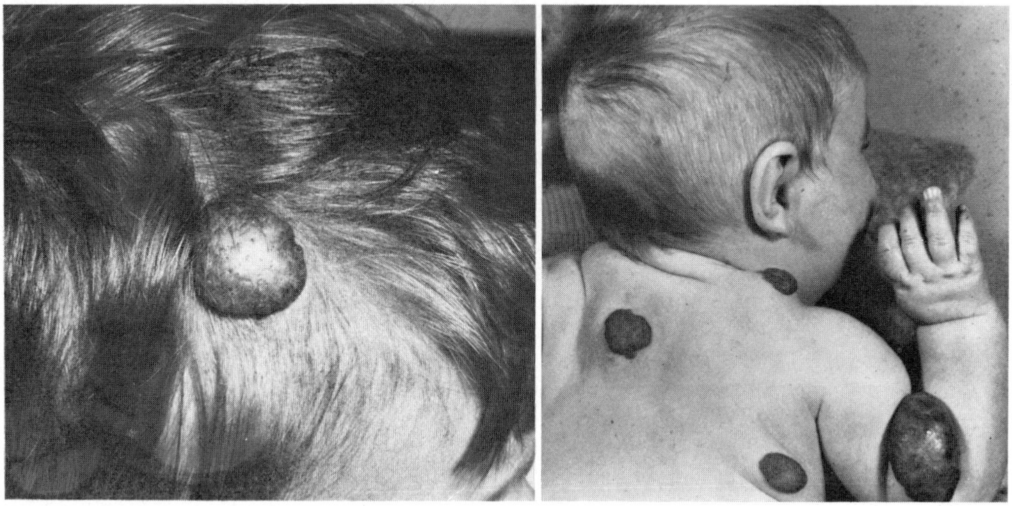

Fig. 11.10A, B Raised capillary haemangiomas (strawberry mark) in a baby.

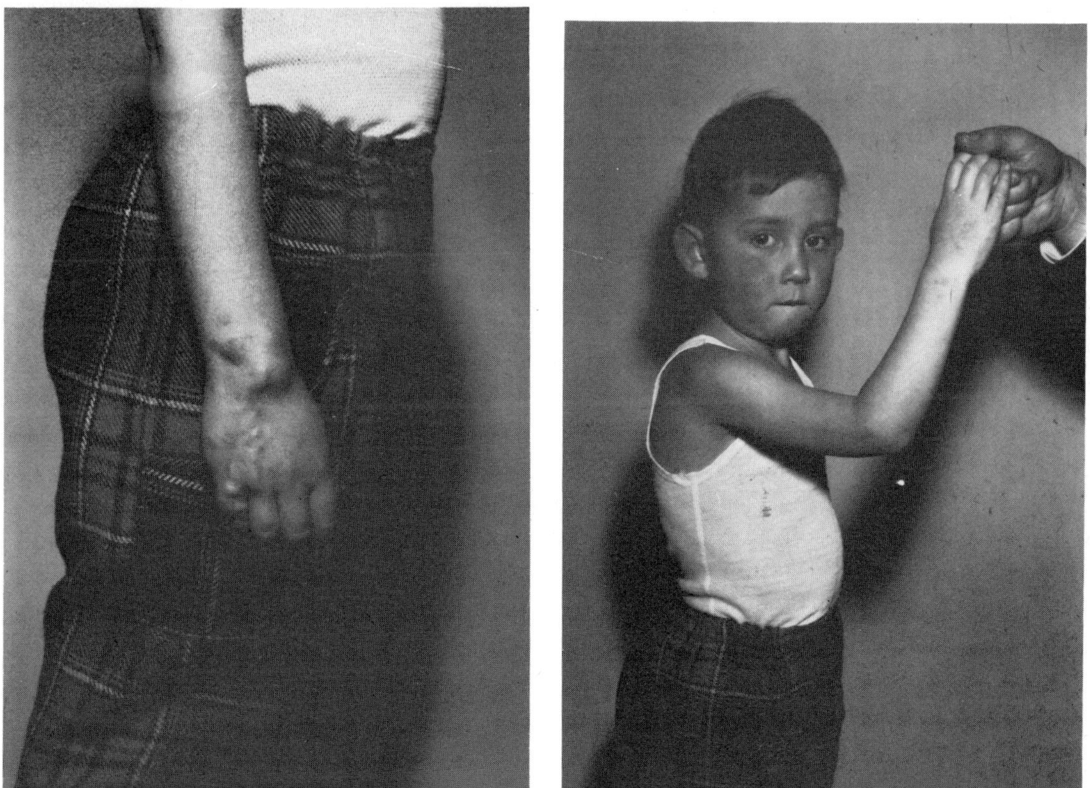

Fig. 11.11A, B Very localised type of cavernous haemangioma of wrist (suitable for surgical excision).

as they nearly all regress spontaneously by the age of about five years.

Cavernous haemangiomas

These are deep-seated masses of venous spaces, which often affect every part of the subcutaneous area over which they occur—subcutaneous fat, muscle, nerve and even bone. The vessel spaces communicate with the normal venous system and so the lesion is compressible and it diminishes in size if the part is raised above the heart (Figs 11.11 and 11.12).

The other important characteristic of these cavernous haemangiomas is the tendency for small tough fibrinous thrombi to form in the vascular spaces. These may calcify and become apparent on an X-ray as multiple 'phleboliths' (Fig. 11.13).

Sometimes, however, when there are large communicating veins to the area these little thrombi may float off to the lungs, forming multiple, recurrent, small, tough pulmonary emboli. One of the authors has seen such a case presenting as gross right-sided heart failure in a young man of thirty-two.

From the point of view of treatment the cavernous haemangiomata may be divided into the *diffuse type* and the *localised type*:

DIFFUSE TYPE

The type 1 and type 2 Klippel-Trenaunay syndromes are good examples of this. (Figs 11.1, 11.2 and 11.3). They are so diffuse that surgical excision is not possible. If an ill-judged attempt is made, it is found that the haemangiomatous process goes right through nerve, muscle and bone, and the operation has to be abandoned.

The only way in which surgery may be of help sometimes is in localising and dividing some of the large communicating veins to the lesion. This can be of considerable benefit sometimes, particularly in the lower limb.

The older treatments of injecting boiling water, and radiotherapy, are *not* recommended—they do more harm than good.

LOCALISED TYPE

Occasionally medium sized quite localised haemangiomas occur on the limbs, of which Figure 11.11 is a good example. A venogram of another is seen in Figure 11.12. They often have one or two very large venous sinuses in them which can be removed successfully by local surgery. Even these cases, however, are considerably less localised than they appear when excisional surgery is undertaken!

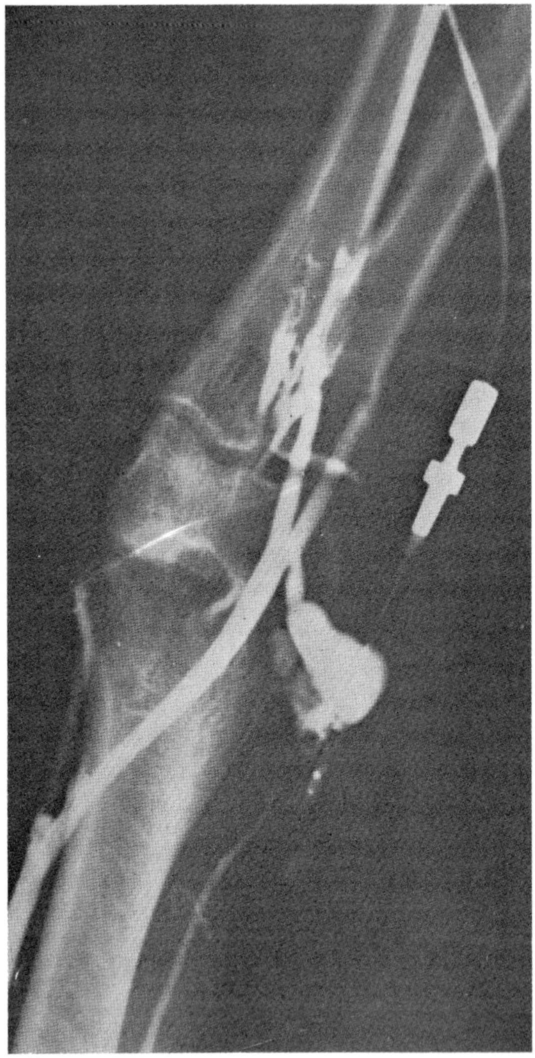

Fig. 11.12 Phlebogram of very localised cavernous haemangioma of arm.

Haemangiomas of meninges and cerebrum

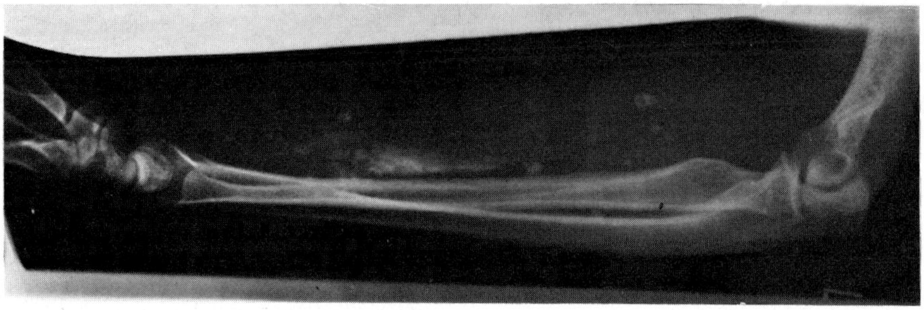

Fig. 11.13 Lateral X-ray of diffuse haemangioma of forearm. This shows the diffuse phlebolith formation, and calci fication which often occurs in these lesions.

and spinal cord also occur as a component of certain rare multiple congenital abnormalities (Sturge-Weber syndrome and Lindau's disease).

THE MID-THIGH COMMUNICATING VEIN

Turning to Chapter 3 (Fig. 3.20) it will be seen that there is normally a very fine communicating vein in the middle of the thigh on the inner side, which connects one of the venae comites of the femoral vein with the long saphenous or one of its tributaries.

Rarely this mid-thigh communicator may be shorter and larger and its valve may be faulty so that it gives rise to a high pressure leak in the middle of the thigh (see Fig. 11.14).

This, however, is a rare phenomenon.

It is very common, however, to find a large branch of the saphenous itself arising at about this level, and *clinically appearing to arise deeply*. (The saphenous vein is situated on the deep fascia at this level and is seldom visible except in very thin individuals.) This appearance is responsible for the frequent *misdiagnosis* of 'mid-thigh communicating vein'. (see Fig. 7.28.)

The incompetent true mid-thigh communicator usually shows itself as a cause of recurrent varicose veins after a successful stripping operation on the long saphenous system. Nearly all the author's cases have presented clinically in this way.

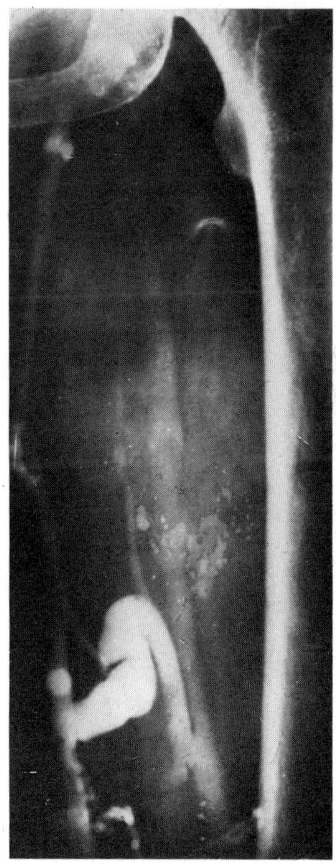

Fig. 11.14 A large incompetent mid-thigh communicating vein, causing the appearance of gross varicose veins at mid-thigh level.

ATHLETES' PROMINENT VEINS

These are only mentioned here because they are an occasional clinical problem. Young athletes who are very spare, and who over-use the muscles of the legs (cyclists, runners, etc.) often appear with prominent hypertrophied superficial veins. It is probable that this is a true hypertrophy due to the greatly increased blood flow from the legs in their frequent periods of strenuous exercise.

In extreme cases they show up almost like an 'anatomical cast of the veins of the leg' they are so visible and prominent.

To many of these people the appearance gradually becomes objectionable, particularly at the age of 25 to 30 when athletic days are finished, and they come asking for surgical treatment.

Most are satisfied when it is explained to them that these are simply hypertrophied normal veins and a legacy of their athletic youth!

They should not be treated.

PURE GRAVITATIONAL STASIS IN OLD AGE

In people with static occupations, a lifetime of standing around with high hydrostatic pressure in the leg veins, results in a slow and gradual dilatation of the venules particularly round the ankle and foot.

Most fit old people show some degree of dilatation of a few veins round the ankle, amounting to a mild 'ankle flare' without any actual valvular incompetence.

Where there is also some additional lesion of the leg such as osteoarthritis of hip or knee, causing extra immobility, this static venous dilatation round the ankle may become marked.

Although normally this does not cause any serious lesion it is of importance for two reasons: (1) diagnostic: the appearance is sometimes mistakenly held to be due to true valvular incompetence, and (2) small, very chronic areas of skin necrosis do sometimes occur over the dilated capillaries round the malleoli which are often due to the too tight application of a bandage over the ankle. If these become infected a serious chronic ulcer can occur.

REFERENCES

Farrer-Brown, G. & Marston, A. (1973) *Peripheral Vascular Surgery*, p. 392. London: Heinemann.
Klippel, M. & Trenaunay, I. (1900) *Arch. Gen. Med.*, **3**, 641.
Lea Thomas, M. & Andress, M. R. (1971) *Amer. J. Roent.*, Vol. 113, No. 4, Dec.
Lindenauer, S. M. (1971) *Ann. Surg.*, **174**, 248.
Malan, E. & Puglionisi, A. (1964) *J. Cardiovasc. Surg.*, **512**, 87.

Part III
Pathology and Surgery of the Deep and Communicating Veins

12. Introduction

During the past half century thrombosis of the deep veins has been recognised as a common and serious complication following accidents, operation, childbirth and severe illness of any sort. More recently it has been recognised that it may occur also quite suddenly, in apparently normal healthy people, not in hospital. It is of great importance for two reasons. *First* because of the danger of pulmonary embolism—fatal or non-fatal—this is well known and dramatic. *Second*, because of the chronic sequelae of thrombosis of the deep veins of the legs. These are less well known and less dramatic. However, up to 75 per cent of people who have had thrombosis of the deep veins of the legs suffer for the rest of their lives from oedema, induration, ulcer or pain in the lower leg. These effects develop gradually during the three, four or five years following the acute thrombosis—and the patient often does not present himself to a doctor until after this latent period has elapsed.

The diagnosis and management of the acute phase of the disease—the phase of *thromboembolism*—has been revolutionised during the past six years by the development of three reliable physical methods for the detection and localisation of thrombus in the deep veins in the very early stages when it is largely unattached to the vein wall and therefore symptomless, silent, and dangerous.

The employment of these methods has led to a great increase in accurate knowledge about the early stages of thromboembolism. This in turn has led to the possibility of much more standard and rational treatment of the disease, based on early, accurate diagnosis. Previously the treatment of this stage of the disease was based on a fog of misty clinical impressions, and statistics based on large series of highly suspect clinical diagnoses. Thus a quiet revolution has occurred in this field.

No less of a revolution has occurred also in our concepts of thrombosis occurring in the major veins—iliofemoral thrombosis. This has been subjected to intensive study from a number of centres, and the significance of major anatomical anomalies and variations at the venacaval bifurcation and also in the deep veins, as an aetiological factor in thrombosis, is now appreciated.

Against this background the treatment of thromboembolism by surgery (thrombectomy and vein interruption methods), by anti-coagulants and by the newer thrombolytic agents (Streptokinase and Urokinase), has been subjected to a new and more intense valuation.

In the difficult field of diagnosing the presence and size of pulmonary emboli which have arrived in the lungs there have been two major diagnostic advances. Pulmonary angiography is now undertaken much more readily—although it is still a more major radiographic procedure than most of the others. Lung scanning, to detect major perfusion defects in the lungs, has been a very significant diagnostic advance, and is an examination which can be undertaken quickly and easily even in a fairly ill patient.

Thus there has been so much advance in knowledge and so much revolution in diagnosis and management in this field that Section III of this book has had to be re-written almost completely.

The aim, however, has been to choose and recommend the best, most simple, and most practical methods of diagnosis and treatment which have emerged from the plethora of recent literature.

The first chapter deals appropriately with the modern methods of investigation.

13. Special Methods of Investigation of the Deep Veins and Pulmonary Vessels

1. Venography—by Michael Lea Thomas
2. Radio-isotope methods—by David Negus
3. Ultrasound methods—by David Negus
4. Pulmonary Angiography—by Michael Lea Thomas
5. Lung scanning—by Desmond Croft

VENOGRAPHY OF THE LOWER LIMBS

Radiographs of the veins after injecting radio-opaque substances into them were first made by Berberich and Hirsch in 1923, using strontium bromide, and by McPheeters and Rice in 1929 with lipiodol, but the method was little, if at all used, until iodine solutions became available for intravenous pyelography. In 1934 Edwards and Biguria reported the use of diodone and this remained the most commonly employed medium until the advent of diatrizoates and iothalamates in the last 20 years.

Allan and Barker (1934) described venograms after intra-arterial injection (*indirect venography*), a method which has found little favour in the lower limbs because of their large bulk and the consequent dilution of the contrast leading to undiagnostic radiographs.

It was not until 1938 that a method was described by dos Santos for outlining the deep, as well as the superficial veins, by making injections into the superficial veins behind the external malleolus, the films being taken as the contrast medium ascended in the leg and thigh with an entirely free circulation. This technique is referred to as *ascending venography*. Since then the value of a tourniquet above the ankle to force the contrast into the deep veins and conducting the examination in the vertical or semivertical position so that gravity helps to fill the deep venous system, have improved the technique and numerous full reports have been published (Bauer, 1940; Dougherty and Homans, 1940; Hellsten, 1942; Dow, 1951; Gryspeerdt, 1953). The disadvantage of these methods is that they are 'blind' involving taking a series of films of the lower limbs with an overcouch tube. When image intensification and small focal spot X-ray tubes for improved detail became available, the use of fluoroscopy, which enables films to be taken when the veins are optimally filled has now become the accepted venographic technique (Lea Thomas, 1970, 1972).

In 1941 Luke injected contrast into the femoral vein and as the contrast medium descended radiographs of the thigh were taken. This method, *descending venography*, later used by Bauer (1948), has nowadays been largely replaced by ascending venography by injection of the contrast medium into foot veins complemented if necessary by injections into the femoral veins or greater trochanters.

Indications for venography

The main indications are:

To detect deep vein thrombosis and especially to find the source of pulmonary emboli. Venograms are carried out as an emergency and are now a standard and essential part of the management of patients with suspected thrombo-embolism. Venography may also be used to assess the effects of treatment of deep vein thrombosis.

To investigate the cause of varicose veins and varicose ulceration. In these patients an evaluation of the deep veins to show the presence or absence of valves, recanalisation or obstruction, is required. Also, combined with this information, the presence and site of any incompetent leg perforating veins can be shown.

To investigate the cause of a swollen leg. This may be due to venous incompetence from recanalisation, or thrombosis with obstruction of the major veins of the caval bifurcation (Chap. 16). The presence and site of major proximal vein obstruction is demonstrated and the collateral venous return shown.

Venographic techniques—general observations

NEWER CONTRAST MEDIA

The modern contrast media (Conray, Hypaque, Urografin etc.) are virtually free of serious complications. The minor reactions consist of flushing due to vasodilatation, occasional nausea and vomiting, and urticaria. These almost always pass off spontaneously but occasionally may need to be controlled with an oral or intravenous antihistamine, or the intravenous injection of hydrocortisone. These minor reactions are not directly related to the very rare major cardiovascular reactions and testing for sensitivity to contrast is not now carried out. The author prefers Meglumine Iothalamate 60 per cent (Conray '280') for ascending venography of the legs, and Sodium Iothalamate 70 per cent (Conray '420') a denser medium, for iliac venography and inferior vena cavography. The maximum safe dose of contrast medium is not known. The amount required for venography in an individual depends on the size of the patient and the number of injections required to clarify the clinical problem. The volume varies from 100 to 400 ml of contrast. No complications from the use of these volumes have been encountered in the author's series of over 3,000 venograms.

THE USE OF IMAGE INTENSIFICATION

The use of image intensification combined with television monitoring has considerably improved the diagnostic accuracy of venography. The direction of flow of the contrast medium, whether from superficial to deep veins or vice versa, important in identifying incompetent perforating veins, can be seen. Furthermore, films can be taken when the veins are seen to be well filled thus avoiding artefacts. The newer, small focal spot X-ray tubes produce as good radiographic detail as was previously obtained by the longer focus-film distance obtained by an over-couch technique. There is now no justification for the use of 'blind' non-screening techniques.

IMPORTANCE OF POSITION OF THE PATIENT

Ideally ascending venography of the lower limbs should be carried out in the vertical position as in this position the deep venous system always fills if it is patent and the position also produces maximum mixing of the contrast medium and blood avoiding artefacts due to streaming which may mimic thrombus. Such a position, however, requires specialised equipment and the position is not readily tolerated by many patients. A 20° to 40° foot-down position is adequate and this can be obtained with a standard screening table. As the contrast medium is heavier than blood, it tends to fill, selectively, the most dependent veins. Thus for iliac phlebography the patient should be in the prone position to show the external iliac and common iliac veins and the inferior vena cava and in the supine position to show the internal iliac system.

THE USE OF THE TOURNIQUET

In a normal leg, contrast injected into a superficial vein of the foot will pass into the deep veins of the leg following the normal route of blood flow. However, when the venous system is pathological, particularly in the post-thrombotic syndrome with occluded or recanalised deep veins, a tourniquet is necessary to direct the contrast medium into the deep system. The tightness of the tourniquet is adjusted to ensure deep venous filling. The tourniquet is applied above the injection needle, that is, just above the ankle. If incompetent perforating veins at the ankles are being sought or ankle ulceration prevents application at this site, the tourniquet may be applied around the forefoot. If too many varicosities fill, these should be cleared by injecting saline and a more proximal tourniquet applied to occlude them. This is more effective than the use of an elastic bandage.

A tourniquet above the knee is also helpful to delay emptying of the calf veins and produce better filling of them.

DIRECTION OF THE NEEDLE

If the contrast is injected in an upstream direction, that is through a needle directed towards the toes, with a tight tourniquet proximal to it, the medium passes directly into the deep venous system through communicating veins on the dorsum of the foot. This produces preferential filling of the deep veins (Halliday, 1968).

THE VALSALVA MANOEUVRE

The Valsalva manoeuvre is performed by asking the patient to take a deep breath closing the lips firmly, pinching the nose and then attempting to blow out hard. This forced expiration with the glottis closed causes a rapid rise in the pressure in the great veins of the thorax which is transmitted to the inferior vena cava producing reflux of blood down the limb veins causing the valves to open. The valve pockets become distended clearly outlining the valve cusps (Fig. 13.5).

This manoeuvre is useful to confirm the presence of valves, to demonstrate incompetent perforating veins, particularly in Hunter's canal, and to distend veins and show tributaries such as the profunda femoris and internal iliac veins.

COMPLICATIONS

Apart from the systemic reactions to the contrast medium mentioned above, the most common complication of venography is thrombosis due to damage of the intima by the contrast medium (May, 1965). To avoid prolonged contact of the contrast medium with the vein wall, the veins should be flushed with physiological saline at the end of the examination and this should be assisted by elevation of the legs, massage of the calf and exercise. In an obstructed venous system contrast medium may be trapped in the foot causing tissue damage (Lea Thomas, 1970). If, using the standard technique described below, the deep venous system does not fill, the examination should be abandoned.

Complications from intraosseous venography include transient pain at the site of injection, osteomyelitis (which should be avoided by a careful aseptic technique) and fat embolism (Lea Thomas and Tighe, 1973) which should be suspected in patients who develop neurological signs following the examination.

In patients with pulmonary hypertension which may occur following massive or repeated pulmonary embolism, cardiac arrest may occur due to reduction in cardiac output because of the vasodilatation caused by the contrast medium. This complication can be minimised by initial vasoconstriction (see pulmonary angiography).

Techniques for ascending venography

A tilting screening table equipped with image intensification, television monitoring and an automatic exposure device is most convenient (Fig. 13.1). A useful film format is a 35·6 cm × 35·6 cm film capable of being split into three. This equipment is not essential, however, and any screening table can be used for the examination.

Both legs and the pelvis are examined in all patients to exclude subclinical thrombosis.

Each leg is examined separately. The patient lies supine on the table and a self-fastening rubber tourniquet is applied around the ankle to distend the foot veins. A 19 gauge (or smaller) butterfly needle is introduced percutaneously into a vein on the lateral side of the foot, to avoid too direct communication with the long saphenous venous system. The needle points towards the toes. Very rarely a cut down on to the known

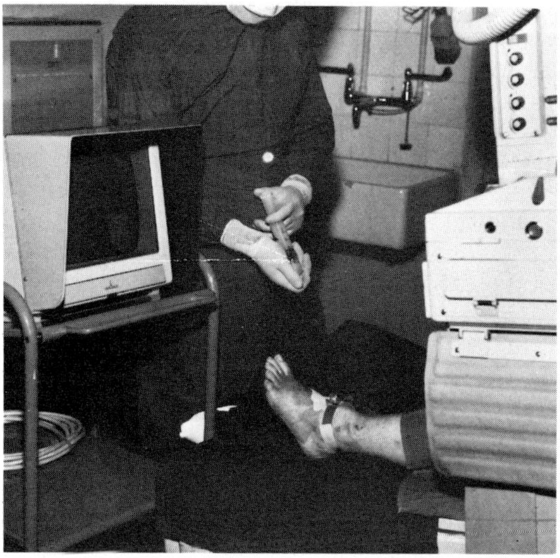

Fig. 13.1 Modern equipment for ascending venography.

position of the lower end of the long saphenous vein is required. A second tourniquet is applied above the knee to trap the contrast medium in the calf. The table is tilted 20° to 40° downwards and the leg internally rotated to separate the images of the tibia and fibula. The needle is connected via an extension tube to a syringe containing the contrast medium and a hand injection is begun under television control. The tightness of the ankle tourniquet is adjusted to ensure deep venous filling. It is not part of the technique to totally occlude the superficial veins as thrombosis and embolism can occur from these veins, but what is more important, contrast from the long saphenous vein may demonstrate the veins proximal to an obstruction in the femoral vein (Fig. 13.2).

Films are taken of the deep veins of the calf in straight and lateral projections. The upper tourniquet is then removed and further exposures are made to show the veins as far as the inferior vena cava. The patient is asked to perform a Valsalva manoeuvre when the common femoral vein and the common iliac veins are filled with contrast in order to show the profunda and internal iliac veins as far as competent valves. Better filling of

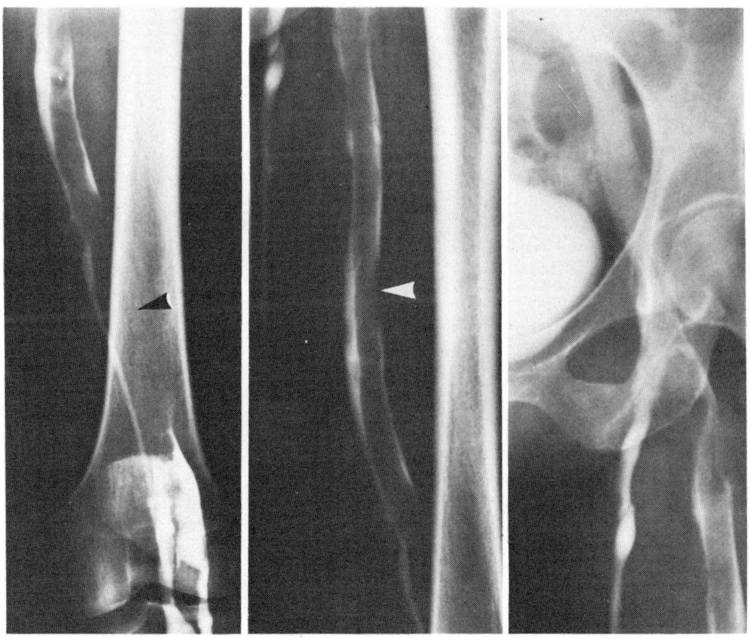

Fig. 13.2 Ascending venogram left leg. There is loose thrombus in the femoral vein outlined by a thin white line of contrast. The thrombus is adherent in part (arrows). Note filling of upper femoral vein and iliac veins from saphenous vein which is not occluded by the ankle tourniquet.

the iliac veins and inferior vena cava is obtained by applying firm pressure, in an upward direction, to the calf, while the exposure is made. No pulmonary embolus has been produced by calf compression, a standard feature of the Doppler ultrasound technique. The reason for this is probably that the pressure rise in the veins produced by calf compression is no greater than that produced by normal muscular contraction.

If an adequate demonstration of the iliac veins and inferior vena cava have not been obtained by this method, the examination is supplemented by the following modification.

ILIAC VENOGRAPHY AND INFERIOR OR VENA CAVOGRAPHY FROM FOOT INJECTIONS

The explorator of the screening set containing a 35·6 cm square film is centred over the upper part of the sacrum and locked in position. A tourniquet is applied tightly above each knee and 50 ml of contrast injected simultaneously through the needles in each foot as rapidly as possible. On completion of the injections the table is tilted slightly head downwards, the tourniquets are removed and immediately firm upward pressure is applied to the calfs while an exposure is made.

In about 5 per cent of patients this method does not adequately demonstrate the iliac veins and lower inferior vena cava, either for technical reasons or because there is proximal obstruction and separate pelvic venography is required.

ILIAC VENOGRAPHY AND INFERIOR VENA CAVOGRAPHY BY PERFEMORAL OR PERTROCHANTERIC INJECTIONS

Perfemoral ascending venography of the pelvic veins is carried out by bilateral simultaneous injection of contrast medium through metal or polyethylene cannulae threaded a short distance into the veins using local anaesthesia. Intraosseous pertrochanteric venography, being painful, requires a general anaesthetic. To facilitate pertrochanteric venography the author has devised a cannula with a 3-faceted drill tip (Fig. 13.3), for easier penetration of the bone (Lea Thomas,

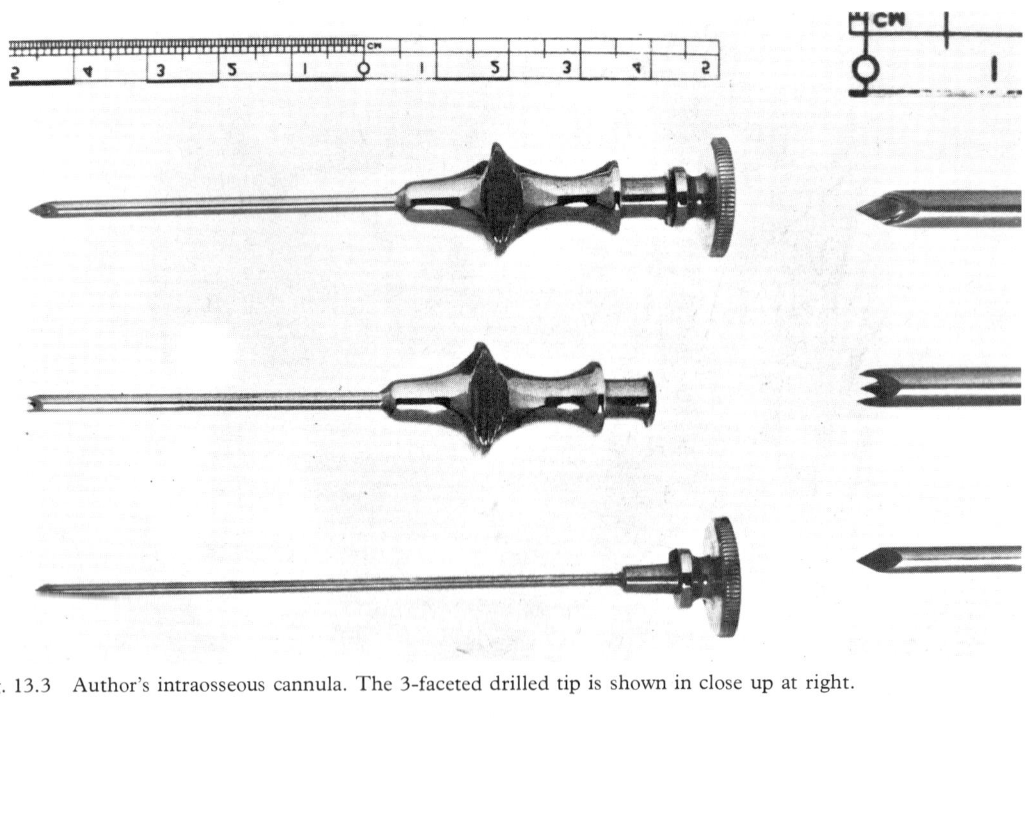

Fig. 13.3 Author's intraosseous cannula. The 3-faceted drilled tip is shown in close up at right.

1969). Often a combined technique is employed with percutaneous femoral injection on the patent side and intraosseous pertrochanteric venography on the obstructed side. Fifty ml of contrast is injected by hand bilaterally in the perfemoral technique and a similar amount of contrast using a pressure pump for the intraosseous method. A series of films of the pelvis and lower inferior vena cava are taken with an A.O.T. automatic serial film changer.

Intraosseous venography (Begg, 1954) whilst most useful in showing incompetent perforating veins can be used to show the deep venous system to exclude thrombosis. An intraosseous cannula 3 cm in length (Lea Thomas et al., 1972) or a bone marrow aspiration needle is introduced into the medial or lateral malleolous using local or general anaesthesia and contrast injected by hand. Films are taken with a screening table as the contrast ascends.

Descending venography

This technique involves injecting contrast medium into the femoral vein in the groin and allowing it to descend by examining the patient in the erect or semi-erect position (Bauer, 1940; Moore, 1951; Luke, 1953). When first described the technique was thought to distinguish between 'competent' and 'incompetent' valves (Bauer, 1948; Lockhart Mummery and Hillyer Smitham, 1951; Boyce, Detar and Vest, 1953) but further experience of the movement of valves by fluoroscopy during the Valsalva manoeuvre (Cockett, 1953; Gryspeerdt, 1953) have shown that contrast flows past normal valves (Fig. 13.5). The degree of retrograde flow in normal veins in the upright position depends partly on the specific gravity of the contrast medium which is heavier than blood, but largely on the force of injection. A forceful retrograde injection will open up the valve cusps so that little of the contrast medium descends in the leg, whereas a slow injection will flow past normal valves. Thus if valves are shown to be present in any deep veins by venography they can be assumed to be normal. Descending venography is more difficult to carry out than ascending venography which, with a Valsalva manoeuvre to show the valves, has now virtually replaced it.

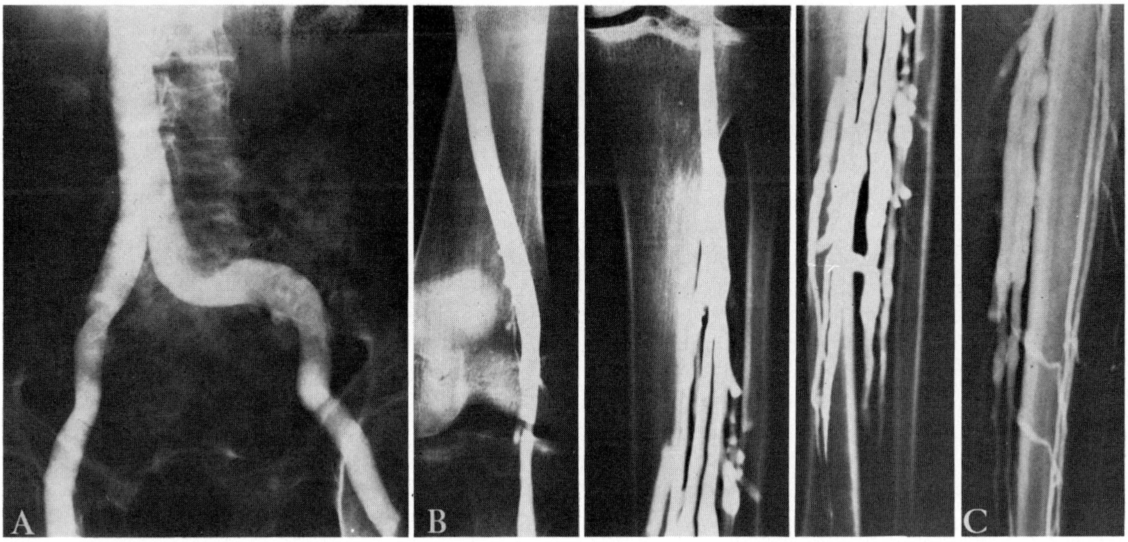

Fig. 13.4 Normal ascending venogram, left leg and pelvis. (a) Iliac veins and lower inferior vena cava demonstrated by foot injection technique. (b) Left femoral and popliteal veins and paired calf stem veins. (c) Lateral veiw of calf veins showing stem and muscle veins.

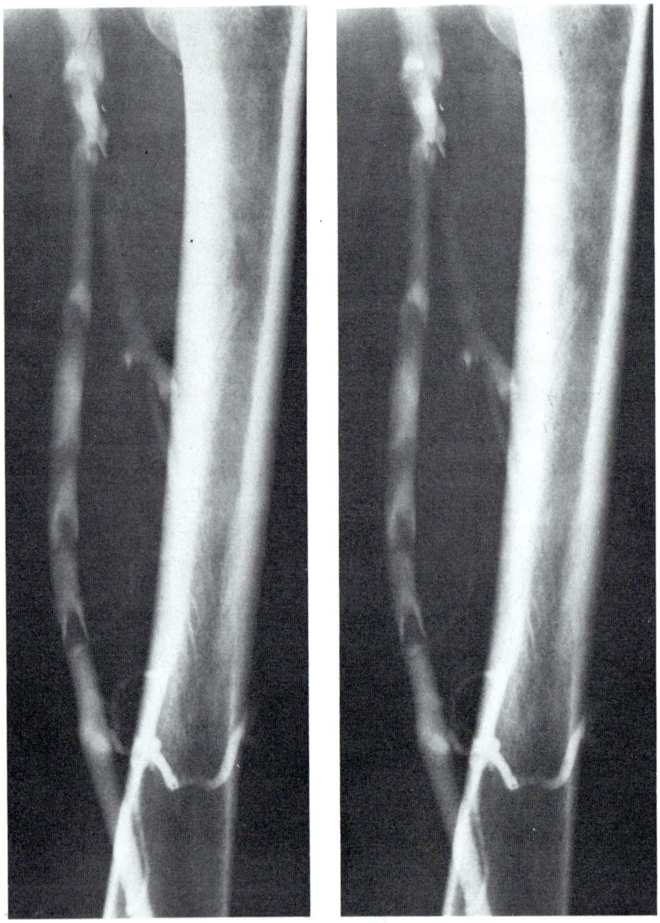

Fig. 13.5 Ascending venogram left femoral vein. Valves are shown clearly by the Valsalva manoeuvre.

Interpretation of venograms

VENOGRAPHIC ANATOMY

The deep veins consist of the deep plantar veins of the foot, the three paired stem veins of the calf which accompany their corresponding arteries, the popliteal vein behind the knee, and in the thigh, the large femoral vein into which the profunda femoris vein drains. The common femoral veins become the external iliac veins at the level of the inguinal ligament and these veins, in the pelvis, drain into the common iliac veins and inferior vena cava. The internal iliac veins are tributaries of the common iliac veins.

The deep muscle veins consist of the soleal veins which drain into the posterior tibial and peroneal veins and the gastrocnemius veins which drain into the popliteal vein (Figs 13.4 and 13.5).

The perforating veins are short vessels passing through the deep fascia which connect the superficial with the deep veins. They are valved, so that blood can only pass from the superficial to the deep veins. Perforating veins are numerous in the foot and at the ankle but become progressively fewer proximally.

The superficial veins which lie in the subcutaneous tissues include the greater and

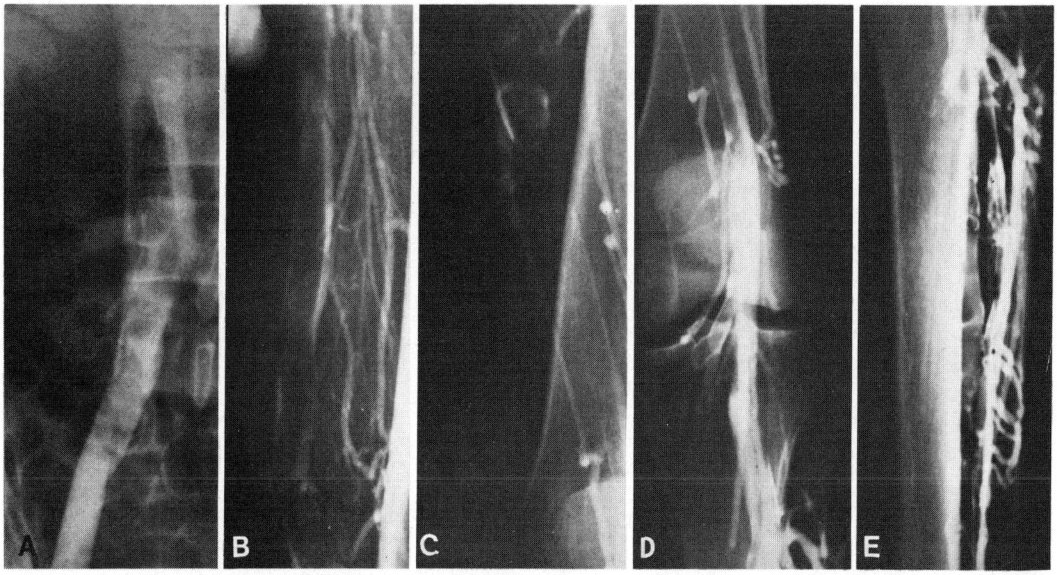

Fig. 13.6 I.V.C., iliac veins and left leg veins demonstrated by ascending phlebogram from foot injections. (Right leg veins normal, not illustrated.) (A) Right external and common iliac veins free of thrombus. The left common and external iliac veins are totally occluded. There is thrombus extending from the left common iliac vein into the inferior vena cava. (B) There is partly adherent thrombus in the femoral vein. Note numerous bypass collaterals. (C) There is partly adherent thrombus in the popliteal vein and lower femoral vein. This thrombus is locked in by the occluded left common iliac vein. A vena comitans functions as a collateral. (D) The popliteal vein is free of thrombus in its distal part. There is recent thrombus in the gastrocnemius veins. There is retracting thrombus shown by thicker rim of contrast medium on lateral aspect in the proximal part of the popliteal vein. (E) There is loose thrombus in the medial peroneal vein. There is adherent thrombus in the lateral peroneal vein. The posterior tibial vein is totally occluded. The anterior tibial veins are free of thrombus.

lesser saphenous systems emptying into the femoral and popliteal veins respectively.

The normal deep veins are smooth, branching and become progressively wider as they pass upwards. Valves are present in them, most numerous in the calf and becoming fewer proximally. Generally no valves are present in the external and common iliac veins or inferior vena cava. The internal iliac venous system is valved. If valves are demonstrated they can be assumed to be normal (Fig. 13.5). Valves may be destroyed by recanalisation following thrombosis or very rarely may be congenitally absent in the femoral and popliteal veins.

VENOGRAPHIC APPEARANCES OF THROMBUS

Unequivocal venous thrombus shown by venography produces a well defined filling defect in an opacified vein, which presents a constant appearance both on screening and on at least two films taken with an interval between them. Loose thrombus is surrounded by a thin white line of contrast medium. Obliteration of this white line indicates adherence of thrombus (Figs 13.2 and 13.6). When thrombus obstructs a vein, or a segment of vein completely, the obstruction is bypassed by contrast filled collaterals (Fig. 13.6). Thrombus which is adherent cannot embolise and loose thrombus distal to it is also prevented from embolising (Fig. 13.6). These are important points in the management of thromboembolic disease.

The proximal end of a loose thrombus frequently forms a tail lying free in the blood stream and if this breaks off to embolise, it leaves a straight upper margin.

The full extent of thombosis must be shown in all patients (Fig. 13.6).

Appearances which may mimic thrombus

Most filling defects due to normal structures such as valves, and artefacts due to underfilling, dilution and streaming of contrast medium can be avoided with the screening technique described above. The Valsalva manoeuvre makes valves easier to identify (Fig. 13.5) and fills tributaries of the main veins where entry of non-opacified blood may mimic thrombus. A series of films of the iliac veins and inferior vena cava excludes artefacts in these veins as thrombus

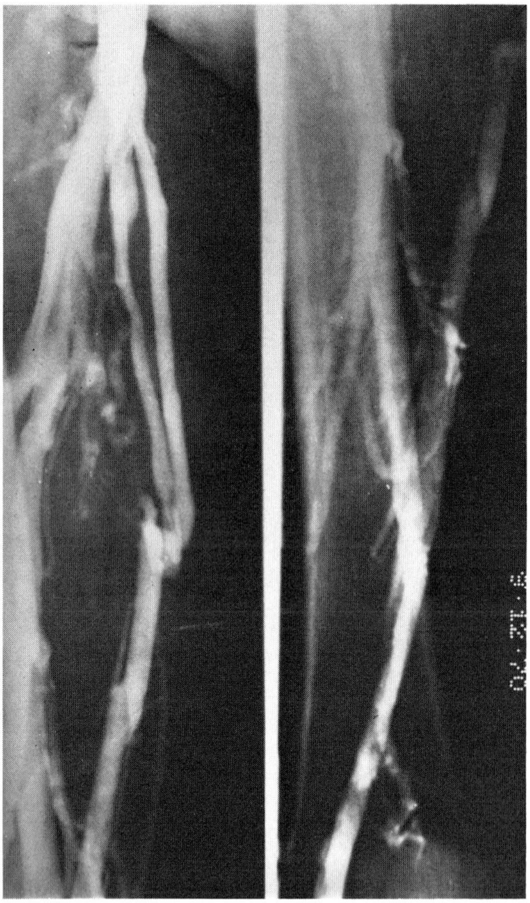

Fig. 13.7 Recanalised right femoral vein shown by ascending venography. The distal part of the femoral vein and the popliteal vein are irregular and no valves are demonstrated. The femoral vein is occluded in the mid-thigh and replaced by 2 venae commitantes functioning as collaterals.

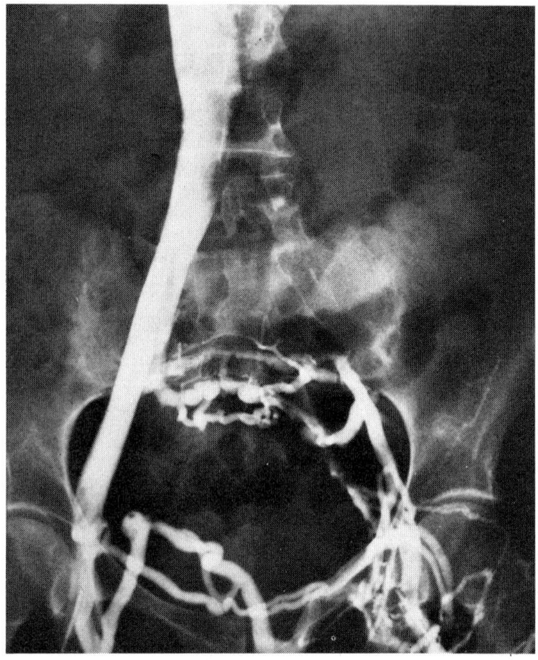

Fig. 13.8 Iliac venogram by percutaneous right femoral injection and left pertrochanteric intraosseous injection. There are recanalisation changes in the upper part of the left femoral vein and the external iliac vein. The left common iliac vein is totally occluded. Note dilated collaterals passing from left to right through the superficial epigastric vein, pubic veins and presacral plexus.

presents a constant appearance in several films.

VENOGRAPHIC APPEARANCES OF RECANALISATION AND INCOMPETENT PERFORATING VEINS

Recanalised deep veins have absent valves and an irregular and sometimes a multiple channelled lumen (Fig. 13.7). Narrowed or occluded veins are bypassed by collaterals (Figs 13.8 and 13.9).

In order to show incompetent perforating veins by ascending venography the superficial veins must be totally occluded by the ankle tourniquet so that contrast can be seen by fluoroscopy to pass from the deep to the superficial venous system through an incompetent perforating vein (Fig. 13.10). Preferential filling of the deep venous system is also achieved by a steep 40° foot-down table tilt. Once the origin of one incompetent

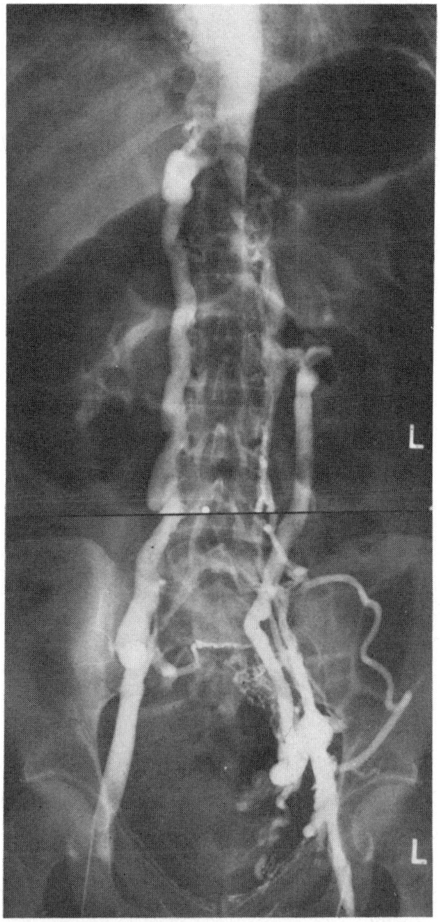

Fig. 13.9 Bilateral perfemoral inferior vena cavogram showing total occlusion of the inferior vena cava and re-canalisation changes in the left common and external iliac veins. The main collaterals are the azygos vein, ascending lumbar vein and ovarian vein. The deep circumflex iliac vein also functions as a collateral. None of these collaterals were clinically demonstrable.

perforating vein has been demonstrated, the contrast medium is flushed away with normal saline and another tourniquet applied above the first incompetent vein so that superficial filling does not obscure the origins of other incompetent perforating veins. This procedure is repeated using television monitoring until all incompetent perforating veins, including any in Hunter's canal, have been displayed. A Valsalva manoeuvre is helpful to display more proximal incompetent perforating veins (Fig. 13.11).

An accuracy rate of 80 per cent for this technique has been claimed (Lea Thomas, McAllister and Tonge, 1972).

Intraosseous injection of contrast medium into the medial malleolus is probably the most accurate method of demonstrating incompetent perforating veins as by this method the medium passes directly into the deep venous system (Townsend, Jones and

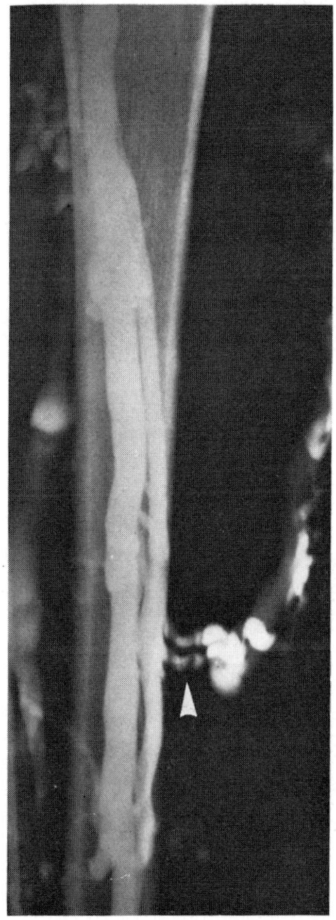

Fig. 13.10 Incompetent perforating vein shown by ascending venography. The incompetent perforating vein arises from the medial posterior tibial vein. On screening the contrast passed from the posterior tibial vein into the incompetent perforating vein (arrow). The incompetent perforating vein is duplicated, dilated, irregular and there is a superficial varix.

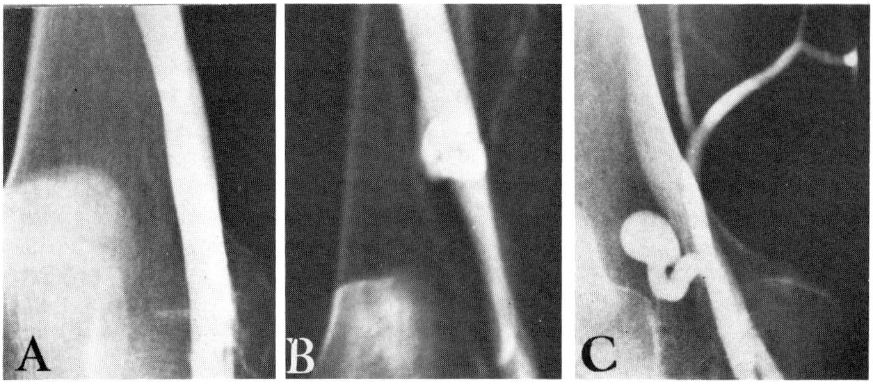

Fig. 13.11 Incompetent perforating vein in Hunter's canal shown by ascending venography with a Valsalva manoeuvre. (A) The incompetent perforating vein is not demonstrated. (B & C) Progressive filling of the vein during Valsalva manoeuvre.

Williams, 1967). Its disadvantage is that being painful a general anaesthetic is usually required. However, the examination can be carried out as an immediate pre-operative procedure in the operating theatre. Care must be taken not to introduce an intraosseous cannula through ulcerated skin because of the risk of osteomyelitis and alternative sites for injection which may be used include the lateral malleolus and the os calcis.

A single straight radiographic projection is usually sufficient, lateral views being confusing due to overlapping of contrast filled veins.

Incompetent perforating veins are frequently paired, tortuous and may have a superficial varix (Fig. 13.10).

To overcome the objection that it is difficult to relate the sites of incompetent perforating veins shown by venography to patients' legs, it is suggested that the radiographs with the incompetent veins marked on them with a grease pencil are placed on the patients' legs and these marks transcribed to the legs with a felt pen.

THE POST-THROMBOTIC SYNDROME OF THE ILIAC VEINS AND INFERIOR VENA CAVA

The following abnormalities may be shown by venography:

(a) Complete occlusion of the whole or part of one or other external or common iliac veins or inferior vena cava (Figs 13.8 and 13.9).

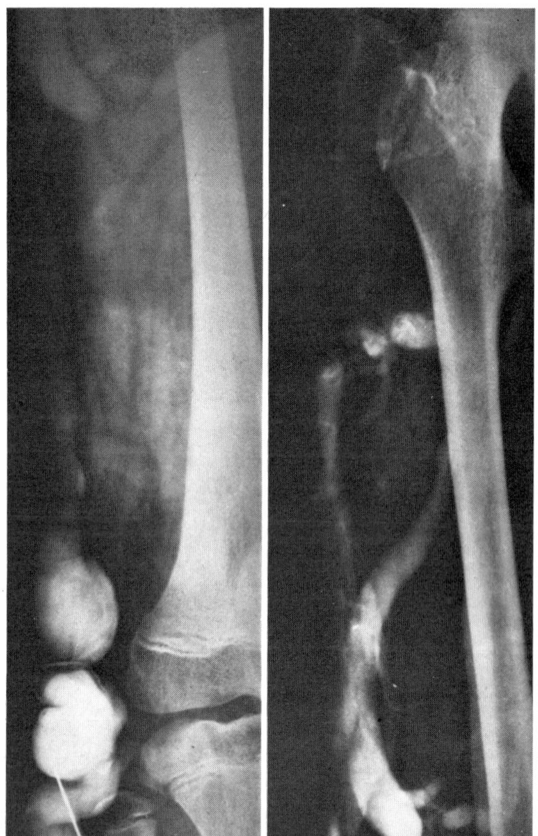

Fig. 13.12 Direct injection venogram in Klippel-Trenaunay syndrome. Injection of the large lateral venous trunk shows its connection with the profunda vein.

(b) Recanalisation of veins (Figs 13.8 and 13.9).

(c) The presence of dilated collaterals (Figs 13.8 and 13.9).

The site of these collaterals depends on the site of obstruction. In localised common iliac vein or inferior vena caval obstruction, the main collaterals are through the presacral and vertebral plexuses whereas only when the obstruction extends down as far as the common femoral vein, do the clinically obvious superficial epigastric and superficial circumflex iliac veins function as collaterals. Hence the importance of venography in the diagnosis of obstruction of the pelvic veins (Lea Thomas and Fletcher, 1967).

VENOGRAPHY IN VENOUS DYSPLASIAS

In venous dysplasias such as the Klippel-Trenaunay syndrome, in addition to ascending venography, it is sometimes helpful to inject contrast directly into the angiomatous malformation to show any connection with the deep veins. Direct injection may also outline the deep venous system which can be difficult to fill by conventional ascending phlebography (Lea Thomas and Macfie, 1974).

RADIO-ACTIVE FIBRINOGEN UPTAKE

The ^{125}I-fibrinogen uptake technique

Human serum fibrinogen labelled with radioactive iodine when injected into the circulation is incorporated into a thrombus and can be detected by an external scintillation counter (Hobbs and Davies, 1960; Atkins and Hawkins, 1965) (Fig. 13.13). 50 to 100 microcuries ^{125}I labelled fibrinogen* is injected intravenously after thyroid uptake of iodine has been blocked with oral inorganic iodine (sodium iodide 150 mg 24 hours before injecting the ^{125}I and continued daily for 3 weeks) and measurement of radioactivity is subsequently made over the right ventricle and at marked points along the main veins of the legs using either a scaler or a ratemeter. A popular ratemeter which is suitable for clinical work is the isotope localisation monitor 235, DA Pitman (Fig. 13.14). Counting points are marked at 4-inch intervals on the skin of the thigh and calf using indelible ink (Fig. 13.15). The count rate at each point is

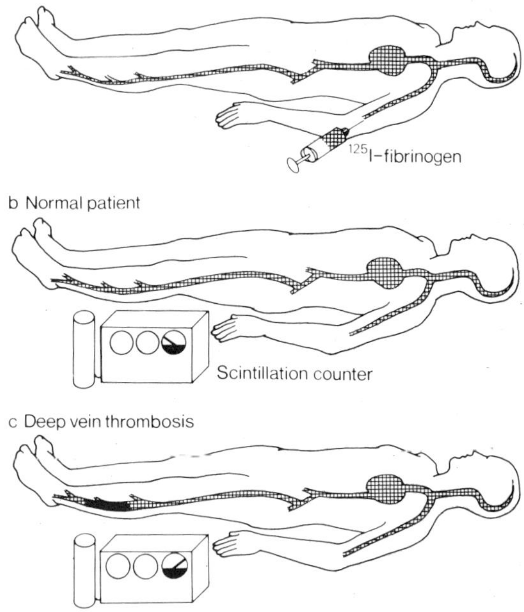

Fig. 13.13 The set up for I^{125} Fibrinogen uptake measurement (diagrammatic).

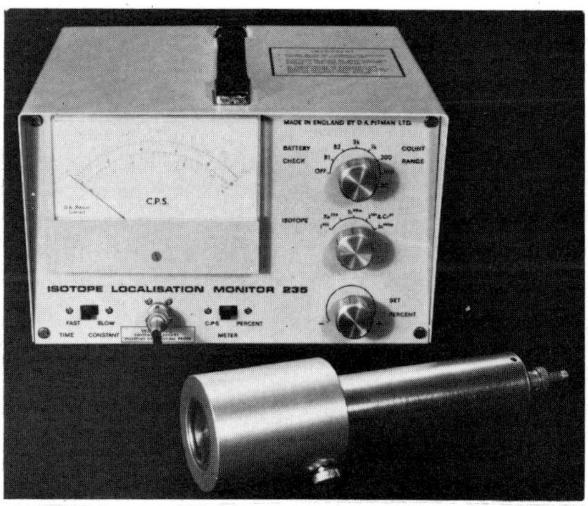

Fig. 13.14 An Isotope localization monitor and scanning head.

* Obtainable from the radio-chemical Centre, U.K. Atomic Energy Authority, Amersham, Bucks.

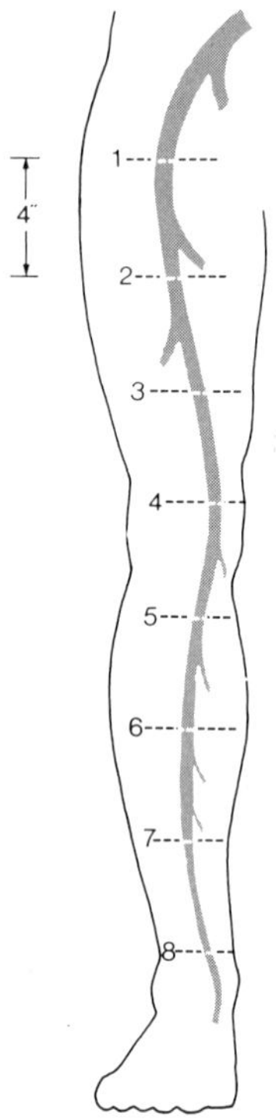

Fig. 13.15 Marked points along the leg and thigh at which count rates are recorded daily.

expressed as a percentage of the heart count measured on the same occasion, and the resulting figure, the 'percentage uptake', is compared with the previous day's figure and those of adjacent sites on the leg. This method of working allows for biological and radioactive decay. Comparison with phlebography has shown that a rise in count rate of 20 per cent at any point which persists and increases on subsequent occasions indicates thrombus formation (Fig. 13.16).

The ^{125}I fibrinogen uptake technique will accurately detect small thrombi in the lower leg and thigh up to within 4 inches of the inguinal ligament but it cannot be used in the presence of healing wounds or haematoma formation and therefore cannot be used following operation to the legs (Flanc et al., 1968; Negus et al., 1968). In the groin and abdomen the blood background is too high for accurate detection of local increases in fibrinogen concentration. The ^{125}I fibrinogen uptake technique should not be used in young or pregnant patients because of the radiation hazard.

As a research tool, the ^{125}I fibrinogen uptake technique has provided much useful information about the incidence and time of development of post-operative venous thrombosis. Studies at several centres show an overall incidence of post-operative deep vein thrombosis in about 28 per cent of middle aged and elderly patients (Browse and Negus, 1970). Most of these thromboses are small, confined to the calf vein and of no clinical significance.

^{125}I fibrinogen uptake studies have shown that these small thrombi are more common in the elderly and that abdominal and thoracic operations carry a higher risk than head and neck or breast surgery. These studies have also shown that deep vein thrombosis is particularly common in patients with malignant disease and in those undergoing splenectomy, hip operations and retropubic as opposed to transurethral prostatectomy (Browse et al., 1974). Fibrinogen uptake has also shown that following severe myocardial infarction a large proportion of

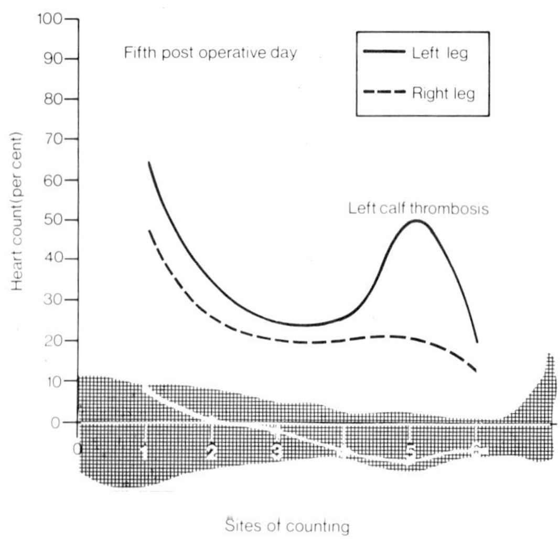

Fig. 13.16 Typical 'percentage uptake graph' in a patient with a left calf thrombosis.

patients develop small deep vein thromboses.

The fibrinogen uptake technique has also shown that the majority of post-operative calf thromboses start *early*, either during or very soon after operation. This observation has stimulated investigation of methods of prophylaxis aimed at the pre-operative and immediate post-operative method, and these methods have been evaluated by the ^{125}I fibrinogen technique. They are fully described in Chapter 15.

Fibrinogen uptake has only a small place in clinical practice. It is an accurate method of screening high risk patients undergoing operation. Although it would seem advisable to screen all high risk patients, the method is little used in practice for two reasons. Firstly it is relatively expensive and more time consuming than Doppler ultrasound, and secondly because most of the thrombi detected with ^{125}I fibrinogen are so small and insignificant as to require no treatment whatsoever.

The fibrinogen uptake test has very little place in the diagnosis of clinically suspected deep vein thrombosis. The method depends on the incorporation of isotope labelled fibrinogen into a forming thrombus, and it is hardly surprising that *formed* thrombus may take up little or no labelled fibrinogen. Browse and others found only an 84 per cent correlation with phlebography as against 95 per cent correlation in prospective trials where the labelled fibrinogen is injected *before* thrombus formation. Similarly, Mavor and his co-workers (1972) found that the fibrinogen uptake technique often failed to diagnose deep vein thrombosis in patients presenting with pulmonary embolism. This is not in the least surprising; indeed it is remarkable that the fibrinogen uptake technique ever detects formed thrombus.

It cannot be emphasised too strongly that the ^{125}I fibrinogen uptake technique is primarily a research tool. As such it has been, and is still, of considerable value in producing information about the natural history and prophylaxis of deep vein thrombosis and it must not be expected to compete with phlebography in the diagnosis of the suspected case.

Summary of present position of this test

1. It is primarily a research tool, and as such has provided useful information about the natural history and prevention of deep vein thrombosis.
2. It may not detect 'formed thrombus', so it is not necessarily accurate in emergency cases in detecting the presence of relatively large amounts of thrombus in the deep veins.
3. It can only be used accurately in the limbs.
4. It cannot be used if there is any wound, injury, or bruise or even oedema in a limb. This therefore puts it out of count in any case of operation on a leg (i.e. a large part of vascular surgery).
5. It is expensive, and needs the specially prepared ^{125}I fibrinogen and it does need special training and experience to work with it accurately.

DOPPLER ULTRASOUND TECHNIQUE

The transcutaneous Doppler ultrasound flow detection method detects changes in the flow velocity, such changes being electronically converted either into sound or into a graphic record (Fig. 13.17). The apparatus consists of a small portable box (Sonicaid D 205 or Parks Doppler model 801 or 802) (Fig. 13.18) to which is connected a light probe. The latter contains two crystals, one emitting, the other receiving high frequency

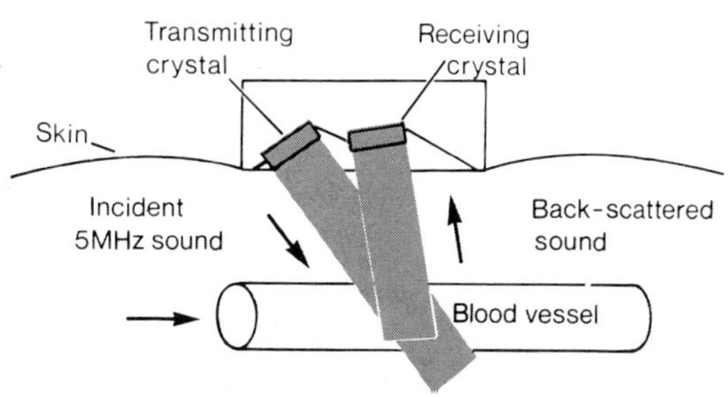

Fig. 13.17 The principle of the ultra-sound probe.

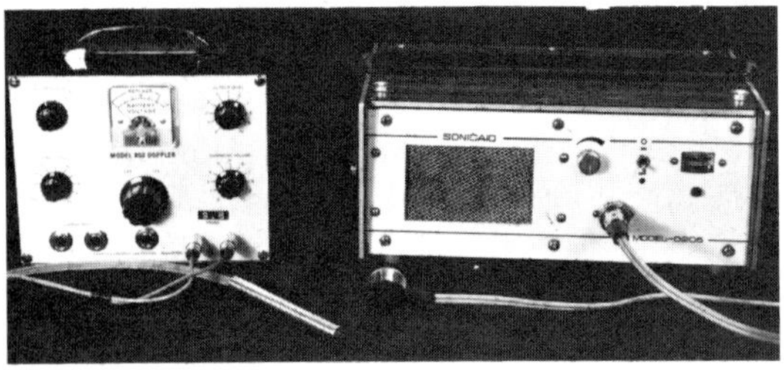

Fig. 13.18 The *Sonicaid D205* model on the right, and the *Parks Doppler 802* on the left.

sound. A change in flow velocity under the probe produces a change in frequency and a signal from the machine. Arterial pulsation can, therefore, be detected but the relatively slow venous flow does not produce a signal. Such a signal can, however, be produced either by squeezing the limb distal to the probe (Strandness et al., 1967; Sigel et al., 1968), or by changes in respiration which alter the flow in the iliac veins and inferior vena cava (Yao et al., 1972).

Technique

The patient is placed sitting up with the legs dependent and the ankles supported in order to encourage blood to pool in the calves. The probe is placed over the common femoral vein and the calf and lower thigh are squeezed by hand in turn. Patency of the distal veins is indicated by a sudden loud noise from the machine. The patient is then asked to take a deep breath and to perform the Valsalva manoeuvre and patency is again indicated by a distinctive wind-like roaring. Obstruction to flow is indicated by silence from the apparatus (Fig. 13.19).

The Doppler ultrasound technique has been established as accurate in detecting thrombosis from the level of the popliteal vein to the inferior vena cava by comparison with phlebography (Evans and Cockett, 1969; Yao et al., 1972).

Advantages and limitations

Doppler ultrasound has the great merits of simplicity, speed and cheapness, and with a little training and experience can be safely and usefully used by medical students or house surgeons. The method is incapable of detecting thrombosis confined to the calf; this disadvantage is less serious than it may at first seem, as calf thrombi, though by far the most common of deep vein thromboses, are unlikely to produce significant pulmonary embolism unless propagation has reached the popliteal vein or above (Evans, 1971).

Doppler ultrasound can be usefully used for routine screening of patients recovering from major thoracic and abdominal surgery. Middle aged and elderly patients should be examined daily. The method can also be used for the rapid investigation of patients with suspected deep vein thrombosis, whether this presents in the leg or as pulmonary embolism.

Loose thrombi may sometimes cause so little obstruction of the vein lumen that they are undetectable by the Doppler ultrasound technique. For this reason a suspicious finding by Doppler ultrasound must be investigated immediately by phlebography This is particularly important in patients presenting with pulmonary embolus, when the thrombus

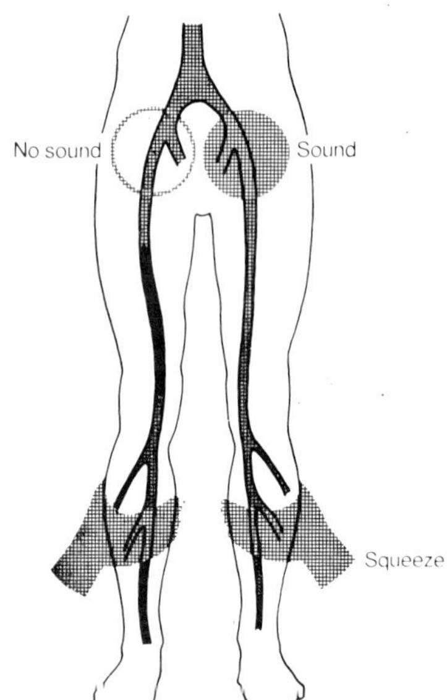

Fig. 13.19 Ultrasound findings in a case with thrombus in the right femoral vein (diagrammatic).

is more likely to be floating and failing to obstruct the venous return.

Summary

Main practical advantages of this method:

1. Cheap, portable, easy, requires no trained personnel.

2. *Will* detect the major thrombi of a size likely to cause serious pulmonary embolism.

3. Will not detect small calf thrombi (which, however, are not a threat for serious embolism).

4. Is essentially a quick screening procedure. Positive or suspicious findings with this method should be followed *at once* by emergency phlebography to get the accurate information.

PULMONARY ANGIOGRAPHY

Indications

Apart from the use of pulmonary angiography to show stenoses of the pulmonary artery and its branches, lesions of the left heart and aorta, or the presence of a left to right shunt, the main indication for pulmonary angiography is in suspected pulmonary embolic disease.

Technique

A No. 7 or 8 NIH angiocatheter, flushed with heparinised saline, is passed from a vein in the right arm through the right atrium, the right ventricle and across the pulmonary valve into the main pulmonary artery under screen control. During passage of the catheter the patient is monitored with an E.C.G. and continuous pressure measurements are recorded. The catheter is positioned with its tip in the main pulmonary artery midway between the pulmonary valve and the bifurcation of the main pulmonary artery and its position checked by a test injection of contrast medium. A control 35·6 cm × 35·6 cm film is taken for radiographic exposure using an A.O.T. serial film changer. The film should be slightly more penetrated than a conventional chest radiograph. Fifty to 60 ml of Urografin 76 per cent is injected at 500 PSI and serial films taken 4 to 5 per second for 2 to 3 seconds followed by a slower rate for a further 2 to 3 seconds. Anteroposterior radiographs alone are exposed as, in the lateral projection, the circulations of the two lungs are superimposed. During exposure of the films the patient holds his breath in deep inspiration as hyperventilation produces better detail of the pulmonary vasculature.

If specialised equipment is not available, a single film of both lungs taken between 2 and 4 seconds after the beginning of a bilateral simultaneous injection of 50 ml of contrast through large bore needles in veins in the antecubital fossa will usually produce a diagnostic demonstration of the pulmonary arterial system.

Complications

The only serious complications, cardiac arrythmias and arrest, occur in patients with pulmonary hypertension. These result from the reduction in cardiac output due to the vasodilatation caused by the contrast medium. It is for this reason that the pulmonary artery pressure should be known before contrast is injected. The vasodilatation can be counteracted by producing vasoconstriction before injection of the contrast. Phenylnephrine 0.3 mg is given intravenously and repeated if necessary until the systemic systolic blood pressure is about 20 mmHg above its original level. Volume overload by the injection of 200 ml of Dextran also helps to maintain the cardiac output.

Even taking these precautions pulmonary angiography carries a significant morbidity in patients with pulmonary hypertension.

Interpretation

NORMAL ANATOMY

The main pulmonary artery which forms part of the left mediastinal border divides into right and left main pulmonary arteries. The right main pulmonary artery is longer than the left and passes behind the ascending aorta and superior vena cava to enter the right lung anterior to the bronchus. The left pulmonary artery arches to the left and downwards and enters the lung slightly from above and behind the main bronchus. The pulmonary artery branches are closely related to the corresponding bronchi and have a similar distribution (Fig. 13.20).

The pulmonary veins, on the other hand, do not accompany the pulmonary arteries or the bronchi, although their drainage corresponds to the bronchial segments. Anatomical variants, particularly of the veins, are common.

As the branches of the main pulmonary arteries pass peripherally they branch and gradually become smaller in calibre. In a normal pulmonary arteriogram it is usually possible to identify the segmental branches as far as the 4th or 5th divisions.

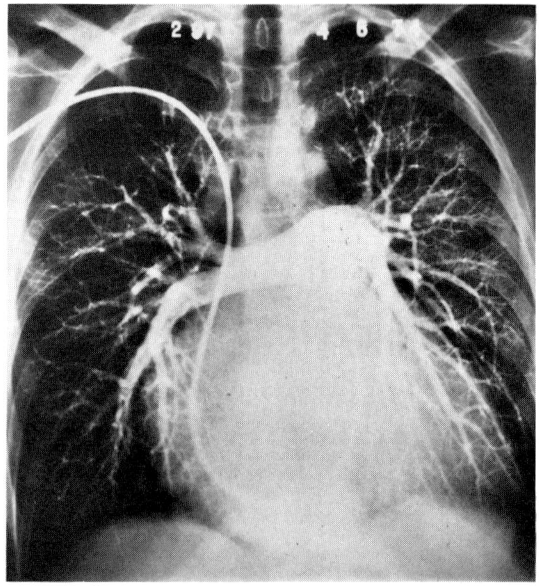

Fig. 13.20 Normal pulmonary arteriogram. The branches of the main pulmonary arteries follow the distribution of the corresponding bronchi. The branches become narrower and divide as they approach the periphery. (Radiograph by courtesy of Dr Ian Kerr.)

PULMONARY EMBOLISM

In acute pulmonary embolism the main pulmonary artery or its branches, show radiolucent filling defects in filled arteries outlined by contrast medium. This is the only absolutely diagnostic feature of pulmonary embolism (Ferris et al., 1967; Williams and Wilcox, 1968; Williams et al., 1968; Hume et al., 1970). Non-filling of vessels, areas of slow perfusion, vascular tortuosity and delay in clearance of contrast medium from affected segments, are secondary signs. (Fig. 13.21).

Multiple peripheral emboli may produce clinical shock, right heart failure and death. Correlation of plain film changes, angiography and the results of isotope lung scanning, may be required to reach a correct diagnosis.

In chronic pulmonary hypertension the central pulmonary arteries are dilated and there is narrowing, tortuosity and pruning of small dilated vessels together with areas of peripheral non-perfusion. Such appearances are not specific to multiple peripheral pulmonary embolic disease and can be seen in patients with other causes for pulmonary hypertension such as congenital heart disease.

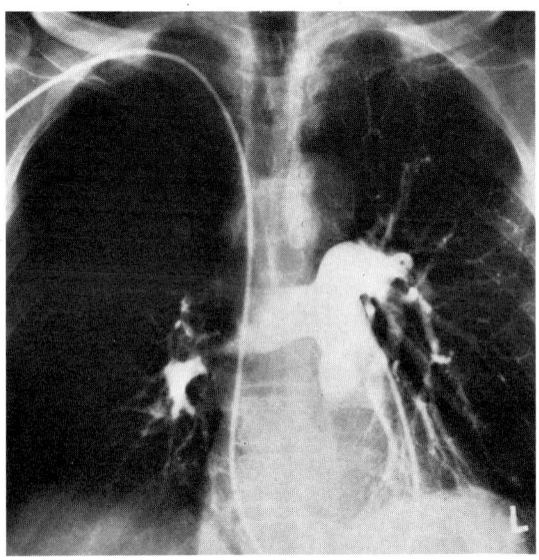

Fig. 13.21 Pulmonary angiogram in major pulmonary embolism. Note the large pulmonary embolus almost totally occluding the right main pulmonary artery. The branches to the left upper lobe are diminished indicating occlusions by other emboli.

LUNG SCANNING

Clinical indications

Lung scans, which detect areas of impaired pulmonary perfusion, are a useful diagnostic technique when pulmonary emboli are suspected in the *presence of a normal chest X-ray* and the *absence of a history of asthma or chronic obstructive airways disease* (Secker-Walker, 1968). They may also detect emboli when the chest X-ray is abnormal, as perfusion defects may be detected in areas other than those abnormal on the chest X-ray.

Technique

Macroaggregated albumin or albumin microspheres are labelled with ^{99m}Tc, ^{131}I or other appropriate radio isotope. The labelling procedures are much simplified by using commercial kits. Before the technique can be used on patients advice is needed from a physicist and pharmacist. The labelled macroaggregates or microspheres are injected intravenously slowly over the course of 2 minutes. During the injection the patient should lie comfortably on his back and take slow deep breaths in order to ventilate the lungs. After the injection has been completed the distribution of radioactivity can be recorded using either a rectilinear scanner or a gamma camera (Fig. 13.22). The latter, which is a more complicated and more expensive piece of equipment, has the advantage that the images can be taken with the patient sitting up. This is useful if the patient is dyspnoeic or has pleuritic pain. The gamma camera produces the result (a lung 'snap') within 5 minutes, whereas the scanner takes 15 to 20 minutes to complete each view.

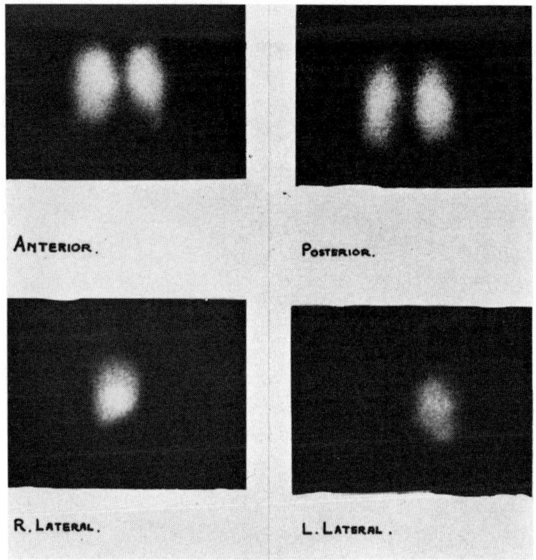

Fig. 13.23 A normal perfusion lung scan showing anterior, posterior and two lateral views.

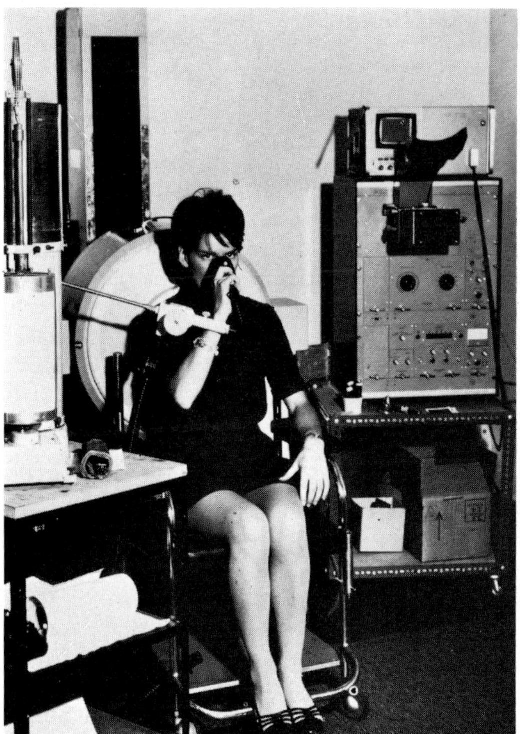

Fig. 13.22 A gamma camera in use during a ^{133}Xenon ventilation lung scan.

The procedure is safe so long as the patient does not have chronic and severe pulmonary hypertension. The particles after injection flood into the pulmonary vasculature and occlude about 1 in 10,000 of the pulmonary capilliaries for a few hours. This has no observable effect on the patient. In the presence of severe pulmonary hypertension, in which the pulmonary vascular bed is greatly diminished, the technique should be used with caution as there are a few recorded deaths (Williams, 1974). Under these circumstances the injection should be given

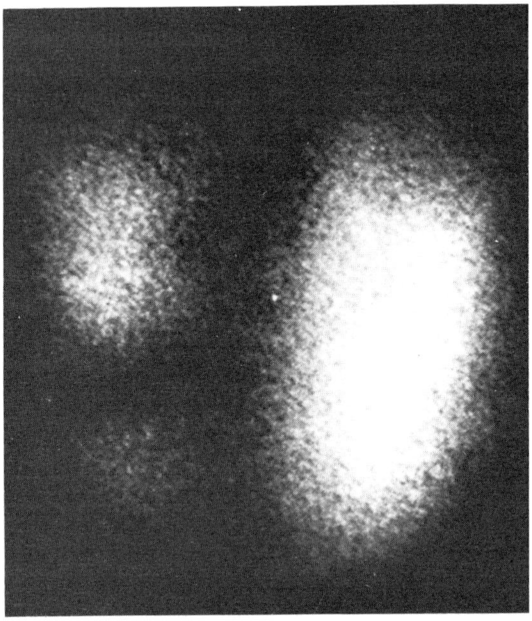

Fig. 13.24 Abnormal posterior perfusion scan showing a large perfusion defect on the left in the mid-zone.

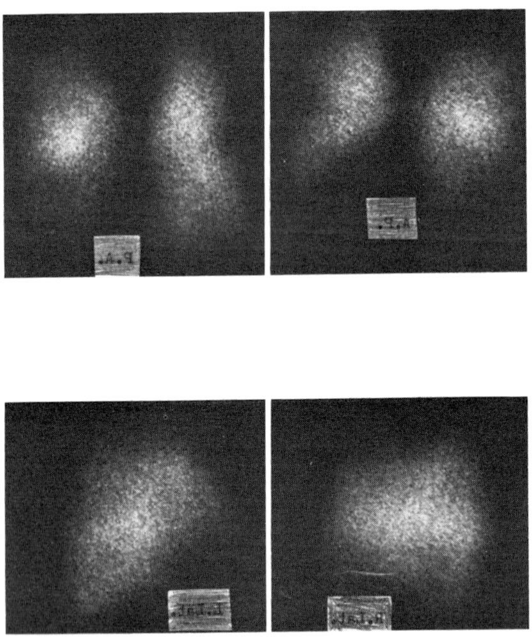

Fig. 13.25 Abnormal perfusion scan showing defects which are obvious on the anterior and posterior views (top of figure, left and right respectively).

very slowly by a trained doctor who has immediate access to resuscitation equipment.

Interpretation (Deland and Wagner, 1970)

NORMAL

Four views are obtained: anterior, posterior, right lateral and left lateral (Fig. 13.23). The posterior view is the single most useful as it visualises most of both lung fields. The heart causes a defect which is visible at the left base under normal circumstances. If it is enlarged there is an increased area of defective perfusion at the left base. In women the breasts may cause decreased activity at both bases on the anterior, but not the posterior, view.

ABNORMAL

Focal areas of impaired perfusion, when associated with a normal chest X-ray and no history of asthma or bronchitis, are virtually diagnostic of pulmonary emboli (Figs 13.24 and 13.25). False-positive results may arise in areas of healed tuberculosis that are not apparent in the chest X-ray, and in areas of radiation damage. Experience is needed for the correct interpretation of lung scans, and it is important to appreciate that areas of impaired perfusion may occur for many reasons other than pulmonary emboli.

In order to overcome the problem created by asthma and chronic obstructive airways disease we have developed the combined ventilation-perfusion lung scan (Williams et al., 1974). In this technique ^{133}Xenon gas is inhaled and the distribution of radioactivity on the lung snap detects areas of defective ventilation. Perfusion is also abnormal in these areas. These perfusion defects are not due to pulmonary emboli but are secondary to the ventilation defect. Pulmonary emboli cause areas of defective perfusion that ventilate normally (ventilation-perfusion discrepancy). This type of defect is highly correlated (85 per cent) with the presence of ^{125}I fibrinogen positive venous thrombosis in the legs, which confirms its value in the diagnosis of emboli (Browse et al., 1974). In order to do ventilation-perfusion lung scans it is necessary to have a gamma camera.

In conclusion lung scanning is a useful aid to the diagnosis of pulmonary emboli. It is safe, does not cause discomfort to the patient and can be completed in a half to one hour. For reliable results it requires a team that is experienced in performing the technique, and in interpreting the result.

REFERENCES

Allen, E. V. & Barker, N. W. (1934) *Proc. Mayo. Clin.*, **9**, 571.

Atkins, P. & Hawkins, L. A. (1965) *Lancet*, **2**, 1217.

Bauer, G. A. (1940) *Acta chir. scand.*, **84**, suppl. 61.

Bauer, G. A. (1941) *Acta med. scand.*, **107**, 136.

Bauer, G. A. (1948) *J. int. Chir.*, **8**, 937.

Begg, A. C. (1954) *Brit. J. Radiol.*, **27**, 318.

Berberich, J. & Hirsch, S. (1923) *Klin. Wschr.*, **2**, 2226.

Boyce, W. H., Detar, J. H. & Vest, S. A. (1953) *Surg. Gynec. Obstet.*, **96**, 471.

Browse, N. L. & Negus, D. (1970) *Brit. Med. J.*, **3**, 615.

Browse, N. L., Clapham, W. F., Croft, D., Jones, D. J., Lea Thomas, M. & Williams, J. O. (1971) *Brit. Med. J.*, **4**, 325.

Browse, N. L., Clementson, G. & Croft, D. N. (1974) Fibrinogen-detectable thrombosis in the legs and pulmonary embolism. *Brit. Med. J.*, **1**, 603–604.

Cockett, F. B. (1953) *Brit. J. Radiol.*, **36**, 339.

Deland, F. H. & Wagner, H. N. (1970) *Atlas of Nuclear Medicine*, Volume 2, Lung and Heart. Philadelphia: W. B. Saunders.

Dos Santos, J. C. (1938) *J. int. Surg.*, **3**, 625.

Dougherty, J. & Homans, J. (1940) *Venography, A Clinical Study.*

Dow, J. D. (1951) *J. Fac. Radiol.*, **2**, 180.

Edwards, E. A. & Biguria, F. (1934) *New Engl. J. Med.*, **211**, 589.

Evans, D. S. & Cockett, F. B. (1969) *Brit. Med. J.*, **2**, 802.

Evans, D. S. (1971) *Ann. Roy. Coll. Surg.*, **49**, 225.

Ferris, E. J., Stanzler, R. M., Rourke, J. A., Blumenthal, J. & Messer, J. V. (1967) Pulmonary angiography in pulmonary embolic disease. *Amer. J. Roentgen.*, **46**, 610.

Flanc, C., Kakkar, V. V. & Clarke, M. B. (1968) *Brit. J. Surg.*, **55**, 742.

Gryspeerdt, G. L. (1953) *Brit. J. Radiol.*, **26**, 329.

Halliday, P. (1968) *Brit. J. Surg.*, **55**, 220.

Hellsten, W. (1942) *Acta. chir. scand.*, **86**, suppl. 73

Hobbs, J. T. & Davies, J. W. L. (1960) *Lancet*, **2**, 134.

Hume, M., Sevitt, S. & Thomas, D. P. (1970) *Venous Thrombosis and Pulmonary Embolism.* Harvard University Press.

Lea Thomas, M. & Fletcher, E. W. L. (1967) *J. Anat. Lond.*, **3**, 627.

Lea Thomas, M. & Fletcher, E. W. L. (1967) *Clinical Radiology*, **18**, 399.

Lea Thomas, M. (1969) *Brit. J. Radiol.*, **42**, 395.

Lea Thomas, M. (1970) *Proc. roy. Soc. Med.*, **63**, 123.

Lea Thomas, M., McAllister, V. & Tonge, K. (1971) *Clin. Radiol.*, **22**, 495.

Lea Thomas, M. (1972) *Arc. Surg.*, **104**, 145.

Lea Thomas, M., McAllister, V., Rose, D. J. & Tonge, K. (1972) *Clin. Radiol.*, **23**, 486.

Lea Thomas, M. & Tighe, J. R. (1973) *Lancet*, **2**, 1415.

Lea Thomas, M. & Macfie, G. B. (1974) *Acta Radiol.*, **15**, 43.

Lockhart Mummery, H. E. & Hillyer Smitham, J. (1951) *Brit. J. Surg.*, **38**, 284.

Luke, J. C. (1941) *Surg. Gynec. Obstet.*, **73**, 472.

Luke, J. C. (1943) *Canad. Med. Ass. J.*, **49**, 86.

May, R. (1965) *Nuclear Energy*, **4**, 120.

McPheeters, H. O. & Rice, C. O. (1929) *Surg. Gynec. Obstet.*, **49**, 29.

Moore, H. D. (1939) *Brit. J. Surg.*, **37**, 78.

Negus, D., Pinto, D. J., Le Quesne, L. P., Brown, N. & Chapman, M. (1968) *Brit. J. Surg.*, **55**, 835.

Secker-Walker (1968) Scintillation scanning of lungs in diagnosis of pulmonary embolism. *Brit. Med. J.*, **2**, 206–308.

Sigel, B., Popsky, G. L., Wagner, D. K., Boland, J. P., Mapp, E. McD. & Feigl, P. (1968) *Surg. St. Louis*, **64**, 332.

Strandness, D. E., Schultz, R. D., Sumner, D. S. & Rushmer, R. F. (1967) *Amer. J. Surg.*, **113**, 311.

Townsend, J., Jones, H. & Williams, J. E. (1967) *Brit. Med. J.*, **3**, 583

Williams, J. R. & Wilcox, W. C. (1963) Pulmonary embolism: Roentgengraphic and angiographic considerations. *Amer. J. Roentgen.*, **89**, 333.

Williams, J. R., Wilcox, W. C., Andrews, G. J. & Burns, R. R. (1968) Angiography and pulmonary embolism. *J. Amer. med. Ass.*, **184**, 473.

Williams, J. O. (1974) Death following infection of lung scanning agent in a case of pulmonary hypertension. *Brit. J. Radiol.*, **47**, 61–63.

Williams, O., Lyall, J., Vernon, M. & Croft, D. N. (1974) Ventilation-perfusion lung scanning for pulmonary emboli. *Brit. Med. J.*, **1**, 600–602.

Yao, S. T., Gourmos, M. D. & Hobbs, J. T. (1972) *Lancet*, **2**, 1.

14. The General Problem of Thrombo-embolism

1. The Clinical Problem
2. Aetiology and Pathology
3. Anticoagulants
4. Thrombolysis and Streptokinase

Thrombo-embolic disease presents itself to the clinician in such a wide variety of ways, and in such a wide variety of patients, that it defies rigid classification. Yet whether it turns up in the young or old, the cardiac patient or the gynaecological one, after operation or 'just out of the blue', it is essentially the same disease with the same basic problems.

The literature of this subject is full of statistical studies purporting to show that it is commoner in one group than another, and often drawing unwarranted conclusions about the cause of thrombosis from 'statistically significant' figures involved. Such figures may give useful indications of the general behaviour of the disease as a whole, but the truth is that there is no one dominant cause of thrombosis. Each patient is an individual problem, and the aetiology of his or her thrombosis may be quite different from that of the next patient. The problem is to define as far as possible the known causative factors, and to search for these in each individual. Moreover the patient may present at any stage of the disease—the acute or chronic stage. Many patients present as a post-thrombotic syndrome of the leg—without having been aware of the early stage of the disease at all (or having forgotten it entirely). There are three important general points to make about thrombosis and embolism before we go on to detailed considerations. These are:

1. The disease is thrombosis *not* clotting. A thrombus is found in flowing blood and is a much more solid and tough structure than clot which essentially occurs in static blood. Most intravascular thrombi are composed of different proportions of thrombus and clot, and their toughness, their susceptibility to lysis etc. depends a lot on the proportion of hard white thrombus and soft red thrombus, the latter being much more like pure clot in consistency.

2. Whenever a patient presents with a venous thrombosis (superficial or deep) one's first thought should bc *'look for a cause'*. There may be a perfectly straightforward pathological cause for the thrombosis. Either a general cause such as a carcinoma somewhere, or a blood disease like polycythaemia vera, or there may be some local pressure on the vein such as an aneurysm, a pelvic mass, or carcinoma of prostate etc. It is most important not to forget this, as about 15 per cent of all cases of deep vein thrombosis are merely a result or complication of some other disease or condition.

3. Thrombosis originating in the iliac veins near the caval bifurcation, and thrombosis originating in the deep veins below the inguinal ligament present such differing clinical pictures, and have such different problems in management that it is convenient to consider them as almost two separate clinical types of deep vein thrombosis.

Thrombosis in the iliac veins (known as iliofemoral thrombosis, white leg, or 'phlegmasia alba dolens'), and peripheral deep vein thrombosis are therefore dealt with in separate chapters in the ensuing text.

This distinction has not always been made in the voluminous literature on this subject up to date, and the inclusion of both types of thrombosis in various series and statistics has led to some confusion. The main clinical features of the two types are briefly summarised in Table 14.1.

Table 14.1

	Iliofemoral thrombosis	Peripheral deep vein thrombosis
Mode of onset	Sudden swelling of *whole* leg with pain or discomfort, often left leg, and always swelling of thigh.	May be *quite silent* in early stage, then tenderness of calf and ankle swelling.
Emboli	May be accompanied by one embolus, at onset of condition, then risk of further emboli is low.	Large or fatal emboli common in early silent stage of disease. Embolism often the only presenting symptom.
Age	Often occurs in a young age group.	More common in the elderly, and in hospital patients.

Most of the discussion in the literature on the incidence of thrombosis and the risk of embolism in hospital patients has centred round peripheral deep vein thrombosis.

THE GENERAL PATTERN OF THROMBO-EMBOLIC DISEASE

In 1966 and 1967 when emergency phlebography had just become established as a diagnostic method in the acute, early stage of the disease, a consecutive series of 76 unselected patients were examined at St. Thomas' Hospital by this method. All these patients were clinically diagnosed as having early thrombo-embolic disease and they came from all parts of the hospital, medical, surgical, gynaecological and outpatients, and so there was no 'bias' towards any one group of patients. Most of the patients had either a suggestive sudden pain in the chest or sudden constrictive feelings or shortness of breath making the clinical diagnosis of early pulmonary embolism likely. Many but not all, had peripheral leg signs—calf tenderness and ankle swelling.

On examining the results of these phlebograms it was interesting to find that the patients sorted themselves out into six rather sharply defined groups.

The findings are summarised in Table 14.2.

Group 1. Fourteen had normal phlebograms. These were patients with very suggestive signs of thrombo-embolism (i.e. tender calf, pain in the chest, and a sudden attack of dyspnoea) yet whose whole peripheral venous systems were proved to be absolutely clear, and who were, therefore, saved from a lot of unnecessary and wrong treatment.

This figure is also interesting in indicating the margin of error in pure clinical diagnosis. This 18 per cent error was made by skilled and experienced clinicians specifically interested in the disease! It once more emphasises the fallacy of case statistics based on purely clinical diagnosis.

Group 2. Six who had a definite and obvious local cause for their thrombosis, such as malignancy or aneurysm pressing on the vein.

Group 3. Eight had a deep vein thrombosis which had spread inwards from a superficial thrombosis of their varicose veins.

This surprisingly high percentage of the total cases (10 per cent) focuses attention on the danger of superficial thrombosis in varicose veins—a condition not generally appreciated as potentially dangerous.

Group 4. Fifteen formed an interesting group who developed peripheral deep vein thrombosis with embolism occurring suddenly 'out of the blue' during their normal life.

Most of these were found reposing in

Table 14.2 Emergency phlebography in 76 patients

Group 1 (14 patients)	Negative result No thrombus seen	18%
Group 2 (6 patients)	*Thrombus positive* Obvious local causes (malignancy aneurysm, etc.)	8%
Group 3 (8 patients)	*Thrombus positive* Spread from superficial thrombosis in varicose veins	10%
Group 4 (15 patients)	*Thrombus positive* Peripheral type thrombo-embolism, 'out of the blue' in normal life. (Usually a fairly mature age group, 40+)	20%
Group 5 (15 patients)	*Thrombus positive* Peripheral type *post-operative* pulmonary embolism.	20%
Group 6 (18 patients)	Anatomical abnormality of great veins (iliac compression type or duplication). Thrombus not always clearly shown.	24%

medical beds with the diagnosis of pleurisy or pneumonia. A few were cardiac cases. But about half of them were otherwise normal middle aged or young individuals who were suddenly incapacitated by an embolus or a swollen leg, while in the midst of their every-day life. A very interesting group, worth more attention.

Group 5. Fifteen post-operative patients, the well known group who develop thrombo-embolic signs 7 to 10 days after operation. In nearly all of them the thrombosis started in the peripheral deep veins: calf, popliteal or femoral.

Group 6. Eighteen forming a sharply defined group of relatively young patients (average age 23) in whom thrombosis occurred in the major iliac veins. In all of this group, whether frank and demonstrable thrombosis was shown or not, there was always present some major anatomical abnormality of the great veins near the caval bifurcation. These abnormalities ranged from numerous cases of iliac compression syndrome to cases of reduplicated or left sided vena cava. Clinically, these young patients presented in one of two ways: as a major iliofemoral thrombosis with or without one small pulmonary embolus at onset, or, more rarely, as a problem of recurrent small embolic episodes. This is the group of 16 patients described under the heading of iliac compression syndrome (see Chap. 16). It is also of interest to note that in 36 per cent of this group there was a family history of thrombo-embolism, suggesting that the anatomical malformation of the major veins is an inherited fault.

This series of 76 patients illustrated well the general pattern of thrombo-embolic disease as seen in a large general hospital dealing with all types of patients.

HISTORICAL ASPECTS

Malpighi (1686) in *De Polypo Cordis Dissertatio* was one of the first to describe macroscopically a pulmonary embolus. He, like Laennec (1846) and Rokitansky (1855), failed to appreciate the origin of emboli, although they wrote about the macroscopical findings in the lungs.

Virchow, in his writings between 1846 and 1856, was the first to describe the peripheral formation of a thrombus and then the breaking off of this to form an embolus. He appreciated that emboli were carried in the venous system to the heart and so into the pulmonary vascular bed. He also postulated

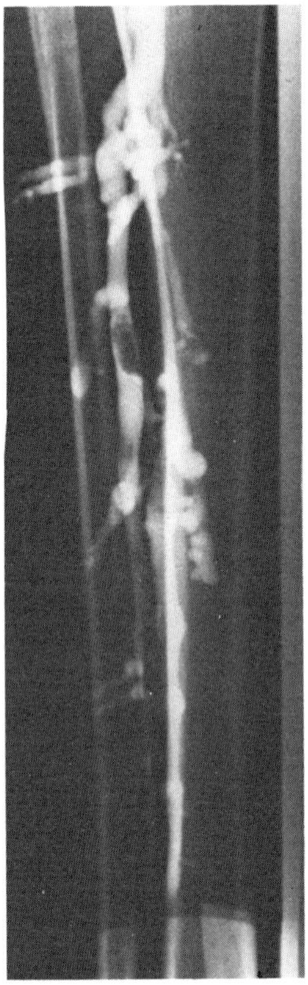

Fig. 14.1 This perfectly fit patient, aged 40, had two pulmonary emboli without any warning and without any signs in the legs (Group 4, in text). Emergency phlebography immediately after the second embolus showed an area of loose thrombus in the peroneal veins. He has had no further emboli after bilateral femoral vein ligation.

the famous three conditions necessary for the formation of thrombus (Virchow's triad), namely:

1. Damage to the wall of the vein.
2. Slowing of the flow of blood in a vein.
3. A change in the constitution of blood.

Following this Cohnheim (1872 and 1875), Welsh (1899) and others described the clinical picture of embolism as we know it today.

Pitman (1864) recorded the first British description of a patient dying from pulmonary embolism when he wrote of 'Obstruction of the Pulmonary Artery by Coagula causing sudden Death'. His patient was a woman of 23 who was admitted with slight febrile symptoms. She developed stiffness and swelling of the left leg just before discharge from hospital. Later she collapsed in a water closet and died within a few minutes. At post-mortem, the pulmonary artery was entirely filled with a partly discoloured clot which extended from the pulmonary valve to beyond the bifurcation of the pulmonary artery. The right femoral vein contained 'thrombus from the mid thigh distally to the ramifications'.

Trousseau (1870), similarly recorded another case of a young woman in 1858, who after delivery collapsed with right sided chest pain. The patient died, and at post-mortem was found to have a pulmonary infarct with an embolus blocking the pulmonary artery to that area.

Bowen (1889), Remfry (1891), and Glenn (1896) recorded case histories of patients recovering from pulmonary embolism following collapse. All the case histories were typical of what we would require today to make a clinical diagnosis. However, Remfry stated that the accuracy of diagnosis might be questioned, a statement just as pertinent now as in 1891.

INCIDENCE OF THE DISEASE

Statistics purporting to give the incidence of early thrombo-embolic disease in large series of cases are apt to vary considerably and be misleading. The reason for this is two-fold: (1) the early symptoms of the disease are protean and often slight and thus (2) the criteria for the diagnosis of deep thrombosis vary widely from one clinical observer to another, depending on how vigilant and 'thrombosis-conscious' he may be. These statistics and their pitfalls have been subjected to analysis and criticism by DeBakey (1954); many of the following figures have been taken from this classic paper. When we attempt to find out the incidence of *fatal* pulmonary embolism we are on surer ground. Matas in 1932 surveyed nearly a million surgical cases from many clinics and found the incidence of fatal pulmonary embolism to be 0·25 per cent (1 in 400 cases). This gave a panoramic view of the incidence up to that time. The Mayo Clinic figures from 1917 to 1926 were 0·28 per cent (1 in 357 cases) (Henderson, 1927), and from 1927 to 1950 were 0·2 per cent (1 in 500 cases) (Barker et al., 1940). Pilcher (1937) surveying 731 cases over the years 1925 to 1934, collected from twelve London hospitals, found an overall incidence of 0·105 per cent (1 in 947 cases) in surgical cases, as against 0·064 per cent (1 in 1,562 cases) in medical cases. But he commented that, in his opinion, a considerable number of cases had escaped diagnosis and the figure was lower than the actual incidence. Murley (1950), studying 1,763 surgical cases, found the overall incidence to be 0·11 per cent (1 in 909 cases), and noted that the incidence of non-fatal pulmonary emboli was five to six times as great. Fowler and Bollinger (1954) found that 0·089 per cent of hospital admissions died from pulmonary embolism.

From 1960 till the present, pathologists have continued to report an increasing incidence of deaths from thrombo-embolism. Morrell et al. (1963) studied the incidence in Oxford hospitals over the period 1952 to 1961. In 1952 there were 33 cases; in 1961 there were 154. As there was a 95 per cent post-mortem rate, this was almost certainly a real increase. Approximately half of the cases were fatal and there were, therefore, four to five times more deaths in 1961 than in 1952. However, there was a steady increase in the age of patients coming to post-mortem during this period as well.

Uhland and Goldberg (1964) reported that 12 per cent of all autopsies during a five-year period had emboli. Many of these were multiple, which suggested that, if the clinical diagnosis had been made earlier, successful treatment might have been instituted. In this group only 9 per cent had been diagnosed before death.

More recently Kakkar et al. (1969) examining 132 consecutive post-operative patients by the I^{125} fibrinogen scan method, showed that 40 of them (30 per cent) developed evidence of minor thrombosis. In 14 patients this lysed in 72 hours, but in the remainder it persisted and in 9 extended into the popliteal or femoral vein. Only half the patients had physical signs suggesting the diagnosis!

Evans (1970) worked out the incidence of deaths from massive pulmonary embolism in St. Thomas' Hospital over the years 1963 to 1968 (Table 14.3).

It is interesting and somewhat discouraging to note that the incidence remained steady despite the increasing campaign for early diagnosis and treatment of thrombo-embolism which was in progress at the time!

These figures, culled from a great variety of sources, give a good overall picture of the disease: namely, the average incidence of death from fatal pulmonary embolism in surgical patients is between 0·1 and 0·2 per

Table 14.3 Incidence of deaths from massive pulmonary embolism in St Thomas' Hospital (1963 to 1968)

Year	Hospital admissions	Hospital deaths	Hospital P.M.'s	% of hospital deaths coming to post-mortem	Number of massive emboli	% of post-mortems disclosing massive emboli as cause of death	Incidence of fatal emboli in ALL hospital admissions
1963		544	375	(69·1%)	15	(4·0%)	
1964		534	388	(72·7%)	27	(7·0%)	
1965	13,085	588	383	(65·1%)	15	(3·9%)	0·11%
1966	14,121	542	373	(68·8%)	21	(5·6%)	0·15%
1967	15,551	590	375	(63·6%)	15	(4·0%)	0·096%
1968	15,000	674	346	(60.3%)	21	(6·1%)	0·14%
Total	57,757	3,372	2,241	66·5%	114	(5·0%)	0·12%

cent (1 in 500 to 1,000 cases). The incidence in medical patients is as great if not higher. The incidence of non-fatal pulmonary embolism in surgical patients is five to ten times as great (at least) although the figures for this are necessarily not so reliable.

Pulmonary embolism is recorded as the cause of death in 4 to 5 per cent of all autopsies at large general hospitals.

MECHANISM AND PATHOLOGY OF THROMBOSIS

The genesis of intravascular thrombosis has been beautifully described by Aschoff (1924) and no better descriptions than his are to be found. Hadfield (1950) re-emphasised the importance of this basic pathology. The stages in the formation and natural history of the intravascular thrombosis are shown in the diagrams of Figure 14.2. Thrombosis is initiated by the fact that the platelets in flowing blood tend to adhere to any irregularity or area of trauma in the vessel wall. Thus the first stage in thrombosis is the formation of a platelet thrombus over a traumatised or irregular area of vein wall (Fig. 14.2A). This is grey, amorphous, semitransparent, and in fact is the natural element with which the blood repairs or smooths over any wound or irregularity of the intima. Whether the process stops here (as it normally would) or progresses into the formation of an occluding thrombus depends on a number of factors, predominant among which are the size of the vessel and the speed of the blood stream and possibly changes in the fibrinogen and clotting factors in the blood.

Figure 14.2B shows the next stage of the process—the addition to the platelet thrombus of the coralline thrombus. This interesting formation consists of a series of upstanding, corrugated, parallel laminae composed of hyalinised platelets, which grow across the stream and are bent in the direction of its flow. The surface of this is traversed by fine, closely set ridges which are the edges of the platelet laminae—these ridges are known as the 'ripple lines of Zahn'. If this structure

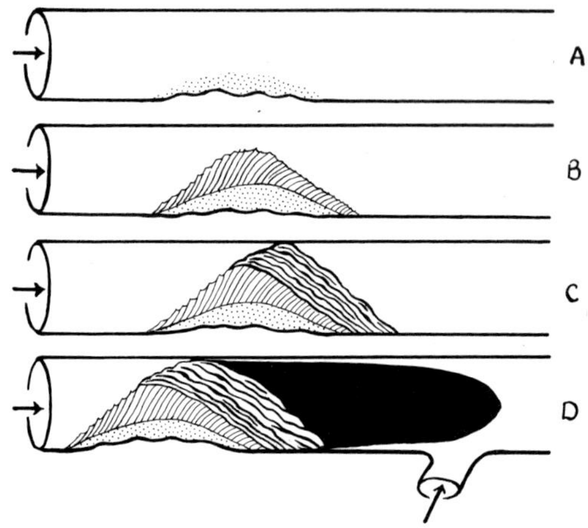

Fig. 14.2 The pathology of thrombosis.

produces significant vascular obstruction, stagnant blood plasma and red and white cells are entangled in the eddy distal to the thrombus and some coagulation occurs, a laminated red occluding thrombus grows—this is shown in Figure 14.2C. When the vessel is completely occluded by the thrombus, the stagnant column of blood up to the next branch clots and becomes organised to form a rather brittle red thrombus (Fig. 14.2D). This is known as the consecutive thrombus. There may also be some retrograde thrombosis to the next branch vein. If the whole of the blood stream in which this process is taking place is still or sluggish, this consecutive thrombosis may occur for a considerable distance along the blood vessel, and is then known as a propagated thrombus which then gradually contracts (i.e. the normal process of clot retraction). The result is that there is at this stage a long contracted thrombus, perhaps a foot or more in length, lying free in the vein lumen, anchored only at the site of initiation of the thrombosis. This is the situation which is fraught with danger—for this long, free thrombus only has to break off to become the fatal pulmonary embolus. (Fig. 14.3)

Now it is important to realise that at this stage of the process (the dangerous stage, with regard to pulmonary embolism) there

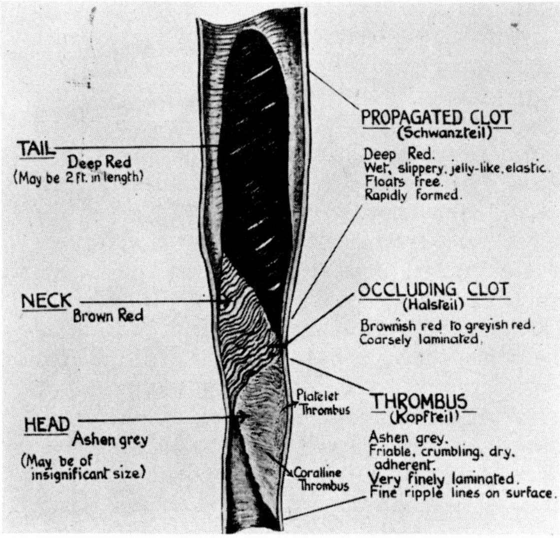

Fig. 14.3 A fully formed occluding thrombus with loose propagated clot, lying in a vein.

may be no detectable clinical signs present. The free consecutive thrombus is not obstructing, so there will be no signs of venous obstruction. The original area of intimal or venous damage which started the thrombus may be too small to give rise to any clinical symptom or sign. This silent, dangerous stage of the process is often referred to as the stage of '*phlebothrombosis*'.

Now the next stage is that the consecutive or propagated thrombus (if it has not broken off and killed the patient) becomes adherent to the vein wall. This may take two to four days to occur. When it does occur it does two things: (1) it obstructs a considerable segment of the vein. (2) it sets up a sterile inflammatory reaction in the vein wall and perivenous tissues. This condition has plenty of clinical signs, and is the second stage of the process, and is called *thrombophlebitis*. The clinical signs will be those of venous obstruction, and of local tenderness over the affected vein, and of general reaction (fever and high pulse rate).

An area of thrombophlebitis in the deep veins of the calf may, if the conditions are right, act as the starting point for a second propagated thrombus. And so it is possible to have thrombophlebitis and phlebothrombosis together in the same limb at the same time. They are simply two stages in the natural history of intravenous thrombosis.

These observations go far to explain many of the anomalous observations on the clinical behaviour of thrombosis and embolism.

All observers and writers on the subject have noted that: (1) peripheral deep vein thrombosis usually occurs in *both* legs, and (2) approximately half the cases of fatal pulmonary embolism and many non-fatal cases, occur unexpectedly, with no preceding signs in the legs. Signs in the legs (i.e. signs of thrombophlebitis) may occur one or two days *after* a non-fatal pulmonary embolus. Remembering, therefore, that deep thrombosis is usually bilateral, we may have the following conditions in the legs of a postoperative patient:

1. Phlebothrombosis in one or both legs—asymptomatic, silent, dangerous.
2. Extensive thrombophlebitis in one leg—numerous signs and symptoms; benign. Recent phlebothrombosis in the other—silent, dangerous.
3. Signs of calf thrombophlebitis, with a propagated thrombus present (i.e. thrombophlebitis and phlebothrombosis present in the same leg. Maybe bilateral).—symptomatic and dangerous.

Small pulmonary emboli (too small to have given rise to any symptoms during life) are found on carefully searching the lungs of almost all patients who have died, in whom ante-mortem clot is found in the leg or calf veins. These studies, and those of Raeburn (1951), have indicated that pulmonary emboli occur much more frequently than one would think clinically. An embolus has to be of considerable size before it produces clinical symptoms and signs (Laufman, 1954).

The most outstanding factor which was observed by Aschoff (and by Virchow before him) to influence the growth of a thrombus was the speed of flow of the blood stream. A second factor of some importance was the size of the vessel concerned. It is obviously much easier to produce an occluding thrombus in a small vessel than in a big one, and it is a prerequisite for thrombus growth in these conditions that the blood stream be sluggish. By an appreciation of this fact we have in our hands the most powerful weapon to combat post-operative thrombosis—to find out and use all the measures which increase the venous return from the legs in bed-ridden, ill, and post-operative patients.

Lastly, in certain anatomical malformations of the veins, where a large vein becomes suddenly constricted, this may produce a change from a laminar flow pattern, to an eddying flow pattern at and just beyond the constriction, leading to deposit of platelets and thrombus formation. This mode of thrombus formation is seen more frequently in the arterial system where it is the usual method of build up of the segmental occluding thrombus near an arterial stricture. In certain anatomical malformations of the veins (particularly the so called compression syndromes at the caval bifurcation and congenital constrictions of the peroneal veins) this may contribute to thrombus formation.

PATHOLOGY OF PULMONARY EMBOLISM

The pathology of pulmonary embolism is a large subject with a voluminous literature—very extensively and well treated by Hume, Sevitt, and Thomas (1970). However, it is so indissolubly bound up with venous thrombosis that we must consider it in some detail here.

To understand the pathology and rationale of diagnosis and treatment of embolism there are two basic points which must be grasped.

1. *Embolism is essentially a repetitive process.*

2. *Emboli vary considerably in their composition.* Some are small and contain a high proportion of white thrombus (and are therefore relatively firm) and others are large and have a higher proportion of soft, red thrombus and clot.

Repetitive embolism

Pathologists have known for years that pulmonary emboli 'occur in series' or 'repetitively' (Sevitt and Gallagher; Morrell and Dunnill, 1968). Even in cases of fatal pulmonary embolism due apparently to a large embolus in the main pulmonary artery, earlier, smaller emboli are often found in the more peripheral pulmonary arteries, blocking a significant proportion of them and contributing to the patient's death. Thus in a case of fatal pulmonary embolism the killing embolus may in fact be the last one and possibly (but not necessarily) the biggest one of a series. The previous smaller ones may have passed completely unnoticed clinically—or their clinical signs may have been so transitory (slight breathlessness, slight tightness in the chest, transient rise in pulse rate, slight pleuritic pain) as to have passed entirely unremarked by both the patient and his attendants.

Surgeons particularly have been slow to grasp this aspect of the disease—as they see the sudden massive embolus and the dead patient clinically and naturally have jumped to the conclusion that this is the fatal and only embolus.

Yet it is only by picking up the signs of the small, early emboli, by great clinical awareness and vigilance, that the later large killers may be detected before they reach the lungs. At this stage various types of vein interruption may be employed to prevent these loose thrombi from ever reaching the lungs (see Chap. 15).

Cause of death in pulmonary embolism

How do pulmonary emboli cause death? When enough blockage of the pulmonary artery has occurred to cause (a) considerable dilatation of the right ventricle and great tachycardia and (b) therefore such a fall in venous return to the left ventricle that the heart is unable to maintain the systemic blood pressure, then the patient is in great danger of death. The final mechanism of death occurs when the heart is unable to maintain enough blood pressure in the aorta to sustain adequate coronary flow—at which point ventricular fibrillation and death is imminent. It therefore follows that clinically, signs of shock and a falling systolic blood pressure are the most important clinical signs of impending death—indicating that urgent action must be taken to save the patient's life.

Resolution of pulmonary emboli

What happens to major pulmonary emboli in the lungs if the patient survives? The answer is that lysis of the embolus occurs—rapidly in the first few days—and then more slowly over the next three or four weeks—leading to eventual recanalisation of the pulmonary vein which was obstructed. This parallels closely what is found to occur in peripheral veins. However, there is considerable lack of uniformity in the degree and types of recanalisation and in the amount of restoration of lung function.

This subject has been studied in three ways:

1. From post-mortem material (Morrell and Dunnill, 1968).
2. By serial pulmonary angiography—following recovery from major embolism (Fred et al., 1966; and Brompton Hosp. work).
3. By serial lung scans in patients recovering from major embolism (Walker, Jackson and Goodwin).

The result of this work seems to show that major emboli which have lodged in the main large pulmonary artery branches may clear remarkably quickly and completely—often resulting in almost complete restoration of lung function. Smaller peripheral emboli and particularly areas of lung affected by small, recurrent emboli recanalise less completely and lung function does not recover so well.

Moreover the large emboli in the big vessels often disappear leaving practically no trace—while those in smaller branches may leave a fibrous web in the vessel, or show the multiple channel type of recanalisation (as often found in the femoral vein after post-thrombotic recanalisation).

The reason for this great variation in the degree of lysis and recanalisation of pulmonary emboli, and in the degree of restoration of lung perfusion and function is not clear. However, it seems likely that it may be related to the composition of the original embolus. Large emboli with a great deal of soft red thrombus would be expected to lyse more quickly and completely than smaller and older emboli containing a higher proportion of hard white thrombus.

SITES OF OCCURRENCE OF THROMBOSIS

The vast majority of peripheral venous thromboses as a potential source of pulmonary emboli occur in the deep veins of the legs. But the *initiation* of the process may be anywhere from the calf sinusoids to the caval bifurcation.

Moreover there are certain other sites of venous thrombosis which may more rarely give rise to pulmonary embolism. These are the right side of the heart, the liver sinusoids in certain types of cirrhosis, and nowadays after certain types of prosthetic heart valves used for replacing the mitral valve. Peripheral venous thrombosis does also occur in the axillary vein but this practically never gives rise to embolism.

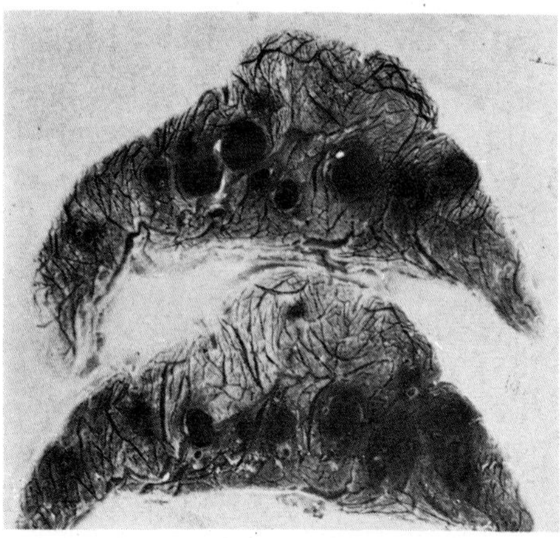

Fig. 14.4 Transverse section through the soleus muscle of a patient who died from pulmonary embolism. Note the thromboses in the large intramuscular venous sinuses.

Sites in the iliac and femoral veins

If a series of post-mortem dissections of the venous system of the leg is carried out on either unselected cases, or patients who have had evidence of thrombo-embolic disease in life, ante-mortem thrombi in the calf sinusoids are found in a high proportion of cases. (Fig. 14.4) Thus Raeburn (1951) in 130 unselected necropsies found calf thrombosis in 35; of these 35 cases, 20 showed large emboli in the lungs. Similar observations have been made by Rossle (1937), Hunter et al. (1945), Greenstein (1945) and ourselves.

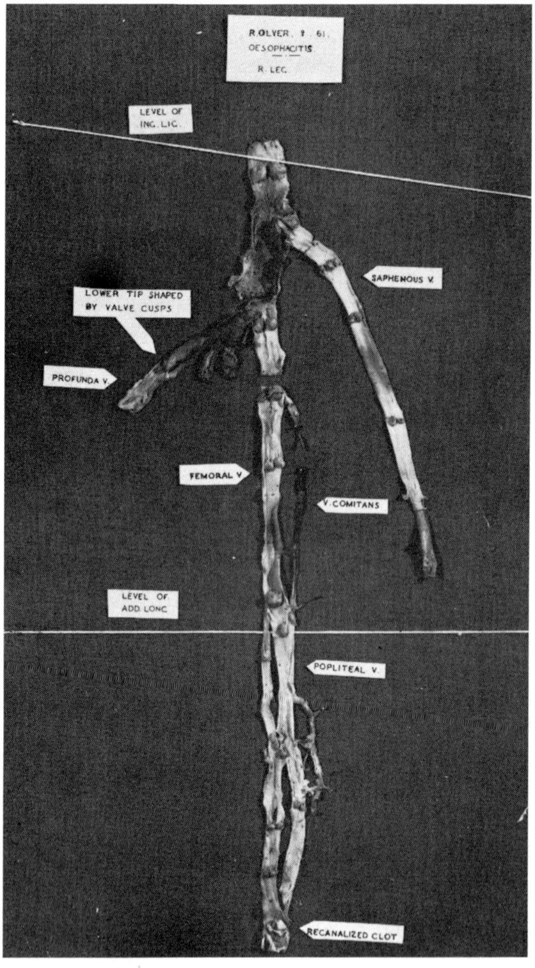

Fig. 14.5 Ante mortem thrombus arising in profunda vein.

However, McLachlin and Paterson (1951 and 1954) have pointed out that this is by no means the only place in the lower limb in which thrombi originate. In a significant proportion of their material, thrombi were found in the thigh veins, and a few in the pelvic veins, with the calf veins clear. Moreover, they point out that many thrombi in the large veins originate in relation to a valve cusp.

Figure 14.5 is the photograph of the vein dissection of a man who died of pulmonary embolism. In this case the embolus originated from a thrombus which started in a valve cusp in the profunda vein. In another case of the author's, a fatal embolus occurred on the tenth day. At autopsy, no sign of thrombosis could be found in either leg despite a complete exploration. In this case the right internal iliac vein was solid with clot and the ragged edge of the thrombus, from which the embolus had broken off, was projecting into the common iliac vein (Fig. 14.6).

Other workers, Carlotti et al. (1947), and Fowler and Bollinger (1954), who have included large numbers of cardiac failure autopsies in their series, draw attention to the fact that thrombus may also be found in the

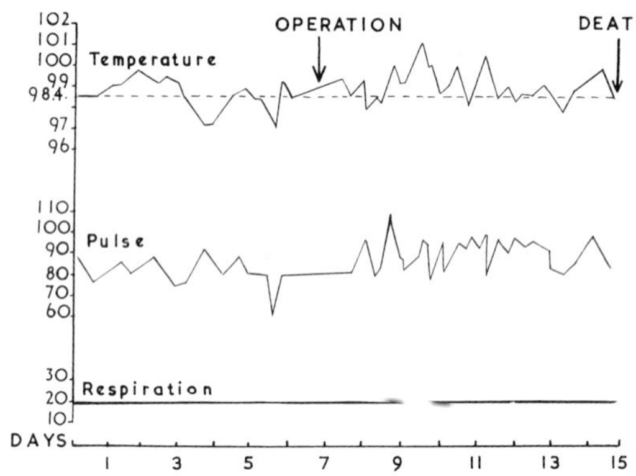

Fig. 14.6 Temperature chart of a patient who died of pulmonary embolism after cholecystectomy. There were no physical signs of thrombosis. The only abnormality was the low intermittent pyrexia, for which no adequate cause could be found. On the ninth post-operative day a fatal pulmonary embolus occurred. At post mortem this was found to have arisen from the left internal iliac vein.

right auricle in these cases, and pulmonary embolism may arise from this source in this group of cases. Fowler and Bollinger considered that the right heart was the source of fatal embolism in 38 of 97 fatal cases studied at post-mortem. They point out that in many cases the embolus occurred soon after auricular fibrillation had been controlled or converted to normal rhythm with digitalis. Miller and Berry (1951) drew attention to this point. However, it was the finding of Carlotti et al. (1947) at the Massachusetts General Hospital that, even in cardiac cases, most of the pulmonary emboli arose from venous thrombosis in the legs.

More recently the work on the major iliac veins (Chap. 16) has demonstrated that thrombi may arise in the common iliac veins and even in the cava itself, usually in association with some degree of the anatomical malformation known as the iliac compression syndrome.

It may also arise as a complication of superficial varicose veins, the thrombus spreading into the deep veins by way of either the saphenofemoral junction at the groin, the short saphenous junction with the popliteal vein, or the ankle perforating veins. These cases represent quite a significant number (10 per cent) of the cases of thrombo-embolism (see Table 14.2).

Thus it would appear that deep vein thrombosis in the legs giving rise to embolism may start in any of the following sites:

1. The venous sinusoids of the soleus muscle.
2. In relation to valve cusps in the main deep channels (femoral, posterior tibial and peroneal veins).
3. In the iliac veins, or lower cava—often in association with congenital anatomical malformations here.
4. Spreading in from superficial thrombosis in varicose veins.

Only an emergency venogram will show accurately the site of early thrombus formation in an individual case, if it is done early in the progress of the disease.

All authors who have studied the subject by whatever means are moreover united upon two other points:

1. Thrombosis of leg veins when it occurs is *bilateral* in a high proportion of cases. Often the thrombosis may be extensive in one leg, and slight in the other (i.e. extensive thrombophlebitis in one leg, clinically manifest, and early phlebothrombosis, clinically silent, in the other).
2. Pulmonary emboli are never found in the absence of a peripheral source (i.e. leg veins, liver veins or right auricle). Primary pulmonary artery thrombosis is an excessively rare phenomenon.

Deep thrombosis in the upper limb

Thrombosis of the axillary vein occurs in two groups of cases:

1. Following trauma to the axillary vein (i.e. during mastectomy) and following compression by malignant glands or growths in the supraclavicular region. This type of thrombosis is referred to as secondary thrombosis.
2. Primary axillary vein thrombosis of young adults. This peculiar and alarming syndrome presents as the sudden appearance of a painful, swollen, blue arm, with distended, superficial veins. Often there is a history of an unusual type of activity such as 'painting the ceiling'. Pulmonary embolism is so *rare* as to be almost unknown in this type of thrombosis (Hughes, 1949). The symptoms and signs (tightness and oedema) usually subside in from two to four weeks leaving the limb asymptomatic—except for occasional discomfort during sustained heavy work (Hufses, 1954).

The aetiology of this interesting syndrome appears to lie in a rare anatomical abnormality whereby the axillary vein as it passes over the first rib and then dips down into the superior mediastinum (to form the subclavian vein), is compressed by the overlying clavicle and tendon of subclavius muscle, so that the vein is converted into a flattened, fibrous band at that point—very similar to the iliac compression abnormality (see Chap. 16). This abnormality can only be shown if the clavicle is completely removed over its inner two thirds (with disarticulation at the sternoclavicular joint). This operation, oddly enough, leaves the patient with no functional disability, and does provide a complete exposure and decompression of the whole region. The author has had three cases in which this 'claviculectomy' has been successful in relieving late pain and congestive symptoms after a primary axillary vein thrombosis.

A much rarer cause is the compression of the axillary vein lower in the axilla by an abnormal rudimentary musculotendinous slip, which forms a 'sling' round the axillary vein at the outlet of the axilla (Fig. 14.7). This slip, called the 'axillary arch' springs from the upper end of latissimus dorsi and crosses the axilla to join the tendon of pectoralis major. It is said to be present in 7 per cent of subjects (Grays Anatomy, 1932).

FACTORS PREDISPOSING TO DEEP VEIN THROMBOSIS

Virchow first recognised that there is no 'single universal cause' of thrombosis, when he postulated his famous triad (p. 198).

Many cases of deep vein thrombosis have a fairly easily defined pathological cause. This may be either *local* (i.e. local obstruction or trauma to the vein wall) or *general* (general change in the composition or coagulability of the blood).. This is called secondary thrombosis.

Local causes

1. *Trauma* to a vein, accidental surgical injury, ligature, etc.

2. Injection of irritating chemicals which damage the intima, e.g. injection of varicose veins, and certain types of drip thrombosis.

3. Obstruction or constriction of a main vein by external pressure—usually from a tumour. In the male—aneurysm, enlarged malignant glands in pelvis or abdomen and spread from carcinoma of prostate are all common causes of iliac or femoral vein obstruction leading to thrombosis. In the female—ovarian, uterine and cervical tumours, and malignant glands are usual.

General causes

Under this heading come:

1. Changes in the blood. The commonest cause is polycythaemia. Rarer causes are thrombocythaemia (post-splenectomy) and possibly paraproteinaemia and various leukaemias. These all cause increase in blood viscosity and cellular content.

Much less well defined are changes in the clotting factors themselves—so far, in spite of a voluminous literature, there is no general agreement on any one significant change in these factors, although the work on fibrin degradation products may well highlight this subject more in the future.

2. The well known fact that primary carcinoma of the lung and sometimes of pancreas or ovary, may be associated with a peripheral leg thrombosis, even in the quite early stages of the disease. This is a well established clinical observation, but its mechanism is unknown.

Primary (or stasis) thrombosis

Many cases of major deep vein thrombosis, however, occur without an easily recognised pathological cause. Most of the cases of post-operative and hospital thrombo-embolism come into this category. The factors leading to this type of thrombosis are more difficult to define, except that we are reasonably certain that venous stasis has a great deal to do with it—in fact this type of thrombosis has been called 'stasis thrombosis' by many authors. Variations in the anatomy of the iliac veins and also of the deep veins of the leg, and of the venous sinusoids in the soleus muscle may also be an important factor.

A more detailed consideration of the factors leading to this type of thrombosis will be found in Chapter 15.

SEPTIC THROMBOPHLEBITIS

The forms of thrombophlebitis dealt with in the preceding sections have been aseptic.

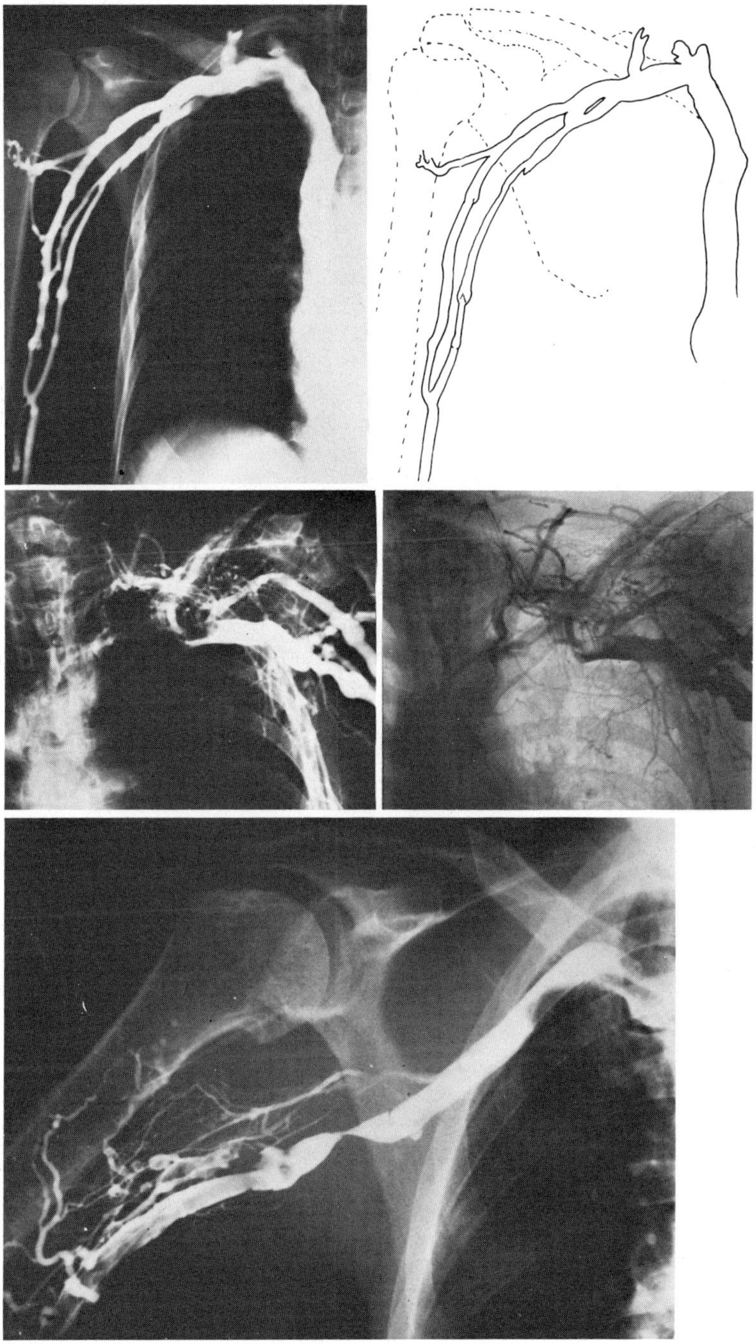

Fig. 14.7
(1) Normal axillary venogram showing the sharp angle and partial deformity of the axillary vein as it passes over the first rib down into the mediastinum.
(2) Primary axillary vein thrombosis. Occlusion of axillary vein at the first rib.
(3) Constriction of axillary vein at lower border of axilla by the 'axillary band'.
Journal of Clinical Radiology

In spite of the fact that the local clinical signs were those of heat, tenderness and swelling, and the appearance of fever, and are all signs of infection, it is a sterile inflammatory reaction. Septic thrombophlebitis does occur, and is different in its onset and clinical signs. In the legs it is rare, being most commonly seen as a result of an infusion into a vein which has become infected. There is intense local pain, redness and tenderness, and unless treatment is started early, spread of the septic thrombosis may occur. The classical sign of septic thrombophlebitis is the occurrence of a *rigor*. The common places for septic thrombophlebitis are:

1. *In the pelvic veins*—following a septic abortion or operation on a septic pelvic condition.
2. *In the lateral sinus*—due to spread from mastoiditis.
3. *In the cavernous sinus*—following a compound fracture of the middle fossa or a facial furuncle.
4. *In the leg or arm*—following a septic intravenous infusion.
5. *Portal pylephlebitis*—classically following an operation on septic haemorrhoids.

Since the advent of antibiotics these conditions have become much rarer, but it is important to recognise them at once when they occur. The most striking, and often the earliest, clinical signs that a septic thrombophlebitis is present is the occurrence of a *rigor*. This should lead to immediate treatment with antibiotics and heparin.

ANTICOAGULANTS AND THROMBOSIS

Modern concepts of the blood coagulation mechanism may be summarised diagrammatically by the following plasma reactions:

1. {Platelets, Antihaemophilic globulin, Christmas factors, Factor V, Factor VII} Ca^{++} Thromboplastin
2. Prothrombin——Ca^{++}——Thrombin
3. Fibrinogen————————Fibrin

Of the three stages represented, the first, by which thromboplastin is formed in the blood, normally occupies a matter of 5 or 10 minutes in vitro, while the last two together only require about 10 seconds for their completion.

The 'prothrombin time' is the time taken for plasma to clot in the presence of optimum amounts of tissue (usually brain) extract and calcium, that is thromboplastin. This time is independent of the platelets, antihaemophilic globulin and Christmas factors, but depends on the concentration in the plasma of factors V and VII and, less critically, prothrombin and fibrinogen. By the one stage method of Quick, it is 12 to 15 seconds.

The Dicoumarol group. The Dicoumarol group includes Dicoumarol, Tromexan, Dindevan, and a number of other new synthetic drugs. All these drugs have essentially similar properties, although their solubility, and therefore the time relations for their absorption and action, differ slightly.

The main action of the Dicoumarol group of drugs is to reduce the plasma concentration of factor VII and, to a lesser extent, of prothrombin. For this reason the 'prothrombin time' is a must useful guide in controlling the dosage of these drugs. Coagulation is not adequately inhibited by them until the concentration of factor VII in the plasma has fallen to less than 20 per cent of normal.

The whole blood clotting time, which, if fibrinogen is present, is essentially an indicator of the state of the first slow phase of the coagulation mechanism (a reaction involving platelets, antihaemophilic globulin and the Christmas factor) is rarely significantly lengthened by these drugs, which do not affect this stage of the process.

Heparin. This is the original anticoagulant discovered and purified by Jorpes. The action of heparin is a complex one. It is an antithrombin, and it also inhibits the formation of blood thromboplastin. Thus it both slows thrombin formation and inactivates the thrombin which is formed. Its dosage is controllable by means of the whole blood coagulation time (a very simple test), which is prolonged by its action.

Table 14.4 Comparison of the properties of the two groups of anticoagulant drugs

Heparin	Dicoumarol group
Must be given by injection, (intravenous or subcutaneous)	Is given by mouth
Action is immediate when given intravenously but may be delayed not more than an hour by the subcutaneous route	Action is delayed; from 12 to 48 hours, according to the drug used
Action lasts 3 to 4 hours only (intravenously) (but up to 12 to 20 hours with concentrated preparations subcutaneously)	Action lasts up to 48 hours or more after cessation of drug
Action certain	Action uncertain; subject to the vagaries of absorption, excretion and patient idiosyncrasy
Antidote: Protamine (dose 0·3–0·5 mgms per kilo. body wt.)	Antidote: Vit. K (by injection) 10–50 mg

Protamine solution must be injected slowly (over 5–10 mins) otherwise it may cause profound hypotension and shock.

Before passing on to a discussion of which drug should be used in the treatment of thrombosis, and how to use it, we must keep clearly before us the objects we hope to achieve by their use. It will be recalled that the essential basic process of thrombosis is:

Platelet thrombus $\longrightarrow$ Vessel occlusion $\longrightarrow$ Propagated clot

Now, all that an anticoagulant drug can do is to stop the formation of the propagated clot, or to stop it from propagating more, if it is already present. There is some evidence that heparin also interferes with the formation of platelet thrombus (Payling-Wright, 1941)—a most important property. Dicoumarol apparently does not have this power. Neither of them has any action on clot or thrombus once it has been formed, i.e. there is no 'dissolving' action. Thus the clinical basis for the use of these drugs is either:

1. The diagnosis of a state predisposing to thrombosis (in which case they can be used prophylactically), or

2. In the presence of an early thrombosis, to prevent the formation of further propagated clot.

In order to attain these objectives the dosage and control of administration must be 100 per cent effective.

Viewed in the light of these criteria, the Dicoumarol and Tromexan group of drugs have certain disadvantages. These are as follows:

1. Delayed action.

2. Extreme variations in absorption, action and excretion rate.

3. Most important, difficulty of control. These drugs have to be pushed to the stage of almost complete disappearance of prothrombin from the blood before an adequate effect on the actual whole blood clotting time is apparent. This entails very close laboratory control, with estimations of prothrombin time (a technical process requiring some experience) once or even twice daily and adjustment of the dose accordingly. In the absence of this strict control it is doubtful if more loosely controlled and probably inadequate dosage has the desired effect. Certainly the long outpatient courses of the drug recommended by some, usually have little effect on the clotting process. Moreover, if pushed to excess for any length of time, toxic effects, such as nausea, purpura and haematuria, may occur.

Recently Wessler (1953) has shown that in isolated vein segments of dogs only very small amounts of prothrombin need be present to produce a fibrin clot. By the same method, he has demonstrated that heparin is considerably superior to Dicoumarol in its anticoagulant effect under these conditions. He also points out an important fact—namely, that there may be a profound dissociation between bleeding and clotting.

To sum up, the Dicoumarol group of drugs probably only achieve the desired effect in near-toxic dosage—which must be closely and expertly controlled under hospital inpatient supervision.

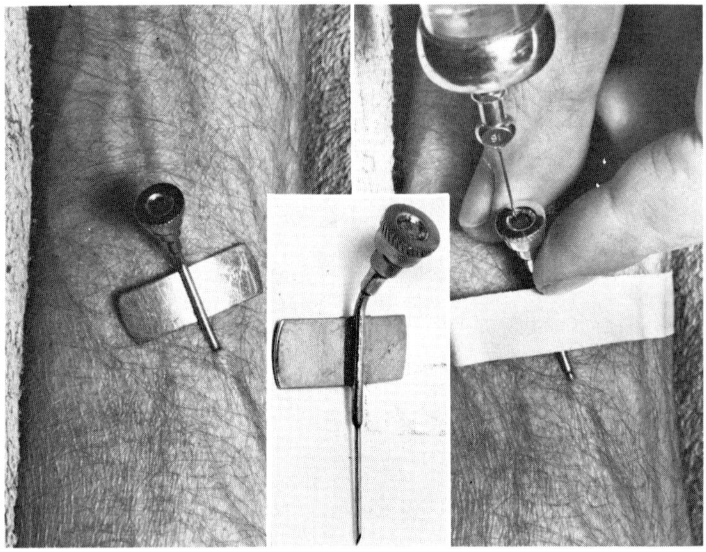

Fig. 14.8 Gordh's needle.

Heparin, on the other hand, has three very considerable advantages. These are:

1. Immediate action; within half a minute of the intravenous injection of a dose of heparin the clotting time has risen considerably.

2. It acts as a direct inhibitor of the clotting mechanism (which is the desired property)

3. Simple control of dosage. (The estimation of the clotting time accurately enough to control heparin dosage is a simple procedure, easily carried out.)

The disadvantage of heparin is that with the preparations in use at the present time it must be given intravenously, and its action wears off in three to four hours. This difficulty can be overcome by the use of Gordh's needle (Fig. 14.8). With this needle in a vein of the arm, three-hourly intravenous injections can be given with ease through the rubber diaphragm over a period of forty-eight hours. After approximately this period it is wise to change the needle to another vein.

The intramuscular and subcutaneous routes of injection with the form of heparin available at present are not practicable for three reasons:

1. They are very painful.

2. Occasionally huge haematomas form (particularly with intramuscular injection) sometimes so big as to endanger life and require transfusion.

3. The vagaries of absorption by these routes are considerable.

The newer preparations of heparin

It has recently been possible to prepare extremely concentrated solutions of heparin with the pure drug. Such preparations (Artz and Pulaski, 1953) are generally available. A dose of 1 ml of a solution containing 200 mg per ml can be given deep subcutaneously on the deep fascia, into the anterior surface of the thigh or chest, and will lengthen the coagulation time adequately (i.e. between 3 and 4 times the normal) for a period of about twelve to twenty hours. *These concentrated heparins must not be given intramuscularly.*

GUIDELINES ON THE CLINICAL USE OF HEPARIN AND THE DICOUMAROL GROUP IN CLINICAL PRACTICE.

1. *Heparin.* Heparin is easily given, is one hundred per cent effective in controlling

coagulation and has a fairly effective antidote. Essentially it should be used for very short term control of the coagulation mechanism. When used for more than twenty-four hours the incidence of serious haemorrhagic complications becomes appreciable. The most serious complication is cerebral haemorrhage —but serious bleeding from lungs, duodenal ulcers, kidneys and large confluent bruises may all occur.

Heparin, although effective, must therefore be regarded as a very dangerous drug except for short term control (i.e. *under twenty-four hours*).

2. *Dicoumarol Group* (warfarin). The use of these drugs in the control of thrombosis has been, and will be for some time the subject of controversy. It has been shown fairly conclusively (Sevitt 1959) that if efficient, closely controlled, oral anticoagulant therapy is used in a small selected group of cases at risk, it is effective in reducing the incidence of thrombo-embolism.

On the other hand all vascular surgeons of any experience have observed thrombosis occurring in patients who are receiving an apparently adequately controlled course of oral anticoagulant. It certainly cannot therefore be relied upon absolutely to control the incidence or spread of thrombosis, once this is present.

At best, therefore the oral anticoagulants should be used for periods up to three months under close laboratory control, and then tailed off gradually.

It is exceedingly doubtful if the very long term use of oral anticoagulants over periods in excess of 3 months and up to several years or more is justifiable. The loose dosage control which is inevitable under such circumstances makes it unlikely to be effective.

The complications of oral anticoagulant therapy are also appreciable. Haemorrhage from duodenal and gastric ulcer, cerebral haemorrhage, and haemoptysis may all occur.

Aspirin, Phenylbutazone, and most antibiotics (particularly Ampicillin), enhance the effect of warfarin, and interfere with accuracy of laboratory control.

THROMBOLYSIS AND STREPTOKINASE

(by Norman Browse)

Plasmin is a naturally occurring enzyme which catalyses the breakdown of fibrin to a number of shorter chain proteins. It is normally present in the plasma in an inactive form called plasminogen. The conversion of plasminogen to plasmin is stimulated by a number of substances, collectively called activators, such as adrenalin and nicotinic acid, and extracts from the streptococcus and urine—streptokinase and urokinase. Streptokinase is a powerful activator which has been available for many years but it was not purified sufficiently for intravenous use until the 1950's. It is the drug most often used for thrombolytic therapy because it is cheaper than Urokinase. Its main disadvantage is that it is an antigenic foreign protein and the body may already have high levels of antistreptococcal antibodies which will neutralise it. Urokinase, which is extracted from human urine and therefore very expensive is not antigenic but has not been studied as extensively as SK. Both substances act in the same manner.

Mode of action

Systemically administered SK will cause the dissolution of thrombus in any part of the body, so it should not be given to patients with a tendency to bleed, e.g. those with peptic ulcers, fresh wounds, recent arterial punctures etc. It works in two ways, firstly it diffuses into thrombus and activates the entrapped plasminogen to plasmin, so producing dissolution of the thrombus from within, and secondly plasmin and plasminogen-streptokinase complexes in the blood around the thrombus seem to be able to swamp the plasma antiplasmins and so dissolve the surface of the thrombus. There is some controversy over which of these mechanisms is the most important. Both require the access of fresh blood containing SK to the thrombus, hence old occlusive adherent thrombus is rarely dissolved. The

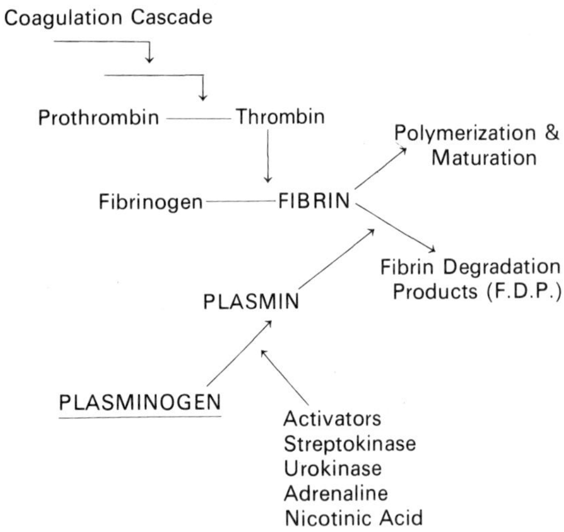

Fig. 14.9 Plasmin cycle.

degree of polymerization of the fibrin also affects the efficiency of lysis, the older the thrombus the less effective the lytic agent. It can be seen from these comments on the mode of action of SK that it is only likely to be effective against fresh (less than 3 days old) thrombus, preferably lying in a stream of blood, i.e. the non-occlusive variety.

Clinical administration of SK

Most clinicians do not measure the anti-streptokinase titre in order to calculate the initial dose but give a standard loading dose of 600,000 units intravenously in the first half hour or hour, followed by 100,000 units hourly for 3 to 5 days. An initial dose of this size is sufficient to overcome the antibodies of 90–95 per cent of the population. In 5–10 per cent where it is inadequate, the first part of the maintenance dose will be neutralised by the circulating antibodies and the patient may not reach a state of fibrinolytic activation for 1–2 hours. If the clinician wishes to be certain that he is getting a therapeutic effect within the first half hour, he must either measure the blood lytic activity or give a bigger loading dose. There is no advantage in giving small doses locally. Effective treatment can only be achieved by whole body thrombolysis. The injection of this foreign protein occasionally causes pyrexia, sometimes sweating, muscle and loin pains, and very rarely an anaphylactic reaction. These side effects can be suppressed by antihistamines and/or hydrocortisone; they rarely cause the treatment to be stopped. The progress of thrombolysis should be monitored by some form of phlebography and the duration of treatment adjusted to the rate of response. Clinical assessment is of no value as the signs of deep vein thrombosis always improve spontaneously.

The only common reason for stopping treatment with SK is the occurrence of bleeding, and consequently most clinicians will not use SK within 72 hours of a surgical operation. If bleeding occurs it is usually sufficient to stop the SK and wait 2–4 hours for its effect to wear off, but the thrombolytic state can be reversed rapidly when the bleeding is severe by giving epsilon-amino-caproic acid, fresh fibrinogen and fresh blood.

The haematological effect of SK can be controlled by measuring the euglobulin lysis time, the dilute blood clot lysis time, the plasma plasminogen and fibrinogen, and the prothrombin time. Many laboratories do not have the facility to do these tests and in practice they are not particularly helpful, as the only indication to reduce the dose of SK is the presence of clinically detectable bleeding. However, if one had to choose the most valuable simple test it would be the prothrombin time. If this is prolonged beyond 45 seconds, it indicates that there has been considerable destruction of the circulating coagulation factors and the chances of spontaneous bleeding are increased. After thrombolysis anticoagulants must be given to prevent re-thrombosis. If re-thrombosis occurs when the plasminogen is low, there will be little plasminogen entrapped within the thrombus and the new thrombus will be resistant to further thrombolytic treatment, Heparin should be started 2–4 hours after finishing the SK. Warfarin can be given before the SK infusion ends, but this is difficult to control.

Clinical indications

Deep vein thrombosis. There is no doubt that SK will dissolve fresh thrombus and so it may reduce the late morbidity of deep vein thrombosis, but there are no long term studies to prove this. SK should probably be reserved for treating fresh non-adherent thrombus, which one knows can be dissolved easily, when there is a chance that removing the thrombus will save the valves. Unfortunately, the commonest variety of thrombus that one sees in clinical practice is old, adherent and resistent to lysis. Treatment with SK should never be advised without phlebographic evidence of the site and nature of the thrombus. The number of times when thrombus in the peripheral veins can be lysed to the clear advantage of the patient is small.

Pulmonary embolism. Thrombus that leaves the legs and reaches the lungs is likely to be relatively fresh and soft. Furthermore thrombus within the lungs, if it does not completely occlude a branch of the pulmonary artery, will have a large volume of blood flowing past it. These two reasons make pulmonary emboli particularly susceptible to thrombolysis.

The effects of pulmonary embolism on pulmonary artery resistance can be divided into three degrees. Massive pulmonary obstruction, which is causing rapid haemodynamic deterioration and where surgery is the only method of removing the obstruction fast enough to ensure survival. Major obstruction, where the raised pulmonary artery resistance causes continuing but non-fatal embarrassment to the right heart, and the third most common degree of obstruction which is either minor in the first instance, or more severe but improves spontaneously. The first group must be treated surgically. In the last group the lungs need no particular treatment but the clinician must ensure that further emboli do not occur. The small middle group are difficult to manage because it is difficult to predict their progress and some may deteriorate. In these patients SK can produce a rapid clinical improvement by reducing the pulmonary artery resistance and increasing cardiac output. However, when a group of this type of patient treated with SK is compared to a similar group treated with heparin it can be shown that, although the haemodynamic status after one to two days is much better in the SK treated group, the results after seven days are almost the same. Thus, although SK can dissolve pulmonary emboli the clinician must decide which patients really need it. At the moment it is usually reserved for those patients who are seriously ill, not quite bad enough to need an embolectomy but who are not showing any signs of spontaneous improvement.

REFERENCES

Aschoff, L. (1924) *Lectures in Pathology*. New York: Hoeber.

Artz, C. P. & Pulaski, E. J. (1953) *Angiology* **4**, 321.

Barker, N. W., Nygaard, K. K., Walters, W., & Priestly, J. T. (1940) *Proc. Mayo Clin.*, **15**, 769.

Barker, N. W. (1940) *Proc. Mayo Clin.*, **16**, 1, 17.

Bowen, O. (1889) *Liverpool Med. Chir. J.*, **9**, 70.

Browse, N. L. (1973) Chap. 5 in '*Peripheral Vascular Surgery*' Ed. M. Birnstingl, Heinemann.

Carlotti, J., Hardy, I. B., Linton, R. R. & White, P. (1947) *Ibid.*, **134**, 1447.

Cockett, F. B. (1970) *Modern Trends in Vascular Surgery*. Butterworths.

Cohnheim, J. (1872) *Untersuchungen uber die Embolischen Processe*. Berlin: Hirschwald.

DeBakey, M. E. (1954) *Surg. Gynec. Obstet.*, **98**, 1.

Evans, D. S. (1970) *M.S. Thesis*, London.

Fowler, E. F. & Bollinger, J. A. (1954) *Surgery* **3**, 650.

Fred, H. L., Axelrad, M. A., Lewis, J. M. and Alexander, J. K. (1966) *J. Amer. Med. Ass.*, **196**, 1137.

Glenn, J. H. (1896) *Trans. R. Acad. Med. Ire.*, **14**, 291.

Greenstein, J. (1945) *S. Afr. Med. J.*, **10**, 350.

Hadfield. G. (1950) *Ann. R. Coll. Surg. Engl.*, **6**, 219.

Henderson, E. F. (1927) *Arch. Surg. Chicago,* **15**, 231.
Hufses, A. H. (1954) *Surgery* **35**, 957.
Hughes, E. S. R. (1949) *Int. Abst. Surg.*, **88**, 89.
Hume, M., Sevitt, S., Thomas, D. P. (1970) '*Venous Thrombosis and Pulmonary Embolism*'. Harvard University Press.
Hunter, W. C., Krygier, J. J., Kennedy, J. C. & Sneeden, U. D. (1945) *Surgery*, **17**, 178.
Jorpes, J. E. (1946) *Edinburgh Medical Journal*, **513,** 222.
Kakkar, V. V., Howe, L. T., Flanc & Clarke, M. B. (1969) *Lancet*, **II**, 230.
Laennec, R. T. H. (1846) *A Treatise on Mediate Auscultation and on Diseases of the Lungs and Heart.* London: Bailliere.
Laufman (1954) *Personal communication.*
Matas, R. (1932) *Univ. Toronto Med. Bull.*, **10**, 1.
Malpighi (1686) in '*De Polypo Cordis Dissertatio*'.
McLachlin, J. & Paterson, J. C. (1951) *Surg. Gynec. Obstet.*, **93**, 1.
Miller, R. & Berry, U. B. (1951) *Amer. J. med. Sci.*, **222**, 197.
Murley, R. S. (1950) *Ann. R. Coll. Surg.*, **6**, 283.
Morrell, M. T. & Dunnill, M. S. (1968) *Brit. J. Surg.*, **55,** 347.
Morrell, M. T., Truelove, S. C. & Barr, A. (1963) *Brit. Med. J.*, **II**, 830.
Payling-Wright, H. (1952) *Brit. Heart J.*, **14**, 325.
Pilcher, R. (1937) *Brit. J. Surg.*, **25**, 42.
Pitman (1864) 'Obstruction of the Pulmonary Artery by Coagula causing sudden Death'. *Lancet*, **1**, 123.
Raeburn, C. (1951) *Brit. Med. J.*, **11**, 517.
Remfry, L. (1891) *Trans. Clin. Soc. Lond.*, **24**, 222.
Rokitansky, C. F. (1855) *A Manual of Pathological Anatomy*. London Sydenham Soc., Vol. 4.
Rossle, R. (1937) *Virchow's Arch.*, **300**, 180.
Secker-Walker, R. H., Jackson, J. A. & Goodwin, J. (1970) *Brit. Med. J.*, **4**, 135.
Sevitt, S. & Gallagher, N. G. (1959) *Lancet*, **II**, 981.
Sevitt, S. & Gallagher, N. G. (1960) *Brit. J. Surg.*, **48**, 475.
Trousseau (1870) in Lecture 31 on 'Gangrene of Lung', *Clinical Medicine*, Vol. **III**, 173.
Uhland, H. & Goldberg, L. M. (1964) *Dis. Chest*, **45**, 533.
Virchow, R. (1846) *Die Verstopfung der Lungenarterie und ihre Folgen. Beitr. exp. Path. Physiol.* Berlin, Traube **2**, 1.
Virchow, R. (1846) Ueber die Verstopfung der Lungenarterie Votizen Gebiete. *Natur. u. Heilk.*, **37**, 26.
Virchow, R. (1856) Neuer Fall von Toedlicher Embolie oer Lungenarterie. *Virchow's Arch.*, **10,** 225.
Virchow, R. (1859) De l'obstruction de l'arterie pulmonaire, Paris, *Union Med.*, **4.**
Welsh, W. H. (1899) 'Embolism'. *System of Medicine*. (Edited Allbutt, T. C.) **6**, 228.
Wessler, S. (1953) *J. Clin. Invest.*, **7**, 650–654.

15. Peripheral Deep Vein Thrombosis and Control of Thrombo-embolism

As described in the previous chapter there are two main clinical groups of lower limb thrombosis:

1. *Ilio-femoral Thrombosis*—which affects predominantly the common and external iliac veins, and may spread a greater or lesser distance down the femoral vein. This type is considered in the next Chapter.

2. *Peripheral Deep Vein Thrombosis*—which arises in the veins *below* the inguinal ligament.

It is true that occasionally thrombosis arising in the peripheral veins may spread upwards and involve the great vessels right up to the cava and thus produce the clinical picture of a severe ilio-femoral thrombosis. However, the slow spread of the thrombosis upwards is usually fairly evident clinically and has a somewhat different history from the sudden appearance of a swollen thigh and leg which characterises the true ilio-femoral thrombosis arising in the iliac veins. (Chap. 16.).

The great importance of peripheral deep vein thrombosis is threefold:

1. It occurs particularly (although not entirely) in hospitals as a complication of any illness (surgical or medical) which involves rest in bed for any length of time, and is often found in *both legs*.

2. It has a slow, insidious onset without signs or symptoms in the early stage, with the attendant danger of repeated pulmonary embolism.

3. It usually involves destruction of the valves in the ankle perforating veins by the thrombosis and therefore the appearance of the post-thrombotic syndrome of the ankle, with or without ulceration, after a period of five years or so in most of the patients.

Peripheral deep vein thrombosis may start anywhere in the deep veins. The common ways in which it may start however, are:

1. In the soleus sinusoids (Fig. 14.4). These large, sinusoids in the soleus are quite peculiar to this muscle. They drain direct into the posterior tibial or peroneal veins by a number of short, straight vessels, entering the tibial or peroneal veins at the same place as the ankle perforators join them.

The degree of development of the calf sinusoids differs considerably from patient to patient and it is possible that here we may have an anatomical cause for the predisposition of some patients to calf thrombosis.

2. Some thrombi arise in the main deep veins usually in association with a valve cusp, (see Fig. 14.5) (McLachlin and Paterson 1951 and 1954).

3. Another group occurs spreading inwards from a superficial thrombosis in varicose veins. The spread into the deep veins occurs either at the sapheno-femoral junction (in the case of long saphenous thrombosis) or at the sapheno-popliteal junction (in the case of short saphenous thrombosis) or in through the direct ankle perforating veins.

As in all cases of thrombosis, one's first thought on being presented with a case, is to ask 'is there a pathological cause?' (Pressure on the vein, carcinoma, polycythaemia, etc.—see Chapter 14.) Only when this has been excluded can one assume it to be a case of 'idiopathic' or 'stasis' thrombosis.

This condition is liable to occur and build up quietly in any patient who is in bed ill, after an operation, or after any illness which entails inactivity and rest in bed. It occurs with increasing frequency in the older age groups particularly (50–70 years) and usually both legs are affected.

Finally, although the condition has acquired the name 'stasis thrombosis' owing to its association with post-operative or post 'illness' bed rest, there is a large interesting group of cases which occur in apparently normal people as a sudden episode, when they are active and not associated with previous illness (see Chap. 14, Table 14.2). These cases of idiopathic thrombosis are obviously not primarily due to stasis. Another odd factor about them is that there is often a family history of thrombosis and embolism. All this points to some other cause being operative in these cases, and there is some evidence that inherited anatomical abnormalities of the deep veins (such as well developed calf sinusoids, and balloon like dilatations of the main deep veins) may be an aetiological factor in some of them.

CLINICAL PRESENTATIONS OF THROMBOSIS

The great difficulty in the diagnosis of this disease is that in its early stage of 'phlebothrombosis' there may be no detectable clinical signs of the disease at all. Small thrombi in calf veins and small pulmonary emboli may occur without any signs or symptoms. It is only when peripheral thrombi or pulmonary emboli reach a certain critical size that they produce clinical signs which may be detected by the careful clinician. This disquieting fact has been known for many years, but its truth was only amply demonstrated when the very sensitive I^{125+} tagged fibrinogen method of detecting small deep vein thromboses in the legs was employed to screen all the legs of a selected hospital population at risk. (Kakkar et al 1968; Negus, 1968). In one series (Kakkar) minor thrombosis was detected in fully 30 per cent of the patients examined. This was confirmed by Browse and Negus, (1969).

However, most of these very small thromboses never develop into a dangerous or significant size, and when they do, certain clinical indications develop. Phlebographic evidence suggests that thrombi do not become dangerous from the point of view of severe or fatal pulmonary embolism until they have reached and begun to grow into the main popliteal and femoral veins. But even at this stage there may be surprisingly few clinical signs.

The fact that a patient has a deep venous thrombosis may be signalled *clinically* in three separate ways:

1. By the occurrence of a detectable pulmonary embolus, fatal, or more usually non-fatal—'out of the blue'.
2. By the persistence of a low grade pyrexia which fails to settle after operation.
3. By the occurrence of local signs of thrombophlebitis in the limbs.

It is important to realise that a patient may present in any one way alone, or in all three ways together, or separated by a greater or lesser time interval. We must now consider these three clinical types in more detail.

1. *An Embolus—unanticipated.* From our consideration of the pathology of thrombosis it is obvious that if a patient is in the stage of phlebothrombosis, there may be a long propagated thrombus floating loose in the leg veins, attached only at its lower end. This may give no signs or symptoms at all until it suddenly becomes detached, is carried to the right heart and plugs the pulmonary artery to become a fatal pulmonary embolus. If only a small piece of it breaks off, the patient may be luckier and the embolus may be non-fatal—that is fittingly called a 'warning embolus'. It is a caution, because it indicates that the patient has phlebothrombosis somewhere—probably in the lower limbs and unless this is treated energetically and urgently the patient may not be so fortunate with the second embolus.

This concept is in accordance with all the observed facts about pulmonary emboli, for nearly all authors (DeBakey, 1954 and Marks et al., 1954) have recorded that approximately half of all emboli, both fatal and non-fatal occur without preceding signs of thrombosis in the legs. Of course there is another possible reason for this, which accounts for some cases, namely that the site of occurrence of the thrombophlebitis (which may be initiating the propagated embolus clot) may not be in the legs at all, but in the hypogastric veins, or profunda femoris vein. In both places, clinical signs of even established thrombophlebitis are slight and undetectable clinically in the early stages. In this type of case, however, the temperature chart usually signals a low remittent pyrexia and this may be the only indication (see Figs 15.1 and 14.6).

What makes the propagated clot break off and become an embolus? An old observation that pulmonary emboli often occur when the patient is straining on the bed pan, or is beginning to be active, has some significance. If the passage upwards in the deep veins of some diodone is watched under the X-ray screen, and the patient is then asked to perform the Valsalva manoeuvre (essentially the same as straining on a bed pan, i.e. holding the breath and straining) the veins will be seen to dilate as blood refluxes into them, ballooning out the valves and distending them. On cessation of the Valsalva manoeuvre the veins deflate and the blood is aspirated upwards again, with the gasping inspiration which follows the straining. Seeing this, it is easy to imagine that this sort of reflux distension, and then sudden relief of distension, would produce just enough force to loosen a fragile, slightly attached, propagated clot. Violent coughing would have the same effect. On the contrary, putting the feet up has precisely the opposite effect. The veins collapse, and if there was a long loose clot in the veins, they would tend to collapse on to it and entrap it more firmly.

At what time does embolism occur? As it occurs just as frequently in medical patients and bed-ridden patients who have not undergone operation, it can obviously occur at any time. However, post-operative embolism does tend to occur at a peak period from the fifth to the tenth post-operative day. Pilcher (1937), in his series, found that they occurred from one day to four weeks after operation, but half of them occurred within the fifth to the

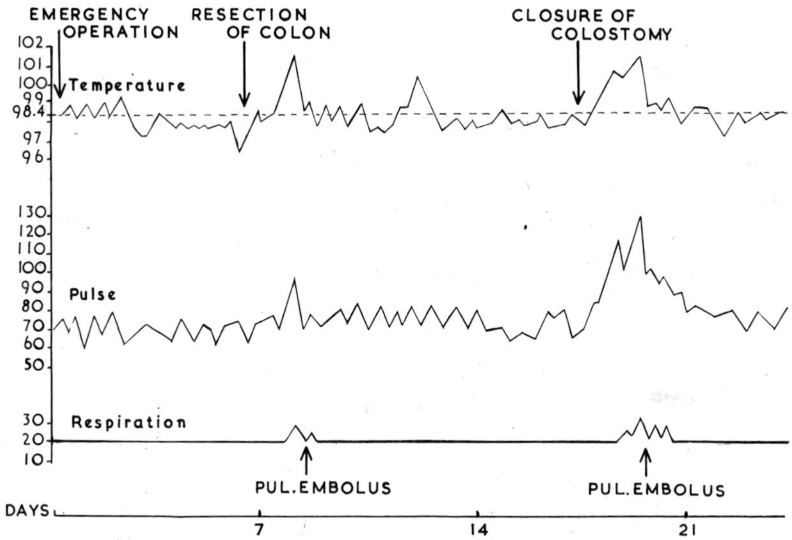

Fig. 15.1 Temperature chart of a patient who had two non-fatal pulmonary emboli. On each occasion the patient had a sharp pain in the chest, followed by haemoptysis. The chart shows the typical 'kick' of temperature and pulse rate which signals an embolus. (Almost exactly the same phenomena accompany an acute lobar or lobular atelectasis.) This patient eventually had a third embolus—and both common iliac veins were then tied. This terminated his embolic episodes. He later left hospital with some residual oedema of his legs easily controlled by elastic bandages. (*By courtesy of Dr. J. Latto.*)

tenth post-operative days. Both of the authors have observed a fatal pulmonary embolus occur on the first post-operative day.

Is it easy to diagnose a pulmonary embolus? Let us consider the fatal ones first. The picture of a post-operative patient who is well one moment, who suddenly has a tense constricted feeling in the chest, and is dead in three minutes or so, is practically pathognomonic and diagnosis is a theoretical exercise only. However, a group of cases exists in whom the embolus is not immediately fatal and the patient may 'hang between life and death' for an hour or two up to 12 or 15 hours. In this group of cases the differential diagnosis between pulmonary embolism and other conditions such as coronary thrombosis, acute ventricular failure, or acute pulmonary collapse, may present real difficulty. It is particularly important to know the diagnosis in this small group, as it is in these rare cases that the possibility of operative removal of the embolus from the pulmonary artery arises, and should be seriously considered. Here an electrocardiogram may be of great use as it always shows right axis deviation in cases of major embolism and it should certainly be done before any operation is contemplated, as the operative exposure of the pulmonary artery in a patient with acute coronary thrombosis would be an error indeed! Another helpful point is that in pulmonary embolism there is always considerable *tachycardia*—this is not so with coronary thrombosis (*see* Fig. 15.1).

Non-fatal pulmonary emboli are not always easy to diagnose. It takes quite a large embolus for it to produce enough pathological change to lead to symptoms and signs (Mathes et al., 1932). Such large to medium sized emboli may produce a sudden 'constricted feeling in the chest' with difficulty in breathing. The patient may sit up, short of breath and alarmed. *There is always a sudden rise in pulse rate with emboli of any size and this is a most important physical sign.* There may be a transient fall in systemic blood pressure and the patient may feel faint or may actually collapse. Recovery from such an episode may be quite rapid, and within half an hour the patient may be easier but the pulse rate remains high for several hours. Such an episode may go almost unnoticed in a busy ward, or may be put down to 'nerves', by unobservant or hard pressed nurses and doctors.

Smaller emboli in the periphery of the lung may give rise to sudden pleuritic pain followed perhaps in a day or so by transient haemoptysis. These are probably the *smallest clinically evident* type of emboli. Laufman (1954) has produced good evidence that this picture of minor pulmonary infarction (i.e. pleuritic pain and blood stained sputum) only occurs when an embolus reaches a part of the lung which is already the site of either collapse or infection. This may explain why this picture is so often seen in post-operative cases.

Rise of pulse rate is a constant and important diagnostic sign with all pulmonary emboli, large or small. This typical 'kick' of pulse rate, together with transient rise of temperature and respiratory rate is shown on Figure 15.1.

X-rays are of little value in diagnosis. With a large pulmonary embolus the straight X-ray may be *practically normal.* In the smaller, peripheral emboli with pleuritic pain and minor infarction, basal fluffy opacities may be seen, with later on a little fluid, but these changes take three to four days to appear.

Occasionally a friction rub may be heard over an area of pleurisy and later coarse crepitations. But these are really late signs of collapse and infarction in the area affected by the embolus. Usually the diagnosis must be made clinically, and in the less severe cases with perhaps a history of transient tightness of the chest and faintness, or a transient pleurisy, the diagnosis must be made practically on suspicion.

Where the facilities exist the only two fairly reliable investigations to prove the existence of a major pulmonary embolus in the lung are the lung scan (Chap. 13), and in the last resort, the pulmonary angiogram.

Recurrent pulmonary emboli

Occasionally small, recurrent pulmonary emboli may occur over a period of time—perhaps over years, producing a gradual plugging of the small pulmonary veins. This may lead to the gradual onset of pulmonary hypertension and the patient may present with signs of right heart failure. (Dyspnoea, cyanosis, enlarged neck veins and persistent tachycardia with right axis deviation on the electrocardiogram.) Such cases occur from the gradual build-up of multiple, small, tough emboli which are often too small to give any dramatic episode on their own. One such case seen by one of the authors, was a young man of thirty-two with terminal right heart failure, who had been feeding small thrombi into his pulmonary circulation for years, from a large, cavernous haemangioma in his leg.

2. *Persistent Low-Grade Pyrexia.* This may occur at the same time as the onset of signs in the legs. It is more properly a sign of the stage of thrombophlebitis than of phlebothrombosis. Its value lies in the fact that when thrombophlebitis is occurring in parts of the venous system not readily accessible to clinical examination (i.e. the pelvic veins, and the deep veins of the thigh) and having, therefore, no other detectable clinical signs, the persistent low pyrexia may be the only clue to its presence. An emphatic illustration of this point is seen in Figure 14.6. In this case the persistent low pyrexia was the only sign of the thrombophlebitis of the pelvic and internal iliac veins which eventually led to the patient's death from embolism.

At this point it may be well to stress that the occurrence of this pyrexia does not necessarily mean that a septic process is going on. True septic thrombophlebitis gives a different clinical picture. (Chap. 14).

3. *Local Signs of Thrombophlebitis in the legs.* Local signs in the legs occur after thrombosis has been present in the legs for some time (3–7 days at least) and is becoming adherent, producing obstruction of the vein and an inflammatory reaction in the vein wall. The signs therefore are the signs of venous obstruction and inflammation. They vary therefore according to the size and length of vein affected.

A rough guide to the clinical signs expected as the thrombosis spreads to involve smaller, then bigger veins is given in the accompanying table, 15.1.

It is extremely important to remember that this type of peripheral deep vein thrombosis is *usually bilateral*, and the process may be at different stages in the two legs. Thus, there may be plentiful signs in one leg (stage of thrombophlebitis, with most of the thrombus adherent) and no signs in the other leg (which might easily have a loose, dangerous, early thrombus in it).

Investigation and appearances on phlebography

The main thing which has hampered diagnosis and rational treatment of thromboembolism, has been the lack of a reliable physical method to detect the presence, and site of loose thrombus in the early and dangerous stage of the disease. Clinical diagnosis in this stage is difficult and open to error which varies considerably with the experience or enthusiasm of the observer until recently. Treatment has therefore been somewhat empirical.

This situation was revolutionised between 1967–1971 by the appearance and extensive use of three new and reliable methods for the detection of early, loose, symptomless thrombus in the deep veins of the legs. These methods are:

1. Emergency phlebography
2. The use of ultrasound
3. The use of I^{125} labelled Fibrinogen.

Full details of the technique and use of these three methods are given in Chapter 13.

The question which we shall try to answer here is *when* should these investigations be used in clinical practice and *which* ones?

No method gives such universal, reliable and accurate information as an emergency venogram and this should always be the final court of appeal on which treatment is based.

The Doppler ultrasound method is simple, cheap, portable and can easily be used by a

Table 15.1 Clinical guide to spread of thrombosis

Stage 1:	Thrombosis confined to calf sinusoids.	Calf tenderness on deep palpation only.
Stage 2:	Spread of thrombosis to involve a length of post-tibial veins, and the ankle perforating veins.	1) Calf tenderness and ? positive Homan's signs. 2) Tenderness and oedema on inner aspect of ankle and lower third of leg. Tenderness is sometimes acute just over the upper and middle internal ankle perforators behind the posterior border of the tibia. (Cohen, 1952). 3) Low pyrexia. 4) Ankle is warm. 5) Duskiness of foot in dependant position.
Stage 3:	Spread of thrombosis to involve whole of posterior tibial veins, and spreading to popliteal.	As above, plus 1) Marked oedema of ankle. 2) Increase in girth of calf. 3) Leg is obviously warm to touch. 4) Pyrexia up to 99°–100°F.
Stage 4:	Spread to involve whole of femoral and iliac veins.	Picture of white leg; phlegmasia alba dolens. 1) Concentric, tense oedema of whole limb (leg and thigh). 2) Limb pale or dusky blue. 3) Limb hot to touch. 4) Fever up to 101°F. 5) Limb heavy; moved and flexed with difficulty. 6) May be pain over femoral vein in groin.

house surgeon at the bedside with minimal training. It will detect early thrombus of a size which is just beginning to form in a major vein such as the popliteal—it will not detect minor calf thrombosis. In other words it will detect large, dangerous thrombi.

The I^{125} tagged fibrinogen method is really a research tool rather than a universal clinical method. It has many disadvantages for routine clinical use. These are: (1) It is far too sensitive, and will pick up the smallest thrombus in the calf veins; (2) For this reason it cannot be used on any patient with a wound, or bruise, or operation on the legs. (This automatically cuts out its use in all peripheral vascular and vein cases—a very large field!); (3) It cannot be used reliably to detect thrombus in the ilio-femoral veins, particularly after any lower abdominal surgery; (4) The apparatus required is expensive and needs trained personnel to use it; (5) It cannot be used as an emergency until the thyroid has been blocked by a preliminary dose of sodium iodide; (6) It may not detect locally 'formed' thrombi as it depends on the uptake of isotope labelled fibrinogen in the 'forming' process. This makes it unreliable when given to a suspicious case. Its real value is when it is given prospectively, e.g. before the thrombus has formed. It is very accurate when used in this way and has a useful place in clinical trials and in the screening of high risk patients, but not, repeat NOT, in the diagnosis of the patient presenting with suspicious tenderness or swelling of the calf, or with signs of pulmonary embolism.

For these reasons, the I^{125} Fibrinogen method is not for routine clinical use and can only be used where trained personnel are available and in hospitals where there is a radio-isotope department.

It is suggested that a practical method of investigation of any case of suspected thrombo-embolism should be:

1. An immediate 'Doppler ultrasound' examination of *both* legs. If this is positive, this should be followed by:
2. An emergency venogram of *both* legs (see Chap. 13). *This will give accurate information about the site and position of the thrombus, on which immediate treatment can be undertaken.*

Even if Doppler ultrasound investigation is negative, an emergency venogram may still have to be done if the clinical suspicion is great enough.

A typical example of how an emergency venogram is used for diagnosis and treatment is shown in Figure 13.2 and in Figure 16.12.

TREATMENT

The treatment of deep thrombosis falls under two headings:

1. The prevention of deep thrombosis (prophylactic treatment).
2. The treatment of the established condition.

Of these two the first, prophylactic treatment, is by far the more important.

PROPHYLAXIS

Prevention is better than cure and the following points are particularly applicable to post-operative surgical cases. If stasis of venous blood in the legs during and after operation is a major factor in the aetiology of this type of peripheral deep venous thrombosis, then a major point in the prophylaxis must be to encourage a fast and even venous return from the legs on the operating table and afterwards during recovery. This also applies to any ill medical patient and to surgical patients in bed *before* operation. Thus the points of importance are as follows:

1. *Gentle handling* of the unconscious patient. Avoidance of trauma to the calves and legs generally when moving the patient. Excessive pressure on the calves as with unpadded lithotomy poles is undesirable. Tight, obstructing bandages round the *thighs* to attach diathermy plates should be avoided.
2. *The legs should if possible, be raised to just above the heart's level, i.e. the foot of the bed, or operating table should be raised about six or nine inches* (Fig. 15.2).

This is by far the most important and simplest anti-stasis measure which can be applied to nearly all patients at risk, both surgical and medical. All surgical cases should have a slight 10° tilt with the feet up before any long operation, and the foot of the bed should be up during the whole of the recovery period (5–10 days or more) but especially so when the patient is unconscious or weak. (Wright and Osborn, 1952).

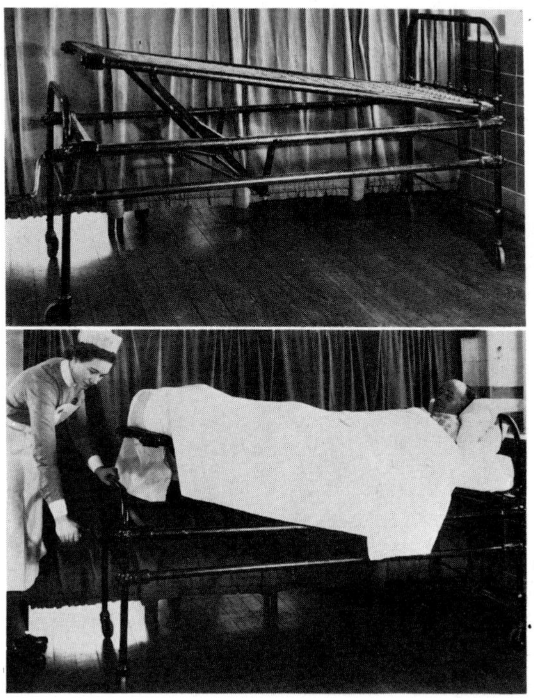

Fig. 15.2 The anti-thrombosis bed.

3. *Activity*. Muscular activity of the calf is of course the best physiological method of speeding the venous return from the legs. Recently papers have appeared advocating simple ways of achieving muscular activity of the calf on the operating table in the unconscious patient, by repeated electrical stimulation. (Coran, F.S.A. & White, H.M., B.J.S., 1967.) (Browse & Negus, B.M.J., 1970), and by pneumatic compression methods; (Hills, Pflug, Jeyasuph, Boardman, Calnan, B.M.J. 1972). There is good evidence that such methods cut down the incidence of small calf thrombi found during or just after operation. However, the routine use of such apparatus in all operations would be a considerable extra undertaking and it is doubtful if going to such lengths is really worthwhile, particularly as much the same result can be achieved by simply elevating the feet above the heart.

However, these studies do pin-point the importance of muscular activity. All patients before and just after operation must be trained to move and exercise the calves and feet in bed. This means steady 'indoctrination' of not only patients but of all who have the day to day care of patients, e.g. house surgeons, nurses, physiotherapists, etc.

4. *Early Activity*. This is not synonymous with the practice of driving the patient out of bed on the day after operation to sit slumped in a chair, with his legs down and inactive, which promotes leg stasis! It means that the patient should get out of bed at the earliest possible moment that he can move actively, walk and exercise his legs. Early activity *out* of bed is the sequel to early activity *in* bed that should have started as soon as the patient came into hospital, and on recovery from the anaesthetic.

5. *Elastic Stockings and Bandages*. It has been claimed that limb compression by elastic hose produces an increased flow velocity through the deep veins by narrowing and compressing the venous bed. (Wilkins et al., 1952; Meyerowitz & Nelson, Flanc et al., 1969, *Lancet*). Whether this is so or not, adequate elastic compression of the calf and leg generally does compress both the superficial and deep veins. This may have an appreciable effect particularly in elderly patients who for various reasons cannot put their feet above their heart for long periods. Elastic compression in bed and during the whole period of inactivity is particularly applicable to older patients, who have dilated varicose veins. Thrombosis in these is a real hazard, in bed, or after operation, or illness, and may well spread to the deep veins. *Such patients should always wear light elastic compression bandages in bed during the whole course of the operation or illness.*

It is significant that in the exhaustive study of the effect of these prophylactic measures by Flanc et al. (*Lancet* 1969), significant reduction of the thrombosis rate was only and particularly demonstrated in the *elderly* undergoing surgery. This again points to the possibility that in younger patients other factors may be operative such as congenital vein malformations. (See Chap. 16)

The place of anticoagulants in prophylaxis

Sevitt (1959) has shown in a classic controlled experiment that if efficient, closely controlled oral anticoagulant therapy is used in a small selected group at risk, it is effective in controlling thrombo-embolism. The particular group used in the trial were a series of elderly patients with fractured femurs, a group notoriously liable to thrombo-embolic complications. Patients were maintained on oral anticoagulants (Dindevan) from admission, before, during and after operation right up to discharge—a good demonstration of the *true* prophylactic use of anticoagulants.

Unfortunately these councils of perfection are not applicable to the hospital population as a whole. One's imagination staggers at the thought of every hospital patient in the country on anticoagulants during the whole of their admission! It is probable that under such circumstances the complication rate of the anticoagulation therapy alone might outweigh the risks of the disease it was supposedly preventing. Moreover, in most operations the added risk and complication rate of operating under anticoagulants would make it unattractive. Finally the maintenance of the required low prothrombin index requires constant and skilled laboratory attention.

Thus for practical purposes in the generality of the hospital population, true and adequate prophylactic anticoagulation is not a practical proposition. It may however, be applied to small, selected groups, but even in these the complication rate is appreciable and nearly equals the risk rate from major thrombo-embolism.

THE TREATMENT OF ESTABLISHED THROMBO-EMBOLISM

As we have seen the disease 'Thrombo-embolism' commonly shows itself in three ways:

1. As an embolism, fatal or non-fatal.
2. As a pyrexia of unknown origin.
3. As deep thrombosis of a limb with local signs.

First we must consider what are the prime aims of treatment. These are, in order of importance:

1. The prevention of death or disability by recurrent pulmonary emboli.
2. The prevention of further spread of the local thrombosis and thus the reduction of long term morbidity (post-thrombotic syndrome).

By far the most useful advance in treatment has been based on the increased awareness and 'suspicion index' of the early warning signs of the thrombo-embolic state, and then the emergency application of the modern, accurate methods of detecting the dangerous, loose thrombus in the peripheral veins. (Ultrasound scanning followed by emergency phlebography).

The procedure should be as follows: The suspicion that the patient has a thrombo-embolic state may be aroused by one of the early warning signs, such as a small warning embolus, or a tender calf with or without slight swelling of the ankle, or a persistent pyrexia. First the ultrasound detector should be employed on both legs. If this shows that both femoral and popliteal veins are clear of occluding thrombus then the patient is not in immediate danger, and a venogram can be arranged within the next twenty-four hours. If however, the ultrasound test is positive, indicating an occluding thrombus in a major popliteal or femoral vein—then emergency phlebography should be undertaken without delay (within 2–3 hours) in both legs, as this indicates the possibility of a large embolus.

The appropriate action to be taken is decided on the result of the emergency phlebogram. Broadly speaking there are three possible results which may be shown (Fig. 15.3):

1. Veins clear.
2. Small thrombi confined to veins in calf or lower leg.
3. 'Floating' thrombus in popliteal or femoral vein.

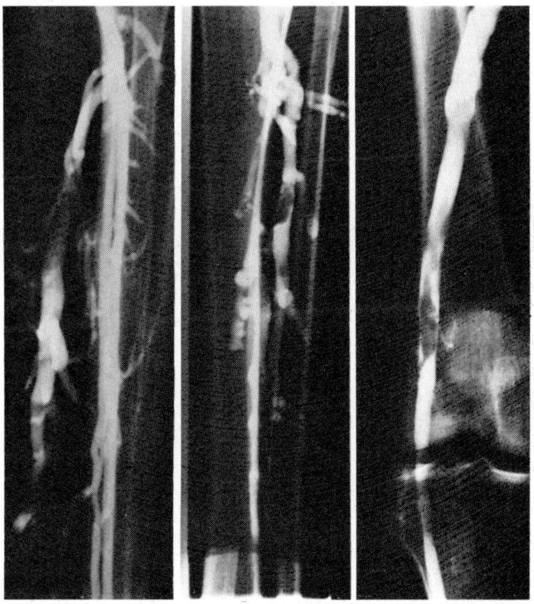

Fig. 15.3 These phlebograms illustrate the three conditions which may be found on emergency phlebography: (1) Normal veins. (2) Small thrombus, confined to calf or leg veins. (3) Thrombus in femoral veins.

Let us consider what action to take in each case.

1. *Veins clear*: No treatment. Continue activity and mobilisation and observation.

2. *Small thrombi* confined to veins in calf or lower leg.

These are not considered an immediate threat to life, although they may give rise to recurrent minor embolism. In general therefore if the patient is recovering from an operation or illness and is being mobilised and will be out of bed and active within a few days, no special treatment need be considered for these cases. Mobilisation and activity should continue, elastic bandages should be used round both calves from the toes to the knees. The patient should be monitored with the ultrasound every two days to guard against the possibility of quiet extension of the thrombus.

However if the patient is *not* in sight of immediate activity and mobilisation of if *he is to undergo another operation*, then the probability is that these thrombi will extend and give rise to repetitive embolism. Such cases are best treated by bilateral ligature of both the superficial femoral veins below the profunda (see below) followed by a short course of oral anticoagulants.

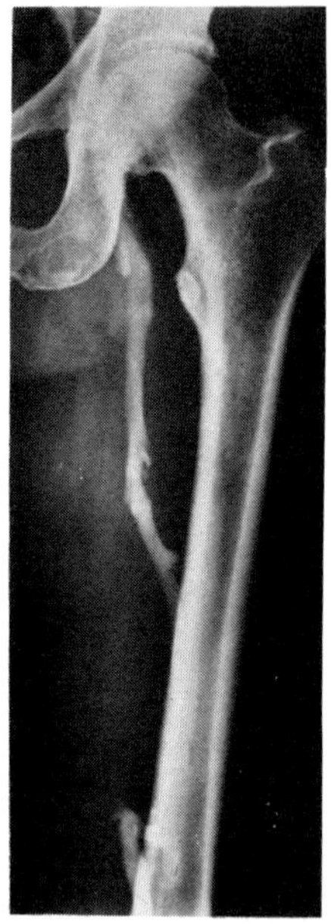

Fig. 15.5 Three months previous to this venogram the femoral vein distal to the entry of the profunda had been tied (as a prophylaxis against embolism). This patient developed no swelling or sequelae of any kind, and the excellent deep collateral circulation via the profunda vein is seen on this venogram, by-passing the short segmental thrombosis which has resulted from the ligature.

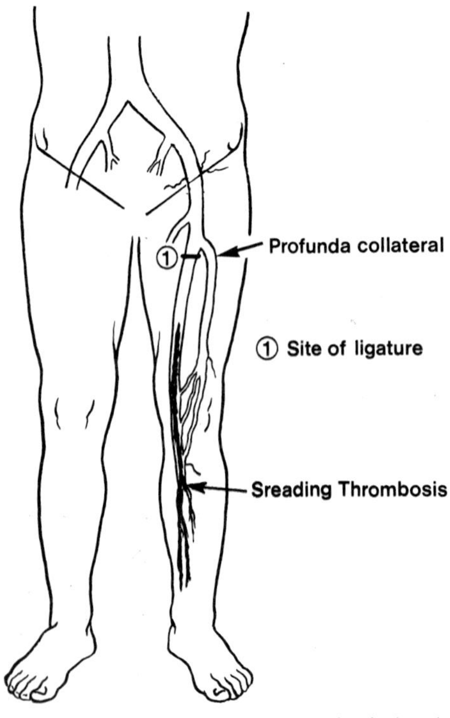

Fig. 15.4 Ligature of superficial femoral vein just below profunda.

(Treatment with oral anticoagulants *alone* in these cases may *not* in fact prevent growth of thrombus and repetitive emboli, see Chap. 14.)

3. *'Floating' thrombus in Popliteal or Femoral Vein* (*see also* Fig. 13.2).

This is the dangerous situation, which calls for immediate effective treatment. The patient in fact may have already had one or more small emboli (silent or with minor symptoms and signs only) and the next embolus waiting in the femoral vein may be the killer.

On seeing this condition on the venogram

the safest course of action is immediate surgery. The patient is taken to theatre and under either a local, (if very ill) or a general anaesthetic, the femoral vein at the profunda junction is displayed in *both* groins. Both femoral veins are ligatured just distal to the profunda junction. If a Fogarty catheter is available the femoral vein may be opened and as much as possible of the loose thrombus extracted. This manoeuvre is facilitated by squeezing the calf and limb vigorously and so massaging loose thrombus up to the venotomy, which is then closed with 0000 silk. A dose of Heparin is then given (6–7,000 International Units) and the wounds are closed with a small 'Readivac' drain in each. The patient is maintained on oral anticoagulants for about one month and is mobilised as soon as possible.

Sometimes phlebograms show a loose tail of thrombus extending above the profunda into the common femoral or even into the external iliac vein or above. In such cases it may be necessary to plicate the common femoral, external iliac or even in certain cases the common iliac vein or cava (see case Chap. 16, Fig. 12).

If it is necessary to interrupt a vein above the entry of the profunda this should always be done by 'plication', (see next Chapter) rather than by ligature. Ligature of the common femoral or of the iliac veins always leaves the limb with some residual swelling and tenseness and discomfort on exercise. Ligature of the superficial femoral vein below the profunda however, is a benign procedure as the profunda collaterals are profuse and there is seldom any swelling or discomfort of the leg other than that which occurs slowly as a result of the destruction of the valves in the ankle perforating veins by the thrombus in the calf (Fig. 15.5).

REFERENCES

Browse, N. L., Clapham, W. F., Croft, D. N., Lea Thomas, M. & Williams, J. O. (1971) *Brit. Med. J.*, **4**, 325.

Browse, N. L. & Negus, D. (1970) *Brit. Med. J.*, **3**, 615.

DeBakey, M. E. (1954) *Surg. Gynec. Obstet.*, **93**, 1.

Doran, F. S. A. & White (1967) *Brit. J. Surg.*, **54**, 686.

Flanc, C., Kakkar, V. V. & Clarke, M. B. (1968) *Brit. J. Surg.*, **55**, 742.

Flanc, C., Kakkar, V. V. & Clarke, M. B. (1969) *Lancet*, **1**, 477.

Hills, N. H., Pflug, J. J., Jeyasingh, K., Boardman, L. & Calnan, J. S. (1972) *Brit. Med. J.*, **1**, 131.

Kakkar, V. V., Howe, C. T., Flanc, C. & Clarke, M. B. (1969) *Lancet*, **II**, 230–233.

Laufman (1954) *Personal communication.*

Marks, J., Truscott, B. M. & Witheycome, J. F. R. (1954) *Lancet*, **2**, 787.

Mathes, M. E., Holman, E. & Reichert, F. L. (1932) *J. Thorac. Surg.*, **1**, 339.

McLachlin, J. & Paterson, J. C. (1951) *Surg. Gynec. Obstet.*, **93**, 1.

Meyerowitz, B. R., Nelson, R. (1964) *Surgery St. Louis*, **56**, 481.

Negus, D., Pinto, D. J., LeQuesne, L. P., Brown, N. & Chapman, M. (1968) *Brit. J. Surg.*, **55**, 835.

Pilcher, R. (1937) *Brit. J. Surg.*, **25**, 42.

Sevitt, S. & Gallagher, N. G. (1959) *Lancet*, **II**, 981.

Wilkins, R. W., Mixter, G., Stanton, J. R. & Litter, J. (1952) *New Eng. J. Med.*, **246**, 360.

Wright, H. P. & Osborn, S. B. (1952) *Lancet*, **1**, 22.

16. Ilio-femoral Thrombosis

DEFINITION

In the past ilio-femoral thrombosis had a number of names according to the severity or supposed aetiology of the condition. These names, i.e. 'milk leg', 'white leg', 'phlegmasia alba dolens', 'phlegmasia caerulaea dolens', are of historical interest only.

The essential feature is thrombosis of the common and external iliac veins above the inguinal ligament. Usually, but not always, the thrombosis extends as far as the vena caval bifurcation. This thrombosis leads to an acute obstruction of the main venous return, causing swelling of the whole limb—thigh, calf and ankle.

The leg may be white and cold for a short period, not more than 12 hours, immediately after the obstruction due to the thrombosis, but this phase of the 'white' swollen leg rapidly gives place to a blue, warm, tensely swollen limb, which is quite painful. The blueness and the warmth are due to superficial dilatation of all the small veins and venules which now open up to partake in the collateral venous return. Collateral veins in the pelvis (ovarian, presacral, ilio-lumbar and numerous superficial and deep veins over the inguinal region) open up gradually, and so the swelling, pain and tenseness subside. When the acute phase is over, the leg enters the chronic phase of the disease with symptoms due to main vein obstruction lasting for the rest of the patient's life.

AETIOLOGY

Thrombosis may spread upwards into the iliac veins from a thrombosis which originally started below the inguinal ligament (**Group 1**), or it may originate in the iliac vein (**Group 2**).

These two groups are somewhat different in their aetiology and clinical presentation.

Group 1:

In these cases the thrombosis reaches the iliac veins by extension of thrombosis which has started peripherally in the calf and femoral veins (see Fig. 16.1). This type usually occurs in older people, often post-operatively or after confinement to bed with some illness. Occasionally serious embolism occurs, as the advancing head of the thrombus may fragment and move up to the heart before it becomes adherent.

Clinical picture:

The clinical history is not so acute as in **Group 2** cases. The appearance of the swollen limb is preceded by the milder symptoms of the calf and femoral thrombosis, namely a little ankle and calf swelling, calf tenderness, a low grade pyrexia, and possibly a small embolic episode. However, when thrombosis reaches the iliac veins and extends up to the caval bifurcation, the end result is similar to that in the bad **Group 2** cases: namely the clinical picture of a severe ilio-femoral thrombosis (see Fig. 16.2).

Group 2:

In this group the thrombosis starts in the common or external iliac veins. It may be initiated by some form of external pathological compression or irritation, such as secondary malignant glands, ovarian carcinoma, prostatic carcinoma, or aneurysm pressing on the vein. This tends to occur in the older age group.

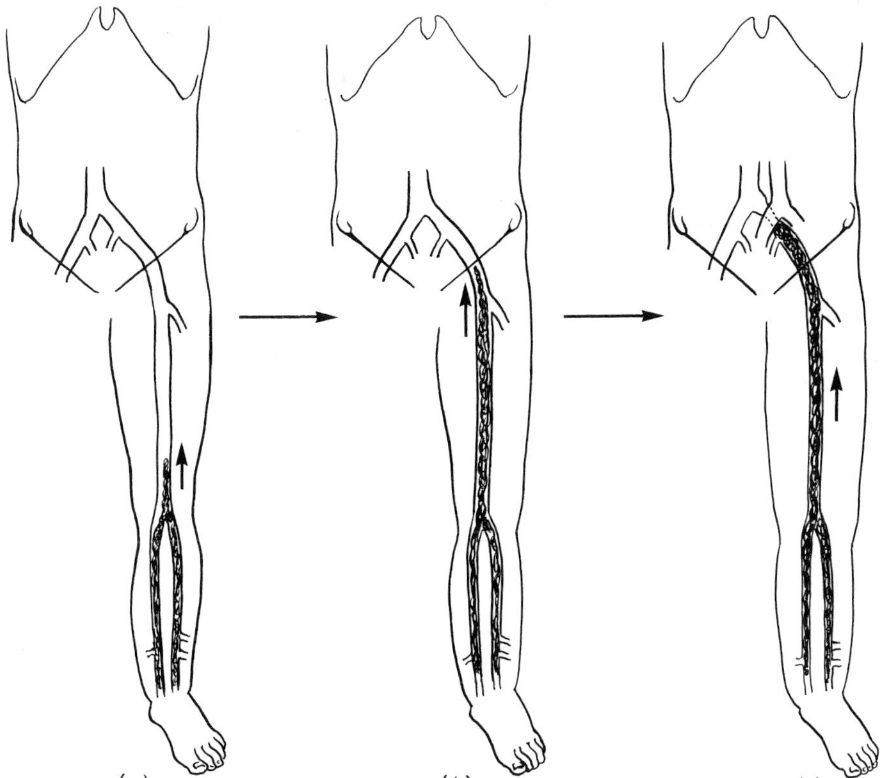

Fig. 16.1 Group 1—thrombosis arising in peripheral veins of leg. (a) Mild calf and ankle swelling only; (b) calf and ankle swelling; (c) full ilio-femoral thrombosis, clot spreading from femoral to iliac veins, the right side is occasionally so affected.

When it occurs in the younger age group however, it is usually due to a developmental abnormality of the caval bifurcation, known as the 'Iliac Compression Syndrome'. In this, the most common type is where the left common iliac vein is severely compressed and partially obliterated by the right common iliac artery stretched over it. This abnormality causes a thrombosis in the obstructed left iliac vein, which makes its appearance suddenly in early adult life (age 15–30), and usually during the course of some minor illness or pregnancy.

Clinical picture:

The thrombosis once it has occurred in the iliac veins may remain localised in the iliac segment above the inguinal ligament. Such cases are referred to as 'segmental ilio-femoral thrombosis'. They do not present such a dramatic clinical picture as when the whole deep venous system is involved, nor do they have such crippling long term sequelae, as the calf vein valves and perforators at the ankle escape destruction.

They are characterised by a very sudden swelling and engorgement of the thigh (usually the left one) in a young person—often during pregnancy or a minor illness. It is accompanied by quite *severe pain in the groin* which often persists in a minor way for some weeks and by a pyrexia of up to 100°F.

With rest in elevation it usually subsides rapidly and typically the patient is com-

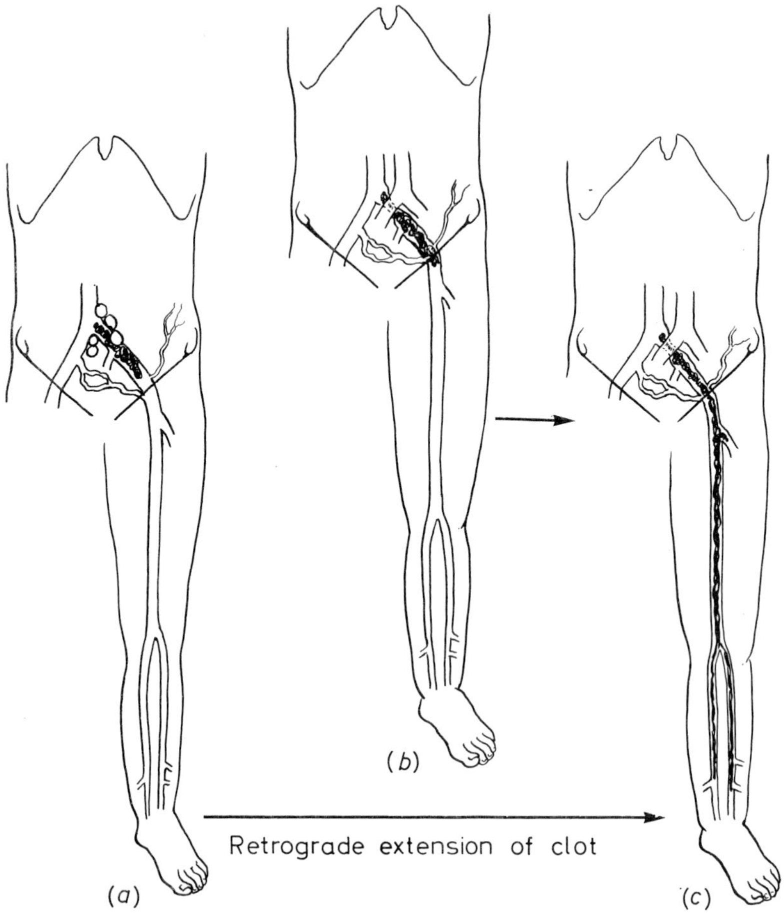

Fig. 16.2 Group 2—thrombosis arising in the iliac veins. (a) Local pathology pressing on iliac veins (glands, malignancy or aneurysms, etc.). Mild swelling → recovery which depends on extent and type of pathology; (b) iliac compression syndrome with thrombosis localised to iliac segment. Mild swelling → rapid recovery with development of profuse collateral channels; (c) retrograde spread involving whole ilio-femoral system. Severe swelling → slow recovery → chronic sequelae (swelling ulcers, etc.).

fortable and without bad swelling or pain in two or three days.

Infra red photography is of great assistance in diagnosis, as it shows up the distended superficial collateral very well (Fig. 16.3).

Severe cases—Phlegmasia Caerulaea dolens:

Where the thrombus spreads retrogradely right down to the femoral, popliteal and calf veins, a more severe clinical picture appears. Once again the onset may be fairly acute (over a few hours) and the whole limb becomes swollen, painful and congested, particularly in the thigh. In the early stage (first 6–12 hours or so) the limb may be white and cold but this rapidly gives place to a dusky blue colour and the whole limb feels warm to the touch, as the superficial venous collaterals open up. At this stage the patient may have a high temperature up to 101°F.

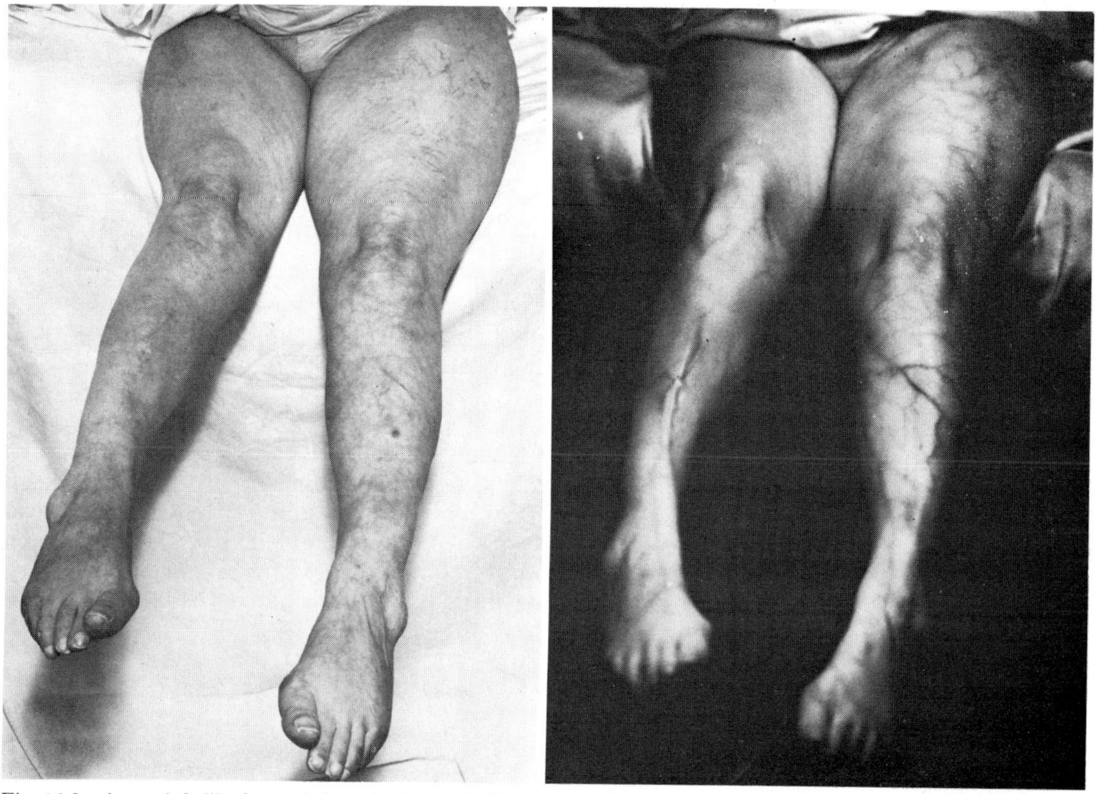

Fig. 16.3 Acute left ilio-femoral thrombosis (probably segmental). On left ordinary photograph; on right infra red photograph. Note swelling is most marked in thigh.

Where the thrombosis is particularly widespread the circulation in the foot may be blocked off almost entirely, and the foot and lower leg may become cold, blue, painful and swollen, with black malignant looking blisters on the toes and foot. The severe type of condition is sometimes referred to as 'Phlegmasia Caerulaea Dolens' or 'Venous Gangrene'.

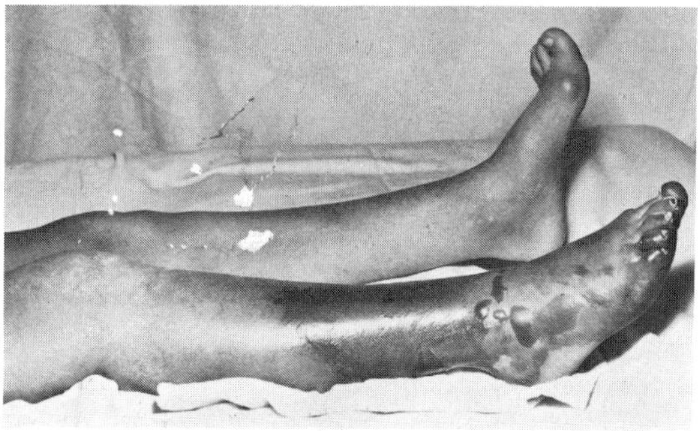

Fig. 16.4 *Phlegmasia Caerulea Dolens.* This patient had had a carcinoma of pancreas resected one year previously. The first evidence of recurrence was the appearance of a white leg on the left side. This subsided, but was rapidly followed by a deep thrombosis of the right leg of a more severe and widespread nature—shown here. As a result of this the patient's toes and forefoot became gangrenous.

So great is the acute loss of body fluid into the big swollen extremity that these cases may even show signs of shock—with high pulse rate and falling blood pressure in the early stage, and *severe pain* in the extremity is a feature. (Haimovici, 1950).

ILIAC COMPRESSION SYNDROME

This name has been given to an abnormality of the vena caval bifurcation which exists to a greater or lesser degree in a small percentage of the population. It consists most commonly of a localised fibrous band across the left common iliac vein where it is crossed by, and compressed by, the right common iliac artery. In most cases this band causes a

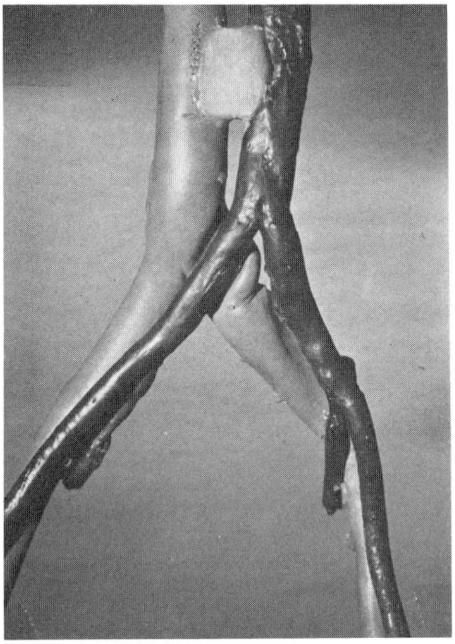

Fig. 16.5 Marked compression deformity of the left common iliac vein where the right common iliac artery crosses it. (From a neoprene corrosion cast prepared by D. E. Negus, Ch.M., F.R.C.S.).

partial stricture in the vein at this point, but, in a minority, the fibrous stricture of the vein is severe enough to occlude more than two-thirds of the lumen and cause significant obstruction to venous return (Figs. 16.5, 16.6, 16.7).

The condition has been extensively studied and documented both in post-mortem examinations (McMurrich, 1908; Ehrich and Krumbhaar, 1943; May and Thurner, 1957; Negus et al., 1968) and in clinical cases (Cockett and Lea Thomas, 1965; Negus and Cockett, 1967). It is probable that a majority of people with lesser degrees of this abnormality go through life with no symptoms attributable to it, or at least with only minor symptoms of aching and tiredness in the left leg. This is suggested by the frequency with which minor degrees of this deformity turn up in iliac venograms of patients with no symptoms referable to it. *However, in those*

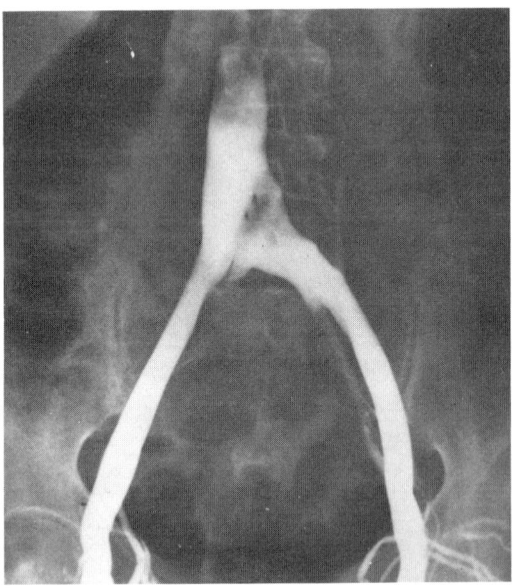

Fig. 16.6 Phlebogram illustrating a typical compression band before thrombosis. Note absence of collateral channels. (Reproduced from Cockett (1967) by courtesy of the Editor of the British Journal of Surgery.)

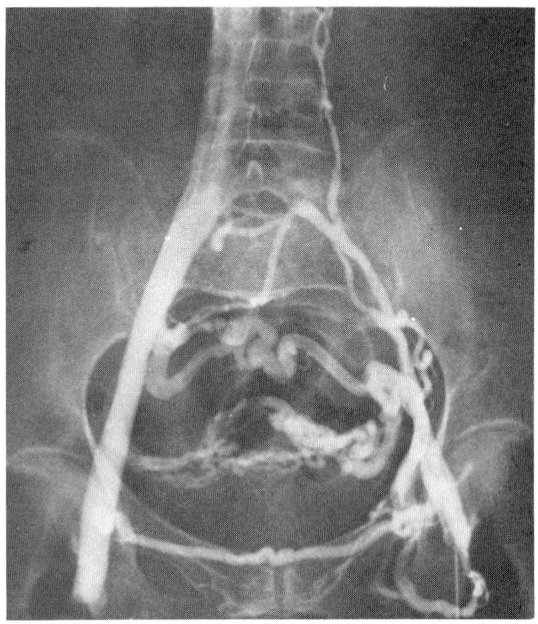

Fig. 16.7 Phlebogram showing the results of an iliac compression band several years after the episode of iliofemoral thrombosis. There is complete obstruction at the caval bifurcation and the profuse collateral channels passing across to the right side of the pelvis; and up the iliolumbar veins are seen.

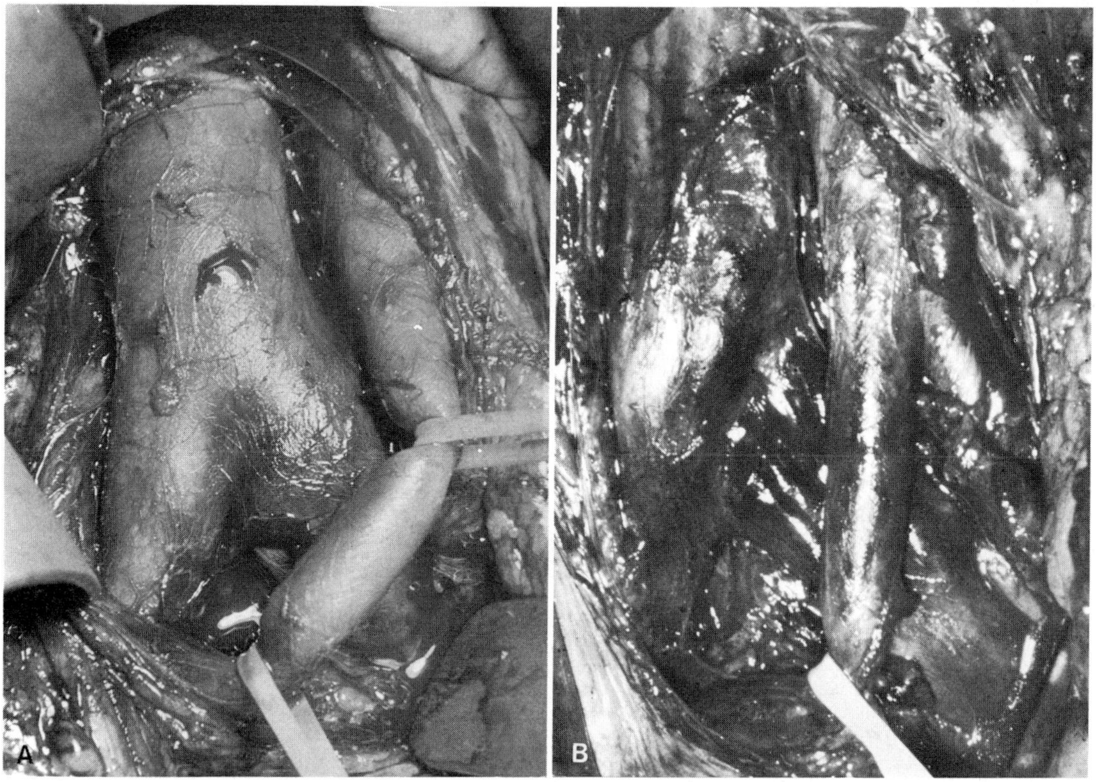

Fig. 16.8 (A) Normal caval bifurcation with right common iliac artery dissected free and pulled over to left; (B) Severe left iliac compression (patient aged 19). Right common iliac artery dissected free and lifted away from the left common iliac vein to show the permanent compression stricture at this point, with multiple channels leading up to it.

with a more marked degree of this abnormality its importance is considerable. It predisposes to iliac thrombosis, usually at an early age, and is responsible for most of the cases of acute ilio-femoral thrombosis occurring under the age of about 30. Once the thrombosis has occurred it sets up further inflammation and fibrosis round the iliac compression band and converts the partial iliac obstruction into a complete one.

Recanalisation then does not occur through this compressed and fibrosed area of the vein and therefore the patient is left with a complete obstruction of the left iliac vein for the rest of his life. This, however, may be compensated by the development of collaterals, the degree of collateral development varying widely in its efficiency (Lea Thomas et al., 1967). Those patients in whom the collateral is inadequate suffer from severe obstructive symptoms in the leg—swelling, venous claudication on exercise, tiredness and eventually severe intractable ulceration in the periphery.

Further study of this condition has revealed that, although the left common iliac vein is the commonest site for a severe compression band, a similar situation may occur at other points in the pelvis. In a small proportion of patients complete overriding of the caval bifurcation by the aortic bifurcation may take place, leading to *inferior vena caval thrombosis.* Also, the right or left external iliac vein may be nipped at the bifurcation of the common iliac artery, or, more rarely, the vein may be compressed as it passes under the inguinal ligament. These two latter varieties account for the rather less frequent *right-sided* cases. These secondary sites of compression are summarized in Figure 16.9.

NATURAL HISTORY

The natural history of acute ilio-femoral thrombosis may be summarized as follows:

Acute phase—Whole limb (particularly thigh) is swollen, tense, painful; high temperature; cold in the first few hours, rapidly becoming warm.

Recovery (2–3 weeks)—Swelling subsides; pain and temperature recede.

Chronic phase (variable) (1–5 years or whole lifetime)—Some swelling of leg, gradual onset of peripheral venous congestion and ulceration. (Except in segmental iliac cases.)

The place of surgery in this condition must be judged against the background of the natural history. In most cases natural recovery in the acute phase is fairly rapid, and there is a tendency to ascribe miraculous recovery during this period to any minor surgical procedure or medical treatment which may have been done.

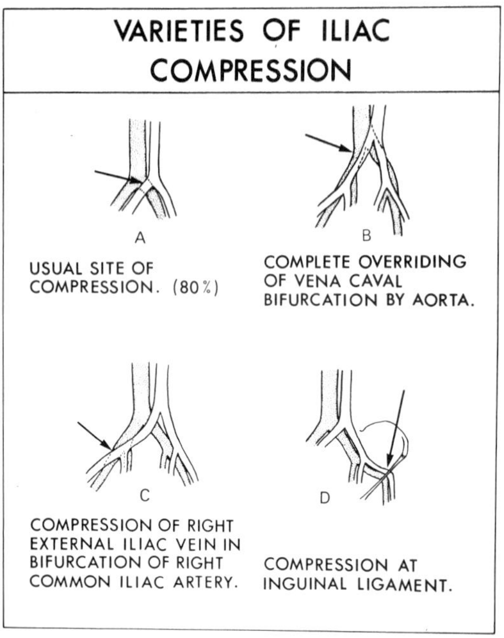

Fig. 16.9 Varieties of iliac compression. (a) Usual site of compression (80 per cent); (b) complete overriding of vena caval bifurcation by aorta; (c) compression of right external iliac vein in bifurcation of right common iliac artery; (d) compression at inguinal ligament. (Reproduced from Cockett, Lea Thomas and Negus (1967) by courtesy of the Editor of the British Medical Journal.)

Recovery in the acute stage depends on the development of collateral venous return. In young people with the iliac compression syndrome there already may have been some pre-existing collateral and, in these cases particularly, recovery in the acute phase may be very rapid and complete and this is especially so if only the iliac segment has thrombosed. Recovery is, of course, more prolonged if the thrombosis has spread retrogradely to the whole of the femoro-popliteal segment and calf.

Recovery in the chronic phase is dependent on two things, the further development of collateral and, as important, the recanalisation of the thrombus. Ever since adequate phlebograms of the femoral and iliac veins have been performed, and surgeons have explored these veins in the post thrombotic syndrome, the remarkable difference in the degree of recanalisation achieved in the leg veins and in the iliac veins has been noted. In all the veins below the inguinal ligament recanalisation is very complete leaving a channel which, although devoid of valves, is adequate for the return of blood from the lower limb without obstruction. In the iliac segment the reverse is nearly always found, namely very poor recanalisation, the veins being reduced to small fibrous cords with very small and inadequate recanalisation channels. This lack of recanalisation is *particularly evident where the vein is pressed on by an overlying artery*, seen in its most extreme form in the iliac compression syndrome already described. Even in most of the cases (*Group 1*) where the clotting has extended into the iliac veins from below, recanalisation is poor, and it would appear that some degree of pressure by overlying arteries in the pelvis, or at the inguinal ligament, is responsible.

Lastly, if the clotting has extended to the calf veins then the valves in the important ankle perforating veins are destroyed, and in such cases the patient is left with *incompetent ankle perforating veins as well as a central venous obstruction* and so venous congestion and ulceration round the ankle is likely and may be severe.

The final condition of the leg after an ilio-femoral thrombosis has occurred, and full collateral development and recanalisation has taken place, is summarized in Figure 16.10. The patient is left with a chronic iliac vein obstruction which is compensated for by collaterals to a greater or lesser degree, with good recanalisation of the veins below the inguinal ligament, but with incompetent ankle perforating veins if the original clotting extended down this far.

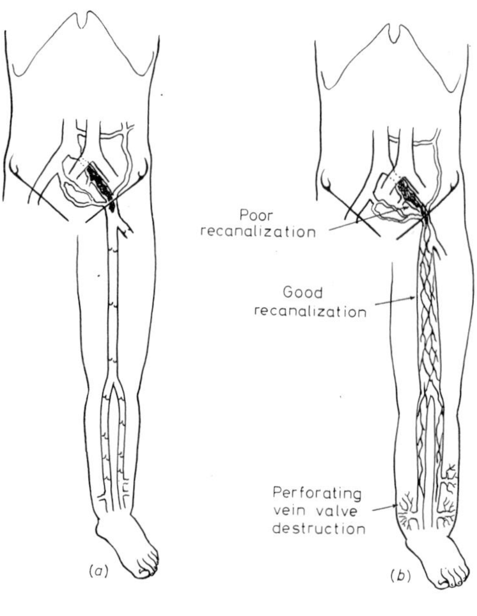

Fig. 16.10 Final stages of ilio-femoral thrombosis. (a) Clotting of iliac segment only. Iliac obstruction with collateral compensation. No destruction of peripheral valves, symptoms mild. (b) Clotting of whole ilio-femoral segment down to calf. Iliac obstruction plus peripheral valve destruction, and destruction of valves in perforating veins. Symptoms severe: swelling, pain, ulceration at ankle, and steady progressive deterioration.

ILIAC COMPRESSION, POST-PARTUM 'WHITE LEG' AND HYSTERECTOMY

In the original clinical investigation into the iliac compression syndrome (Cockett and Lea Thomas) it was noticed that many cases presented as an acute ilio-femoral thrombosis after either a hysterectomy or after confinement. Further experience with numerous venograms and clinical cases in young females revealed the presence of a special condition of the uterus and ovaries due to the development of venous collateral in these cases with obstructed left iliac veins. (Cockett, 1968).

The condition is shown dramatically in the venograms in Figure 16.11.

It will be observed that where the left common iliac vein or caval bifurcation is obstructed, the bulk of the venous collateral goes through the uterus and parametrium and through the ovarian veins. The uterus may become very vascular and full of large, congested, tortuous veins. (The condition known to gynaecologists as 'varicose veins of the parametrium'), and the ovarian veins may become very large and thin walled.

Thus in these patients the bulk of the venous return from the left leg may be going through the uterus and left (and right) ovarian veins.

This state of affairs may have certain interesting and important consequences:

1. *Menorrhagia and Pelvic Pain.* The venous congestion of the uterus may lead to gradually increasing menorrhagia in young adults. This may become so bad that eventually hysterectomy may be advocated. The distended parametrium may also give rise to chronic left groin pain.

2. *Post-Hysterectomy Ilio-Femoral Thrombosis.* If hysterectomy is performed in one of these cases, removal of the uterus and left ovarian vein may in fact remove the bulk of the collateral venous return from the left leg—precipitating a state of considerable venous obstruction and stasis which may lead to ilio-femoral thrombosis.

If hysterectomy has to be done in such cases, considerable care should be exercised

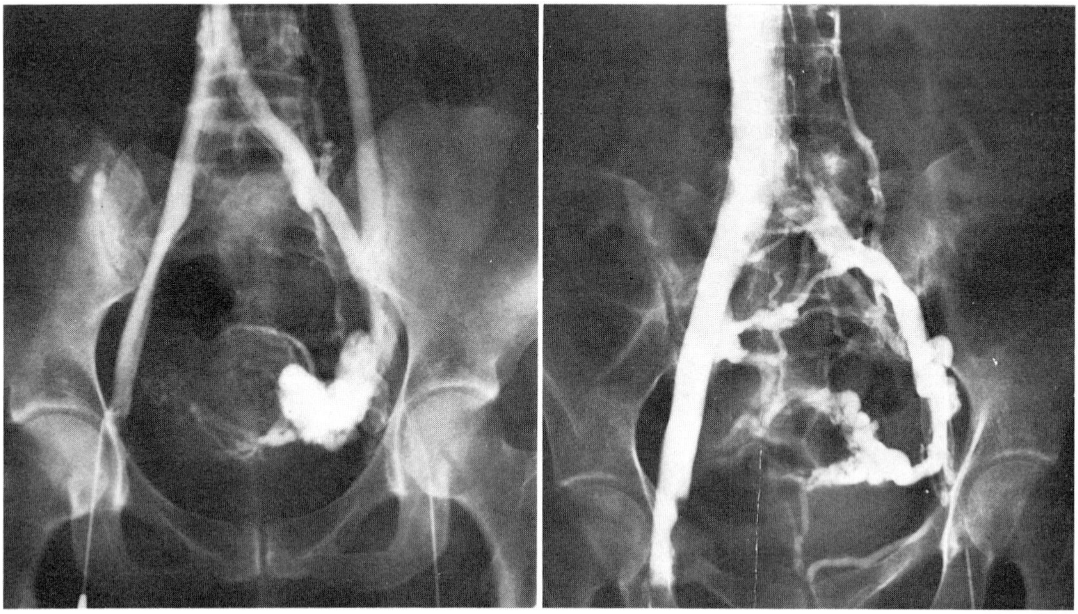

Fig. 16.11 Venograms of two patients with iliac compression syndrome, with large dilated collateral veins in the uterus and adnexae. In the case on the left, the ovarian vein is taking a large amount of the venous return from the left leg.

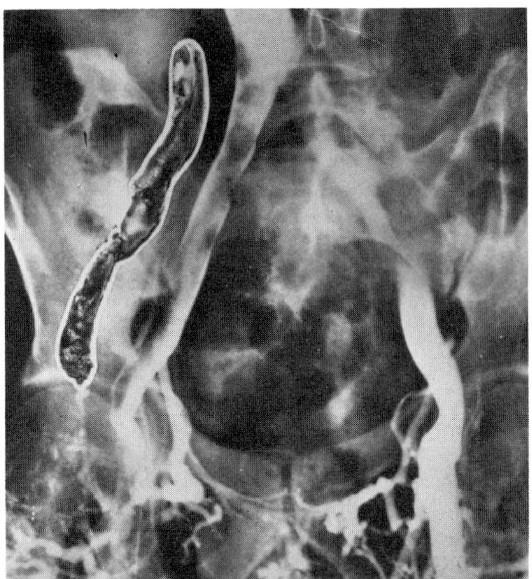

Fig. 16.12A (A) The emergency phlebogram in a doctor, aged 60, done after a second pulmonary embolus. It shows loose extension thrombus in the right iliac vein, propagated upward from a femoral thrombosis. The loose thrombus removed from this site is shown inset.

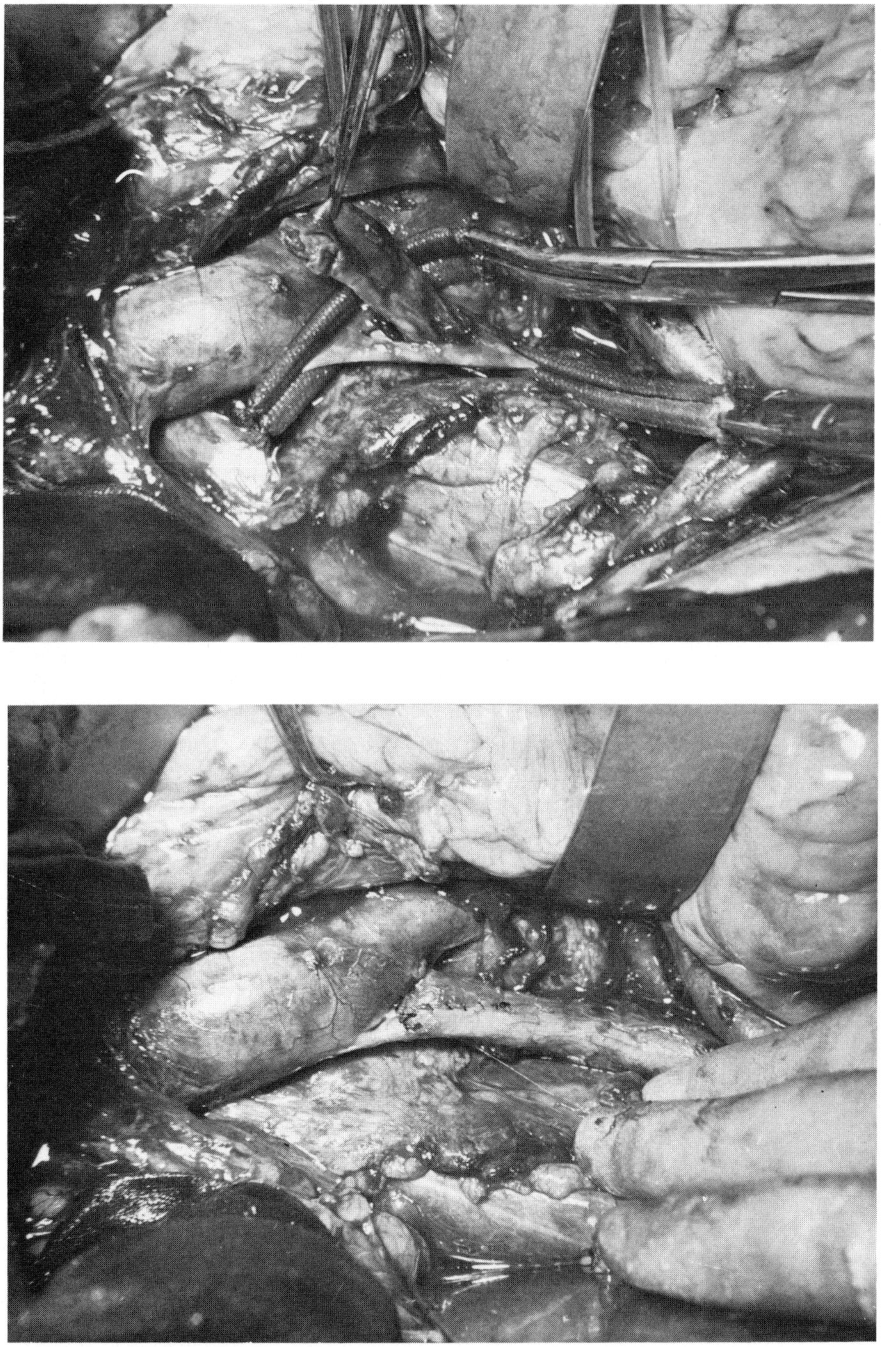

Fig. 16.12B, C The operation on the patient. (B) Extraction of the thrombus from the right common iliac vein; (C) plication of the right common iliac vein, above the thrombus, at its junction with the cava. This patient then had his femoral vein ligated on the other side.

to leave the ovarian vein intact and to keep as close to the uterus as possible.

3. *Post-Partum White Leg.* An almost exactly similar state of affairs may occur just after childbirth in young patients with an iliac vein compression syndrome.

During pregnancy, the enormous size of the uterus and ovarian veins is adequate for the collateral return from the left leg. But soon after childbirth as the uterus shrinks rapidly—a state of relative venous obstruction may develop in the left leg—resulting in a post-partum ilio-femoral thrombosis.

The existence of quite a severe iliac obstruction, well compensated for by collaterals in uterus and ovarian veins, and with practically no symptoms (except sometimes a deep seated pain in the left groin, and transient aching of the left leg) is not uncommon. Its presence may be undetected and unsuspected until a major ilio-femoral thrombosis, or pulmonary embolus occurs.

It is a hazard not only to the patients, but also to the interpretation of statistics on female thrombosis purporting to show the possible thrombogenic effects of the contraceptive pill.

PULMONARY EMBOLISM IN ILIO-FEMORAL THROMBOSIS

Pulmonary embolism is occasionally a problem in ilio-femoral thrombosis, and there are three definite groups of cases:

1. In *Group 1* cases (p. 227) where the thrombosis is advancing from below—the advancing head of the thrombus may break off to become a large pulmonary embolus. A good example of this is seen in Figure 16.12.

In such cases the large threatening embolus usually comes from the *right* side.

2. In cases of left ilio-femoral thrombosis due to the iliac compression syndrome, there is sometimes one minor embolic episode at the beginning, then no more. The reason for this is shown in Figure 16.13.

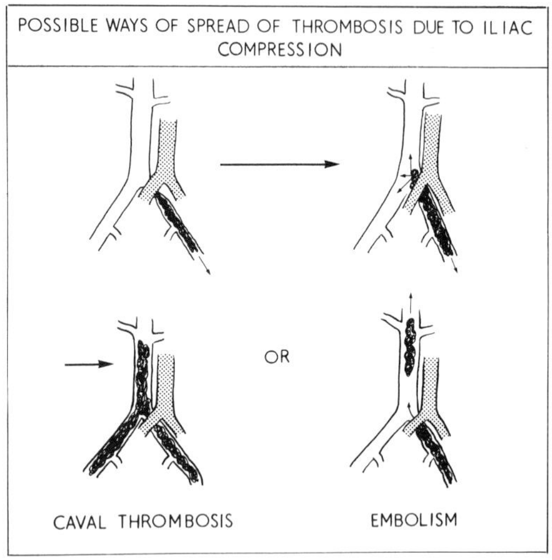

Fig. 16.13 The fourth diagram shows the way in which a single large embolus may arise at the first thrombosis, and then no more (from the left side).

Once clotting has occurred and become adherent around a left iliac compression band then the vein becomes almost completely obstructed and no embolus can get through from below. The only possibility of further embolism lies in the patient's *right* side.

3. Occasionally cases occur who have serious trouble with repeated small emboli after an ilio-femoral thrombosis. They are often found on phlebography, to have some major deformity of the caval bifurcation. Flow abnormality in this region may then give rise to thrombus formation which is repeatedly dislodged by the abnormal flow pattern. Such cases often suffer from many minor episodes of embolism, with repeated attacks of pleurisy and increasing destruction of lung function.

Occasionally, as shown in Figure 16.14 some gross abnormality is found on phlebography, such as a left sided vena cava.

Treatment:

Treatment in all these three types of cases should be decided upon the result of a good iliac venogram.

If the venogram shows a large, loose, threatening thrombus (as in Fig. 16.12), there should be no hesitation in plicating the vena cava above the thrombus, or the common iliac vein as was done in the case illustrated.

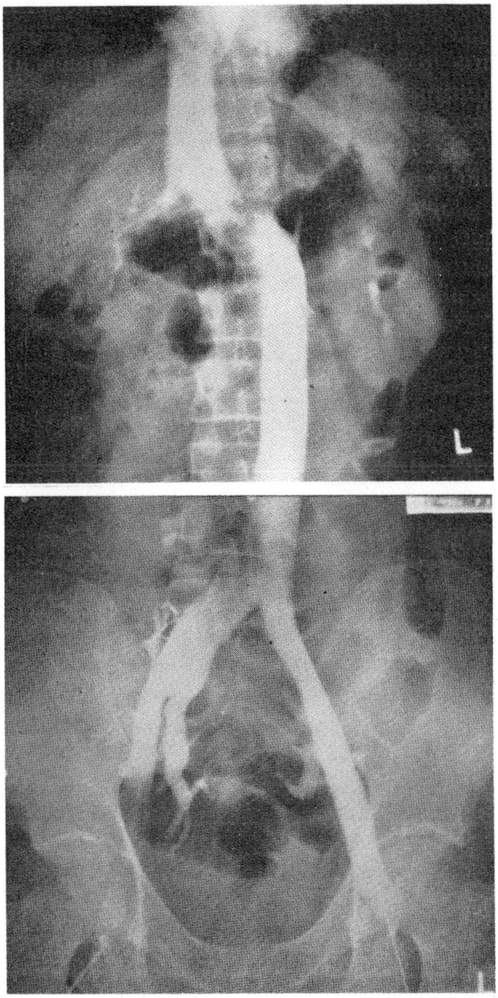

Fig. 16.14 This young patient, aged 26, presented with a problem of recurrent small emboli. His phlebogram showed a left sided vena cava, crossing behind, and compressed by the aorta at the level of the hepatic veins. It is likely that his small emboli are coming from this compressed and deformed area, the rest of his peripheral venous system being clear.

In cases of repetitive embolism, provided there is unequivocal evidence from the lung scan that embolism has taken place, these also should be considered for caval plication. In many of these cases the iliac venogram merely shows a gross abnormality of the caval bifurcation region, without definite evidence of loose thrombus on the venogram. However, the combination of repeated embolism positive lung scan and some abnormality on the venogram, is enough evidence for surgical plication and in the author's experience this operation is usually effective in these difficult cases.

Caval plication

There are three methods of caval interruption; by ligature, plication by suture or external prosthesis, and by silk suture filter.

All these methods require operative exposure of the vena cava by either a transabdominal (long right paramedian incision) or by a right retroperitoneal approach. The latter is easier for the patient, but more difficult for the surgeon! These are major operative procedures, unsuitable for very ill patients, and not to be entered into lightly.

Recently a small 'umbrella-like' filter, which can be placed in the cava, via a long catheter has been developed by K. Mobbin-Uddin (1969).

Ligation of the normal vena cava, in the opinion of the author, should practically never be done. The many cases in the past which have been reported with apparently negligible sequelae have probably been cases of left iliac compression syndrome with an *already preformed* collateral venous circulation. In patients who have no such preformed collaterals the obstructive sequelae of caval ligation are profound. *In the immediate post-operative phase there may be excessive fluid retention in the legs and the patient may go into a shock-like state. If he recovers from this, permanent gross swelling and congestion of both legs is usual.*

If the cava or a major vein has to be attacked, *plication* is the operation of choice. Spencer (1959)—(see also Spencer and Quattlebaum, 1962)—devised this method of dividing the inferior vena cava into several small channels which would allow normal blood flow, but which would not allow thrombi of any size past. Various modifications of this technique have appeared, particularly the silk suture net technique of De Weese (De Weese and Rogoff, 1958), and

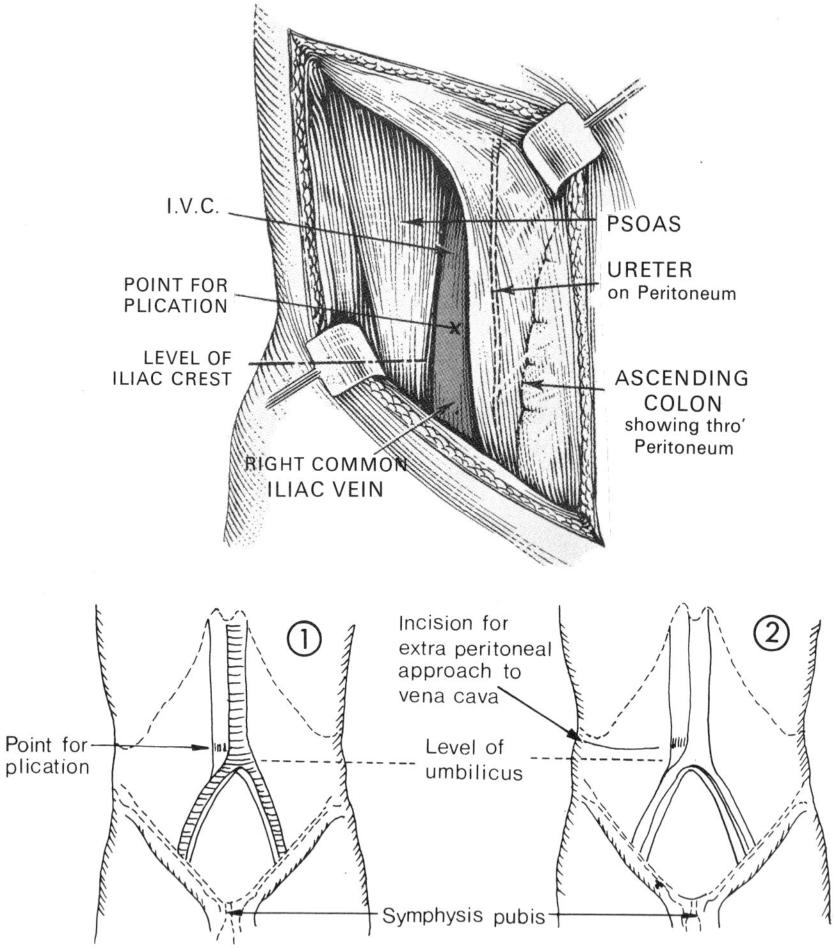

Fig. 16.15 A & B The approach and site for plication of the inferior vena cava.

the use of external plastic clips of various designs (Moretz, 1959; Miles, 1964).

In our experience, straightforward plication of the cava by three or four silk sutures passed straight across the cava, whilst it is temporarily occluded by two fine DeBakey clamps, is a simple, quick, easy and effective method (Figs 16.15 and 16.16).

TREATMENT OF ILIO-FEMORAL THROMBOSIS

Acute phase

Most cases settle down and recover quite adequately with no treatment other than rest in elevation, and with active movements of the limb. The question arises as to whether treatment in the acute phase can either hasten recovery or diminish the late effects of valve destruction by the process of clot organisation and recanalisation. There are two possible means of treatment in the acute phase; heparin or thrombectomy. A third method of treatment—by thrombolytic drugs such as streptokinase or urokinase, is under trial at various centres, but at the present time it is doubtful whether it has great practical value.

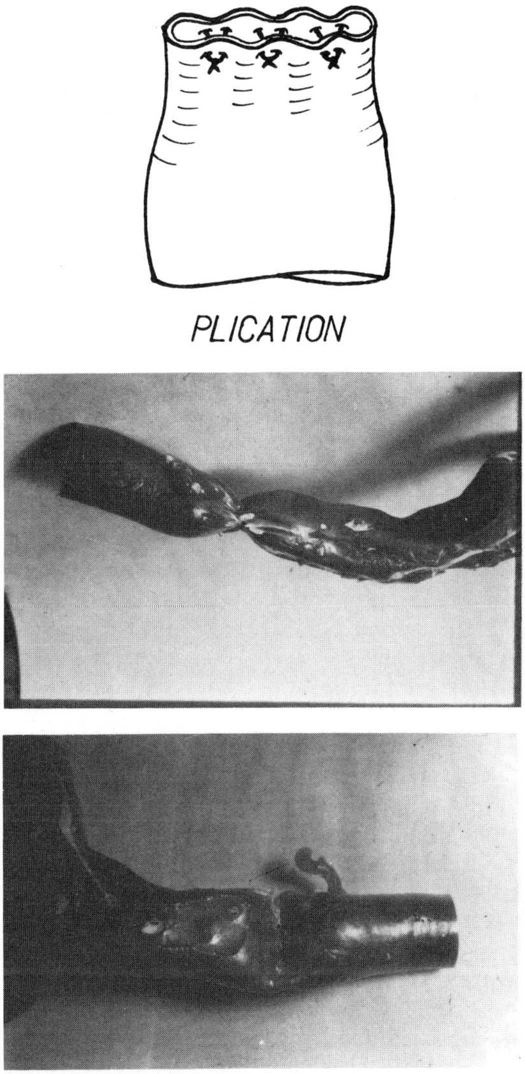

Fig. 16.16 *A*. Diagram of plication of cava. *B* & *C*. Neoprene casts of the cava of a patient who died after a plication.

Any treatment, if it is to have much effect, must be carried out within approximately the first 48–72 hours after onset of the condition. After this time the clot is becoming organised and is beginning to adhere to the vein wall, and secondary inflammatory changes in the vein wall are just appearing. By this time, any treatment—surgical or medical—is unlikely to influence the natural history of the condition very much.

Treatment by heparin

In the milder type of case, without very much swelling or pain, surgery has little to offer and it is better to put the patient on heparin for a short initial period of about one or two days. The benefits of early heparinisation are twofold; the prevention of further extension of the clotting, and, as some evidence from the work of Dos Santos (1966) and others suggests, more rapid and efficient clot recanalisation.

Treatment by thrombectomy

In the more *severe* cases, however, with sudden onset of severe swelling, pain, and blueness of the limb and toes, thrombectomy followed by heparinisation should be considered. It must be done within three days of the onset of symptoms to obtain maximum benefit, as it is only the early, loose, non-adherent clot which is easily and completely removed by thrombectomy. Thrombectomy is a comparatively minor and safe operation, and in cases of doubt it is on the whole better to proceed with it than to hold back.

It is carried out by exploring the femoral and common femoral veins at the groin through an oblique incision (Fig. 16.17). Although best done under general anaesthesia it can be done under local. After the common femoral vein has been exposed right up to the inguinal ligament, the dissection is carried distally for about two inches to expose the profunda femoris and an inch or so of the femoral vein. These three veins are controlled by plastic tapes passed round them. The common femoral vein is then opened by a longitudinal incision, and clot is removed from the distal segment first by vigorous pressure over the whole length of the vein down to the calf. If this fails to produce a lot of clot and a vigorous flow of blood, it means that the distal clot is already organising and adherent, and it is unlikely that suction or the use of a Fogarty catheter will produce further results. As soon as a free

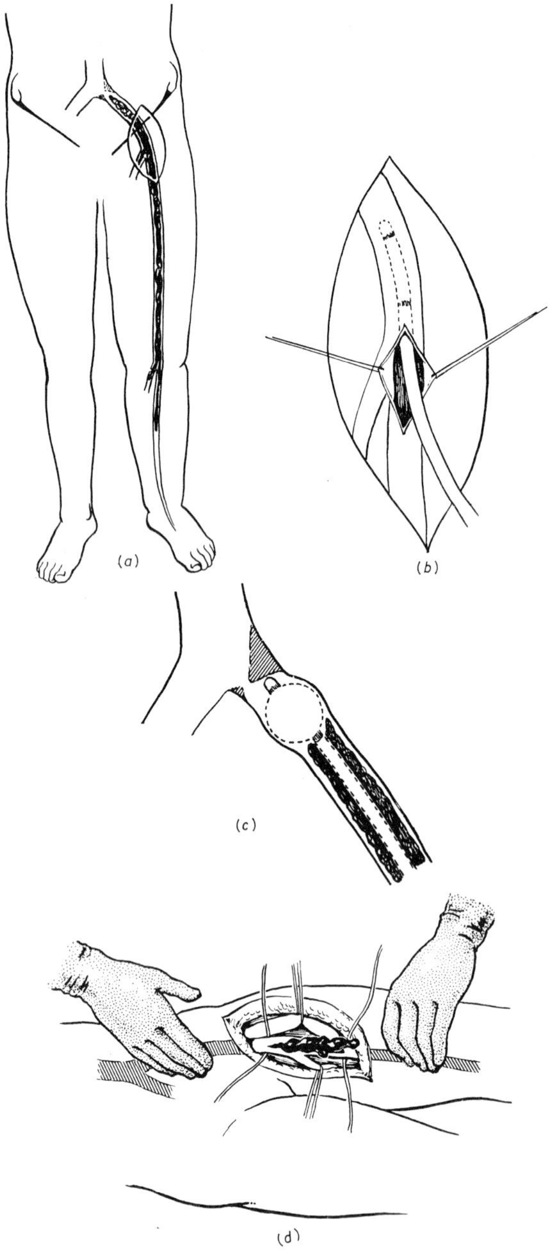

Fig. 16.17 Thrombectomy. (a) Site of incision; (b) insertion of Fogarty catheter alongside the clot; (c) inflation of the balloon just distal to the iliac compression band where resistance to outward passage of the catheter is often encountered; (d) the way in which a clot can be 'milked' out of the venotomy by manual pressure over the line of the distal vein.

flow of blood has been obtained a full dose of heparin (5–6000 international units, 50–60 mg) is given intravenously to prevent further clotting.

The upper part of the thrombus is then best removed by sliding a Fogarty catheter up as far as the caval bifurcation and withdrawing it with the balloon blown up while at the same time gently applying manual pressure to the vein just above the inguinal ligament. Some care is necessary in manipulating the Fogarty catheter, because as it approaches the caval bifurcation from the left it may meet a complete or partial obstruction due to an iliac compression stricture in the vein. The Fogarty catheter balloon may have to be deflated a little to slide past it and through the narrowed, compressed area of iliac vein here. Clot can only be removed up to this point, and no further, in such cases. The venotomy is then closed with 5·0 mersilk, and the wound closed in layers over a small suction drain.

This technique appears to be free of the danger of producing an embolus according to the accumulated experience of many authors (Haller, 1967; De Weese et al., 1960).

After the operation heparinisation is maintained for 24 hours, followed by a period of two weeks on oral anticoagulants (Warfarin), or until the patient is thoroughly mobile again.

Results—The immediate result of early thrombectomy in severe cases of ilio-femoral thrombosis is striking, with relief of pain and swelling. More important, however, is the fact that if adequate removal of the distal clot is achieved the patient may escape the crippling sequelae caused by the post-thrombotic destruction of valves in the deep and perforating veins (De Weese et al., 1960). Embolism is seldom a problem in these cases, probably because the iliac vein is closed or narrowed at the top end by a compression stricture.

Chronic phase

Surgery may have an important part to play in the management of the chronic phase. Symptoms in this phase, which usually take about five years after the acute episode to reach such a degree that the patient seeks advice again, are referable to two main lesions. These are: (1) The chronic obstruction of the iliac vein, which causes a chronic venous hypertension in the whole limb, and (2) The destruction of the valves in the ankle perforating veins, which is the main proximate cause for the development of induration, swelling, and ulceration of the ankle.

Surgery has an important part to play in this second group because, if incompetent perforating veins and other incompetent superficial veins (long or short saphenous), are eliminated early by the appropriate radical surgery before chronic intractable ulceration has taken place, then this may prevent or delay serious deterioration of the ankle skin for a long time.

If there is serious general venous hypertension due to iliac obstruction one cannot expect such good results from peripheral vein surgery as in a limb with peripheral valve destruction only. In such cases the surgery must be backed up with efficient elastic support and, in some cases, intermittent periods of rest in elevation. If there are collaterals in the groin in these cases a flush saphenous ligation should not be done, as this would remove some of the collaterals, but an incompetent saphenous vein should be tied below the groin collaterals and stripped.

The whole question of the management of these cases is dealt with in more detail in Chapters 17 and 18.

SURGERY OF CHRONIC ILIAC VEIN OBSTRUCTION—ILIAC COMPRESSION SYNDROME

In recent years, since the recognition of this lesion, various attempts to alleviate the obstruction by surgery have been made. *It must be pointed out, however, that the mere demonstration of an obstructed iliac vein by phlebography is no indication for surgery in itself.* Many of these iliac obstructions, particularly the very localised ones in the left common iliac vein only, are very adequately compensated by the natural collaterals. Only when the obstruction is functional, that is, collateral compensation is inadequate, is the lesion damaging to the limb by causing chronic venous hypertension. These patients are characterised by two particular symptoms: *swelling* of the whole limb, including the thigh, and *venous claudication*, which is an aching or bursting pain felt in the calf mainly on a certain degree of exercise. In these patients there is a raised resting venous pressure in the femoral vein below the block which rises rapidly to very high levels on exercising the limb (Fig. 16.18). The method of measurement of these femoral venous pressures and their significance has been described by Negus and Cockett (1967).

In those cases in which there is gross functional obstruction in the iliac veins,

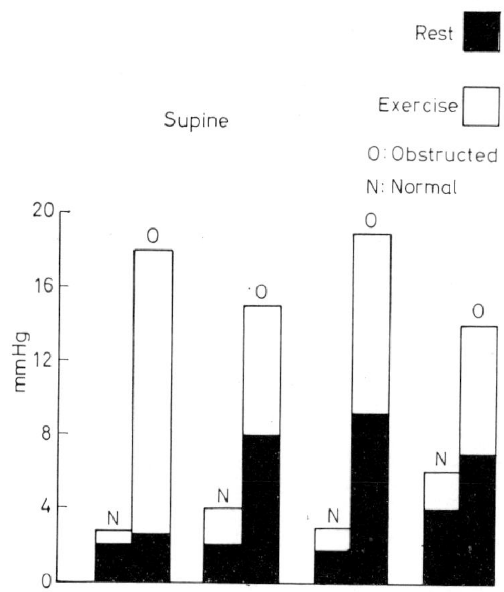

Fig. 16.18 Four observations of the resting and exercise venous pressures in the main femoral vein just below the inguinal ligament. On the left in each figure is the normal unobstructed leg, and on the right, the leg with the iliac vein obstruction. It is seen that even if the resting femoral pressures are nearly equal on the two sides, the slightest exercise sends the pressure up on the obstructed side. Collaterals may not be adequate to handle the increased flow on exercise.

attempts at relief by surgery have been attempted. These operations have fallen into two classes:

1. Attempts at bypassing the obstruction, and
2. Direct surgery at the site of obstruction.

Bypass operations

These have been described by Dale (1966), Palma (1966) and Cockett (1967). Most of the procedures utilize the long saphenous vein either as a free graft or as a suprapubic graft (see Fig. 16.19).

In the author's experience (Cockett, 1967) these venous grafts are unsatisfactory for two reasons, first because the vein is not big enough, and, second because obliteration of the graft at the anastomosis nearly always takes place owing to the lack of sufficient intra-luminal pressure to keep it widely open. All small venous graft anastomoses suffer from this defect, as has been shown by Kunlin (1966).

More recently, attempts have been made to bypass severe obstructions by using a stretch of normal femoral vein taken from below the profunda on the normal side, and using an external Dacron splint to keep the anastomosis open. This technique has given promising early results.

Direct operations

Experience of 30 operations on the occluded segment has recently been described (Cockett, 1967). They have been of two kinds.

In the first group of patients the vena caval bifurcation and the overlying adherent right common iliac artery have been extensively

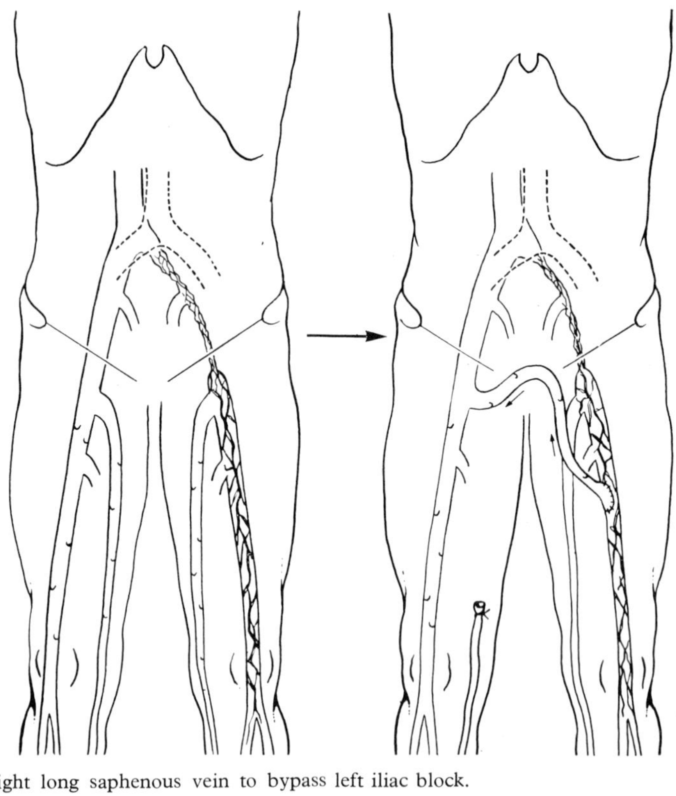

Fig. 16.19 Use of right long saphenous vein to bypass left iliac block.

mobilised, pressure by the artery relieved, and the fibrous tissue round the vein dissected away. The artery is then held away from the vein by a small peritoneal sling passed between the vein and artery. This fairly extensive surgical manoeuvre seems to have produced some relief of symptoms in about half the patients.

In the second group, after mobilising the two bifurcations, a direct attempt at dealing with the stricture in the vein has been made. This has been done either by incising the stricture and inserting a saphenous vein patch to widen out the narrower iliac vein at this point, or by resecting the left common vein across the stricture and reimplanting the vein lower down, into the right common iliac vein.

All these procedures are major abdominal operations of some considerable technical difficulty, and, in the author's opinion, the results obtained do not really justify such a major procedure. Moreover, in a proportion of those explored, the whole of the common and external iliac vein on the left side was found to be so compressed and fibrosed that no worthwhile direct surgical procedure was found to be possible. In the author's opinion, therefore, the direct surgery of iliac obstruction in the chronic phase is unsatisfactory at the moment. The possible further approach to this problem probably lies along the lines of using a large vein as a bypass, with an improved technique of external support to the venous anastomoses.

ASSOCIATED LYMPHATIC OBSTRUCTION IN ILIAC COMPRESSION SYNDROME

Figure 16.20 is a lymphangiogram of a normal person, showing how the whole of the lymphatic drainage of the limb converges into a plexus which runs up to the caval bifurcation, closely applied to the external and common iliac veins. It is thus at these points (i.e. round the common iliac vein and at the caval junction) that the *whole* lymphatic drainage of the limb is susceptible to obstruction.

Clinically in some iliac compression cases there is associated lymphatic obstruction. Occasionally this may be severe enough to cause a well marked lymphoedema as well (Fig. 16.21).

Oddly enough the combination of severe venous obstruction and severe lymphatic obstruction is somewhat rare clinically.

Many of the young girls who develop lymphatic obstruction of the lower limb early in life (lymphoedema praecox) show a definite iliac compression picture on their venograms. It is tempting to postulate that there may be a 'lymphatic defect syndrome' in this area as well as a venous one, which might account for the many 'lymphoedema praecox' cases!

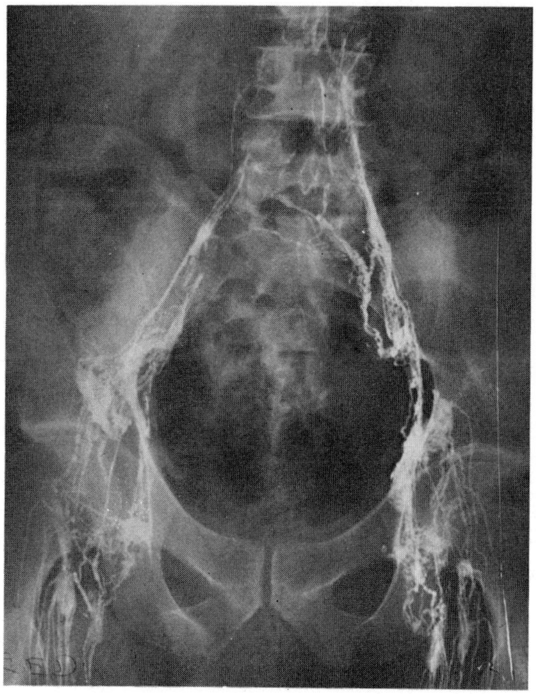

Fig. 16.20 Normal lymphogram, showing how the lymphatic drainage from the legs converges to a local plexus surrounding the common iliac veins and caval bifurcation. Local obstruction of lymphatics here could produce lymphoedema of the lower limb.

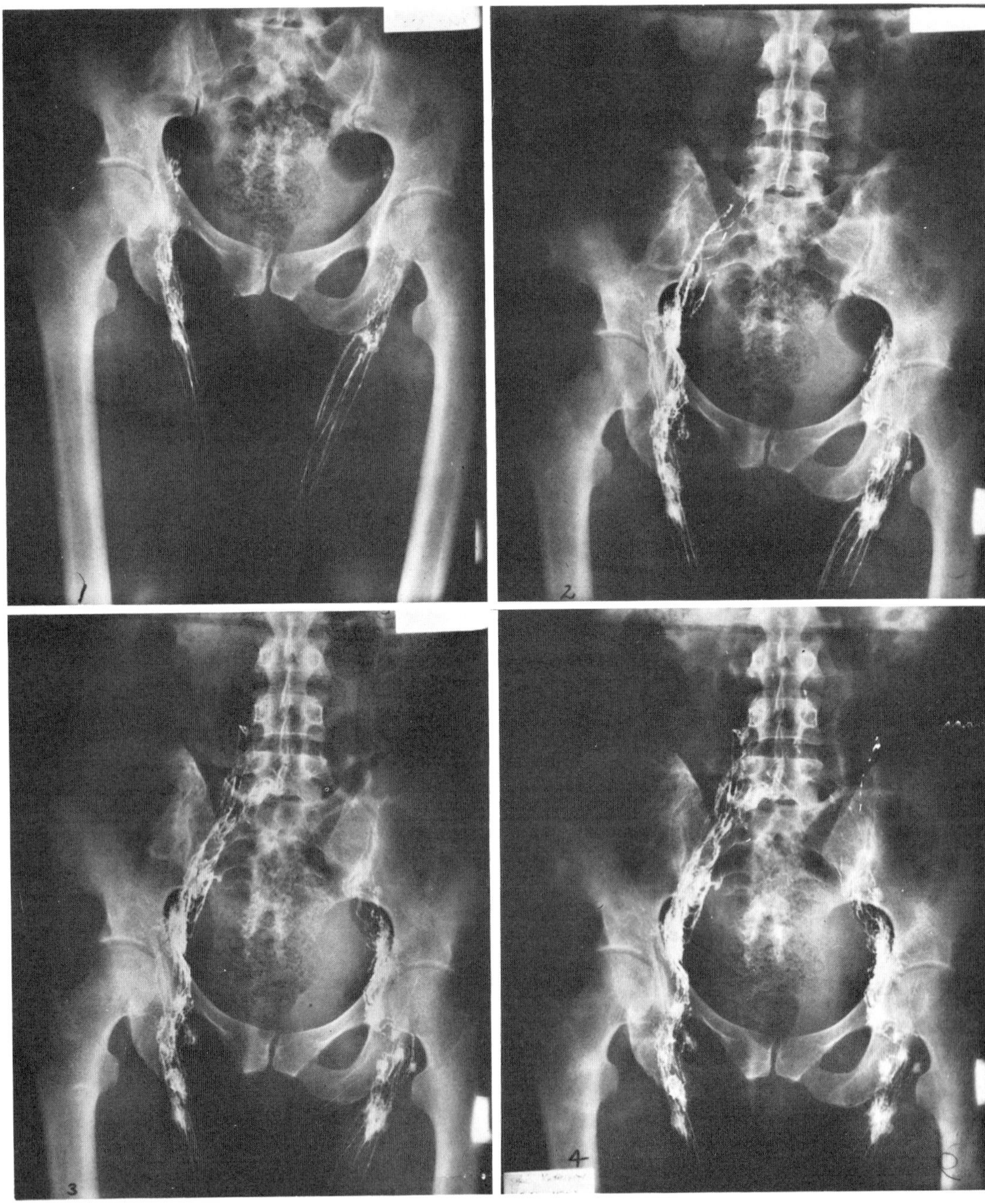

Fig. 16.21 Timed lymphangiograms showing delay and obstruction in the left iliac region in the area of the iliac compression band.

REFERENCES

Cockett, F. B. (1967) *Brit. J. Surg.*, **54**, 892.
Cockett, F. B. (1968) *J. Obstet. & Gynec. of British Commonwealth*, **75**, 12, 1316.
Cockett, F. B., Lea Thomas, M. (1965) *Brit. J. Surg.*, **52**, 816.
Dale, W. A. (1966) *Surgery*, **59**, 117.
De Weese, J. A., Jones, T. L., Lyon, J. & Dale, W. H. (1960) *Surgery*, **47**, 140.
De Weese, J. A. & Rogoff, S. M. (1958) *Angiology*, **9**, 268.
Dos Santos, J. C. (1966) *Unpublished Lecture* (London).
Ehrich, W. E., Krumbhaar, E. B. (1943) *Am. Heart J.*, **26**, 737.
Haimovici, H. (1950) '*Circulation*', **1**, 225.
Haller, J. A. (1967) '*Deep Thrombophlebitis*'. London: Saunders.
Jackson, B. T. (1972) 'The Lumbar Lymphatics'. *Thesis for London, M.S.*
Kunlin, J., Lengua, F. & Richard, S. (1966) *J. Cardiovascular Surg.*, **7**, 520.
Lea Thomas, M., Fletcher, E. W. L., Cockett, F. B. & Negus, D. (1967) *Clin. Radiol.*, **18**, 403.
May, R., Thurner, J. (1957) *Angiology*, **8**, 419.
McMurrich, J. P. (1906) *Brit. Med. J.*, **II**, 1699.
Miles, R. H., Chapel, F. Y. and Rener, O. (1964) *Ann. Surg.*, **30**, 40.
Mobbin-Uddin, K., *et al* (1969) *Arch. Surg.*, **99,** 711.
Moretz, W. H., Rhode, C. M. & Shepherd, M. H. (1959) *Ann. Surg.*, **25**, 617.
Negus, D., Cockett, F. B. (1967) *Brit. J. Surg.*, **54**, 522.
Negus, D., Cockett, F. B., Fletcher, F. W. L., Lea Thomas, M. (1968) *Brit. J. Surg.*, **55**, 369.
Palma, E. C., Passano de M. M. & Guevara, A. (1965) *Reuta. Cirug. Urug.*, **35**, 11.
Spencer, F. C. (1959) *Surg. Forum*, **10**, 680.
Spencer, F. C. & Quattlebaum, J. (1962) *Ann. Surg.*, **155**, 827.

17. The Post-thrombotic Syndrome and Venous Ulceration

It is now well known that most patients who have had a deep vein thrombosis develop over the next few years a post-thrombotic syndrome of the leg. According to the site and extent of the original thrombosis this post-thrombotic syndrome may vary between relatively slight (with minor aching, swelling and congestion), and extremely severe, even crippling (venous ulceration, pain, swelling and induration of the lower leg).

The most well-known and troublesome component of this syndrome is the *venous ulcer* of the ankle. For many years these lesions were known as varicose ulcers—although it was repeatedly pointed out that they were not usually associated with gross superficial varicose veins. This name has been responsible for many of the old misconceptions in pathology and treatment. It is only during the last forty years that the relationship of these ulcers to old deep vein thrombosis has been established, and it is only during the last twenty years that the important role of valve destruction in the ankle perforating veins in their pathology has been demonstrated.

History:

The history of the growth of knowledge about these ulcers and their relation to disorders of the venous system was dealt with admirably by Anning (1952), and the following short summary is taken from this source.

Hippocrates first noticed the association of varicose veins with leg ulcers. However, not until Harvey's discovery of the valves and the part they play in the circulation, did further progress occur. Wiseman (1676), writing about venous thrombosis, dilatation of veins, and the results of these conditions on the valves, seems to have been the first to consider that these ulcers might be due to a circulatory defect. As a result of the writings of many distinguished men of the late eighteenth and early nineteenth century, (Home, 1801; Hodgson, 1815; Brodie, 1846; Chapman, 1853; Astley Cooper, 1837; Hunt, 1859; Hilton, 1861; and Critchett 1848) the emphasis was placed on the varicose veins and the term varicose ulcer was adopted.

However, in 1867, an outstanding investigation on the aetiology of ulcers of the leg was published by Gay (1867–68, Chap. 2). The work was the first painstaking scientific investigation of this condition in England. He pointed out, as did Nunn (1852), that severe long-standing varicosity may exist without ulceration—and that it is in fact the rule rather than the exception—a most important observation, neglected until comparatively recent years (Lockhart-Mummery and Smitham, 1951). He noted that with ulcers there were other serious lesions of the deep veins, and he wrote: 'Ulceration is not a direct consequence of varicosity, but of other conditions of the venous system of which varicosity is not infrequently a complication.' A most penetrating observation. He described the pathological condition of the deep veins in the post-thrombotic leg, and he gave an accurate anatomical description of the ankle perforating veins. *The term venous ulcer was first introduced by him.*

Since the time of Gay little advance was made until Homans (1917) presented his study of the pathology of thrombosis of the deep veins of the leg and showed that recanalisation with destruction of valves was probably very common after deep thrombosis, and that ulcers of the leg followed and were closely related to this deep venous pathology.

The introduction of venography by Dos Santos (1938), and the study of venous pressures in the veins of the leg and foot at rest and exercise added a great deal to our knowledge of the normal physiology of venous return from the leg, and the effects of thrombotic disease on this. Finally, a re-study of the venous anatomy of the leg, particularly the anatomy to the direct ankle perforating veins has made it possible to build up a clear picture of the pathology of venous ulcers and the post-thrombotic syndrome.

Interest was further stimulated in the subject by Gunnar Bauer in the early 1940's and he initiated the appearance of a number of statistical clinical studies on the relationship between deep vein thrombosis and the post-thrombotic syndrome and venous ulcers.

Some of these studies are given in the table below.

Table 17.1

Author	No. of cases of ulcer	Percentage giving a definite history of previous thrombosis
Bauer, 1952	38	87 per cent
Birger, 1947	432	40 per cent
Nilzen, 1945		41–56 per cent
Anning, 1952	715	80 per cent
Dodd, 1954	121	30 per cent

The extreme variability of these figures must be expected, for there are two variable factors in compiling each series: (1) the criteria as to what constitutes a history of deep thrombosis may vary widely among even well-qualified observers, and also among the patients themselves. (2) The type of clinic from which these statistics are compiled. Thus Anning's very high figure comes from a skin clinic, and cases with obvious varicose veins may not have been referred to it.

However, from these figures it appeared that in approximately forty to fifty per cent, (at least) of the patients complaining of ulcerated leg, a previous history of deep vein thrombosis could be obtained.

Another and more fruitful line of clinical research was pursued by Bauer (1942) and Højensgard (1952). These authors followed up over a number of years a group of patients known to have had deep thrombosis in the past from their hospital records. Bauer's findings are given in the following table:

Table 17.2

No. of years after thrombosis	Percentage of cases with induration of the lower leg	Percentage of cases with actual ulcers
5	45 per cent	20 per cent
10	72 per cent	52 per cent
later	91 per cent	79 per cent

Højensgard (1952) published the results of a follow-up study of 89 unselected extremities from 57 patients in which deep thrombosis had occurred from 6 to 36 years previously. No fewer than 89 per cent of these legs had developed serious sequelae. 87 per cent had heaviness and fatigue, 78 per cent had chronic oedema, 27 per cent had present or past ulcer, and 45 per cent had to wear a supporting bandage all the time.

These figures are impressive, showing that within five years of occurrence of deep thrombosis of the leg about half the patients have developed indurative lesions in the gaiter area with or without actual ulceration. *As time goes on this proportion gets higher.* These figures call special attention to the time factor, which was also stressed by Homans. Between two and five years after a deep thrombosis is the peak time for the appearance of ulcer and induration. In a series of twenty patients with a definite previous history of post-partum white leg studied at St. Thomas' Hospital (Cockett, 1953), ten (50 per cent) first noticed the ankle lesions two to two-and-a-half years after the deep thrombosis.

Thus, from these clinical studies, there was indisputable evidence of the great importance of previous deep thrombosis in the ulcer and induration syndrome of the lower leg.

Investigation in the years 1950–1960

During this period the more detailed pathology of these mysterious venous ulcers was gradually worked out by a series of investigations by many workers, which fall into three main groups.

1. The investigation of the deep veins in ulcer cases by the newly emerging and rapidly developing method of venography.

2. The investigation of the behaviour of the venous pressure in the deep and superficial veins.

3. A further study of the exact anatomy of the ankle perforating veins and their role in the venous drainage of the skin and subcutaneous tissues round the ankle (see Chap. 3).

Venographic studies. Although peripheral deep phlebography was first introduced by Dos Santos in 1938; to Gunnar Bauer (1942, 1950), the credit must go for establishing that after a main deep vein thrombosis, the deep veins recanalise, and once again become adequate conduits for venous flow, but the valves are destroyed. This was confirmed and his techniques amplified by many subsequent workers—Luke (1943); Linton and Hardy (1948); Dow (1951); Højensgaard (1952); Bowen (1964); Pratt (1964) to mention but a few.

For a time attention was focused on this valve destruction in the main deep veins as the main cause of ulceration.

However, at St. Thomas' Hospital Cockett (1953) presented a venographic investigation of three groups of cases with ulcer of the leg. (1) Cases with venous ulcer and varicose veins; (2) Cases with venous ulcer, no varicose veins, but a definite history of post deep thrombosis; (3) Cases with venous ulcer, no definite past history of thrombosis and no demonstrable superficial varicose veins (Fig. 17.1).

The site and clinical appearance and behaviour of the ulcer was the same in the three groups of cases. The venographic findings were that in group (2) cases there was complete recanalisation with valve destruction in the whole popliteal and femoral veins. In groups (1) and (3) however, (patients who had exactly similar ulcers) valves in the popliteal and femoral veins were present and normal.

These findings thus tended to show that post-thrombotic valve destruction in the popliteal and femoral veins was not necessarily the prime cause of induration and ulceration in the lower leg.

As a result of this study attention was

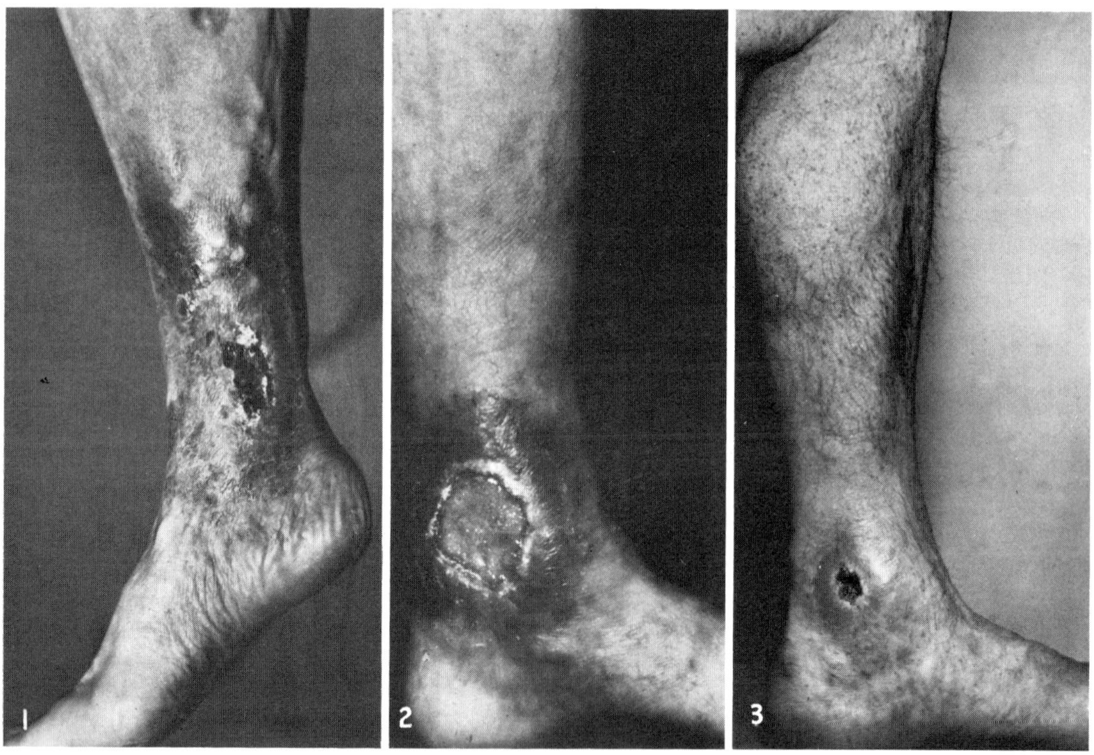

Fig. 17.1 The three legs depicted here are the three major clinical types of venous ulcer 1. Group 1. A chronic ulcer, with obvious and grossly incompetent veins of the great saphenous system. 2. Group 2. A chronic ulcer, with no superficial veins visible on the leg. This woman gave a clear history of a deep femoral thrombosis or 'white leg' two years before her ulcer appeared. 3. Group 3. A chronic ulcer, in a young man. He had no incompetent superficial varicose veins. He denied all history of previous thrombosis. Note that all three ulcers occupy the same position. An incompetent ankle perforating vein was found at operation in all three apparently different types of ulcer.

focused on the valves in the ankle perforating veins whose detailed anatomy had just been studied afresh (Cockett, 1953, Linton 1952).

It began to be appreciated that the essential local cause of ulceration lay in the destruction of the valves in these ankle perforating veins which were shown to be the direct route of venous drainage of the ankle skin (the so-called 'gaiter area') in the erect exercising limb. This thesis was supported by a consideration of the situation of venous ulcers.

The situation of venous ulcers

Homans (1938) writing on post-phlebitic ulcers, noted that there was little specific about them and that they tended to occupy the same part of the leg as the so-called varicose ulcers. Looking again at Figure 17.1, it is striking that the situation occupied by, and the appearance of, all these ulcers of apparently different venous pathology is the same. Hanschell (1949) stated 'The great majority of patients with varicose veins, at all ages, have and have had no leg ulcers; while the great majority of patients with leg ulcers, at all ages, have and have had no varicose veins; yet in its clinical features, under all conditions, there is no discernible difference between ulcer with, and ulcer without varicose veins'.

Turning back to the section on anatomy it will be appreciated that the lower leg and ankle, the gaiter area, is the area which is drained by the direct ankle perforating veins, which empty straight into the deep veins (posterior tibial and peroneal) (*see* Fig. 17.2).

The ulcer precursor state, the ankle flare and fat necrosis

In many patients an ulcer precursor state can be observed (Cockett and Elgan Jones, 1953). This consists of a fine dilatation of the venules in the region above, behind and below the internal malleolus, disappearing as a marked flare of dilated venules into the thick skin of the heel pad. This may also be observed, though less often, on the outer side of the ankle. This dilatation is the result of sustained high venous pressure transmitted

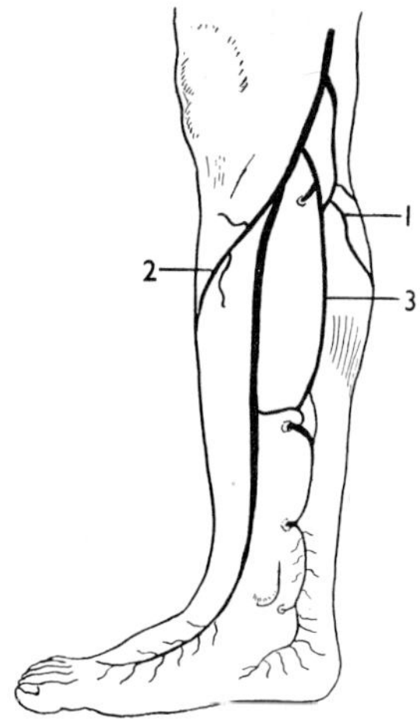

Fig. 17.2 Diagram of main perforating veins of the leg. The figures refer to the three groups of branches which usually arise at knee level (see Anatomy chapter). The vein marked 3 is the large constant posterior arch vein which descends to anastomose with the ankle perforators.

to the fine venous arches which connect the ankle perforating veins and is called the *Ankle Flare*. (Fig. 17.2). We have had the opportunity of watching this state develop in a patient, whose picture and history is given in Figure 17.3. Figure 3, Chapter 19, shows another example of this fine venular dilatation in the ankle area.

In many female patients with a fair thickness of subcutaneous fat in this area this venular dilatation may be masked, and instead the whole of the area becomes the seat of a tight brawny oedema which rapidly gives place to the familiar 'induration' of the gaiter area. This induration is due to *subcutaneous fat necrosis.* Figure 17.4 shows the venogram and clinical photograph of the lower leg in such a case, and shows the early pathology of this lower leg induration. Figure 17.4 also shows the later stage, a case in which the ulcer and induration syndrome had been present for many years.

The essential pathology of venous ulcers and induration

The essential pathology of the syndrome appears to be a sustained local ambulatory

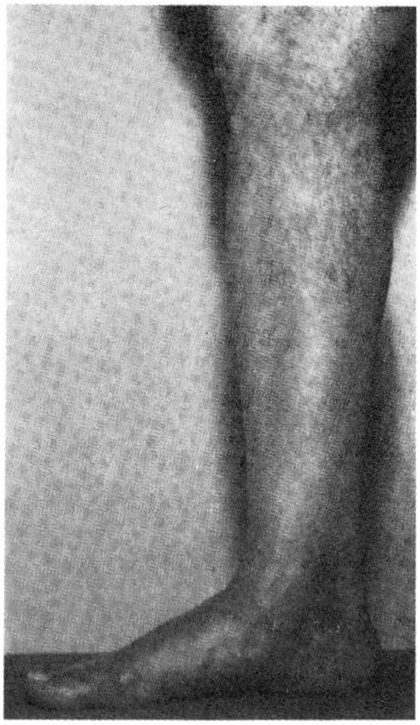

Fig. 17.3 Eighteen months previous to this picture this patient had a normal leg. At this time he was admitted to hospital with a saphenous thrombophlebitis. His common femoral vein was ligated. Following this he developed a retrograde deep thrombosis (proved venographically). After the swelling had subsided, at his follow up visits, the gradual appearance of the 'ankle flare' of dilated veins and pigmentation in the area shown was seen to appear. One year after the deep thrombosis an enlarged upper internal ankle perforating vein could be felt. He has been on continuous treatment with a firm webbing elastic bandage which has prevented him from developing an ulcer so far. If ulceration threatens he will have this perforating vein ligated.

venous hypertension (i.e. during exercise) concentrated in the area of the ankle drained by the direct ankle perforating veins.

Thanks to the work of numerous investigators who have measured the venous pressure in the superficial veins of the foot, and the deep veins, under conditions of rest and exercise, in normal limbs and in limbs with venous incompetence, we have a clear picture of the venous haenodynamics of the leg.

The results of these investigations must now be considered.

Venous pressure measurements

In a normal leg the pressure in the subcutaneous veins of the foot at rest in the erect position is equal to the pressure of a column of blood extending from the foot to heart level. This is equivalent to a pressure of between 85 and 90 mmHg, according to the height of the individual. As soon as the calf muscles are put into action this pressure falls at once to between 0 and 10 mmHg. Thus the efficiency with which the subcutaneous venous system of the foot and ankle is drained by action of the calf pump in the erect position is truly remarkable.

This fact has been repeatedly observed by many workers, including ourselves.

Venous pressure in the foot and ankle in the erect posture is a result of the relative rates at which blood flows into the veins from the arteries, and is removed from them by the muscle pump. During vaso-dilation induced by *heat* (Henry and Gauer 1950) or by *lumbar sympathectomy*, (Edwards 1954) vigorous walking movements failed to reduce the venous pressure much below 70 mmHg. However, when the limb is *cooled*, even involuntary postural muscular movements reduce the venous pressure.

If the venous system or the calf pump is pathological in any way the efficiency of this venous drainage of the subcutaneous tissues via the calf pump mechanism is impaired and this is shown by the fact that the fall of venous pressure in the subcutaneous veins of the erect exercising limb is less than normal, or does not fall at all.

Several fairly extensive studies of these venous pressure changes have been made, notably by Smirk (1936), Pollack and Wood (1949), Pollack, Taylor, Myers and Wood (1949), Walker and Longland (1950), DeCamp, Ward and Ochsner (1951), Warren, White and Belcher (1949), and Højensgard and Sturup (1949 and 1952). The basic behaviour of the venous pressure in the superficial veins of the leg in cases of pure incompetence of superficial veins, in postphlebitic legs, and in the normal have been established by these authors.

There have been several differences in technique used by them. Pollack and Wood used the saphenous vein itself in front of the

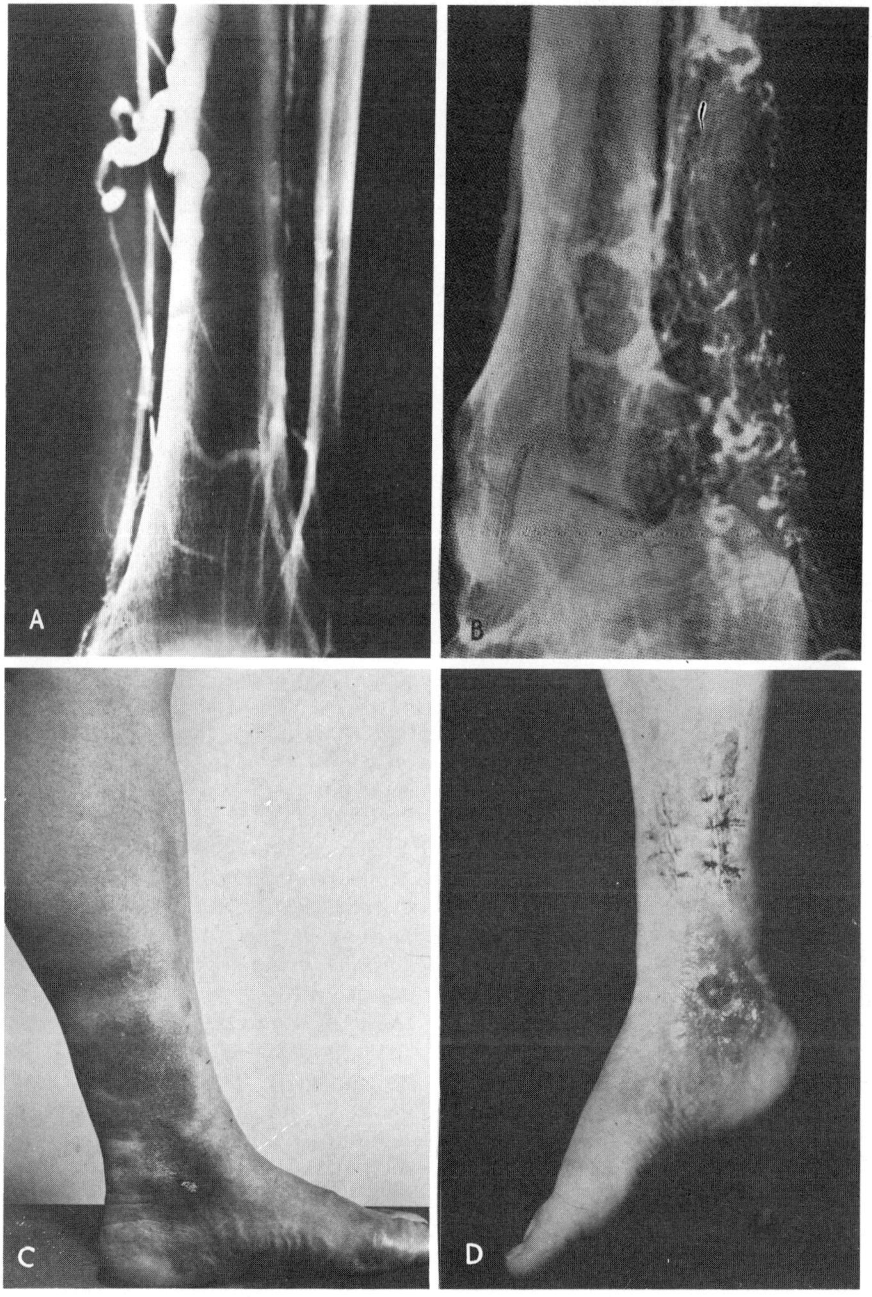

Fig. 17.4 The pathology of post-thrombotic induration and ulceration of the ankle (A and C—early; B and D—late). A and C are the venogram and photographs of the ankle of a patient who had a deep thrombosis one and a half years previously. She now complained of an indurated, red, scaly area well shown in the photograph, which ached, and was painful after being on her feet. No veins were visible or palpable. The venogram revealed the large incompetent perforating vein. Notice particularly the fine venular dilatation in the subcutaneous tissues—leading down from the perforating vein. B and D are the venogram and photograph of a patient who had her deep thrombosis twelve years previously. This is the fully developed post-thrombotic syndrome of the ankle with ulcer and induration. Once again the venogram revealed the incompetent perforating vein, and the fine spray of dilated venules arising from this and permeating the subcutaneous tissues of the ulcer area.

internal malleolus; Warren, White and Belcher used 'a branch of the saphenous vein in the calf' (their illustration shows one high up the calf, being used); DeCamp, Ward and Ochsner used a vein of 'foot or lower leg'; Walker and Longland used a vein of the dorsum of the foot. These facts are mentioned because the particular vein chosen for the pressure recording may have a bearing on the result. Warren, White and Belcher particularly mention this point, and even show different exercise falls of venous pressure in different veins from the same limb.

However, there has been basic agreement on the following facts:

1. In normal legs, with the patient erect, the venous pressure in the subcutaneous veins of foot and ankle falls rapidly on exercise to between 0 and 30 mmHg, and then rises slowly (31 seconds according to Pollack and Wood) on cessation of exercise to its previous height of 90 mmHg.

2. In patients with primary incompetent superficial varicose veins, the pressure falls to a value of 45–60 mmHg, rising rapidly (within three seconds) to the initial figure of 90 mmHg on cessation of exercise.

3. In post-phlebitic cases there appears to be some variation. Most authors find that there is either no fall of pressure on exercise, or a slight fall—to a value of 75 or 80 mmHg, with an immediate return to the pre-exercise level on cessation of exercise. DeCamp et al., actually recorded a slight rise in pressure on exercise in four cases.

In the deep veins, popliteal and femoral, however, there is no great change of pressure on exercise in any of the three groups. Veal and Hussey (1940) and Sturup and Højensgard (1950) showed that although there were fluctuations in pressure in these veins during exercise there was no change in the mean pressure, in normal legs or in legs with varicose veins or a history of deep thrombosis, during rest and exercise.

	Standing pressure	Exercise pressure	Time of return to standing pressure
Normal superficial veins	90 mmHg	0–30 mmHg	31 seconds
Primary varicose veins	90 mmHg	45–60 mmHg	3 seconds
Post-phlebitics	90 mmHg	75–90 mmHg or actual increase	Immediate

Højensgard and Sturup have carried their investigations a step farther during 1952 and 1953. By simultaneous catheterisation of superficial and deep veins, in normal subjects, and in patients with post-phlebitic legs, and measurement of the fluctuation in venous pressure with the Tybjaerg Hansen manometer, they have been able to study accurately the fluctuations in venous pressure in the deep veins and the superficial veins concurrently.

They found that the mean pressure in the big deep venous trunks, the popliteal and femoral, was consistently higher than that in the superficial veins in a normal exercising limb. In the calf, during walking, the pressure fluctuations of the deep veins and the superficial veins followed a similar curve. These curves showed that at a certain phase of walking (the phase of relaxation of the calf, or diastole of the calf pump) the pressure is momentarily somewhat lower in the deep veins. During this phase blood can flow inwards, through the perforating veins. When the calf contracts, the pressure within it rises, and blood is prevented from flowing outwards by the arrangement of the valves in the perforating veins (already noted in the section on anatomy).

These elegant studies by Højensgard and Sturup have been confirmed more recently by Arnoldi and Linderholm (1968) and by Fegan, Fitzgerald and Milliken (1964).

After similar studies in varicose limbs and in post-thrombotic limbs, these authors came to a very important conclusion. They state: 'The abnormal function of the deep veins in the post-thrombotic syndrome is due not so much to a difference in the valvular equipment of the popliteal and femoral veins as to the destruction of valves in the deep lower leg veins'. This conclusion agreed exactly with the conclusion that we arrived at, at St. Thomas' Hospital in 1953 and which Linton had arrived at in Boston at the same time.

Thus the normal calf pump is a remarkably efficient mechanism. It not only forces the blood out of the lower leg upwards, at every contraction, with considerable force, but also during a phase of diastole 'sucks in' the venous blood from the subcutaneous tissues round the ankle, via the direct ankle perforating veins.

Barcroft and Dornhorst (1948) have shown that the calf pump can overcome a resistance greater than 100 mmHg. Moreover, from the work of Wells, Youmans and Miller (1938) and of Ludbrook (1966), we have good evidence that the pressure within the calf on contraction is greatest in the lower third, where the ankle perforating veins go in. These investigations measured the rise in intramuscular pressure on contraction, by a method involving placing a needle in the muscles at various levels. They found a great difference in the pressure in muscles which were not invested by a tight fascia, such as the rectus femoris, and those that were, such as the soleus. The maximal rise of intramuscular pressure on contraction of rectus femoris was 18 mmHg. In the lower third of the soleus, the rise of pressure on contraction was 90 mmHg and the contraction pressure fell gradually to between 30 and 40 mmHg as the needle was put in higher and higher in the calf. Thus there is unequivocal evidence from this work that on contraction of the calf there is a considerable rise of pressure within it, particularly in the lower third.

Turning now to Figure 17.5, it will be seen that the effect of incompetence or destruction of the valves in one or more of the direct ankle perforating veins will be to transmit the high exercise venous pressure within the lower third of the calf during contraction of the soleus, directly to the mesh of fine subcutaneous venules in the gaiter area. This will lead to their gradual dilatation (see Fig. 17.3) including the small subcuticular venules leading down to the heel (the ankle flare).

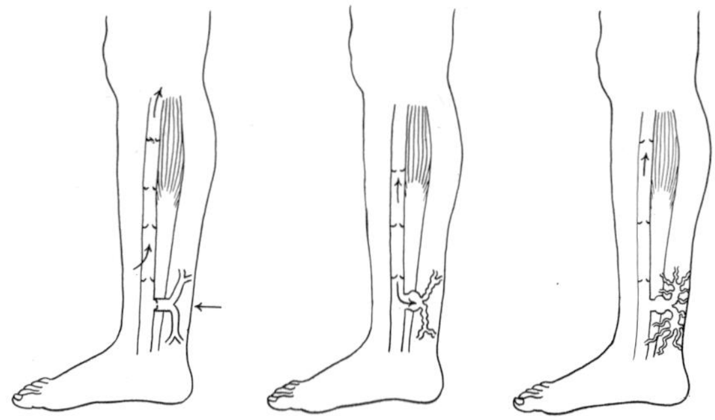

Fig. 17.5 Diagram to illustrate the effects of destruction of the valve in the ankle perforating veins. Via these short wide veins, if their valve was rendered incompetent, the great rise of pressure in the deep veins of the leg on every calf contraction could be transmitted straight out to be delicate venous mesh with which they are connected. The result of this would be a gradual dilatation of all the small venules in this area, a condition which is seen frequently as a pre-ulcer phenomenon and occurs under every established venous ulcer.

Moreover, this localised high venous pressure and dilatation is occurring over an area of remarkably slight arterial supply. The effect on the subcutaneous tissues and skin of the area is to impair their nutrition very considerably, with the production of local swelling and tissue necrosis. This is the essential and basic pathology of venous ulcers and induration of the ankle.

That sustained local venous hypertension can in fact cause ulceration is shown conclusively in Figure 17.6. The patient shown here had a traumatic arterio-venous fistula between a branch of the subclavian artery and vein in the supraclavicular fossa. This had led to widespread local venous dilatation and hypertension in the subcutaneous tissues of the shoulder. Eventually a large chronic venous ulcer appeared over the shoulder, which persisted until the fistula was closed (*see also* Chap. 2, on Ulcers of the leg due to congenital arterio-venous fistulae).

The role of the ankle perforating veins in patients with long or short saphenous varicose veins

From Figure 17.2 it will be seen that there is a direct connection between the great saphenous vein and the fine venous arches

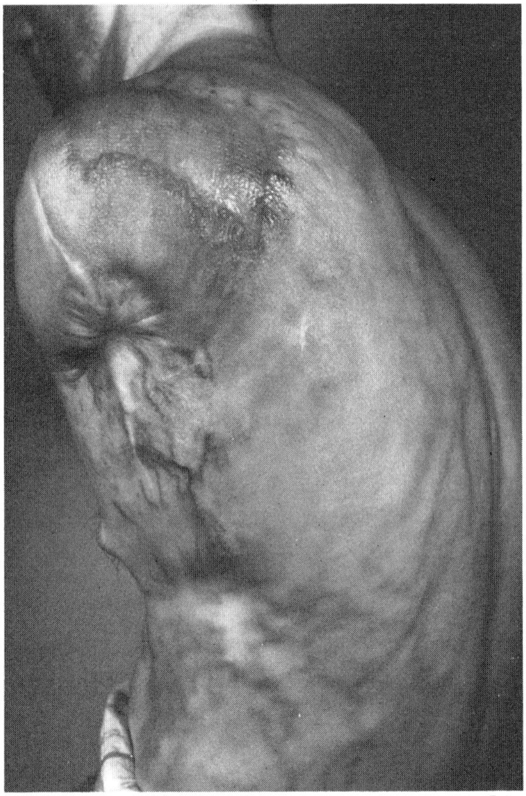

Fig. 17.6 A 'venous ulcer' of the shoulder. This patient had a traumatic arterio-venous fistula between a branch of the subclavian artery and vein in the left supra-clavicular region. His arm had been lost at the time of the original injury. He sought further treatment because of the development of a large shallow surface ulcer of the shoulder. This looked just like a venous ulcer, and responded to pressure dressings in exactly the same way as venous ulcers of the leg do.

connecting the internal ankle perforating veins, by means of the posterior arch vein (Leonardo's vein) arising from the great saphenous vein at knee level. Thus in great saphenous incompetence, the high venous pressure transmitted down this vein may eventually reach the ankle perforator area. But if the ankle perforators are competent, this high venous pressure will be 'sucked off' into the deep veins by the muscle pump. Varicose veins of the great saphenous system must therefore be of considerable size, before they exert an appreciable effect on the venous mesh in the gaiter area.

However if valve failure in one of the ankle perforators should occur, the addition of this source of venous hypertension to that caused by the already incompetent long saphenous vein causes a greatly increased venous hypertension locally, and this is signalled by sudden severe deterioration of the ankle skin, with possible ulceration. *This sequence of events is seen frequently in varicose vein patients who may go on for years with large varicose veins and no ulcer, then suddenly within six months or so a marked deterioration of the ankle skin sets in with aching, congestion, ankle flare, and eventually ulceration.*

Exactly the same remarks hold true for incompetence of the small saphenous vein and incompetence of the lateral ankle perforating veins, except that in this case the maximum effect tends to be on the outer side of the ankle.

One further point is of importance. The direct ankle perforating veins are quite large veins. When they become incompetent and dilate their size is considerably increased. It is not uncommon to find a dilated ankle perforator half a centimetre in diameter in the vicinity of a venous ulcer. This factor of relative size is very important, as the degree to which venous pressure effects can be transmitted without 'damping' increases very rapidly with vessel size. A short wide vessel, such as these incompetent ankle perforators become, is ideal for transmitting high venous pressure.

How the valves in the ankle perforating veins are destroyed

It is our experience that by far the commonest way in which the valves of the perforating veins are destroyed is by thrombosis. One of the commonest varieties of thrombosis, as we have seen (Chap. 15) is calf thrombosis. This starts in the large venous sinuses in soleus and then spreads via the numerous veins draining soleus into the posterior tibial venae comites and thence upwards for a greater or shorter distance.

Now reference to Figure 3.25 and Figure 3.26 in the anatomy chapter will show that if clot spreads down the lower two veins draining soleus it has a direct path of spread into the upper and middle ankle perforating veins. This has been seen to occur at post-mortem dissection several times by us. There is also clinical evidence for this. In an early case of calf thrombosis the sign of tenderness in the lower calf may be elicited; if the fingers are then moved gently up and down the line of emergence of the ankle perforators, often the site of either the upper perforator or the middle one will be found to be exquisitely tender. This early sign of calf thrombosis has also been commented upon by Cohen (1952). During the subsequent months this clot recanalises. Then not only is the segment of deep vein formerly occupied by this clot rendered valveless and incompetent, *but the perforating vein also*. It takes between six months to a year for effective recanalisation of deep veins to take place. Thus the lesions only begin to appear one to two years after the original episode of thrombosis.

Not only the upper two inner ankle perforating veins but also the external ankle perforating veins and mid calf perforator may be rendered incompetent in this way.

An analysis of which ankle perforators are most frequently found incompetent at operation

At operation it is possible to tell whether the valve in a perforating vein is competent or not by a simple and definite test which was first described by Turner Warwick (1931). When a normal perforating vein is cut across at operation, the end which is left disappearing through the hole in the deep fascia to connect with the deep vein does not bleed. This is because its valve, at the junction with the deep vein, is held shut by the venous pressure in the deep veins. This can be shown if a probe is gently inserted down the lumen of the perforator and the valve held aside. Bleeding immediately occurs. Now, if an incompetent perforating vein is cut across, the result is very different—profuse steady bleeding occurs outwards from the deep vein. Moreover, if the calf is suddenly squeezed opposite the incompetent perforator, a jet of blood is ejected from it with surprising force. This is a practical demonstration of what happens in normal circumstances when the calf pump is put into action. This test is known as the 'bleed-back' or 'Turner Warwick's' test.

During 1952 and 1953, ankle perforator exploration was done on 135 limbs with early and late indurative lesions and ulcers of the ankle (at St. Thomas' Hospital). This group of cases did not have grossly incompetent superficial veins of the great saphenous system. Incompetent ankle perforating veins were found, proved incompetent by Turner Warwick's test, and tied in ninety-six of these cases. The veins found incompetent in this series are shown in the following table:

Table 17.3 Ninety-six limbs

Upper internal ankle perforator incompetent only	24
Middle internal ankle perforator incompetent only	55
Both internal ankle perforators incompetent	4
Lower internal ankle perforator (just *below* malleolus) incompetent	0
Lateral ankle perforator incompetent usually with short saphenous incompetence	12
Mid calf perforator	1
	96

This series of cases was most instructive, showing which perforating veins were most likely to be found incompetent in such cases. Three significant facts emerged:

1. Either the middle or the upper internal ankle perforator is most likely to be incompetent. It is less common for both to be found incompetent in the same leg. This may be related to the anatomical fact already noted that they tend to vary inversely in size. Thus when the upper one is large the middle one is small and vice versa.

However in all severe venous ulcers of the leg, it is recommended that the site of both the upper and the middle perforating veins should be explored and both tied, as the bleed-back test is not always easy to carry out and reliable, specially in the smaller size perforators.

2. The lower ankle perforating vein located just below and posterior to the internal malleolus is hardly ever found to be incompetent. This is because it is never, in contact with thrombus occupying the calf veins, so its valve is *very rarely* destroyed.

3. The lateral ankle perforator was found incompetent in just over 12 per cent of the cases and the possibility of this vein being at fault even when most of the pathology is on the inner side of the leg must be kept in mind. By means of a vein passing behind the tendo-Achillis the effects of incompetence of this lateral perforator may be distributed to the internal surface of the ankle as well as the external surface.

During the same period, fifty-four cases with obvious incompetence of the great saphenous system and indurative lesions of the lower leg of varying degrees of severity were also operated upon. These cases had a routine high saphenous ligation, often a stripping of the great saphenous vein, and an exploration of the ankle perforators. The findings in this group were:

Table 17.4 Findings

Fifty-four patients with incompetent veins of the great saphenous system and a lower leg ulcer.	
Cases in which no incompetent perforators in the lower leg could be demonstrated	18
Cases in which either the upper (eight cases) or the middle (twenty-eight cases) ankle perforators were found incompetent	36
	54

Thus, from these figures it would appear that in a high proportion of cases with varicose veins and a lesion in the lower leg, an incompetent ankle perforating vein is also present, and is contributory to the lower leg lesion. It was noticeable that those with the most severe lesions *always* had an incompetent perforating vein as well. This is the main reason why so many varicose ulcers recur after an efficient operation on the great saphenous system only. The incompetent perforator near the ulcer is left behind and perpetuates the ulcer-forming process as soon as normal activity is resumed.

The association of short saphenous incompetence with lateral perforator incompetence

Turning to Figure 7.6 it will be seen that the lateral ankle perforating vein usually joins either the main trunk or a large branch of the small saphenous vein in the lower third of the leg (see also Chap. 3). Incompetence and dilatation of the small saphenous system is rarer than that of the great saphenous system, and it is more difficult to diagnose. The main area affected by small saphenous incompetence is the skin area below and behind the *lateral malleolus*. However, so common are the anatomical variations, and particularly so common is the venous connection with the arch connecting the internal ankle perforators that in over half the cases skin lesions appear behind the internal malleolus also. In a few cases they appear predominantly here.

The small saphenous vein, being a relatively shorter vein and with fewer tributaries than the great saphenous, valvular incompetence or destruction at its union with the popliteal vein allows the high ambulatory venous pressure here to be transmitted down to the ankle region relatively easily. Ankle lesions—venular dilatation, eczema, swelling and ulceration tend to be a much more common accompaniment, and appear earlier with incompetence of the short saphenous vein. If the lateral ankle perforating vein is competent this acts as a safety valve constantly 'sucking off' the accumulating high venous pressure at the lower end of the small saphenous vein. If this lateral perforating vein is incompetent it adds its quota of high venous pressure at every contraction of the calf, to that in the lower part of the small saphenous drainage area. This combination (small saphenous incompetence and lateral perforator incompetence) is found to be the cause of severe eczema or ulceration behind both malleoli in many cases and appears to be a highly destructive combination, comparable in every way with the combination of great saphenous incompetence and internal perforator incompetence.

The factor of variable tissue response to venous stress

The main channels through which a local raised venous pressure may be brought to bear on the capillaries and tissues around the malleoli have been discussed. But this is only half the story in the pathology of these indurative and ulcerative lesions around the ankle. Anyone seeing a large number of patients with venous lesions in various stages of evolution cannot fail to be impressed by the fact that the tissues of different patients react in very different ways to a given degree of venous stress. Thus the hairy, well nourished average male ankle with relatively little subcutaneous tissue will show a considerable degree of venular dilatation before any surface ulceration becomes apparent and even then it may only be slight (see Fig. 7.22B). At the other end of the scale is the fat, hairless, erythrocyanoid type of female ankle. Here nutrition of the large amount of fatty subcutaneous tissues is poor and the addition of an increased local raised venous pressure may precipitate another tissue necrosing reaction. This consists of a relatively sudden *massive fat necrosis* of the subcutaneous tissues. Figure 17.7 shows the clinical appearance of such a case. Dusky, red, indurated, painful areas appear in the subcutaneous tissues of the gaiter area, as shown. Venography shows it is infiltrated by dilated venules, arising from an incompetent ankle perforator. This acute lesion may do one of two things: (1) it may slowly resolve on rest and supportive treatment leaving an indurated plaque in the gaiter area which is always liable to ulcerate; or (2) it may break down and ulcerate. In this case a chronic, ischaemic looking ulcer with blue edges is formed, which being an ischaemic lesion, is intensely painful—particularly at night when the limb gets warm. This type of ulcer may take months to heal even under skilled care. Every variation between these two extremes of reaction may be seen.

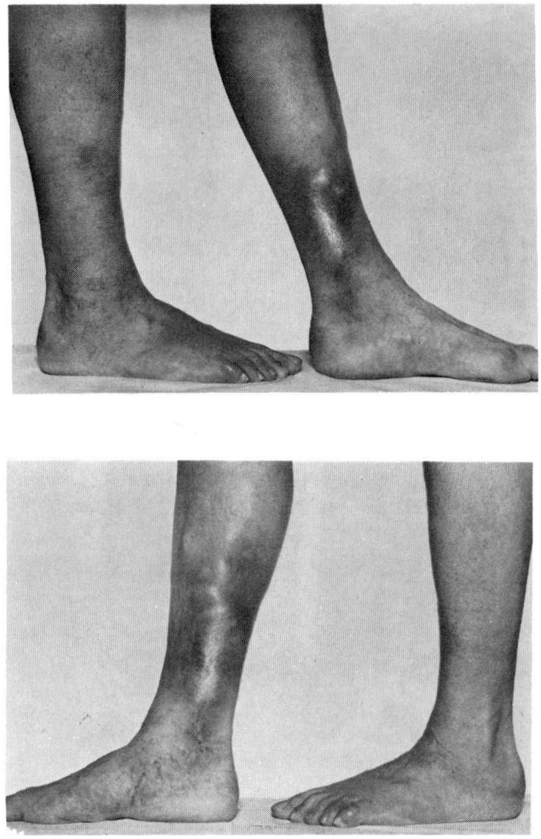

Fig. 17.7 Bilateral fat necrosis and ankle flare in early post-thrombotic perforator incompetence.

Another interesting reaction of the skin and subcutaneous tissue to local venous stress is the occurrence of purpura or ecchymosis. Certain patients seem to react particularly in this way, as shown in Figure 17.8. Senile patients, particularly, may react to even the increased venous pressure occasioned by long standing, by the development of a purpuric rash or ecchymosis around the ankle. These sometimes break down and form ulcers. This 'senile purpura' (so called) is unassociated with any demonstrable blood abnormality, although it may be associated with chronic undernutrition and Vitamin C deficiency, and it is always worth while treating these patients with ascorbic acid. This purpura is one of the important factors in many senile ulcers.

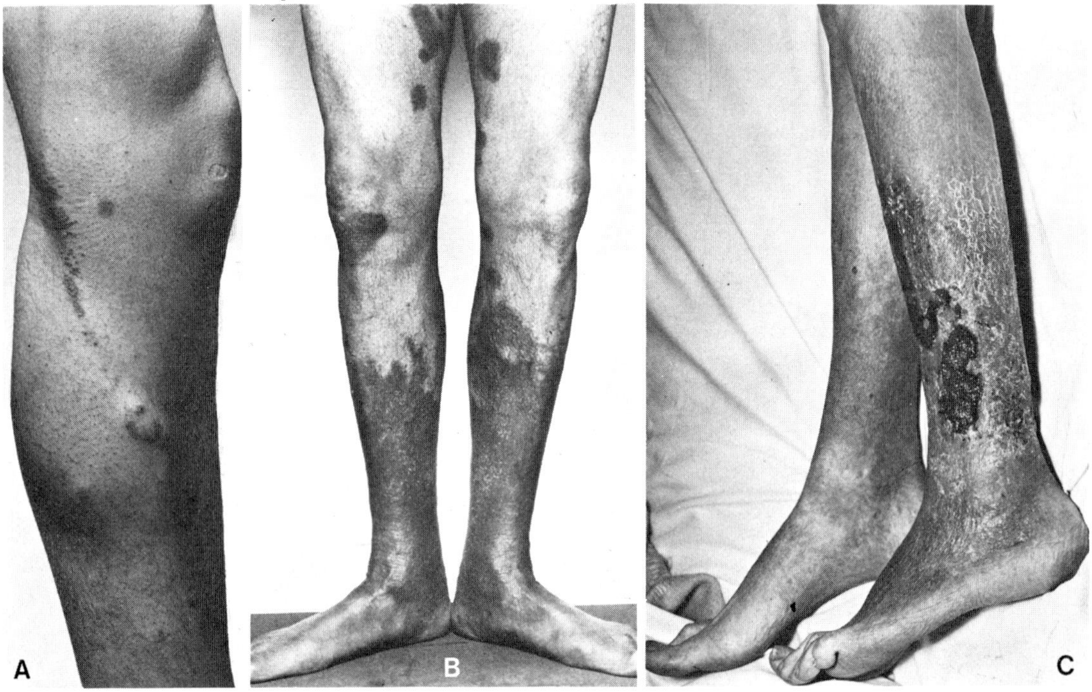

Fig. 17.8 *Purpuric Reactions.* A.—Purpuric reactions of the skin over an incompetent great saphenous vein in a young man. This disappeared after a high saphenous ligation. B.—Ecchymosis of the whole lower third of the legs in a senile patient—the so-called 'senile purpura'. Patients with Cushing's syndrome often develop a similar reaction in the skin of the area. The skin is very poor, and may break down forming numerous ulcers as in C. C.—The senile purpuric ulcers.

The histology of venous ulceration and induration

To appreciate the histological abnormality seen in sections of these lesions it is necessary to be aware of the arrangement of the minute venous drainage and arterial supply of the skin of the area. This is shown diagrammatically in Figures 17.9 and 17.10 and is of great interest, and we are indebted to Dr. Whimster for permission to publish his work here for the first time.

It will be seen that immediately below the epidermis there is a papillary venous plexus, which sends tufts of capillaries into the interpapillary spaces. This subpapillary venous plexus is drained by a number of small veins into the larger veins which lie deep in the subcutaneous tissues. In the dermis these collecting veins anastomose freely, but as they pass through the layer of subcutaneous fat they receive a small number of veins, each one of which drains its own area of fatty subcutaneous tissue and is an end vein (that is to say, it does not anastomose with other venules draining adjacent fat lobules). Thus if one of these veins is thrombosed, or if flow from it is hindered by local venous hypertension, the result can only be swelling and eventual necrosis of the lobule of fat drained by it. This is the essential pathology of the acute fat necrosis seen so often in fat ankles with venous lesions. The effect of the local rise of venous pressure on the subpapillary venous plexus and venules in the dermis is to cause dilatation of the plexus over the affected area and dilatation of the capillary tufts. These changes are shown in Figures 17.11 to 17.16.

The lymphatics in venous ulceration

Kinmonth (1952 and 1954) investigating

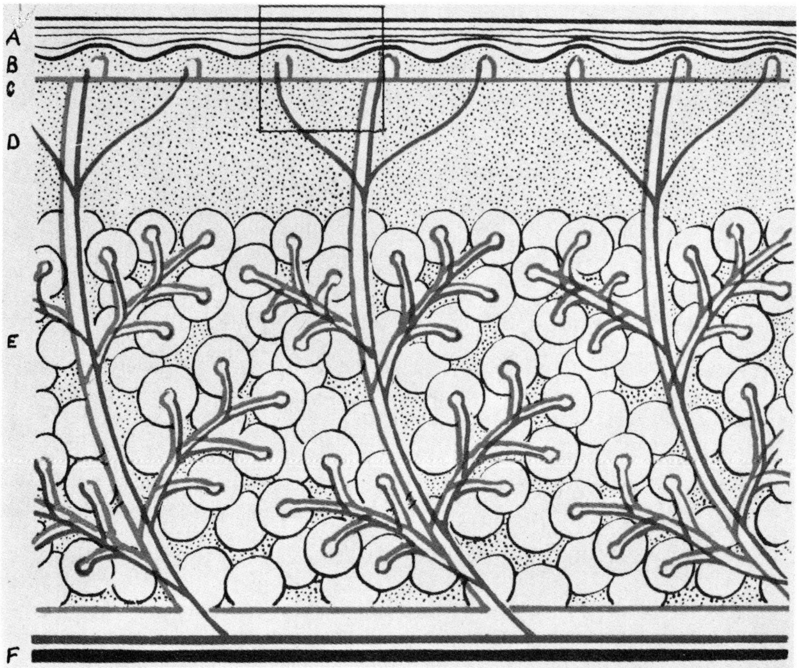

Fig. 17.9 Diagram to illustrate the difference in mode of blood supply between the superficial layer of the dermis and the deeper layers of the dermis and subcutaneous fat. It is not intended to be an accurate representation of the vessels concerned but simply to show the difference between the venous drainage of the two capillary beds. The superficial layer is supplied by a capillary bed draining into a horizontal, reticular venous plexus, which is in turn drained by vertical veins connecting with the main veins running deep in the subcutaneous fat and in the plane of the deep fascia. The capillary bed supplying the deeper layers of the dermis and the fat do not drain into a plexus but into lobular veins which run directly into the vertical veins. The sub-epidermal venous plexus and its capillary bed act as an escape valve for general rises in venous pressure in the skin and a diffuser of local ones, by distension of the plexus and proliferation of the capillary bed. The lobular vascular supply of the deeper layers has not this ability to expand and if venous pressure rises severely in this field due to spasm or thrombosis, circulation ceases and necrosis occurs. (A—epidermis; B—superficial zone of dermis; C—sub-epidermal venous plexus; D—deep zone of dermis; E—fat; F—deep fascia).

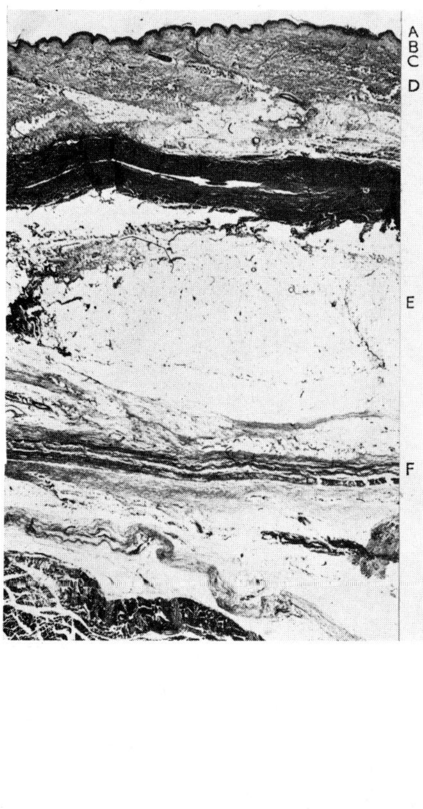

Fig. 17.10 Section through the full depth of the skin of normal leg. (The dark band running across the upper part of the fat layer is a large vein.)

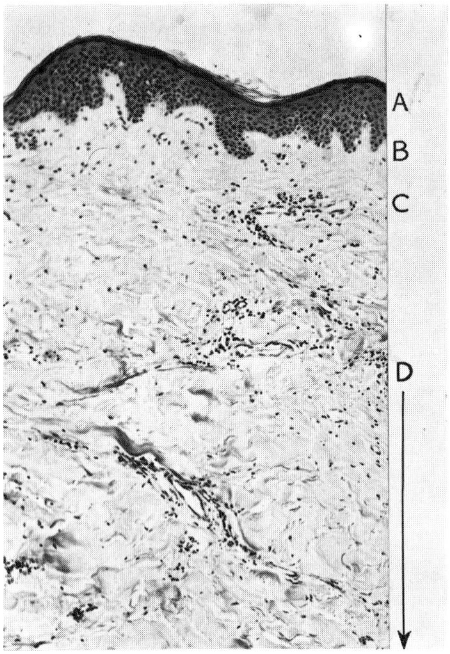

Fig. 17.11 Section through the superficial zone of normal skin.

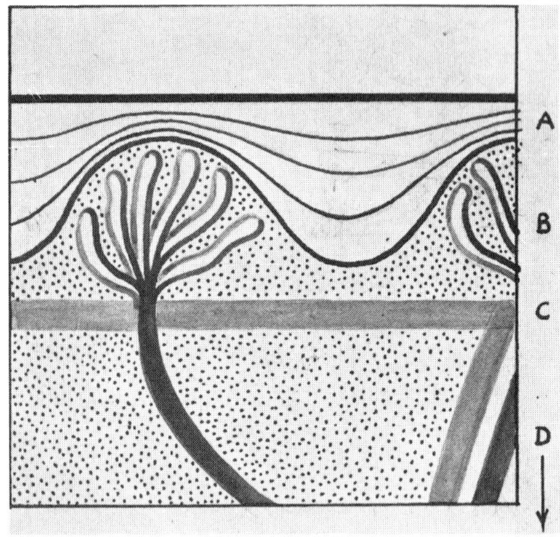

Fig. 17.13 Diagram to show the proliferation of the sub-epidermal capillary bed in chronic venous congestion. Key: A—epidermis; B—superficial zone of dermis; C—sub-epidermal venous plexus; D—deep zone of dermis.

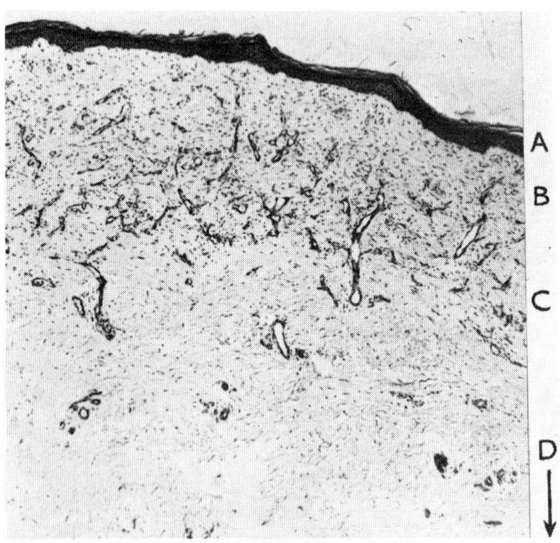

Fig. 17.12 Skin from a leg with chronic non-ulcerated venous congestion showing moderate proliferation of the sub-epidermal capillary bed.

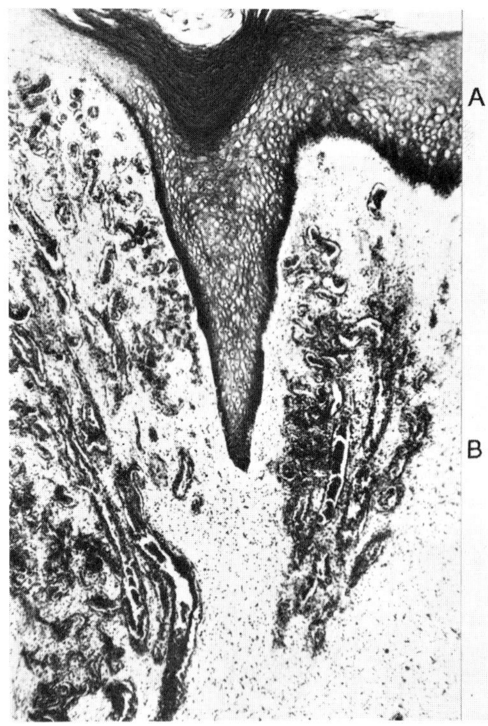

Fig. 17.14 Gross proliferation of the sub-epidermal capillary bed from a chronically congested non-ulcerated leg.

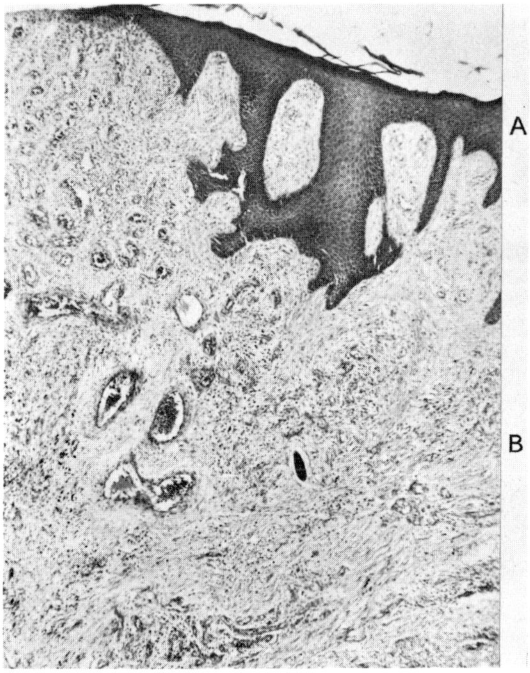

Fig. 17.15 Capillary bed proliferation in the edge of a venous ulcer. Key: A—epidermis; B—superficial zone of dermis.

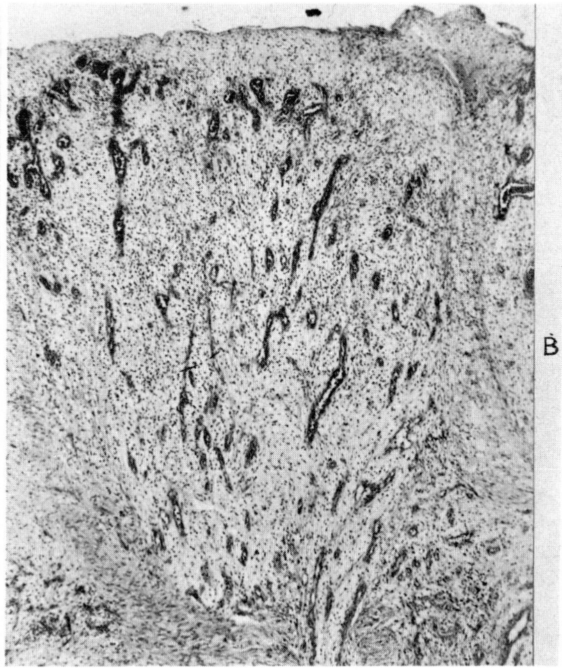

Fig. 17.16 Capillary proliferation in the floor of a venous ulcer.

the lymphatics in post-phlebitic limbs by his standard technique of lymphangiography, showed that in most of these limbs the lymphatic trunks were present and appeared to be normal.

On the other hand there is some evidence that where there is widespread severe fat necrosis and induration round the inside of the ankle, this may in fact obstruct some of the lymphatic drainage coming from the foot and cause a secondary lymphoedema of the dorsum of the foot.

The secondary effects of induration and ulceration on the mechanics of the foot

1. *Tourniquet effect.* The gradual necrosis of the subcutaneous tissues followed by induration and fibrosis of the gaiter area may progress to such an extent that the whole of the gaiter area is encased in a sort of tight fibrous tourniquet. This appearance has been aptly described clinically as 'beer bottle' or 'champagne bottle' legs, according to the taste of the particular writer! This fibrous tourniquet, once formed, further obstructs venous and lymphatic return and contributes to the oedema of the ankle and foot beneath it, and in these cases gross oedema of the foot and ankle may be a serious problem.

2. *Shortening of the tendo-Achillis and secondary effects on the mechanics of the foot.* In a small proportion of cases a contracture of the calf muscles takes place during the active painful phase of ulceration, leaving the patient with a foot in marked equinus. This contracture tends to occur especially in those women with the erythrocyanoid type of limb in which the ulcer is very painful. The ankle is held immobile in the equinus position, as this is the position of maximum comfort.

When the ulcer heals or gets less painful, the contracture may persist and the patient is left with an equinus foot. This equinus deformity may be such that the patient can only

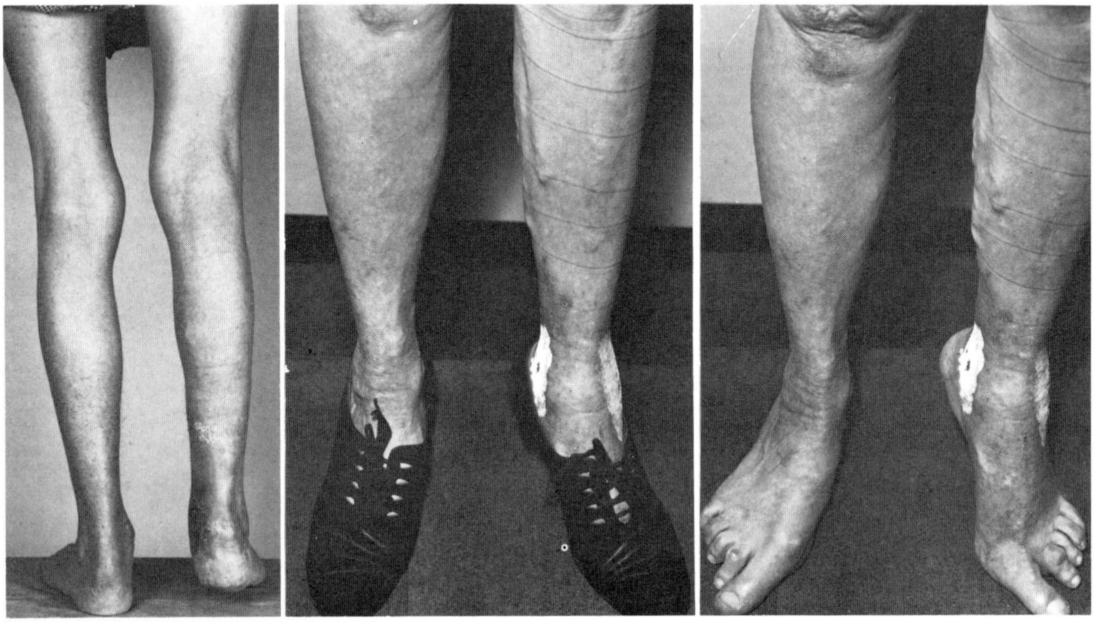

Fig. 17.17 A. This patient with a small chronic venous ulcer could not get her heel to the ground. B.—She was quite comfortable in a high-heeled shoe. C.—Another example of the equinus deformity in a chronic venous ulcer.

walk normally in high-heeled shoes, being quite unable to get the heel to the ground (Fig. 17.17). Minor degrees of the deformity are common in post-phlebitic cases.

This disability soon brings into being a whole train of secondary deformities in the foot. The intrinsic muscles of the foot atrophy and contract and gradually the picture of pes cavus with claw toes and hallux valgus develops. Figure 17.18 is an illustration of this established deformity in an old case of post-phlebitic ulceration.

It is essential to correct this equinus deformity at an early stage to prevent complete deterioration of the foot. In most cases of relatively slight shortening of the tendo-Achillis, adequate treatment to the ulcer, plus exercises under the supervision of a physio-therapist, and insistence of wearing low-heeled shoes will be enough to overcome the deformity. Where gross shortening of the tendo-Achillis has taken place, operative lengthening of the tendon by a subcutaneous tenotomy technique may be necessary. This

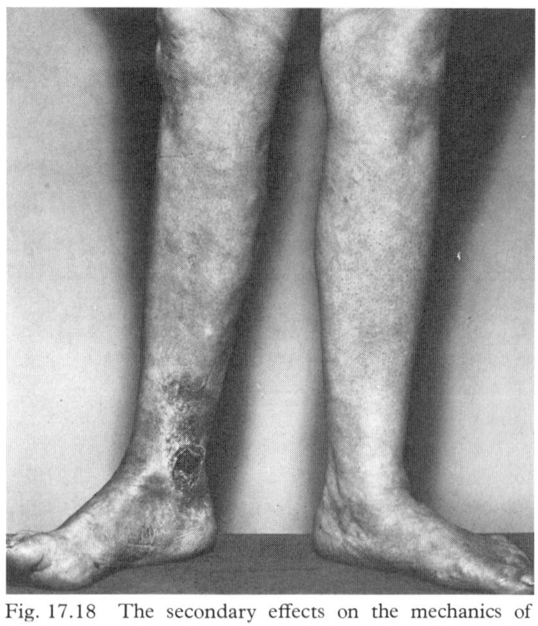

Fig. 17.18 The secondary effects on the mechanics of the foot, caused by ulceration, and shortening of the tendo-Achillis. The slight pes cavus, claw toes and short tendo-Achillis on the ulcerated leg are in marked contrast to the normal foot on the outer side.

shortening of the tendo-Achillis further reduces the efficiency of the calf pump, which is another reason why it must be corrected at the earliest possible moment.

RECENT WORK ON POST-THROMBOTIC SYNDROME

Most of the work prior to 1960 concentrated on the effects of post-thrombotic recanalisation in the popliteal, femoral and ankle perforating veins. During the last ten years or so the aetiology of thrombosis in the iliac segment and cava has been worked out much more thoroughly and in particular the effect of post-thrombotic obstruction in these big veins on the post-thrombotic syndrome is now appreciated. (Cockett and Negus 1967.)

It has been shown that when thrombosis occurs in the ilio-femoral segment, post-thrombotic recanalisation is very poor or absent in some cases, and therefore the limb is left with some degree of permanent obstruction at the main venous outflow in the iliac veins.

In Chapter 16 we have dealt with the aetiology of this iliac vein obstruction in some detail, but its effect on the leg is to cause a generalised venous hypertension of the whole limb, particularly on exercise, when the venous return from the limb increases and the obstructive effect is therefore intensified.

Thus we now know that there are *three* important types of post-thrombotic syndrome, which differ markedly in their severity, course and symptomatology and reaction to treatment. (Cockett 1971).

1. *The below inguinal ligament type.*
2. *The above inguinal ligament type.*
3. *The combined type.* (The most severe and intractable.)

These three types are shown diagrammatically in Figure 17.19.

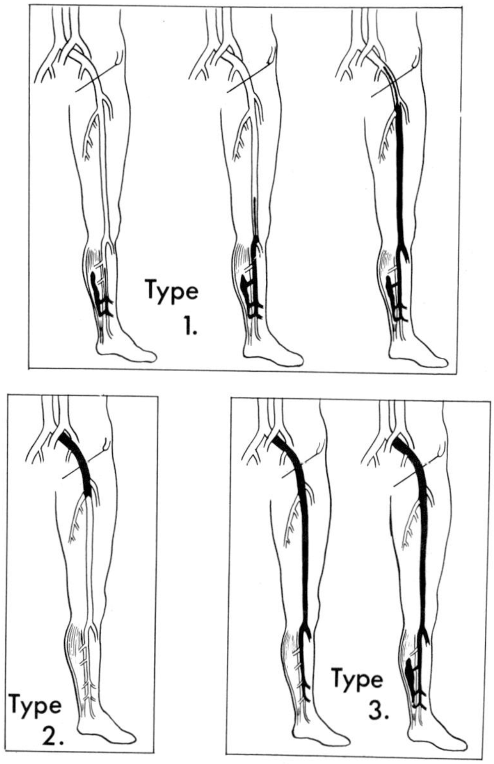

Fig. 17.19 The three main types of post-thrombotic syndrome.

Type 1: Below inguinal ligament type. Here the original thrombosis involved the calf veins, and perhaps the popliteal and femoral veins, but did not extend above the inguinal ligament. In these cases, which fortunately constitute the majority, the main deep veins recanalise well, and the most important lesion is the destruction of the valves in the direct ankle perforating veins. These incompetent ankle perforators, constitute a high pressure leak at the bottom of the calf pump and (often assisted by an incompetent long or short saphenous vein as well) they are the main cause of the *localised* venous hypertension at the ankle, which in time produces the tissue necrosis which we call a venous ulcer.

Type 2: The above inguinal ligament type. Here the original lesion was the so called 'segmental ilio-femoral thrombosis', (see Chap. 16) in which a segment of iliac vein from inguinal ligament to caval bifurcation has thrombosed. These iliac thromboses do not recanalise well (probably owing to the pressure of the overlying arteries on them) and the main trouble therefore is a permanent obstruction of the main venous outflow from the limb. The original thrombosis did not extend below the inguinal ligament so the valves in the main deep veins, and the ankle perforating veins are intact. In other words the peripheral calf pump mechanism is intact, and this forces the venous return through an extensive collateral system back to the heart, by passing the obstructed segment of iliac vein.

Thus the type of post-thrombotic syndrome that these patients get depends largely on the profuseness and availability of collaterals. In the female, the veins of the uterus and parametrium and the ovarian veins are available, and phlebograms of these patients often show amazing collateral systems (see Fig. 16.11). Men seem to have less available collaterals, and their main symptoms are sometimes more severe.

These patients usually complain of a slight swelling mainly of the thigh, but sometimes of the calf also. On exercise the symptoms are exacerbated, increased aching and tenseness of the thigh and calf occurring. They sometimes complain of a 'bursting feeling' in thigh or calf on exercise. Some give a story very similar to intermittent claudication—with quite severe *venous claudication* in the calf on exercise. *As the calf pump and perforating veins are normal, they escape the venous ulcer,* and the ankle skin is usually normal. Another rather odd symptom, which is sometimes very troublesome in women, is a chronic deep seated ache in the left inguinal region, exacerbated at period times. This may be associated with congestion of the left ovary and ovarian vein which is often very large and

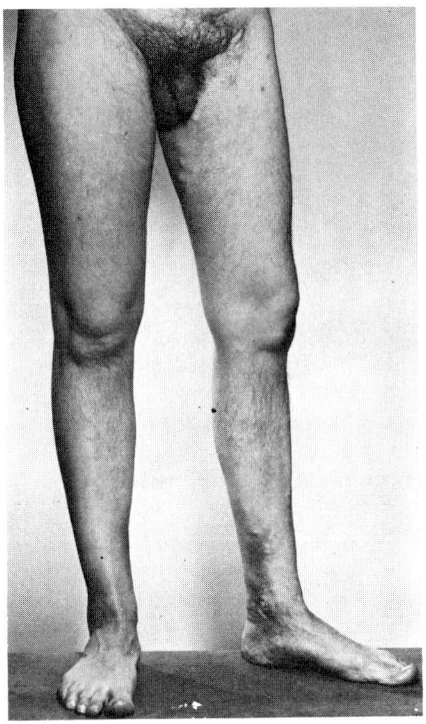

TYPE 1
(Below ligament)

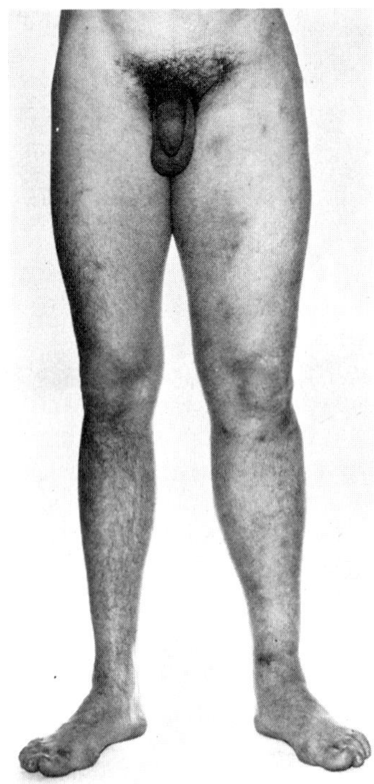

TYPE 2 & 3
(Above ligament)

Fig. 17.20 These photographs show the essential differences in clinical appearance of the Type 1 below ligament, ankle perforator incompetence only. On the right is the early appearance of the Type 3, with marked swelling of thigh, pseudohypertrophy of calf and venous congestion over whole thigh and extending up over the lower abdomen. Early induration and pre-ulcer changes at ankle.

part of the collateral venous return from the left leg.

Type 3: The combined type. Here the original thrombosis involved the whole deep venous system both above and below the inguinal ligament. (Iliac veins, femoral, popliteal and calf veins and perforators.) Most of these patients give a clear history of 'white leg' or severe ilio-femoral thrombosis, often when young and many of them are examples of the iliac compression syndrome and affect predominantly the left leg.

These are the most severe types of post-thrombotic leg and the most difficult to manage. They have both perforating vein incompetence (causing the local venous hypertension in the ankle skin) and iliac vein obstruction causing general venous hypertension throughout the whole limb. *The combination of these two causes of venous hypertension may cause severe intractable ulceration fairly early,* as well as all the other symptoms listed under Type 2 (i.e. swelling, pain on exercise, bursting feeling etc.). But it is predominantly the severe tissue necrosis which takes place in the 'gaiter area' which is the hallmark of this group.

Clinical differentiation of types 1, 2 and 3

Good phlebograms of course will always sort out which type of post-thrombotic syndrome one is dealing with, but apart from this a fairly accurate idea can be obtained by quite brief clinical examination (see Fig. 17.20).

In Type 1 (below ligament) cases nearly all the pathology in the limb is below mid-calf level. Swelling and ulceration and venous congestion (ankle flare) confined to the ankle region. The limb above the knee is normal and not swollen apart from the occasional presence of an incompetent long saphenous vein.

In Types 2 and 3 (above ligament) two important extra physical signs are usually present (Fig. 17.20).

1. The presence of dilated veins coursing over the lower abdomen, usually just above the pubis. These are collateral veins and their presence invariably indicates that the iliac veins have been involved.

2. The second physical sign is that the thigh usually shows some slight general swelling or hypertrophy and very often the calf as well appears rather large and hypertrophied by comparison with the other side. This is due to chronic intramuscular oedema deep to the deep fascia and is highly typical of iliac vein obstruction.

Importance of differentiating the three types of post-thrombotic syndrome

It is essential to know which of the three types one is dealing with when it comes to treatment and management. Their natural history, rapidity of deterioration, tendency to ulceration, all differ and the treatment and prognosis of the three groups is essentially different. This is dealt with in detail in Chapters 16 and 18.

A note on swelling in the post-thrombotic syndrome

One of the remarkable things in the iliac vein obstructions is that although there may be some general swelling of the limb, which is mostly accounted for by the subfascial intramuscular oedema and pseudo hypertrophy, there is usually very little oedema of the subcutaneous tissues of calf and thigh. When there is marked swelling of the subcutaneous tissue envelope, this usually means that there is some associated lymphatic obstruction (see Chap. 16).

REFERENCES

Anning, S. T. (1952) *Lancet*, **2**, 789.
Arnoldi, C. C. & Linderholm, H. (1968) *Acta. Chir. Scand.*, **134**, 427.
Barcroft, H. & Dornhurst, A. C. (1948) *J. Physiol.*, **108**, 391.
Bauer, G. (1942) *Acta. chir. scand.*, **86**, 1.

Bauer, G. (1950) *Brit. Med. J.*, **2**, 318.
Bowen, F. H. (1964) *J. Miss. St. Med. Ass.*, **5**, 187.
Brodie, B. C. (1846) *Lectures Illustrative of Various Subjects in Pathology and Surgery.*
Chapman, H. T. (1853) *The Treatment of Obstinate Ulcers and Cutaneous Eruptions of the Leg, without Confinement.* 2nd edn. London.
Cockett, F. B. (1953) *Pathology & Treatment of Venous Ulcers.* London, Thesis.
Cockett, (1954) *Post-Grad. Med. J.*, **30**, 512.
Cockett, F. B. & Elgan Jones, D. E. (1953) *Lancet*, **1**, 17.
Cockett, F. B. & Negus, D. (1967) *Brit. Med. J.*, **2**, 14.
Cockett, F. B. (1971) *Brit. J. Hosp. Med.*, **Dec.**, 767.
Cohen, S. (1953) *Management of Abdominal Operations.* London: Lewis.
Cooper, A. P. (1837) *Lectures on the Principles and Practice of Surgery.* 8th edn. London.
Critchett, G. (1848) *Lancet*, **2**, 397, 416, 469, 546, 601, 661.
DeCamp, P. T., Ward, J. A. & Ochsner, A. (1951) *Surgery*, **29**, 365.
Dos Santos, J. C. (1938) *J. Int. Chir.*, **3**, 625.
Dow, J. D. (1951a) *J. Fac. Radiol.*, **2**, 180.
Edwards, W. S. (1954) *Surg. Gynec. Obstet.*, **99**, 726.
Fegan, W. G., Fitzgerald, D. E., Milliken, J. C. (1964) *Ir. J. Med. Sci.*, **363**.
Gay, J. (1867) *Lettsomian Lectures.*
Hanschell, H. M. (1949) *Brit. Med. J.*, **1**, 869.
Henry, J. P. & Gauer, O. H. (1950) *J. Clin. Invest.*, **29**, 855.
Hilton, J. (1861) *Lancet*, **2**, 245.
Hodgson, J. (1815) *A Treatise on the Diseases of Arteries and Veins*, London.
Højensgard, I. C. & Sturup, H. (1950) *Acta. chir. scand.*, **99,** 133.
Højensgard, I. C. (1950) *Acta. chir. scand.*, **99,** 527.
Højensgard, I. C. (1952) *Acta. physiol, scand.*, **27,** 49.
Højensgard, I. C. (1952) *Acta. derm.-venereal Stockh.*, **32,** 169.
Homans, J. (1917) *Surg. Gynec. Obstet.*, **24,** 300.
Homans, J. (1938) *J. Int. Chir.*, **3,** 599.
Home, E. (1801) *Practical observations on the treatment of ulcers on the leg, considered as a branch of military surgery.* 2nd edn. London: Bulmer.
Hunt, T. (1859) *A Guide to the Treatment of Diseases of the Skin.*
Kinmonth, J. B. (1952) *Clin. Sci.*, **11**, 13.
Kinmonth, J. B. (1954) *Ann. R. Coll. Surg. Engl.*, **15,** 300.
Linton, R. R. (1952) *Angiology*, **3**, 431.
Linton, R. R. & Hardy, I. B. (1948) *Surgery*, **24**, 452.
Lockhart-Mummery, H. E. & Smitham, J. H. (1951) *Brit. J. Surg.*, **38**, 284.
Ludbrook, J. (1966) '*Aspects of Venous function in the lower limbs*'. Charles C. Thomas, Springfield, Illinois.
Luke, J. C. (1943) *Canad. Med. Ass. J.*, **49**, 86.
Nunn, T. W. (1852) *Varicose Veins and Varicose Ulcers*, London.
Pollack, A. A., Taylor, B. E., Myers, T. T. & Wood, E. H. (1949) *J. Clin. Invest.*, **28**, 559.
Pollack, A. A. & Wood, E. H. (1949) *J. Appl. Physiol.*, **1**, 649.
Pratt, G. H. (1964) *Surg. Gynec. Obstet.*, **118**, 284.
Smirk, F. H. (1936) *Clin. Sci.*, **2**, 317.
Stürup, H. & Højensgaard, I. C. (1950) *Acta Chir. Scand.*, **99**, 526.
Veal, J. R. & Hussey, H. (1940) *Amer. Heart J.*, **20**, 308.
Walker, A. J. & Longland, C. J. (1950) *Clin. Sci.*, **9**, 101.
Warren, R., White, E. A. & Belcher, C. D. (1949) *Surgery*, **26**, 435.
Warwick, T. (1931) '*The rational treatment of varicose veins and varicocele*'. London: Faber.
Wells, H. S., Youmans, J. B. & Miller, D. G. (1938) *J. Clin. Invest.*, **17**, 489.
Wiseman, R. (1676) *Severall Chirurgicall Treatises*, London.

The Management of Venous Ulcers

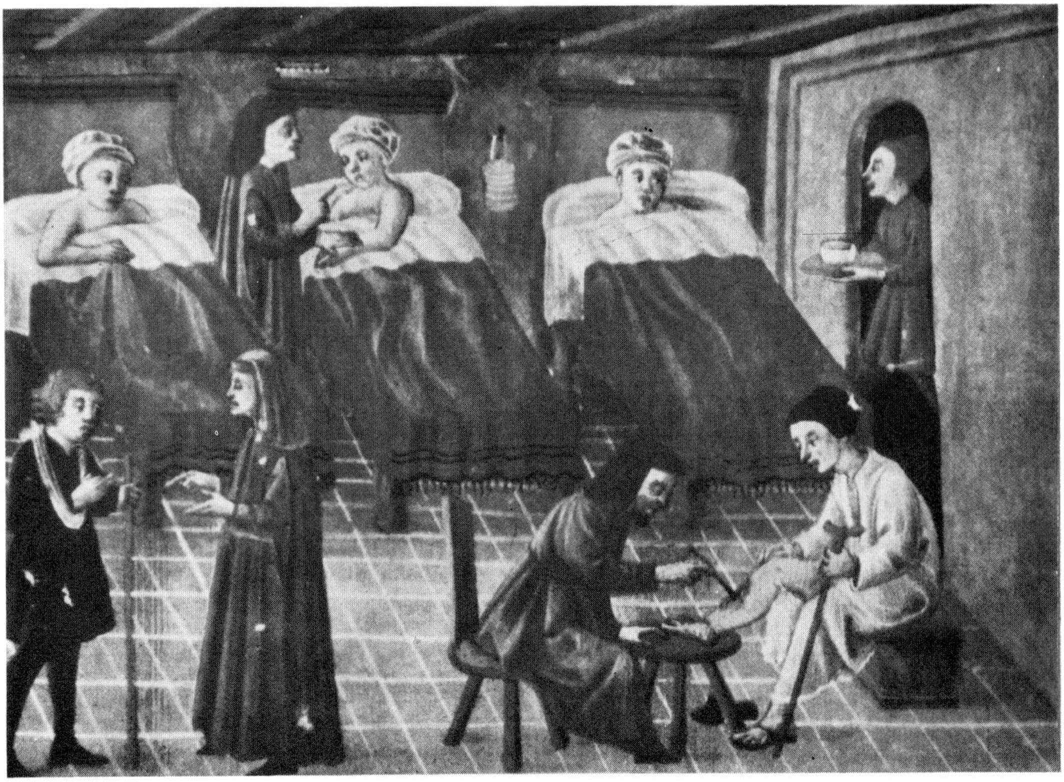

A Mediaeval Hospital
(15th Century Ferrara Manuscript).
The orthopaedic clinic is bottom left, and the venous-ulcer clinic bottom right!

18. The Management of Venous Ulcers

In the preceding chapters it has been shown that after a deep vein thrombosis most veins recanalise and once more become adequate conduits for venous return. This process may take a remarkably short time (two–four months). However, the valves in the main deep veins and in the important ankle perforating veins are permanently destroyed.

This means that when walking the high venous pressure in the calf (100 mmHg or more) is transmitted straight out into the delicate venules and capillaries of the ankle region. In the normal limb this pressure cannot leak out into the skin and subcutaneous tissues, owing to the presence of the valve in the perforating veins. This steady abnormal venous hypertension acting over a number of years causes gradually increasing capillary dilatation, swelling, discomfort, and eventually tissue necrosis (the lesions clinically known as post-phlebitic or venous ulcers).

Owing to the anatomical arrangement of the perforating veins this venous hypertension is particularly concentrated on the inner aspect of the ankle and so the worst tissue necrosis often starts here, the classic site of the venous ulcer (Fig. 18.1).

We have also seen that when the iliac veins are involved in thrombosis they do not recanalise so efficiently as the peripheral veins and there is usually some permanent degree of obstruction of the main venous outflow above the inguinal ligament, which of course contributes further to the venous hypertension in the limb.

Thus the two really important things to grasp about the pathology of venous ulcers and the post-thrombotic syndrome are as follows:

1. The swelling, venous dilatation round the ankle, discomfort and eventually the induration and ulceration are all basically due to the abnormal venous hypertension in the ankle skin and subcutaneous tissues, which occurs when the patient is erect and exercising.

2. The effect of this venous hypertension is *slow* and *progressive*. There is steady deterioration of the tissues round the ankle. It may take three–five years before an ulcer threatens.

Venous ulcers in patients with varicose veins

We have seen in the previous chapter that an identical venous ulcer (occurring in the

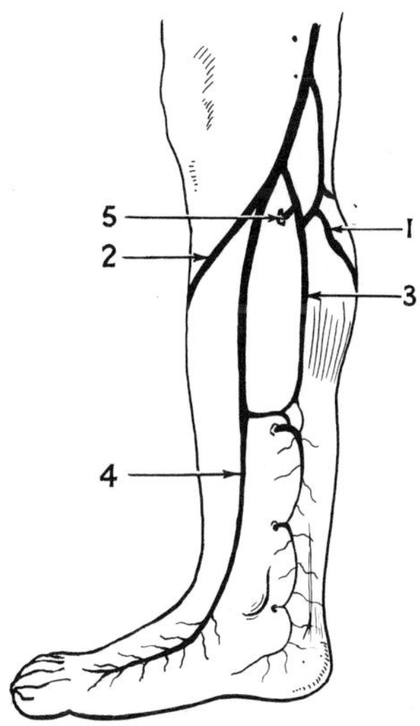

Fig. 18.1 The long saphenous vein and the internal ankle perforating veins. 1. The connection with the short saphenous vein 2. A tributary from the anterior surface of the leg. 3. The posterior arch tributary which also links the three internal ankle perforating veins. 4. The internal saphenous vein. 5. A constant direct communicating vein.

same place and of exactly similar pathology) may occur in some cases of long standing varicose veins. It has been shown that in these cases one or more of the ankle perforating veins have become incompetent, causing a sudden and considerable increase in the localised venous hypertension at the ankle region.

Thus the combination of long saphenous incompetence and perforator incompetence can produce an exactly similar venous ulcer at the ankle region.

We have also seen that the combination of short saphenous incompetence, and either mid calf perforator or lateral perforator incompetence can produce similar venous ulceration round the lateral malleolus, or indeed anywhere round the ankle region and even on the dorsum of the foot.

Principles of management

Once a patient has acquired a post-thrombotic limb or venous hypertension at the ankle with varicose veins, the aim of management is to slow down or prevent the deterioration of the tissues, by controlling (by one means or another) this abnormal venous hypertension.

Broadly speaking there are three main ways of achieving this:

1. Posture
2. Elastic Compression Bandaging
3. Surgery.

Each of these methods play their part at various times in the long, life-time, management of the syndrome. According to the *type* of post-thrombotic syndrome, surgery in particular may have a greater or lesser part to play. But in any case it must be remembered that surgery of whatever type, is really just one episode or part of the long-term, overall management problem.

The most important and worthwhile aim of management is to prevent the patient from developing a post-thrombotic or venous ulcer.

Let us now consider these three methods and their application in greater detail.

1. POSTURE

As long as the legs are at, or just above, the level of the heart, the venous pressure in all the ankle tissues falls to nearly zero. The crucial thing is to have the legs above heart level; this can only be achieved by having the patient lying flat or reclining with not more than two pillows, and the foot of the bed raised about one foot. There are also on the market special tilting 'varicose vein chairs', which achieve this object very well. In this position all lesions that are directly due to venous hypertension (ulcers, eczemas, phlebitis, pain, swelling) rapidly resolve and venous ulcers, even very large ones, will commence healing *with no other treatment.*

This effect of resting the leg just above heart level is so rapid and obvious that it can be used as a *test* as to whether a doubtful ulcer is really primarily of venous origin or not. Arterial and ischaemic ulcers in particular get *more* painful with the legs up and do not heal.

Posture has a part to play in many situations, particularly in pre-operative preparation for surgery in cases of venous ulcer. Also in retrieving the situation, in an ulcer which is just about to break down, a few days off work with the feet up may just get the ulcer into a healing phase.

2. ELASTIC COMPRESSION BANDAGING

This works by controlling the abnormal surface venous hypertension by applying an equal and opposite elastic pressure over the whole of the surface of the leg and ankle and foot.

This is the oldest, most widely used and most universally applicable method of controlling venous ulcers. However, to be successful this method must satisfy two criteria:

1. When used to cure or control a venous ulcer at the ankle, the bandage must be strong enough to counteract the very high venous pressure efficiently. (80–100 mmHg). A light elastic stocking is no good for this, only a heavy webbing elastic bandage of the blue line or red line type (see Fig. 18.2), will really achieve this. Moreover all elastic bandages and stockings lose their elasticity with time

and need renewal after about two months at the most.

2. The bandage must be applied evenly and firmly from the toes to just below the knee. It is extremely important to achieve even pressure all around the bony prominence of the ankle, and this requires a good deal of skill in bandaging, which must be taught to the patients. Small pads of several layers of dry gauze or felt placed under the bandage around the ankle and below the malleoli, are helpful in attaining this even pressure.

A common fault of bandaging technique is to leave the heel out (some bad elastic stockings are made with a hole at the heel). This means that a large part around the malleolus, which *particularly requires the external elastic pressure,* is left out of the bandage and this fault often perpetuates or even causes ulcers at the ankle, which may get worse the tighter and more grimly the patient bandages himself (see Fig. 8.1).

Warning about bandages. On no account must heavy, tight webbing elastic bandages be used in old people with delicate skin. In patients over 70 years of age, even without overt ischaemia, such bandages may produce small ulcers on the tips of the malleoli—pressure-necrosis ulcers, which are very difficult to heal. If there is definite arterial insufficiency in the limb, due to blockage of a main artery, such bandages may produce much pain and even widespread pressure-necrosis of the ankle and foot, leading to frank gangrene. In such patients a light crêpe bandage carefully applied is the most that is allowed.

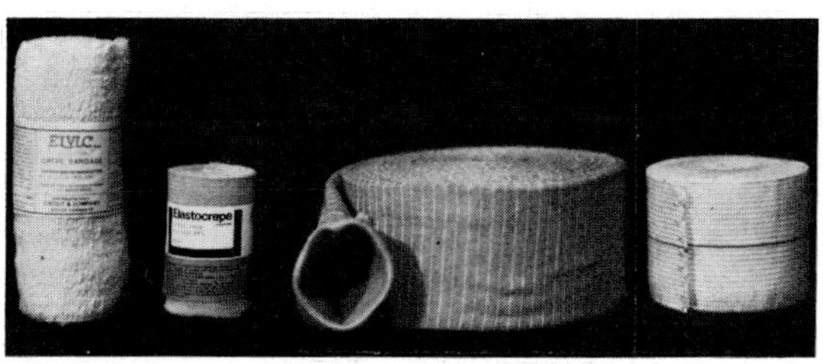

Fig. 18.2 Four types of elastic bandage in common use. Reading from left to right they are: 1. The crêpe bandage; 2. Elasto crêpe; 3. 'Tubigrip'; 4. Red or blue line heavy webbing elastic bandage (sometimes called a 'Bisgaard' bandage). The first three exert light pressure only, and are inadequate to heal venous ulcers. Only the last one has the necessary strength to exert the continuous high counter pressure required to heal a venous ulcer.

Techniques of pressure bandaging

In general there are two ways of applying the principles of pressure bandaging:

1. *The continuous occlusive method.*
2. *The intermittent method.*

The continuous occlusive method

Here a bandage is applied by the doctor—according to the particular type and technique which he favours, and the bandage is then left on continuously for two or three weeks or even longer, until it is changed by the doctor again.

This is the time honoured and historical method. The technique used, the 'mystique' of the occlusive bandage, was gradually built up over the centuries when large infected, uncontrollable ulcers were common-place in all hospitals. Its use is particularly associated with the names of Richard Wiseman (see historical chapter), of Thomas Baynton of Bristol (1797), and in later and more modern times of Arthur Dickson Wright, of St Mary's Hospital, London.

Modern knowledge of the part played by the *elastic pressure* and by posture, and the control of infection by antibiotics, has made these time honoured methods out of date. 'Unna's Paste'; 'Zinc impregnated bandages'; 'Diachylon bandages', are disappearing from clinical practice.

These older techniques were very useful in their day—they gave some external support and pressure to the ulcer area round the ankle and even more important *they protected the ulcer itself from well meant but often misguided local applications,* which really retarded healing, and encouraged infection and skin sensitivity.

However even nowadays a form of continuous occlusive bandage is occasionally of use. In refractory or careless patients, or in patients of low intelligence and application, who are not really capable of learning how to bandage their own leg, this method may be used for a short time.

If this method is to be used there are certain rules:

1. Sticky or medicated bandages of any sort should *never* be applied directly to the skin. Before applying an occlusive bandage to the leg—a layer of tube gauze or light stockinette should clothe the leg, and the bandage is applied over this (see Fig. 18.3). The reason for this is that the skin around ulcers, or in an ulcer precursor area, has a very high likelihood of becoming sensitive to any medicated, external application and reacting by a violent eczema. Once the patient has acquired a sensitivity eczema *as well as* his venous ulcer, the therapeutic problem is much worse (*see* frontispiece).

2. If the patient complains of increasing pain or discomfort under the bandage, it must be at once removed. This may indicate either increasing infection, or pressure necrosis of tissue.

3. On the whole an occlusive bandage *should not be left on for more than two weeks at a time*. By this time it is usually smelly, the skin is irritating, and the patient is uncomfortable, and it has ceased to be effective.

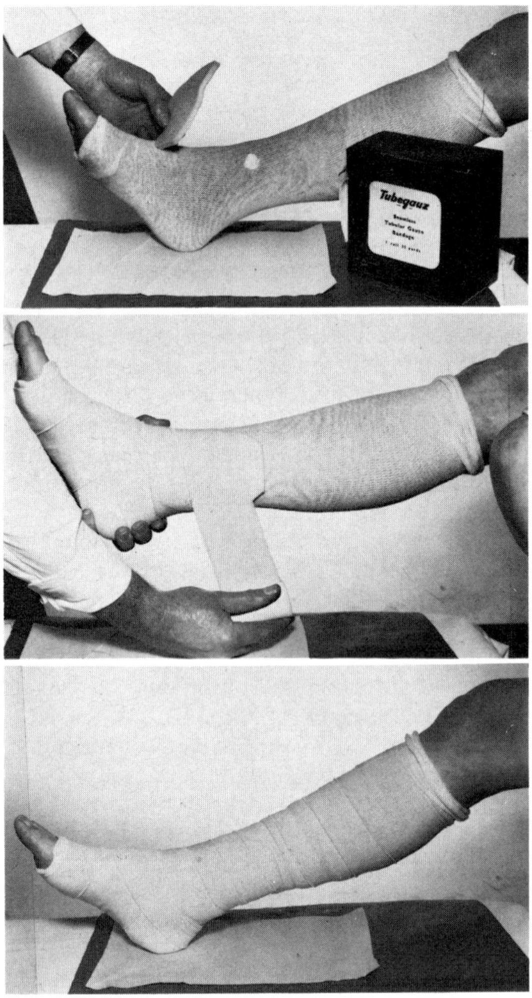

Fig. 18.3 *Continuous occlusive bandaging technique*. Note that the occlusive bandage is applied *over* a tube gauze stockinette. *Nowhere* is it allowed to come in actual contact with the skin. A large felt or gauze pad is put under the bandage, big enough to give pressure over the whole area of the perforating veins. In the example shown here elastoplast is being used. If elastoplast is applied *direct* to the skin severe dermatitis would almost certainly occur.

The intermittent method

In this method a strong elastic cotton, or elastic silk bandage (the red or blue line webbing bandage) is applied to the foot, leg and ankle during the day while the patient is up and about. *It is not worn during the night* when the patient is simply instructed to rest with the foot of the bed slightly raised.

This means that the patient must be taught how to apply the bandage himself and must be aware of why he is using an elastic bandage. He must put it on each morning before the day's work, and take it off when he goes to bed. At night a light tube gauze stockinette is worn—possibly with a light crêpe bandage, or even no dressing at all—and the skin is allowed 'to breathe'.

We have found after twenty years of experience with this method, that nearly all patients can be taught to use these bandages intelligently and satisfactorily, and the skin round the ulcer remains in much better condition, when it is exposed to the air every night.

The routine used in our clinics is adequately shown in Figure 18.4 and the types of bandage in Figure 18.2.

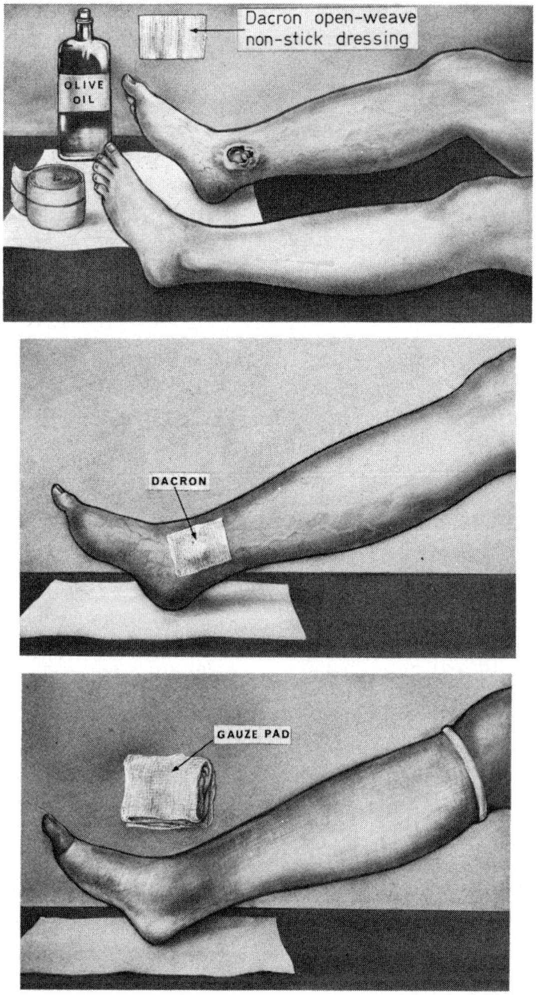

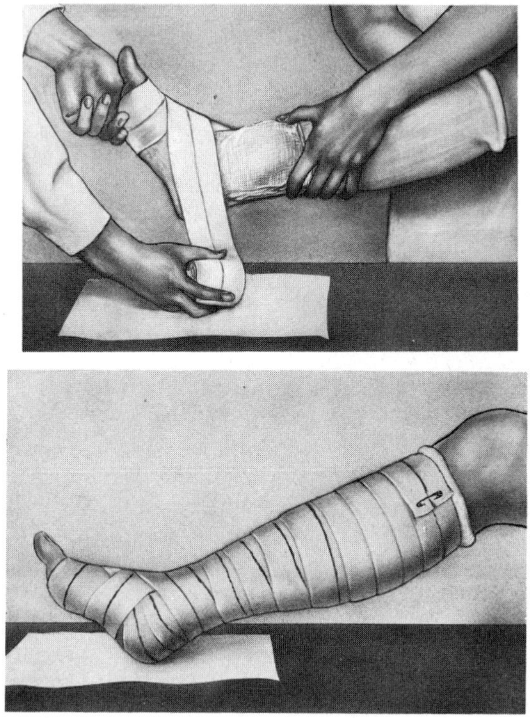

Fig. 18.4 The steps in the intermittent pressure bandaging method.

What to apply to the ulcer itself

The only safe and satisfactory application to a venous ulcer is a pad of ordinary, dry absorbent gauze and nothing else.

Once the skin has been breached in an ulcer precursor area and the open wound which we call an ulcer has appeared, then there is an important new factor requiring control, namely *infection.*

Pain in a venous ulcer or rapid increase in size, is almost always due to infection, and it is almost always those two old offenders the Staphylococcus and the Streptococcus (more rarely) which do the damage.

Thus in treating a venous ulcer the two main objects are:

1. To clear and control infection.
2. To keep the venous hypertension under control by adequate external elastic pressure.

Active sepsis must be controlled by an adequate course of *oral antibiotics, NOT* by local applications. (Strong local antiseptics such as 'Eusol' may occasionally be used as cleansing agents—but *never as dressings.*) An oral antibiotic which is active against the Staphylococcus and Streptococcus is desirable (either the combination of Ampicillin and Cloxacillin, or Erythromycin, have, in the author's experience, been the most useful). Ideally this should be chosen after culture of the ulcer. However—a word of warning—it is often quite difficult to culture the original offenders in an ulcer, particularly if it is chronic, as they get overgrown by many secondary and unimportant organisms. Thus a negative swab does *not necessarily* mean that the Staphylococcus is not there, and it may be necessary to take a culture from under the wound edge to get it.

Regime for treatment of a venous ulcer

Almost all ointments, creams, powders, and local dressings are actively harmful to ulcers; if continued for any length of time they set up a skin sensitivity problem which adds to and complicates the difficulties already present. Under occlusive dressings, which exclude air, the ulcer gets wet and soggy and in this circumstance infection flourishes and spreads.

Thus our rules for the treatment of ulcers may be summed up as follows:

1. Treat sepsis by an adequate course of an oral antibiotic, not local antibiotics.

2. Don't put any medicinal application of any sort on the ulcer. The instructions are simply:

1. Clean around the ulcer with a dab of gauze moistened with ordinary olive oil; this is to rub off scales, caked serum, and so on.

2. Sterilize the skin around by wiping with spirit.

3. Place a square piece of open work terylene gauze (the so-called non-adherent or NA dressing) over the ulcer.

4. Place about four layers of dry gauze over this.

5. Put on the webbing elastic bandage from the toes to just below the knee. The patients must be taught how to do this carefully. The patient is then comfortable for the day (Fig. 18.5).

At night the patient repeats the cleansing of the ulcer with oil and spirit and then simply covers it with a light 'pull-on' of tube-gauze, to allow the air to get at it as much as possible during the night, the foot of the bed being put up.

This excessively simple regime will successfully heal most ulcers, but it is very difficult to restrain patients, and doctors and nurses, from 'putting things on ulcers'. Firm, even pressure, and adequate control of the Staphylococcus and Streptococcus are the *only* two requisites for the control of most ulcers (see Fig. 18.6).

Perhaps we should end this section by repeating and emphasising three big 'don'ts'!

Don't use dressings which completely exclude air, such as 'oiled silk' and 'Melolin non-stick' dressings. These completely stop evaporation from the underlying skin, which gets moist and soggy and is then the ideal culture medium for bacterial growth. This is why ordinary gauze is such an excellent dressing—it allows evaporation from the skin, and is absorbent and porous.

Don't ever use antibiotic creams or paraffin gauze impregnated with 'sulpha-drugs' (Sofra-Tulle) or Balsam of Peru (Tulle-gras). Explosive, widespread allergy is far too common and once present is very difficult to control.

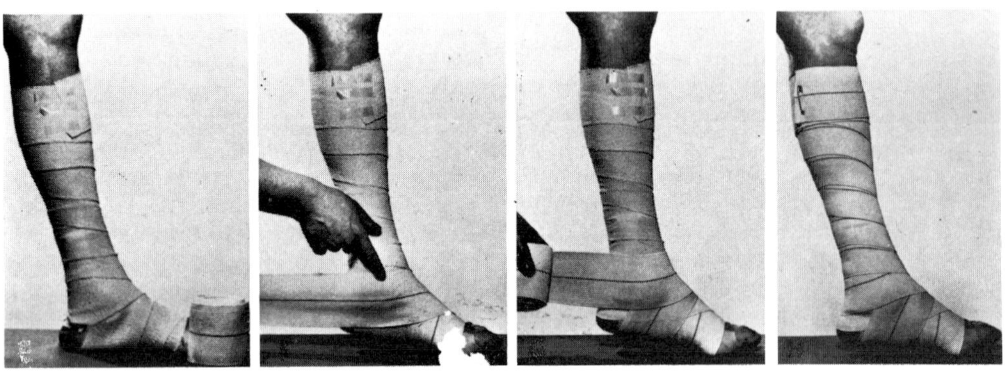

Fig. 18.5 These pictures show the steps in the application of the webbing bandage. Note the extreme care taken to apply pressure by turns of the bandage below the internal malleolus; also note that the bandage must go up to just below the knee and is fixed by a pin. (Tapes allow the bandage to loosen and slip down quickly.)

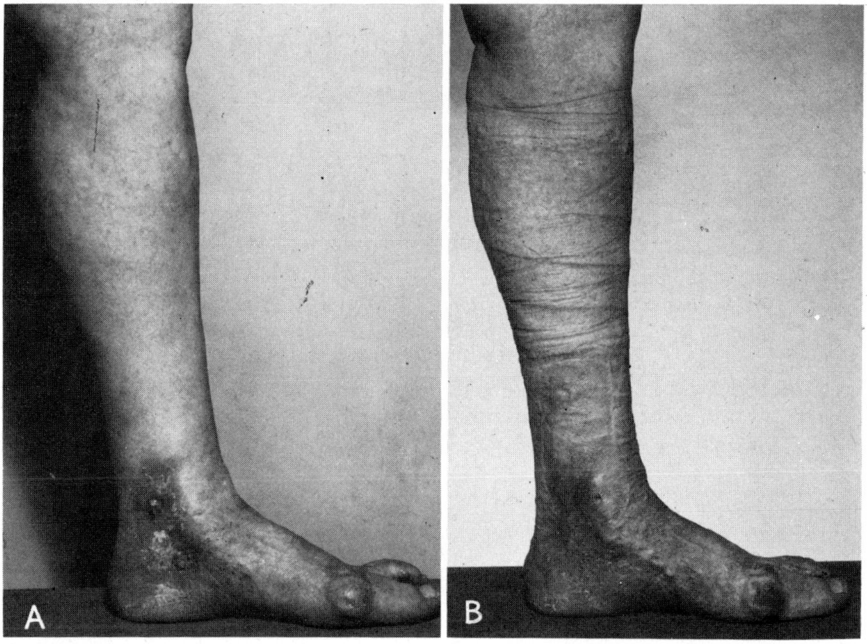

Fig. 18.6 A. A typical post-thrombotic venous ulcer. Note the eczema around the ulcer itself and the ankle flare of dilated venules below, and the slight oedema of the ankle. B. After two months pad and bandage. Note the area of the pressure pad is outlined on the skin. The ridges of the firm pressure bandage which has just been taken off are seen, also the ankle oedema is completely controlled.

Don't use any ointment containing steroids, they prevent healing.

A final note about skin allergy

There is almost no skin application to which a patient may not in time become allergic if it is applied for a considerable length of time.

In patients with chronic venous troubles this is a continuous worry. In addition to the substances listed above, remember that many patients may become allergic to *rubber* which is an essential component of all elastic bandages and stockings. For this reason it is always wise to interpose a layer of linen or cotton stockinette (Tube gauze) between the bandage and the patient's skin, in those whose skin has shown signs of allergic reaction.

Also it is not widely appreciated that allergy to 'lanoline', (wool-fat) which is a common basis for many ointments, is very prone to occur. Zinc allergies to the *Zinc ointments* (which have been widely used in the past) is another common offender—particularly as it occurs in many of the sticky plasters made, such as *Elastoplast* and many adhesive tapes. Elastoplast—containing both Zinc and rubber is particularly 'allergo-genic' and many patients react to it violently.

In the author's experience *olive oil* or its substitute *arachis oil* are the safest applications for routine cleansing of flaky or dry skin round a venous ulcer.

3. THE SURGERY OF VENOUS ULCERS AND THE POST-THROMBOTIC SYNDROME

The main aim of surgery in both the post-thrombotic syndrome and in cases of ulcer with varicose veins, *is to prevent the occurrence of ulceration.*

The idea that you only turn to surgery when an ulcer has appeared and become chronic and unmanageable by other means, is a complete misconception of the role of surgery in management.

However, even when surgery is undertaken correctly, radically and early, it is necessary to have a good idea of what it may be expected to achieve.

Early radical surgery in cases of primary varicose veins complicated by perforator incompetence in the lower leg, may be expected to achieve the best possible results. Usually resulting in complete elimination of the risk of ulceration, and return of appearance and function to near normal.

In the post-thrombotic syndrome however, the problem is not quite so simple and one must have an accurate idea of the particular type of post-thrombotic syndrome one is dealing with.

As we have shown in the previous chapter, there are three possible factors in the post-thrombotic syndrome which may contribute to venous hypertension in the ankle region, either singly or together.

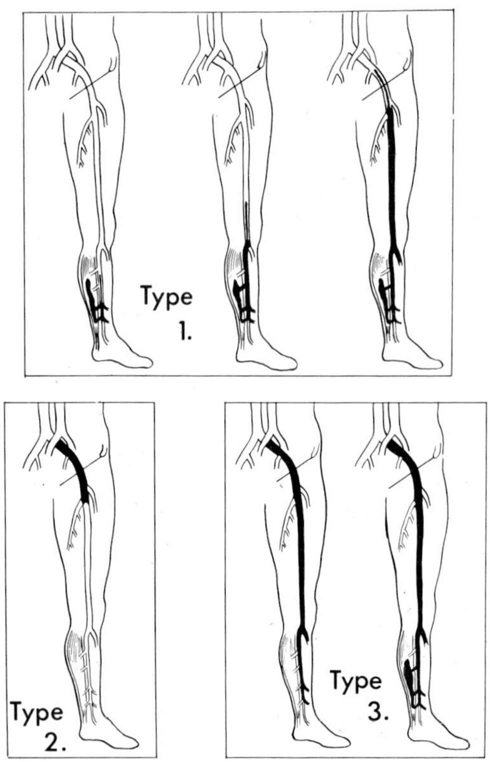

Fig. 18.7 The three main types of post-thrombotic syndrome.

These are:

1. Valve incompetence in the ankle perforating veins.—Amenable to surgery.
2. Valve loss in main deep veins.—Not amenable to surgery.
3. Post-thrombotic obstruction, particularly of the large iliac veins.—Not at present amenable to surgery.

Thus when considering the place of surgery in post-thrombotic patients it is essential to recognise the three important groups of post-thrombotic syndrome (Fig. 18.7) which we have already defined in Chapter 17.

Type 1. The below inguinal ligament type (see Fig. 18.7). In this type, the original thrombosis involved the calf veins and perhaps the popliteal and femoral veins, but did not extend above the inguinal ligament. In these cases, which constitute the majority, the main deep veins recanalise well, and the really important lesion is the destruction of the valves in the ankle perforating veins. These incompetent ankle perforators, often assisted by an incompetent long or short saphenous vein, are the main cause of the localised venous hypertension at the ankle, which in time produces the venous ulcer.

It is in this group of cases that early radical surgery of the incompetent perforating veins, and associated long or short saphenous incompetence, produces the best and most lasting results. Ulceration may be prevented, ankle skin changes regress towards normal and many of the limbs do not need any long term elastic support.

Of course the best results are attained with early operation (i.e. within 3–6 years of the original thrombosis) and preferably just *before* a venous ulcer has actually become established.

Trying to treat a long established ulcer of 10–15 years standing, with chronic infection and induration, by simply tying the perforating veins which originally caused it, may be compared to 'bolting the stable door after the horse has gone'.

Type 2. The so-called segmental ilio-femoral

thrombosis. Here a segment of iliac vein from the inguinal ligament to the caval bifurcation has thrombosed. These iliac vein thromboses, unlike the femoral and popliteal veins do not recanalise well (see Chap. 4). The main trouble here is, therefore, a permanent obstruction to the main venous outflow from the limb, *without destruction of the peripheral valves in the perforating veins of the calf.* Thus these patients usually complain of slight swelling, mainly of the thigh, and discomfort, or a congested or bursting feeling after exercise, or just before periods in women. *They do not tend to develop venous ulcers, as the peripheral calf pump mechanism is intact.*

The degree of symptoms depends on the efficiency of the collateral venous return which is developed to bypass the permanent iliac obstruction. In women, in whom this syndrome is more common, there is usually a profuse collateral circulation through the uterus and ovarian veins revealed on phlebography (see Chap. 16). In men the collateral circulation is often less efficient and they have more symptoms.

In this particular type of post-thrombotic syndrome there is usually little or no place for surgery of the superficial and perforating veins, and the main emphasis is on a supporting stocking to control the gravitational congestion and aching which is often the main symptom.

Type 3. The combined above and below inguinal ligament type. This is the most severe type of post-thrombotic syndrome and needs careful and vigorous management throughout the patient's life to prevent the appearance of crippling severe ulceration. In these patients the original thrombosis involved the whole deep venous system from iliac veins to calf and perforating veins and the patients always give a clear history of 'white leg' or 'severe thrombosis' when relatively young. Many of them are examples of the iliac compression syndrome (Chap. 16) which affects predominantly the left leg.

The important point as regards their management is to remember that in the post-thrombotic period they suffer from both *iliac vein obstruction* (that is obstruction of the main venous outlet of the limb) *and perforating vein valve incompetence.* In other words these unfortunates have two potent causes of venous hypertension operating in the limb; one general (iliac vein obstruction) and one local (incompetent perforators).

Thus operation on peripheral perforating veins in this type of case, even if performed early, does not give the same successful and striking results as in Type 1 and varicose vein cases. Nevertheless operations on peripheral incompetent perforating veins and on large incompetent long or short saphenous veins *do help* in retarding the rapid deterioration of the ankle in these patients, if performed early enough and radically. But the point is that in these cases such operations *do not cure the general venous hypertension of the limb* caused by the iliac vein obstruction, and therefore such operations must be followed up by continuous strong elastic support throughout the patient's life, and even occasional periods of retirement to bed with the feet elevated. Ancillary measures such as elevation of the foot of the bed at night, and getting into the habit of resting always with the feet above the heart (the 'varicose vein chair'), are particularly useful in these cases.

Thus peripheral vein surgery does play an important and worthwhile part in the management of these cases, particularly in the prevention of severe local ulceration, but it must be followed up by continuous efficient elastic support, and postural measures.

The question of relieving the chronic iliac vein obstruction by various forms of direct operation and venous grafting procedures has been under much investigation in recent years (Chap. 16). Suffice it to say that these are somewhat major operations and do not give consistently good results as yet, although this matter is currently under investigation at a number of centres.

The principles of surgical treatment of venous ulcers

This resolves itself into two problems:

1. The treatment of the ulcer itself.

2. The eradication of the incompetent veins causing the ulcer.

As was discussed in Chapter 17, in a large proportion of ulcers the main culprit is one or more incompetent ankle perforating veins. The long or the short saphenous veins may also add their quota of incompetence, and very occasionally may be the main and sole cause of ulcers. However, well over three-quarters of all ulcers (whether associated with saphenous incompetence or not) have an incompetent ankle perforating vein near them, which is the main factor causing the ulcer.

The surgical cure of the ulcer therefore often involves an operation in the immediate vicinity of the ulcer itself, and so the technique of these operations is closely bound up with adequate pre-operative measures to control infection in the ulcer, and either heal it or bring it into a healing phase.

General plan for surgical treatment

The actual operation is only one part of the surgical programme. In dealing with these lesions the pre-operative preparation and post-operative treatment are all important. The programme of surgical treatment is divided into four parts:

1. *The diagnosis* and assessment of which groups of veins are incompetent (i.e. great saphenous, small saphenous, or ankle perforators—or all!)
2. The pre-operative treatment of the ulcer or lesion of the lower leg.
3. The operation.
4. The post-operative management.

1. Diagnosis

Many of the failures of surgery are simply due to a faulty diagnosis as to which groups of veins are defective, and therefore a failure to operate on these.

2. Pre-operative treatment

As an incision near the ulcer and through indurated, poor skin, is often the essential part in the surgical treatment of these conditions, it is very important to get this skin as near normal as possible before operating on it.

The essential pre-operative treatment is (1) a period of efficient elastic compression with the patient ambulatory and at work, or (2) if necessary, a period of complete rest in bed with the foot of the bed raised. These measures will bring about rapid healing or 'near healing' of most ulcers.

3. The operation

Broadly speaking, ulcerated legs fall into two groups from the point of view of operative treatment: Group 1, in which the ulcer is fairly localised, in which induration is not excessive, and in which the subcutaneous tissues just above and around the ulcer are fairly normal, except that they may contain a bog of dilated veins (see Fig. 17.1). Group 2, in which induration of a large part of the gaiter area is a prominent feature, and the subcutaneous tissues are replaced by a plaque of fibrous tissue which is welded to the deep fascia (Fig. 17.7). Over this indurated area there may be a large shallow ulcer of considerable area.

Group 1 is usually fairly easily and quickly controlled by one of the treatments mentioned, and pre-operative preparation may be complete in a few days or weeks.

Group 2 is usually more of a problem but a period of pressure bandaging possibly finishing off with a period of rest in high elevation, will always produce steady healing even in these. It is in these cases that a choice has to be made between (1) Complete excision of the ulcerated area down to the deep fascia—combined with ligation of perforators—followed by skin grafting, or (2) Straight operation on perforators after healing of ulcer, and trusting that removal of incompetent veins will maintain healing, possibly combined with light support.

The choice of which of these operative procedures to pursue in an advanced case is a matter of some experience. (See later—Skin grafting in large ulcers.)

Principle.—The essential part of the operative treatment is the exposure and ligation of the incompetent veins.

The following are the main groups of veins

which have to be considered in the surgical treatment of a venous ulcer:

1. The great saphenous system.—This system need only be considered as a definite or contributory cause of venous ulceration in the lower leg if it is quite obviously enlarged and incompetent. Unless a cough impulse can be felt along the course of the veins, it is unlikely that incompetence of this vein is a contributory cause of the venous ulcer. Venous ulcers associated with incompetence of this system are usually associated with gross dilatation and incompetence which has been present for many years, and usually there is a boggy mass of large veins to be felt near or beneath the ulcer.

The only adequate way of eradicating this source of venous incompetence is by high saphenous ligation, and stripping (as described in Chapter 8).

2. The small saphenous system.—Incompetence of this vein is more common than is generally supposed. There is no easy test for its incompetence (like the cough impulse) and, as it lies deep to the deep fascia in the upper third of the calf, its incompetence can often only be suspected by very careful palpation along the course of the vein, when its enlargement can be detected. Often when the back of the leg is inspected in a good light the enlarged vein can be seen (Fig. 7.6). Its association with enlargement and incompetence of the lateral ankle perforating vein and the mid calf perforator is common. In a fat leg its incompetence may be entirely overlooked until, on exploring the region of the ankle perforating veins, a large vein is found leading up to and connecting with an enlarged small saphenous vein.

When it is incompetent, it should be stripped from below and behind the external malleolus to the popliteal fossa (Chap. 8).

3. The direct ankle perforating veins.—The anatomy of the direct ankle perforating veins will be found in Chapter 3. Most ulcers in the gaiter area are mainly due to valve incompetence or destruction in one or more of these veins.

There are only four which have to be considered and their anatomical position is remarkably constant (Fig. 18.8). They are (1) The Upper internal ankle perforator; (2) The Middle internal ankle perforator; (3) The Mid calf perforator; (4) The lateral ankle perforator.

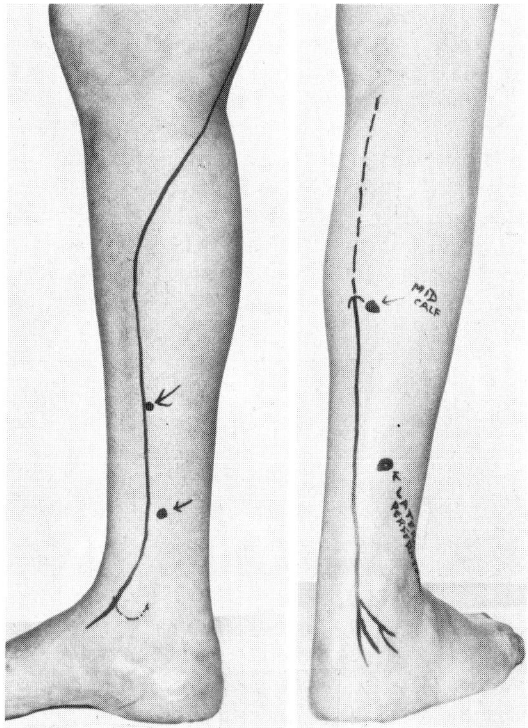

Fig. 18.8 The four main direct perforators of the lower leg which have to be examined and assessed when operation for venous hypertension in the ankle area is to be undertaken.

The upper and middle internal perforators are by far the commonest affected and these are usually always explored together through the same incision. However, the site of the external ankle perforator and mid calf perforator must be inspected in every case, and a decision made as to whether these also need exploring through separate incisions.

Ligation of ankle perforating veins

They can be approached by an operation through the subcutaneous tissues, the perforators being ligated as they penetrate the holes in the deep fascia, *the extrafascial operation.* They can also be ligated beneath the deep fascia—*the subfascial operation.*

If the subcutaneous tissues are reasonably normal (this means *early* cases, the best time for this operation) the extrafascial approach is preferable: if there is extensive induration of the gaiter area (late cases and advanced post-thrombotic ulcers) the subfascial approach is preferred, because in these the subcutaneous tissue plane is scarred and obliterated and has poor vitality.

In the extrafascial approach an *accurate incision over the line of penetration of the perforating veins is necessary* (see Fig. 18.9). Too much lateral dissection in the subcutaneous fat away from the incision, particularly in indurated or ill prepared legs, may lead to skin necrosis in the incision. Lateral dissection must be carried out right down on the deep fascia. The main advantage of this approach is that it allows a fairly complete removal of all the enlarged tortuous veins in the subcutaneous tissues about the ulcer area. The removal of these, when present, is nearly as important as tying the perforating vein from which they arise.

In contrast, wide exploration laterally can be carried out in the *subfascial* plane without risk of skin necrosis, hence its suitability for indurated leg. These two operations will now be described in detail.

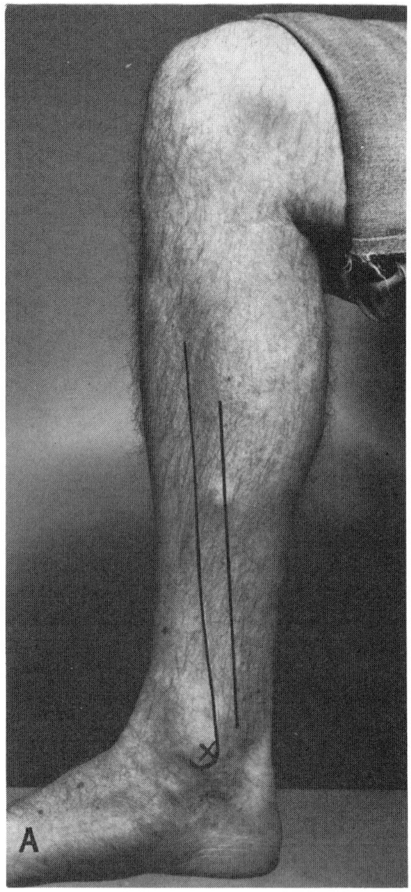

Fig. 18.9 The skin incision of extra-fascial ligation of the ankle perforating veins. A straight incision. Note that the anterior line indicates the posterior border of the tibia.

Extrafascial Operation: (Fig. 18.10)

The pre-operative skin preparation of the whole leg and foot is carried out with hibitane in spirit. It is important not to use iodine or flavine on these cases as a certain number react to these agents by an extensive eczema. The patient lies on his back with the legs apart and externally rotated. The operator sits at the foot of the table. A slight Trendelenburg tilt to bring the feet just above heart level will effectively diminish bleeding.

The incision is a straight one, which starts nearly half-way up the leg, one finger's breadth behind posterior margin of the tibia, and is carried straight down to a point an inch *above* and behind the internal malleolus (Fig. 18.9). It is carried straight down to the deep fascia. Lateral dissection *right down on the fascia* may then be carried out safely by sweeping the tissues off the deep fascia with a gauze swab. The orifices of the perforating veins may come into view in this way, or any large veins in the subcutaneous tissues are dissected out and followed up and down; they lead the operator to one or other of the perforating veins. Usually either the upper or the middle perforator is found to be enlarged or sometimes both. They are then ligated at the site of their penetration into the foramina in the deep fascia, and the plexus of subcutaneous veins is removed. Often a small artery is seen emerging through the same foramen. Any large veins which go off from the area around towards the back of the ankle to join the small saphenous system or lateral ankle perforator must be carefully followed, particularly if no satisfactory incompetent perforator has been found on the inside of the ankle. These may lead one to a clinically unsuspected incompetent small saphenous vein and/or incompetent lateral perforating vein or mid calf perforator. These are dealt with through separate incisions.

The whole dissection is carried out behind the line of the great saphenous vein (see Fig. 18.11). All ligaturing is done *with fine catgut. Unabsorbable sutures should never be buried in this region.* After haemostasis has been secured the skin is drawn gently together with fine silk sutures. All tension must be avoided.

If the patient has gross incompetence of the great saphenous vein as well, after the perforators have been dissected out the great saphenous vein is sought anterior to the line of emergence of the perforators. It is divided and the vein stripper is passed to the groin. Thus this same incision can be used for the lower part of the long saphenous stripping operation.

If an ulcer has been excised during the course of the operation the area is covered with gauze. It has been our practice to wait for four or five days for early granulations to appear before placing a split skin graft at a second operation.

If either the lateral ankle perforator is suspected to be at fault clinically or if no incompetent internal ankle perforator is found then the lateral perforator may be explored through a separate incision. The patient is turned over and a short vertical incision is made over the position of this perforator. If both explorations (lateral and medial) are negative, the final veins to remember are the small saphenous vein and the mid calf perforator. This vein may present a number of anomalies (see Anatomy chapter), but one of the most interesting and important is that in which it passes into the soleus in the midline half-way down the leg—constituting a large mid-calf perforating vein (see Anatomy chapter). When this is incompetent it can be responsible for severe ulceration. We have met this anomaly several times, in each case causing severe trouble (Wright, 1953).

Points of importance in the extra-fascial operation

1. In this operation the deep fascia surrounding the lower third of the soleus is left intact. This firm investing layer is an integral part of an efficient calf pump in this region, and its opening is unnecessary in this operation.

2. A straight incision, going precisely to the line of penetration of the perforating veins, is important. In this way all excessive undercutting of skin is avoided. Undercutting of skin in the subcutaneous plane in this region leads to the possibility of skin necrosis, and all lateral dissection must be done right down on the deep fascia. Linton (1953) also insists on the necessity of using a straight incision for this procedure.

3. In ligating the incompetent perforating veins it is important to ligate them flush up against their foramen in the deep fascia.

4. The bleed-back test (Turner Warwick).

The one sure way of telling whether a perforating vein is incompetent is by the fact that, on cutting across it, smart back bleeding from the deep veins occurs. If a normal competent perforating vein is cut, no bleeding occurs from the cut end which goes into the posterior tibial veins, as its valve effectively prevents the egress of blood. If a probe is gently pushed into its lumen and the valve is held aside, then smart bleeding occurs until the probe is withdrawn. This has been observed at operation many times by us. On the other hand, an enlarged and *incompetent* perforating vein bleeds back smartly as soon as it is cut.

The demonstration of this at operation is not always quite clear cut, as the vein tends to go into spasm when handled.

However if the patient is well vaso-dilated (as occurs in a warm operating theatre) and

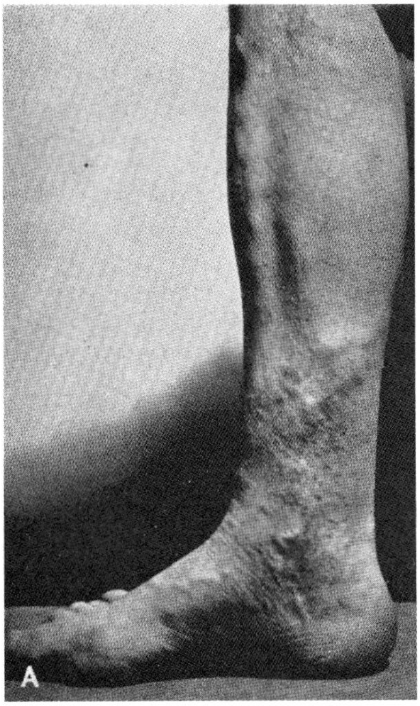

the leg is temporarily put below the heart to fill the deep veins with blood, then the calf is pumped vigorously by flexing and dorsiflexing the foot, a jet of venous blood may be ejected from a perforating vein, in a very convincing manner!

5. Sometimes a perforating vein may divide just below fascial level, and penetrate the fascia as two separate veins, rather close together. It is important to look for this anomaly and tie *all* the veins.

6. The incision must always stop about half an inch *above* the internal malleolus. A vertical incision should never be carried down behind the malleolus, as this lower part always gives trouble in healing. This is of course, only a part of the old surgical rule that one never takes a skin incision across 'Lange's Lines'.

If small veins have to be excised at or below ankle level small separate *transverse* incisions should be used.

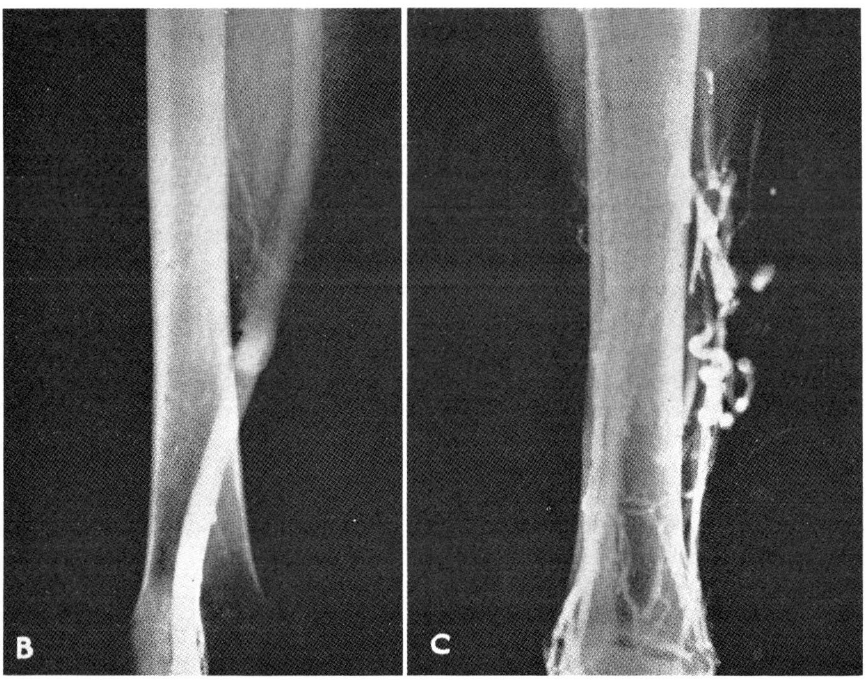

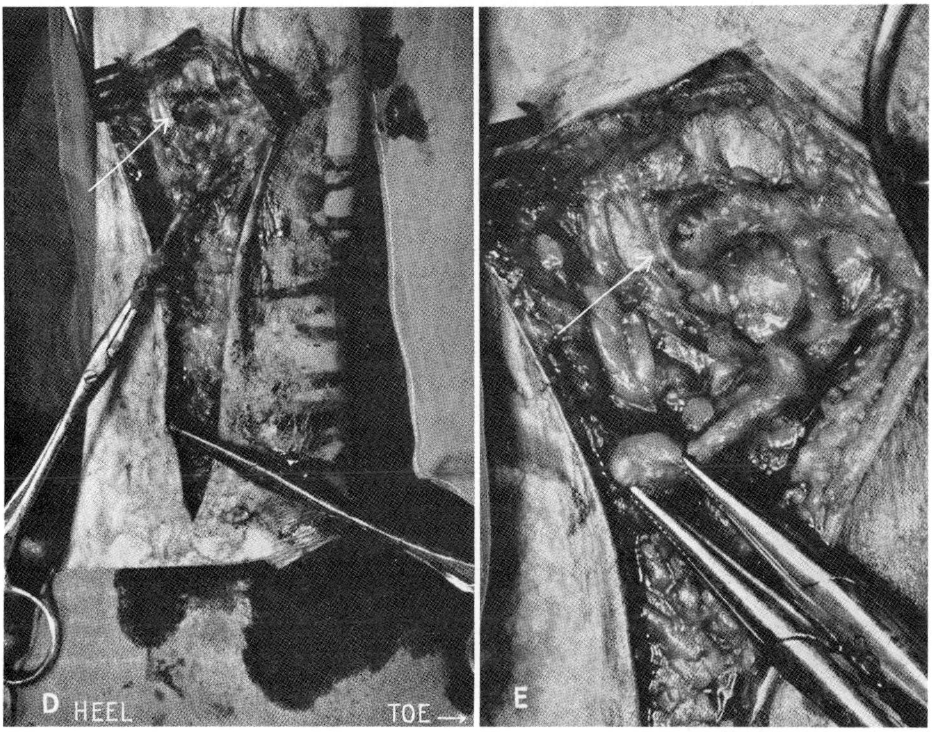

Fig. 18.10 The extra-fascial operation. For three years Mr G. T. had complained of pain, swelling, eczema and irritation over the lower and inner third of the right leg. There were no varicose veins of the great or small saphenous system. Ascending venography showed the popliteal and femoral veins to be patent and normal (B). In the lower leg under the eczematous area, a localised mass of varices could be seen and felt (A). At operation they were found to be arising from a large incompetent internal ankle perforating vein, shown in the accompanying photographs (D and E). Three years later the wound was soundly healed and there was no sign of recurrence. No support was worn. A. Shows eczema, swelling and varices about the inner ankle. B. Venogram showing normal femoral and popliteal vein with valves. C. Venogram showing localised subcutaneous varices about the ankle. D. Shows area of inner ankle perforating veins exposed at operation. Note large upper perforator (arrow). E. Closer view of large perforator. F. 'Leg recovered.'

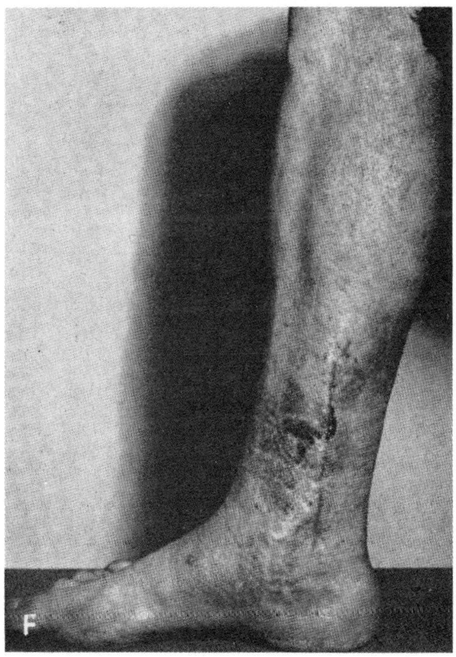

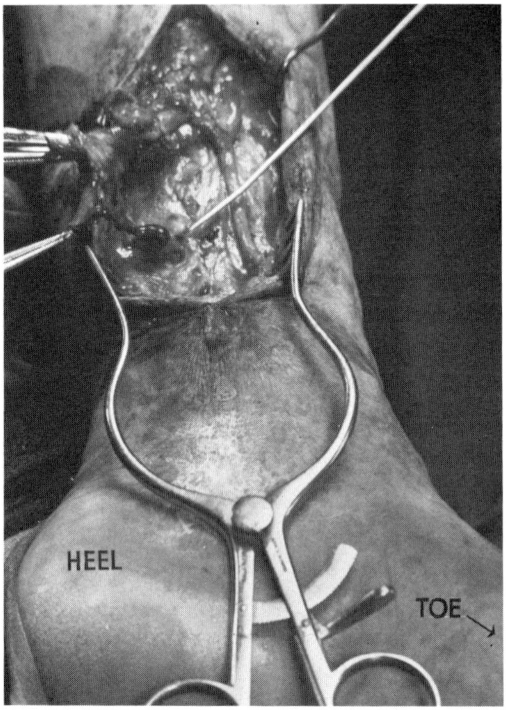

Fig. 18.11 The extra-fascial operation. An operative photograph showing the site of the middle perforating vein which is incompetent in this case. Note its position is behind the great saphenous vein, which can be seen running anteriorly. It is connected with the mass of thrombosed varices which are being held out of the way by artery forceps on the left of the plate. Note the Traver's refractor.

Sub-fascial operation (Linton's operation)

This operation has been developed by Linton of Boston (1953), and is the operation of choice in the advanced case with woody induration. Again it must be emphasised that adequate pre-operative preparation with firm bandaging—to reduce oedema and either heal the ulcer or get it to a healing phase—is absolutely necessary.

The incision is an inch posterior and parallel to the posterior border of the tibia. It is carried straight down to the muscles, through the deep fascia. It is important that it should be a long incision. It should start more than half-way up the leg, and should stop just short of the internal malleolus, as the lower part of the incision may give rise to delayed healing, if carried too far into the post-malleolar groove. The perforating veins are sought by lifting the whole of the anterior flap (consisting of skin, subcutaneous tissue and deep fascia) by retractors, and burrowing gently forwards in the sub-fascial plane until the internal perforating veins are seen passing into the muscles. The anterior flap of deep fascia is raised until the posterior border of the tibia is seen, as the upper perforating vein is close to the bone. They are divided and ligated with catgut. By burrowing under the posterior flap in the same way to the postero-lateral aspect of the leg the small saphenous vein can be inspected (and stripped if necessary) and the 'mid calf' perforator sought for. Even the lateral perforator can be reached if necessary.

Linton then recommends that a sheet of the deep fascia should be excised. This has not been our practice, however. We have either gently approximated the fascia with a few interrupted fine catgut stitches or frequently left it open and then closed the skin. In closing the skin it is important that a large number of small sutures close to the skin edge should be used. If large bites are taken with the sutures there is an added risk of causing necrosis of the skin edges. Turner Warwick (1931), Sherman (1949) and Wright (1954) have also described similar operations.

Complications of operation

The most upsetting complication of this operation is necrosis of the skin edges of the incision. Our cases of serious necrosis of the skin were early in the series, before the importance of the pre-operative preparation of the leg, and of undercutting the skin too widely had been appreciated. One case took four months to heal her necrotic skin incision. After this salutary lesson a good deal more attention was paid to (1) the choice of case; (2) the pre-operative preparation of the leg; (3) the operative technique; and (4) the meticulous after-care. Since that time there has been no case of serious skin necrosis. Minor skin necrosis confined to a part of the edges of the incision occurs in less than one-

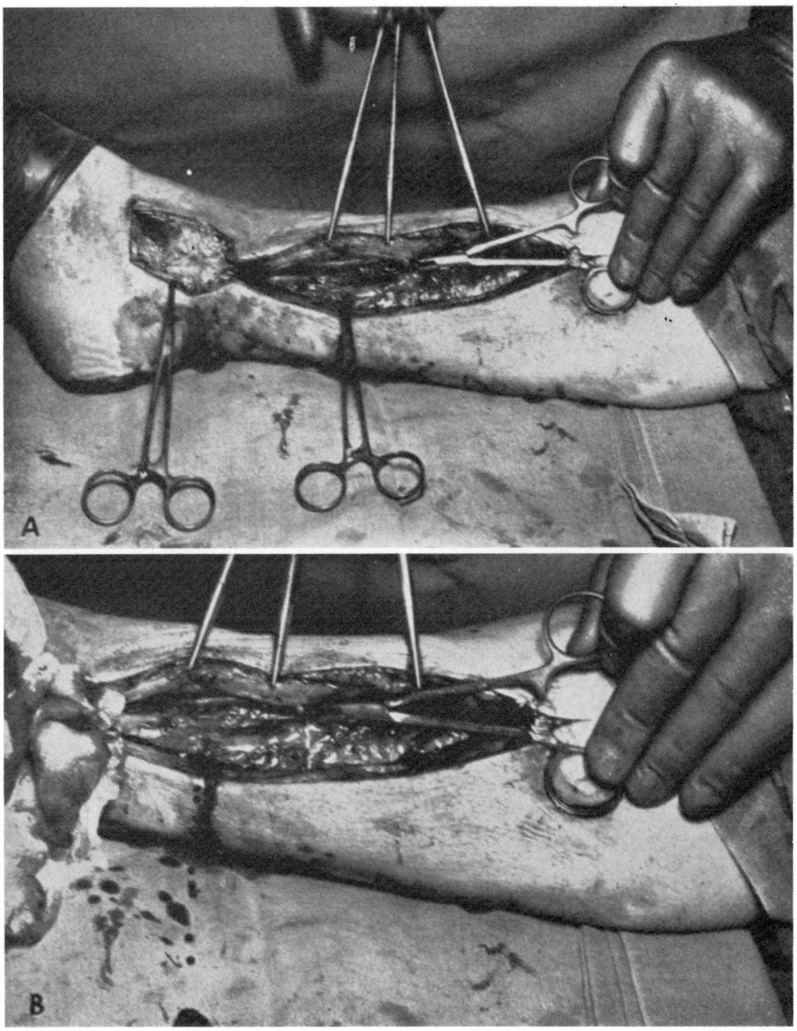

Fig. 18.12 The sub-fascial operations. A. The ulcer has been excised; a straight incision has been made down to the muscles. The anterior flap of deep fascia (dissected up from the muscles) is shown held up by three artery forceps. The upper internal perforating vein is shown emerging from the medial border of soleus with an artery forceps thrust behind it. The middle perforating vein is about two inches distal to it with an artery forceps on it. B. The bleed-back sign: The artery forceps have been removed from the middle perforator, and smart bleeding back from the deep veins has occurred (a gush, with the drops of blood falling on to the towel). C. The upper internal perforator has now been divided between artery forceps, and the middle perforator has been secured again, ready for tying with fine catgut. D. The deep fascial layer is loosely approximated with fine catgut. E. The skin is closed with silk sutures, and tulle gras is placed over the bare area from which the ulcer was excised (this will be grafted in 5–6 days' time). F. Firm bandaging of leg from toes to knee at the end of the operation, with strong crêpe bandage. Note, foot of the table is up. G. The leg two months after the operation to show the sound healing. The patient is at work with a firm stocking only at this stage.

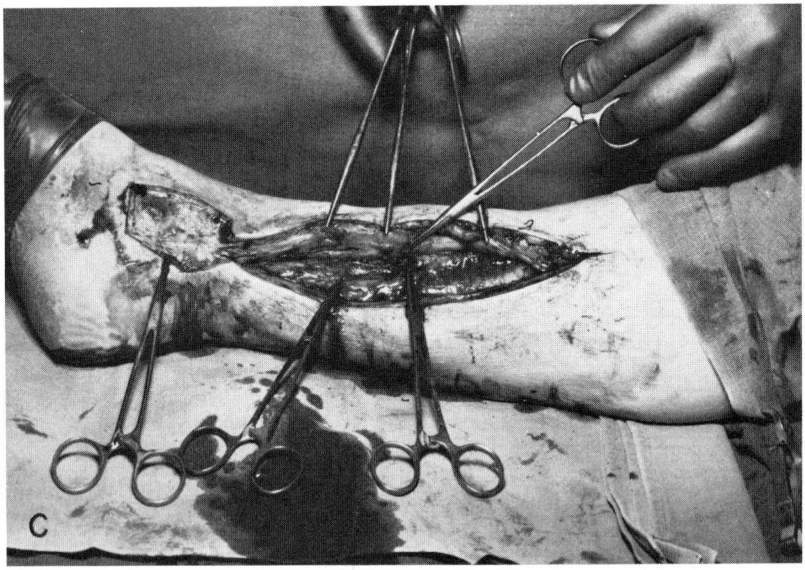

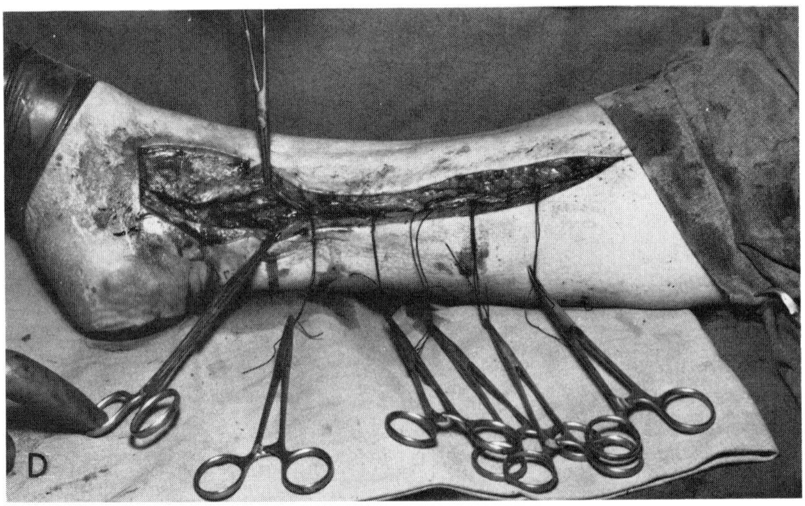

Fig. 18.12 (*contd.*) see p. 285.

fifth of the cases; beyond the fact that it delays healing and requires a regime of firm elastic support for a little longer than normal, it in no way affects the result. The incidence of skin necrosis rapidly decreases with the care and experience of the operator. Very few other complications have been observed. There have been a few cases of sepsis (as opposed to skin necrosis), which have responded to drainage and antibiotics. There have been a few cases of post-operative calf thrombosis, which settled on a regime of elevation and support followed by exercise.

No case of pulmonary embolism occurred in the St Thomas' series reported in Chapter 17. We believe that this has been due to the post-operative measures to combat venous stasis in the legs (post-operative elevation, exercises, and early ambulation with firm support).

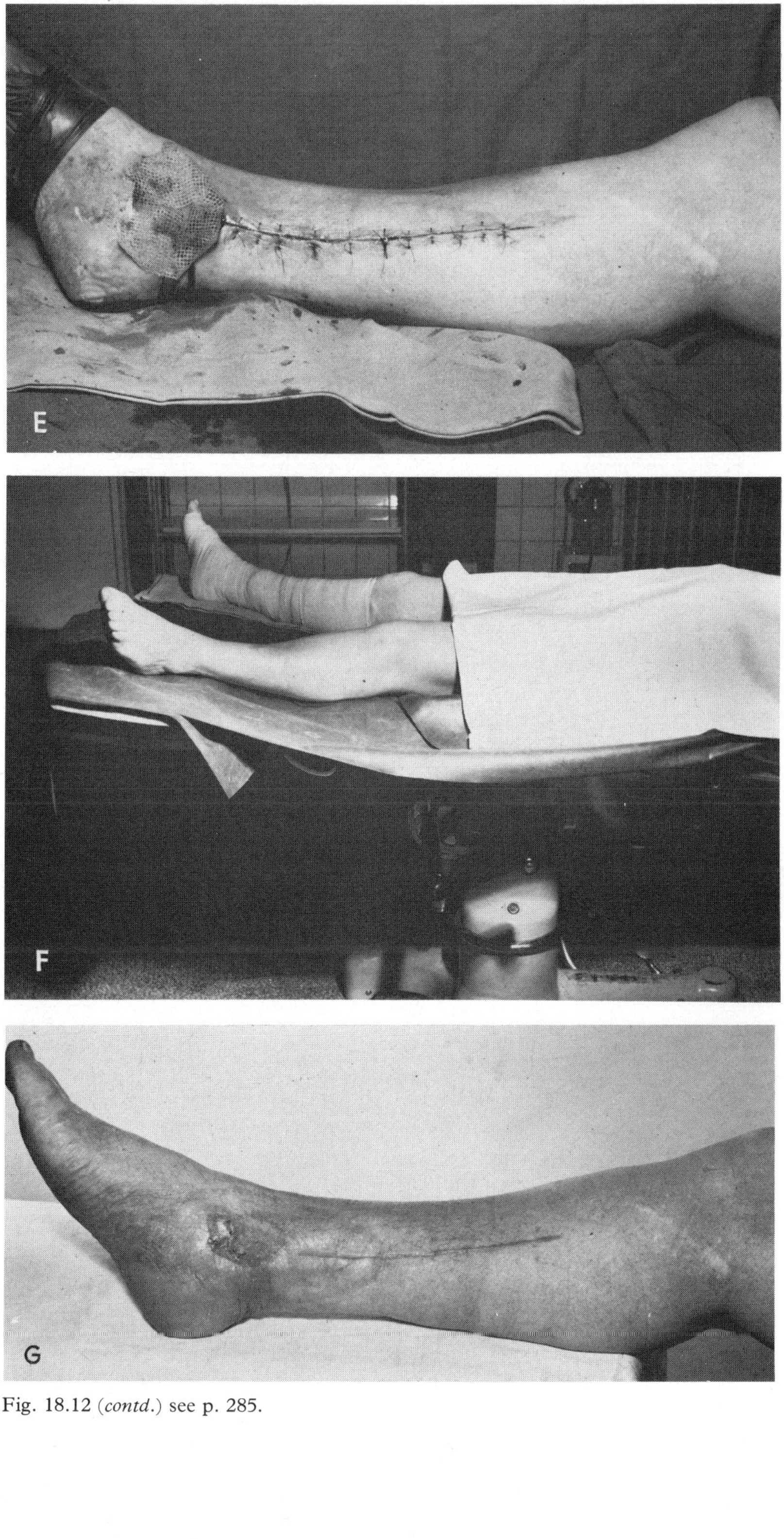

Fig. 18.12 (*contd.*) see p. 285.

4. POST-OPERATIVE MANAGEMENT

The most important point in the post operative management is to relieve the area from all 'venous hypertension' in the immediate post-operative period (i.e. for about three to four weeks). The following points are important:

1. A firm crêpe bandage is applied from toes to knees, including the ankle, immediately on completion of the operation.

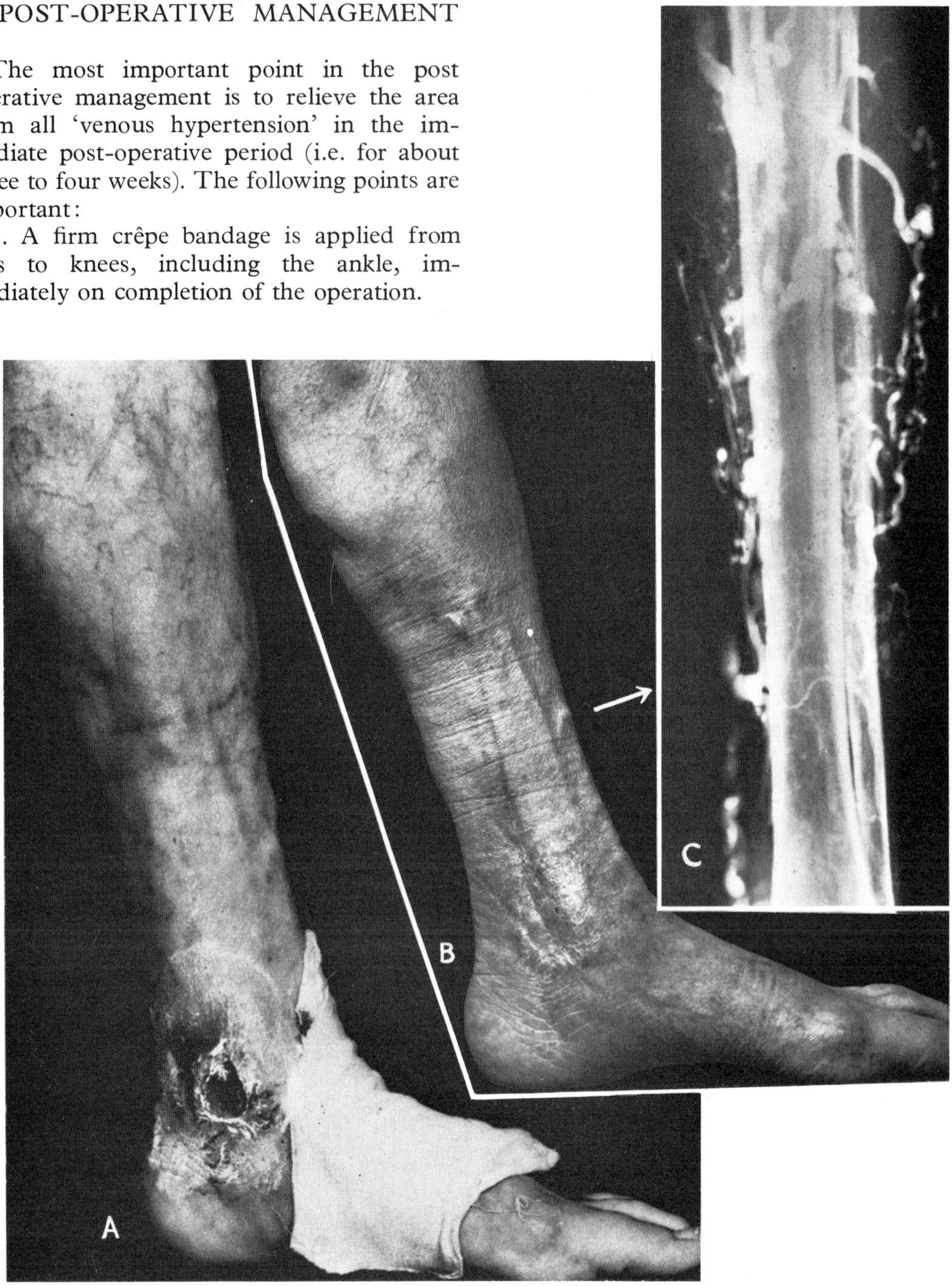

Fig. 18.13 The cause and treatment of a recurrent varicose ulcer. Mrs E. G. (aged 57) had had this varicose ulcer for fifteen years when first seen. A high saphenous ligation, and several operations which had controlled the varicose veins of her great saphenous system, had failed to have any effect on the ulcer. A venogram showed a large internal ankle perforating vein just above the site of the ulcer (indicated by the arrow). This was exposed and tied by the extra-fascial operation, and the ulcer excised and grafted in April, 1952. When last seen in June 1955 (over three years after the operation) the ulcer was completely healed and she had worn no bandage or support of any kind for over two and a half years. She had 'forgotten' about her ulcer. A. Before operation; B. Six months after operation; C. Venogram (pre-operative).

2. The foot of the bed must be raised or put on blocks for the first forty-eight hours to lessen the venous congestion of the operative site (and it is desirable to have the foot of the bed raised during the whole of the patient's stay in hospital).

3. Active leg and foot movements are instituted at once, to prevent venous stasis.

If there has been merely a straight incision, without excision and grafting of an ulcer, the patient is allowed up for 'active walking periods' from the second post-operative day. Before getting up for these walking periods the legs are firmly bandaged and supported by an extra elastic webbing bandage from toes to just below the knee, put on over the crêpe bandage. The walking periods are gradually increased until by the seventh to eighth day the patient is having three or four fifteen minute walking periods per day.

The stitches are removed on about the eighth to tenth day.

The patient is then discharged but he is instructed to wear his firm webbing elastic bandage for at least three weeks after operation during the day while he is up and about—not at night when his leg is up.

Just exactly how much longer elastic support is needed is decided at the first or second follow up inspections, which should be at three and six weeks after discharge from hospital. The more severe cases may need continuous elastic support for several months, but most can dispense with it after a period of four to six weeks.

If an ulcer has been skin grafted however, a rather longer and more careful regime of post-operative support is necessary.

Results

Venous pathology produces lesions which progress slowly and steadily over a period of many years. By the same token the results of surgery cannot be assessed by a short follow up period. In assessing the permanent value of operation a follow up period of *at least five years* is necessary.

The results of many types of treatment (i.e. injection, operation, etc.) are influenced by the elastic support, rest in elevation, and sepsis control which are carried out as a part of the general plan of treatment.

The authors have now had over twenty years experience with these operations, and there is no doubt that the curative effects of radical operation carried out early enough are long lasting.

In the majority of cases of varicose veins with perforating vein incompetence in addition, the patient eventually returns to normal life without elastic support at all. The same is true of most of the type 1 post-thrombotic cases. Some become occasional elastic stocking wearers (i.e. they wear elastic stockings at housework or work during the day, but discard them during the evenings or for outings).

Even in the 'hard core' Group 3 type of post-thrombotic limb it has been striking how operation has helped to maintain ulcer healing and make the leg feel 'easier', although of course these patients have to continue with full elastic support throughout life.

The place of skin grafting in venous ulcers

Venous ulcers, large and small, once the surface has been cleaned, take split skin grafts extremely well. However, the follow up results of grafts alone (where perforating veins or varicose veins have not been dealt with) are extremely poor. As the basic venous cause of the condition has not been dealt with, the grafts either re-ulcerate or 'crumble away' in a few months, even if firmly supported.

Most venous ulcers heal so rapidly and well in the pressure bandage routine, that we now hardly ever have to skin graft the average case.

There are certain types of ulcer however, in which skin grafting is necessary if a permanent cure is going to be achieved. These largely concern ulcers which have been allowed to become chronic, and have been allowed to remain open for roughly five years or more.

Turning back to the section on the pathology of venous ulcers (Chap. 17), it was shown that once the skin was breached, chronic infection occurred. Thus once an ulcer is established the two factors (1) Venous hyper-

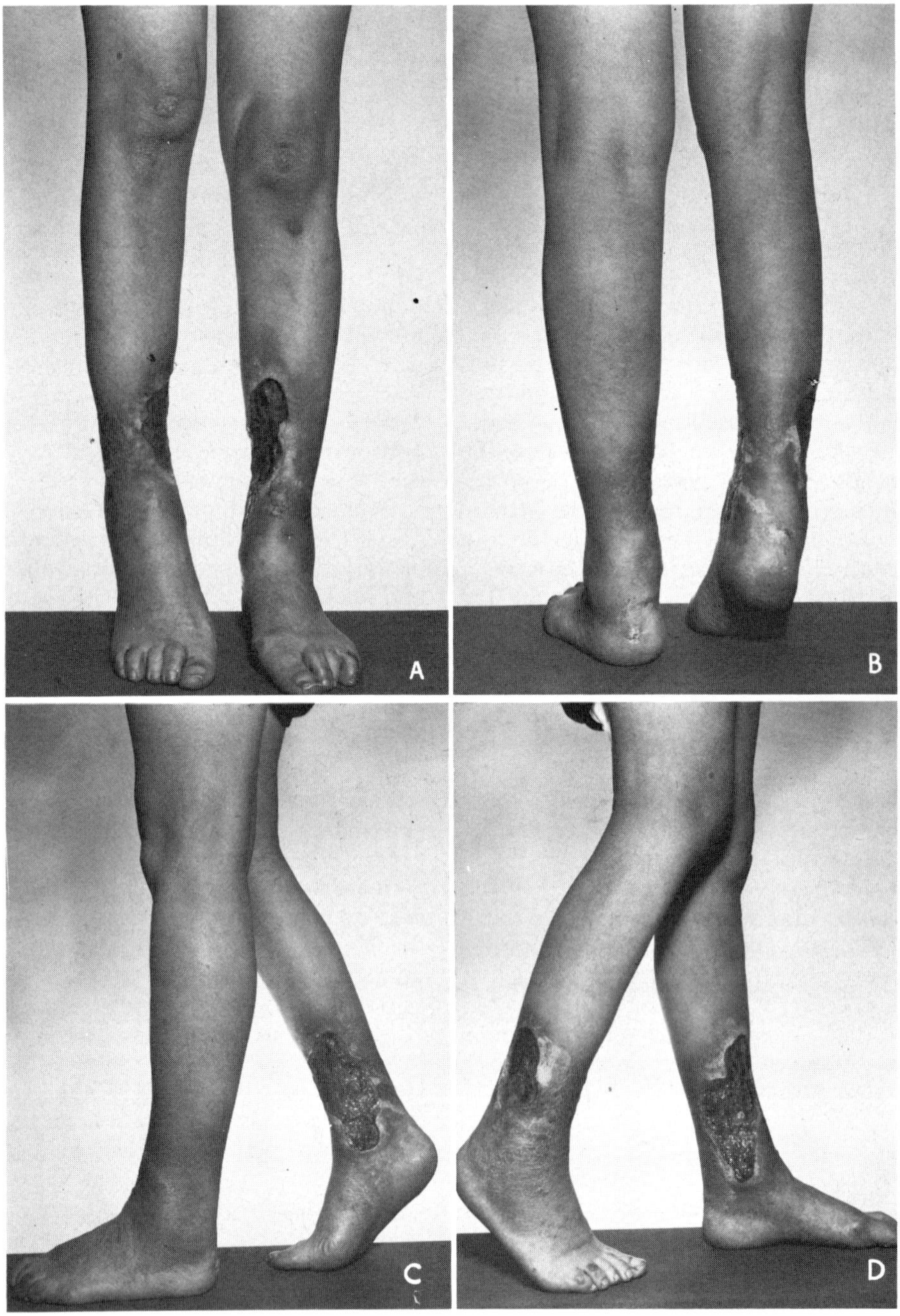

Fig. 18.14 The steps in the management of a severe post-thrombotic syndrome with venous ulceration. A, B, C & D. Shows the patient as she presented. She was a young woman of 38, and the legs had reached this state five years after a post-partum white leg. They were oedematous, very painful, she could not get her right heel to the ground and she was completely incapacitated. E. & F. After a period of rest in elevation, and compression bandaging, this amount of healing was achieved. However, they continually threatened to break down with conservative treatment. G. & H. A Sub-fascial ligation of the ankle perforating veins (internal and external) was performed, and this photograph shows the result six months after the operation. The patient wears elastic stockings only now, and does a full day's housework.

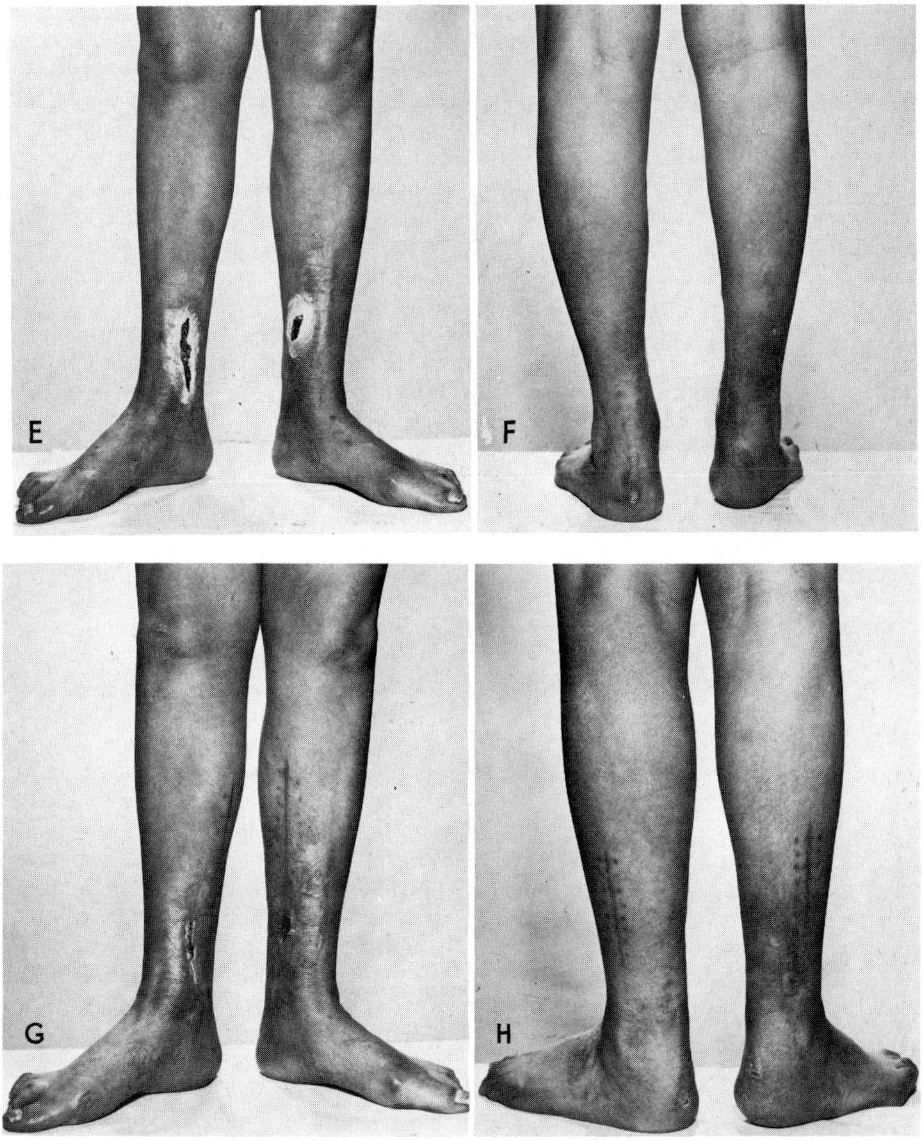

Fig. 18.14 (*contd.*) see p. 290.

tension, and (2) Infection, work together making the ulcerated area of the skin *hyper-vascular* (see Chap. 17). As the years go on the whole of the area of the ulcer becomes more fibrous and more vascular. To put it another way: '*These indolent looking, chronic, fibrous ulcers are not ischaemic lesions, they have too much blood in them at too high a pressure*'.

The surface of such ulcers receive skin grafts very easily indeed, but as soon as the patient gets up and the local venous hyper-tension and hyper-vascularity is re-established, the skin grafts crumble and re-ulcerate. This takes place usually within a year or so, and unfortunately the literature is full of short term reports of the glowing success achieved by split skin grafting large chronic ulcers. A year or two more follow up would have revealed the true situation.

Thus the message is that if a really chronic ulcer (i.e. one of approximately four or five years standing) is to be treated surgically by grafting, *then the whole ulcer area plus subcutaneous tissue right down to deep fascia must be excised widely*. The area is then allowed to granulate for a few days, and then a sheet of split skin, preferably cut with an electric dermatone is laid over the area in the usual way (Fig. 18.15).

Thus the suggested routine for surgical cure of a large chronic ulcer, above the internal malleolus would be:

1. *Pre-operative.*

Period of rest in bed with high elevation of legs—about one week.

The ulcer is cultured and a course of systemic antibiotic is instituted. *Whatever the result of culture, an antibiotic which is effective against Staphylococci and Streptococci is chosen.*

2. *Operation.*

The ulcer is widely excised down to deep fascia. If necessary the incision is extended to explore and tie perforating veins, and to strip incompetent long or short saphenous veins if present.

The whole area is dressed with dry gauze in large quantity and firmly bandaged with crêpe bandage.

3. *Grafting.*

Three to five days later the patient is taken back to theatre. The dressings are removed. If possible a single sheet of split skin, cut with an electric dermatone is laid over the area and sewn into place with a few fine silk sutures. The graft is pressed into place with a paraffin gauze pad and the whole area is pressure bandaged again.

4. *Post-operative.*

In all big grafts of the lower extremity it is important to protect the graft area against venous congestion or hypertension until it is firmly consolidated. *This means that these patients need continuous rest with elevation of the legs for at least three weeks.* This is very important because if the patient is allowed up before this time even with support, the high venous pressure tends to cause ecchymosis under the graft and graft necrosis. During the latter two weeks, exposure of the graft during the day for short periods without dressing, is a good thing.

After three weeks elevation the graft is fairly solid and the patient can start getting up for walking periods over a week or so *with gauze pad and elastic bandage support for the graft area.*

After about four weeks the average patient can then be discharged home on gauze pad and firm elastic bandage support—which is usually necessary for two or three months.

5. *Late Post-operative Instructions.*

The late care of the graft is very important. There are two main points: (1) The graft itself and the surrounding skin always tends to become dry and scaly, and if these scales are not continuously wiped away then they accumulate, become horny and infection occurs beneath them leading to re-ulceration. Therefore every patient is provided with a bottle of olive oil and some gauze and instructed how to descale the graft and surroundings every other evening, by firm olive oil massage. (2) The area is protected during the day by a few thicknesses of ordinary gauze worn as a protective pad under a light elastic stocking (Fig. 18.16).

Comment:

It is evident from the above that the decision to treat a large chronic ulcer by surgery and skin grafting entails a great deal of patience on the part of both surgeon and patient. The time in hospital is seldom under five weeks. After the operation the full time, intelligent cooperation of the patient is necessary to maintain the good result.

If all these prerequisites are followed carefully however, some brilliant long term results

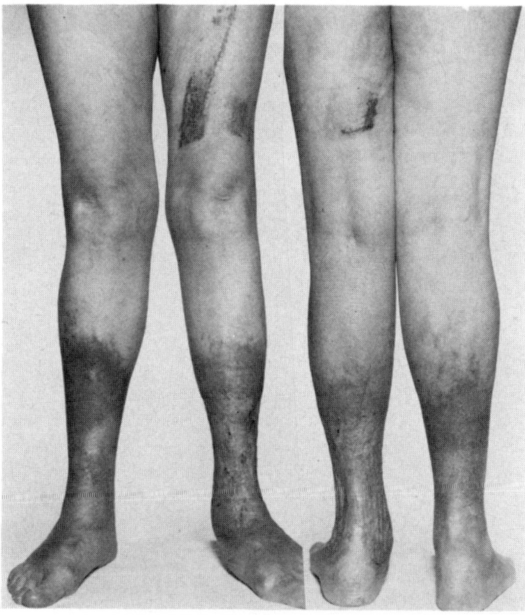

Fig. 18.15 Result of excision of large, nearly circumferential chronic venous ulcer and replacement by split skin dermatone sheet graft. The left leg had been the site of a very large chronic indurated ulcer for about seven years. The patient was in hospital for six weeks but the final result was worth it, and the patient has been free of ulceration during her five year follow up.

in apparently hopeless cases can be achieved, (see Fig. 18.15).

Grafting in localised small sub-malleolar ulcers

There is a type of small, localised, very fibrous and chronic ulcer which sometimes occurs just behind and *below* the internal malleolus. These are very difficult to deal with, because split skin grafts do not do so well in this area, owing to the graft being right over the joint line and subject to much flexion and extension stress.

These ulcers can often be excised completely and given full thickness skin cover by the technique shown in Figure 18.17. A full thickness flap of normal skin from the front of the lower leg and ankle is pulled laterally to fill in the gap left by excision of the ulcer. The split skin graft is then put on the normal tissues in the triangular gap left on the dorsum of the foot, where it does very well.

This technique needs considerable care, and the flap of full thickness skin which is transferred over must have a very wide base as shown, to ensure its blood supply.

This technique gives good long term results for these difficult little sub-malleolar ulcers.

Deep vein ligation in the post-thrombotic syndrome

As we have seen in Chapter 14 after an acute peripheral femoral thrombosis complete

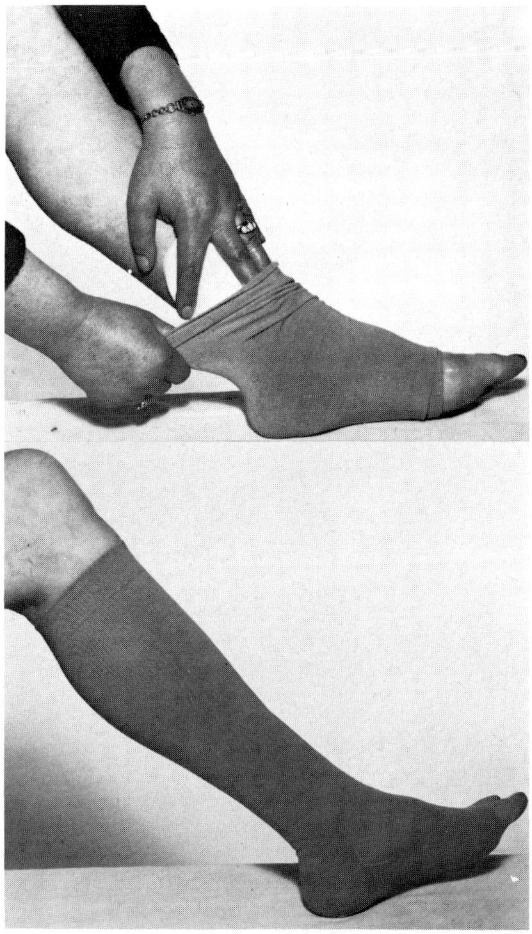

Fig. 18.16 Late care of a grafted venous ulcer. A large felt pad is worn under an elastic stocking to support it and protect the area from further trauma.

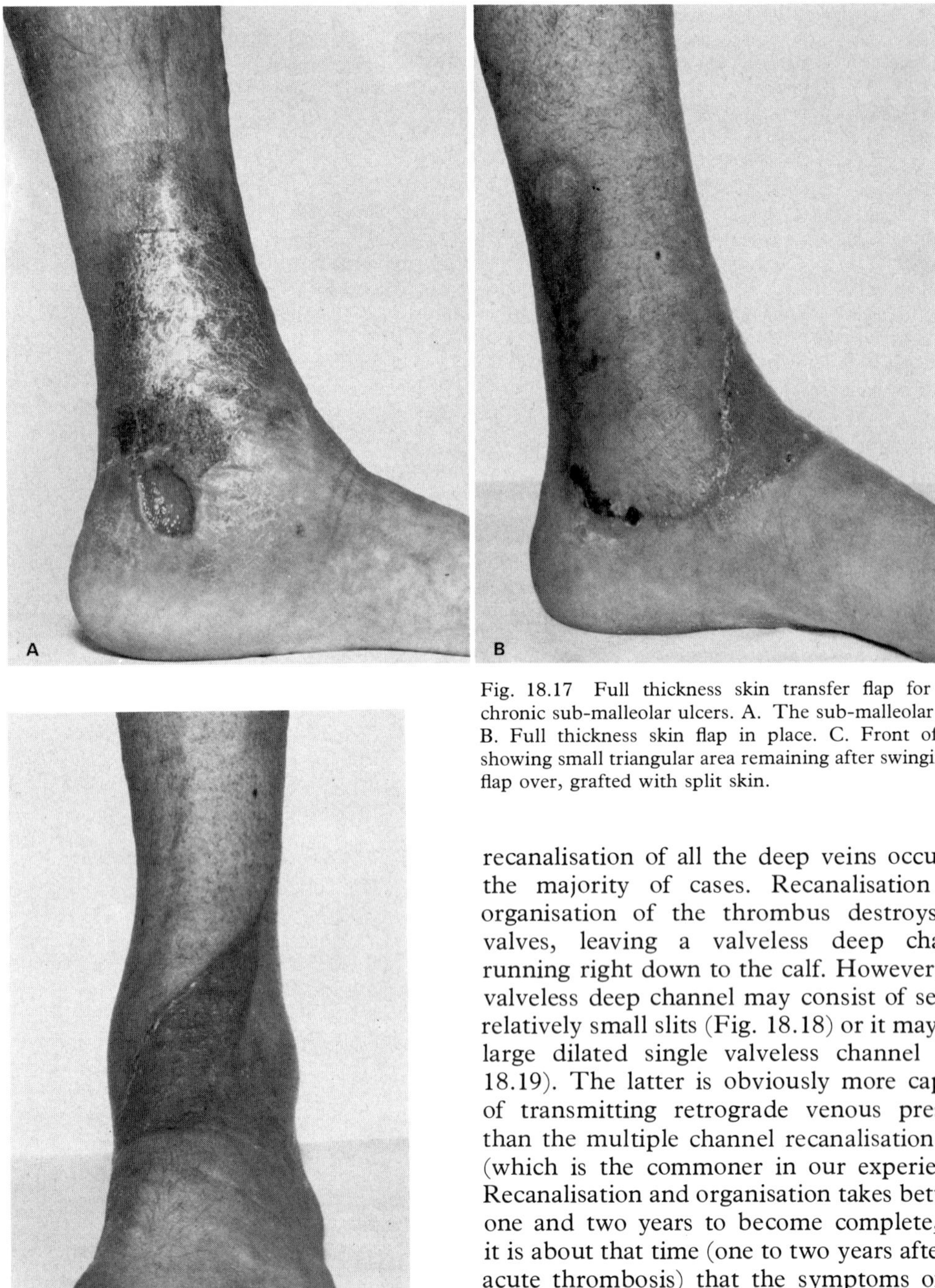

Fig. 18.17 Full thickness skin transfer flap for small chronic sub-malleolar ulcers. A. The sub-malleolar ulcer. B. Full thickness skin flap in place. C. Front of foot, showing small triangular area remaining after swinging the flap over, grafted with split skin.

recanalisation of all the deep veins occurs in the majority of cases. Recanalisation and organisation of the thrombus destroys the valves, leaving a valveless deep channel running right down to the calf. However, this valveless deep channel may consist of several relatively small slits (Fig. 18.18) or it may be a large dilated single valveless channel (Fig. 18.19). The latter is obviously more capable of transmitting retrograde venous pressure than the multiple channel recanalisation type (which is the commoner in our experience). Recanalisation and organisation takes between one and two years to become complete, and it is about that time (one to two years after the acute thrombosis) that the symptoms of the post-thrombotic syndrome may begin to make their first appearance.

For many years it was believed that it was

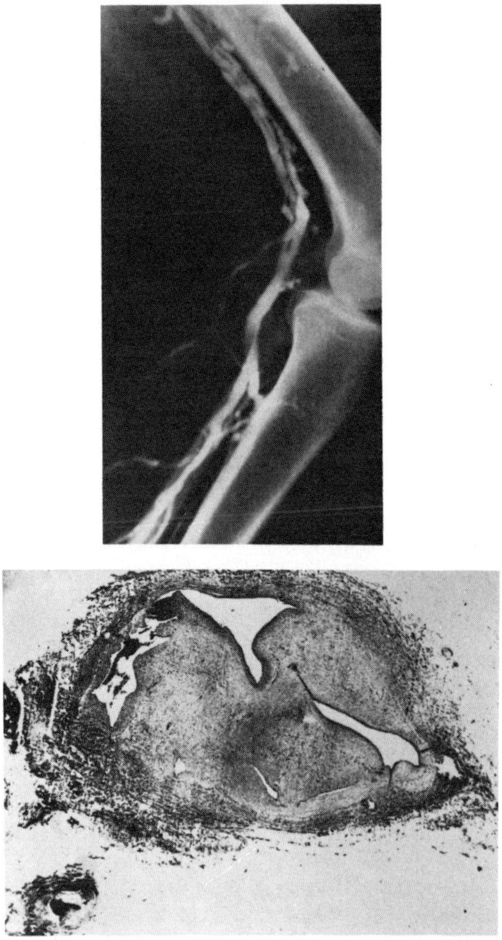

Fig. 18.18 The ascending venogram (Valsalva technique) of a woman, aged 48, who had had a white leg fourteen years previously, and who presented with post-thrombotic induration and ulceration of the lower leg. Note the abnormal appearance of the deep veins—no valves are seen. The femoral vein was tied in Hunter's canal. A cross section of it shows multiple channel canalisation of an old thrombosis. Note that the channels appear as mere slits in the section, but in life these are large, thin-walled venous spaces.

this valve destruction in the main deep veins (femoral and popliteal, etc.) that was primarily responsible for the onset of the ulceration and induration syndrome of the ankle. (Bauer 1948). This reasoning led to large-scale attempts to cure or ameliorate the syndrome by ligating these valveless deep veins (either the popliteal or the femoral). Now, as we have shown in Chapter 14, destruction of valves in the main femoral and popliteal veins is not a prerequisite for the development of induration and ulceration of the ankle, and in fact we have found that many of the so-called post-thrombotic ulcers have normal valves in the popliteal and femoral veins. Højensgaard and Stürup (1949, 1952) came to the same conclusion from a study of venous pressures in the leg.

Thus modern work indicates that valve destruction in the main deep veins (popliteal and femoral) plays a relatively minor part in the development of the post-thrombotic

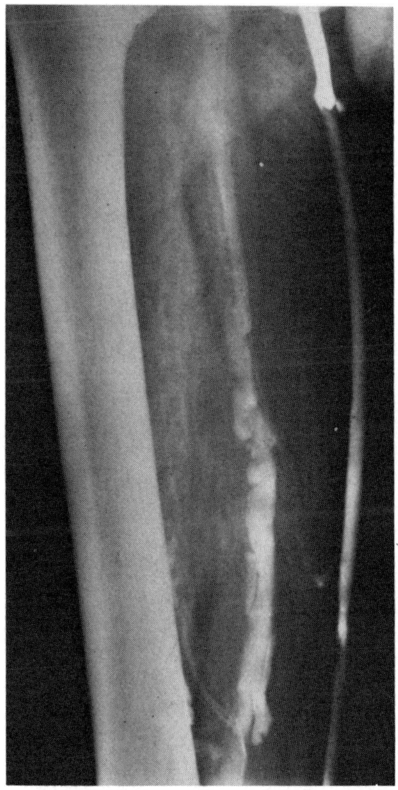

Fig. 18.19 Ascending venogram. Valsalva technique, of a young man of 28 who had a chronic ulcer of the skin for six years. Note the irregular 'moth-eaten' appearance of the femoral vein, without any normal valve cusps. A piece of this vein taken for section at operation showed it to be an old thrombosis. This is an example of valve destruction, leaving a large single channel.

ankle. However, post-thrombotic obstruction does occur in the iliac veins after thrombosis at this level (Chap. 16). *Most of the theorising on the role of incompetent deep veins was done before the modern work on ilio-femoral thrombosis, which has now made these old theories largely untenable* (see Chap. 17). Ligature of the deep recanalised vein for relief of the post-thrombotic syndrome was first suggested and carried out by Homans. However, it was not until Bauer published his glowing reports of the results, in a large number of cases, of ligating the popliteal vein, that this procedure really caught the surgeon's imagination and was fairly widely taken up. Disappointment in the results of the operation quickly followed. It is highly probable that any good effects on the ulcer which accrued were the result of the ancillary treatment that was carried out at the same time, i.e. bed rest and firm elastic bandaging of the ankle. Reports recently published from a number of different sources (Linton 1953, Moore 1953, Goligher 1953, Cockett 1953 and 1955, Boyd et al. 1954) make it clear that deep venous ligation *in itself* has little effect on the course of ulceration and induration of the lower leg. This is only to be expected from a consideration of the pathology, because the basic cause of this part of the post-thrombotic syndrome is the destruction of the valves in the ankle perforating veins.

The place of sympathectomy

Increasing experience both in our clinics and from Linton (1948) makes it clear that sympathectomy is definitely *contra-indicated* in pure venous ulcers of all sorts. As we have already seen in Chapter 5, venous ulcers are not ischaemic lesions, they are *hypervascular* lesions with venous and arteriolar dilatation and considerable venous hypertension. Sympathectomy by further dilating all these vessels, and increasing the blood flow into the part merely exacerbates all these factors and usually makes the ulcer appreciably worse and more difficult to handle.

This is most noticeable clinically and the few 'post-sympathectomy, post-thrombotic cases' we have had to deal with have been considerable problems.

Hot weather, hot climates and anything which leads to prolonged vaso-dilatation and increased flow through the skin of foot and ankle has a noticeably deteriorating effect on all chronic venous ulcers.

Thus we may leave this section by once again emphasising that *sympathectomy is definitely harmful* in all pure chronic venous lesions of the leg.

REFERENCES

Bauer, G. (1948) *J. int. Chir.*, **8**, 937.
Baynton, T. (1797) *A new method of treating old ulcers of the legs.* Bristol: Biggs.
Boyd, A. M., Catchpole, B. N., Jepson, R. P. & Rose, S. S. (1953) *Lancet*, **2**, 113.
Cockett, F. B. (1953) Pathology and treatment of venous ulcers of the leg. London, *Thesis*.
Cockett, F. B. (1954) *Postgrad. med. J.*, **30**, 512.
Cockett, F. B. (1955) *Brit. J. Surg.*, **Nov.**
Goligher, J. C. (1953) *Lancet*, **1**, 96.
Høјensgaard, K. & Stürup, H. (1949) *Acta chir. scand.*, **99**, 133.
Høјensgaard, K. & Stürup, H. (1952) *Acta physiol. scand.*, **27**, 49.
Linton, R. R. (1952) *Angiology*, **3**, 431.
Linton, R. R. (1953) *Ann. Surg.*, **138,** 415.
Linton, R. R. (1953) *Arch. Surg.*, **67,** 2.
Linton, R. R. & Hardy, I. B. (1948) *Surgery,* **24,** 452.
Moore, H. D. (1953) *Lancet*, **1**, 23.
Sherman, R. S. (1944) *Ann. Surg.*, **120**, 772.
Sherman, R. S. (1949) *Ann. Surg.*, **130,** 218.
Warwick, T. (1931) '*The rational treatment of varicose veins and varicocele*'. London: Faber.
Wiseman, R. (1686) '*Severall chirurgicall treatises*'. London.
Wright, A. Dickson (1930) *Brit. Med. J.*, **2**, 906.
Wright, R. B. (1953) *Lancet*, 2, 1273.

19. The Differential Diagnosis of Ulcers of the Leg

In this book a detailed consideration of lesions of the toes, forepart of the foot, and sole of the foot is not undertaken. Ulcers and lesions of these regions are almost never caused by venous pathology. The reason for this is probably best stated in Gay's own words. In his Lettsomian Lectures of 1867 he said 'The veins of the foot anastomose so freely, and such are the means of escape for its blood through either the deep or superficial system, that embarrassment to its venous circulation is hardly possible. It is not so however with regard to the superficial veins of the leg between the ankle and calf. In this part of the limb the venous circulation is exposed to greater difficulty and risk of obstruction than in any other part of the limb, if not in any other part of the body.' To this might be added the fact that the sole and toes of the foot have a profuse arterial supply as compared with that of the skin and subcutaneous tissues of the ankle as has been seen in the section on anatomy (Chap. 3).

Ulcers and lesions of the foot are usually associated with pathology of either the arterial or the nervous system, or are due to the various fungus diseases and other diseases which affect the skin of the toes and feet. These factors are summarized in Figure 19.1 and need not further detain us.

VENOUS ULCERS

Of the ulcers of the leg and ankle, those due to pathology of the venous system form by far the greater part. These ulcers have had various names in the past—varicose ulcers, gravitational ulcers, post-phlebitic ulcers—but in this book the term originally suggested by Gay for them, *venous ulcers*, will be used. Such ulcers occur over the area of the leg shown in the diagram, called appropriately the 'gaiter area' (Fig. 19.2). It will be noted that this gaiter area extends below and behind both the malleoli and very nearly half-way up the legs and on to the dorsum of the foot. Ulcers of purely venous origin are rare outside this region. Moreover, although most venous ulcers start in the small area cross-hatched on Figure 19.2, above and behind the internal

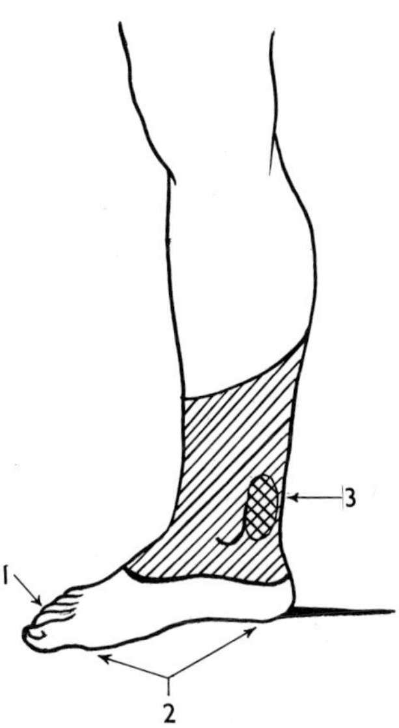

Fig. 19.1 Diagram of the main causes of ulcer of the toes, foot and ankle. 1. Chronic sores or ulcers of toes are due to: (a) Peripheral arterial disease (arteriosclerosis), diabetes, Buerger's disease; (b) Chilblains; (c) Chronic fungus infection; (d) Trauma and bone infection. 2. Ulcers of sole of foot are due to: (a) Nerve lesions; Tabes dorsalis, peripheral neuritis (diabetes), sciatic nerve lesion; (b) Peripheral arterial disease. 3. Gaiter area, over which venous ulcers occur.

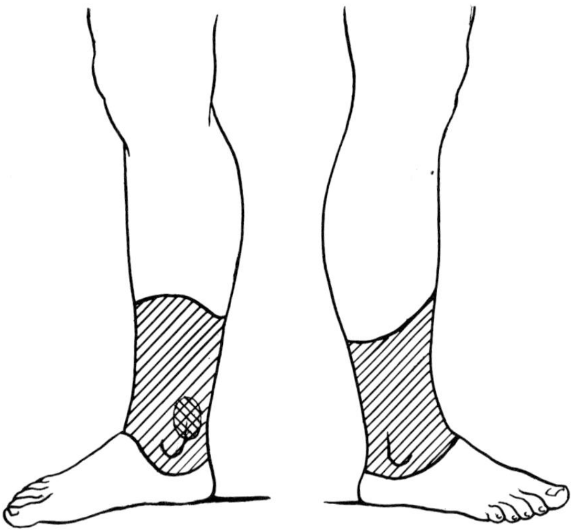

Fig. 19.2 The Gaiter Area. Venous ulcers occur anywhere within this area, but the place where most of them start is shown cross-hatched.

malleolus, they may occur anywhere in this area, both on the outside and the inside of the leg.

Although venous ulcers are by far the commonest here, a number of other types of ulcers occur on the leg and many of them encroach on this gaiter area, and so the problem of differential diagnosis is a real one. In the St Thomas' Hospital Ulcer Clinic during the years 1951 and 1952, 234 new cases of ulcer of the leg were sent up under the diagnosis of venous ulcer. Of these approximately 31, or nearly 13 per cent, had no connection with pathology of the venous system. This is a high figure in a clinic which was at that time especially for so-called varicose ulcers, and the figure would certainly be higher in a general clinic or in a skin clinic.

Clinical characteristics of venous ulcers. Venous ulcers occur twice as frequently in women as in men. Some authorities claim that they have a predilection for the left leg. Their most important diagnostic point is their occurrence within the 'gaiter area'.

They are not necessarily associated with the presence of visible varicose veins and are usually associated with venous hypertension due to incompetent perforating veins. They are shallow ulcers involving skin and superficial layers of subcutaneous tissue only.

When considering the appearance of a venous ulcer it must be remembered that one is looking at one particular stage of a very chronic disease, and the manifestations in the gaiter area in the early years are less severe and widespread than after the disease has been present for twenty years or more. Moreover, these manifestations, their speed of onset, symptoms, and signs vary considerably from patient to patient according to the form and type of leg which is the subject of the disease. Thus the well developed, warm, hairy leg of the average male is far more resistant to ulceration than the adipose, smooth skinned, hairless, cold leg possessed by some men and many women.

Bearing these variations in mind there are certain signs and symptoms which are characteristic of venous ulcers. These are:

1. Situation. Within the gaiter area, with a predilection for the site above and behind the internal malleolus.

2. Association with visible signs of venous pathology, **'The Ankle Flare'.** The most constant sign of venous pathology associated with ulcers is a flare of small subcutaneous dilated venules seen with the patient standing up and occupying the area immediately below and behind the internal malleolus. This is shown in Figure 19.3. There is often a similar flare below and behind the external malleolus as well, when the ulcer may be situated on the outer side of the leg. This characteristic 'ankle flare' is a sign which occurs before actual ulceration takes place, and may then be observed over the whole of the inner side of the ankle (Fig. 19.4). Once ulceration and its attendant infection and oedema has occurred the swelling and fibrosis of the subcutaneous tissues often obliterates this sign, except in the area just above the heel pad (Fig. 19.3). In legs which are fat, or oedematous, this sign is not well marked, as the subcutaneous fat tends to cover the dilated venules.

This 'ankle flare' may be the only visible sign that the ulcer is indeed venous in origin, there being few or no visible superficial

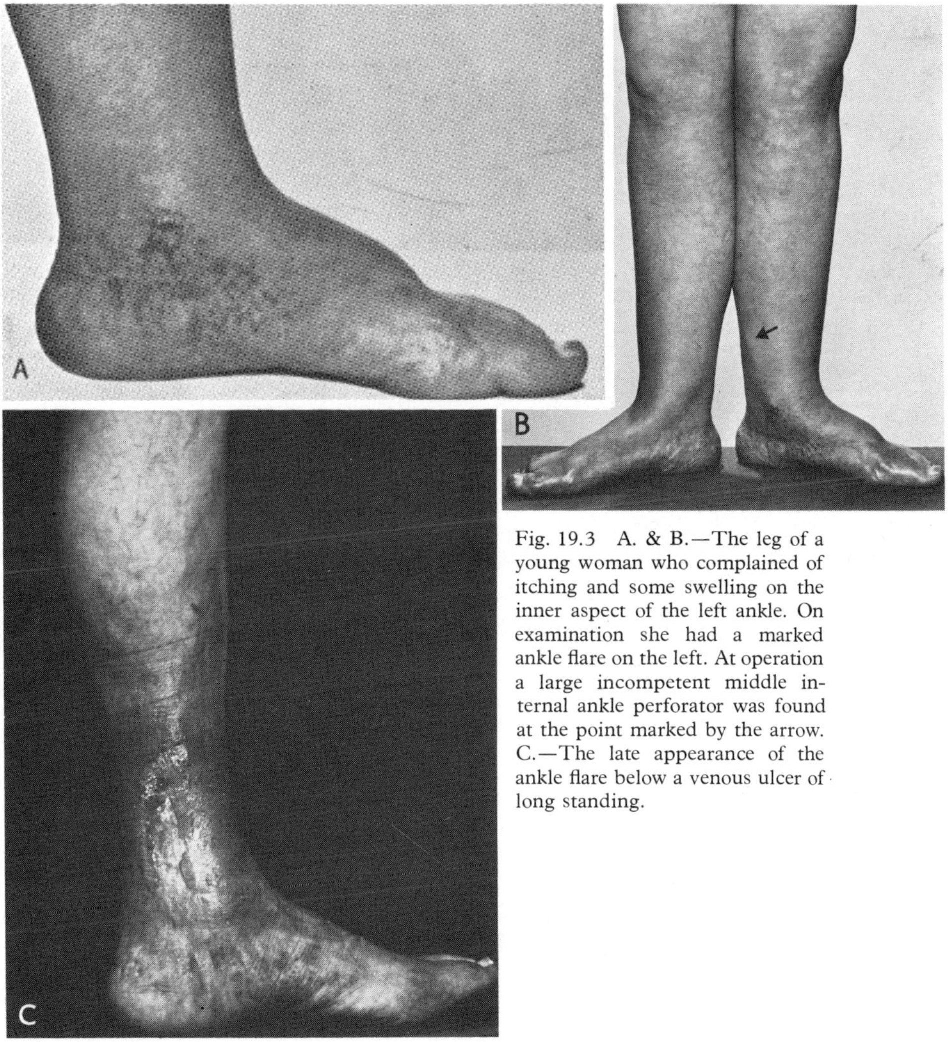

Fig. 19.3 A. & B.—The leg of a young woman who complained of itching and some swelling on the inner aspect of the left ankle. On examination she had a marked ankle flare on the left. At operation a large incompetent middle internal ankle perforator was found at the point marked by the arrow. C.—The late appearance of the ankle flare below a venous ulcer of long standing.

varicose veins in the limb. More usually, however, there are signs of obvious venous pathology in the limb—varying from a few so-called superficial varices above the ulcer region to complete and obvious incompetence and varicosity of the great or small saphenous systems or both.

3. Association with Eczema. Although any ulcer of the leg may be associated with eczema, venous ulcers are particularly prone to this association. The whole of the skin of the ulcer-bearing area may react by a dry, scaly, itching dermatitis. This is particularly so in those who already have a constitutional tendency to eczema or skin disease. When, however, actual ulceration has taken place the skin around the ulcer is always precarious and tends to react by an exudative eczema in the early stages. Local sepsis and the application of local medicaments (particularly penicillin creams, flavine, or sulpha drug creams) are the important precipitating causes for this eczema. Once present, unless controlled early, it may become violent and widespread in the leg. It

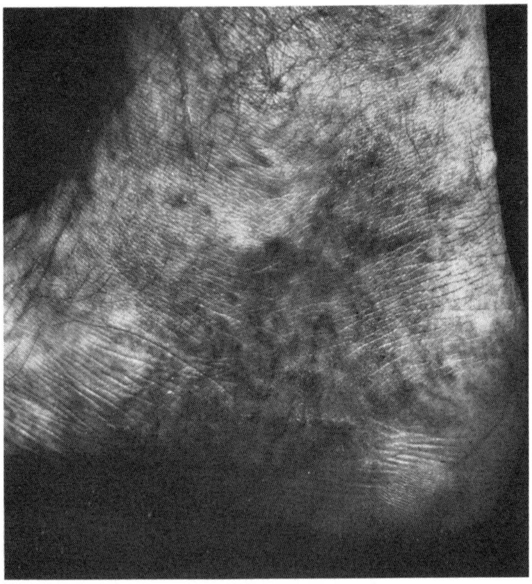

Fig. 19.4 Pre-ulcerous venular dilatation around the ankle. (The Ankle Flare.)

may even 'generalise', the patient then appearing in a miserable state, with eruptions on the face, body and arms.

4. Pigmentation. Pigmentation is the sign which is typical of a long standing venous pathology in the gaiter area. Its degree varies from case to case, but it is particularly noticeable in the older patients. Considerable pigmentation may occur without ulceration, although more usually it is associated with old ulcers. It is dark brown and is due to the deposition of haemosiderin in the subcutaneous tissues, derived from the breakdown of extravasated blood.

5. Induration. In certain cases with and without ulcer, the whole or part of the gaiter area becomes indurated. That is to say, the subcutaneous tissues instead of being of normal thickness and soft, and the skin being freely mobile over the deep fascia, the whole skin, subcutaneous tissue and deep fascia become welded into a firm, solid mass, and contracts. This change is usually maximal above and behind the internal malleolus, but it may spread throughout the gaiter area, and is due to widespread fat necrosis. Thus the larger erythrocyanoid type of leg, and those with a lot of fatty subcutaneous tissue tend particularly to develop this change. The contraction of the fibrous tissue may in time give the appearance of a tight constricting band round the ankle region with a tourniquet effect. These legs have been graphically described as 'inverted champagne bottle' legs, which is a very true description of their clinical appearance. The skin over the indurated area is in a precarious state of nutrition, and any infected surface trauma tends to spread widely forming a vast shallow ulcer, which may become circumferential.

6. Oedema. Venous ulcers are usually associated with some slight degree of oedema of the ankle and foot. This oedema is in fact an integral part of the post-phlebitic syndrome. It varies considerably according to the extent of the post-phlebitic destruction of the valves in the deep and perforating veins, and according to the type of leg. Where there is merely destruction of valves in one perforating vein and minimal destruction of deep vein valves, the oedema may be minimal or absent. Increase in oedema round the ulcer is also seen as a result of acute infection. Gross oedema usually means lymphatic obstruction.

7. Pain. Pain is a variable symptom. At one end of the scale are the small acute necrotic-looking ulcers which typically occur in the erythrocyanoid type of leg of women, in which severe unremitting pain is the presenting symptom. At the other end are the large chronic ulcers, which have been present for years, some of which appear to be completely painless.

Clinically there are three relevant points in regard to the pain of ulcers:

1. Acutely infected ulcers are very painful and most of the pain is relieved by controlling the acute infection.

2. Pain is usually prominent in the ischaemic leg (due to arterial disease) and the erythrocyanoid leg. In these, the pain has the qualities of ischaemic pain, that is to say it is usually better when the limb is dependant or moving, and is bad at night when the limb is up and warm under the bedclothes (rest pain).

These patients often get extremely ill and depressed through lack of sleep.

3. Pain is usually worse during the early stages of ulceration. As the ulcer becomes more chronic, pain tends to become less prominent as a symptom. Most ulcers are painful to some degree, depending on the mentality of the patient; it is a congested, burning sort of pain, not very severe. In contradistinction to group (2) above, it is usually relieved by rest with the foot up, or by tight bandaging.

These then are the main clinical characteristics of venous ulcers.

Next, the other ulcers which may occur on the leg which are not directly associated with venous disease must be considered.

NON-VENOUS ULCERATION OF THE LEG

Ulcers associated with erythrocyanosis frigida :—Lynn (1954), states 'Chilblains' the pernio syndrome, dermatitis hiemalis, erythrocyanosis frigida, nodular vasculitis, erytheme induratum, and Bazin's disease are all terms which have been applied to various stages in the progress of a single disease entity'. There is no reason to retain more than the simplest of these many terms.

Erythrocyanosis frigida or the pernio syndrome are the names of choice for a clinical condition of the legs and ankles seen almost exclusively in women and usually *young* women. The ankles are swollen and bulbous and lose their normal contour. The skin is hairless and in cold weather has a chronic mottled blue tinge, which is maximal to the outer side and posterior aspect of the ankle. This becomes bright red and painful on warming. In the subcutaneous fat of this region many small painful hard areas may develop. These are actually patches of fat necrosis and the skin over them may ulcerate. These ulcers occur usually either on the back of the ankle or to the outer side, and are typically multiple. These patients often suffer from chilblains on the toes as well.

Boyd, (1950), has pointed out that these cases are merely severe examples of a common type of leg, which he has termed the erythrocyanoid limb. This type of limb is seen frequently in women. It is characterised by its smooth, hairless skin, a tendency to cyanosis round the ankle and chronic oedema even in the absence of any other pathology. In general, the severity of these symptoms is greater with increasing thickness of subcutaneous fat (the so-called erythrocyanoid lipoidaemia). One of the basic defects in these limbs appears to be that the arteries are of small calibre, and the arteriolar supply of the thick fatty subcutaneous tissues is not quite adequate. This leads to an anoxia in the subcutaneous tissues, with chronic anoxic dilatation of the skin capillaries and oedema. The whole pathology is greatly accentuated by cold, causing vasoconstriction of the superficial arterioles and further diminution of an already inadequate blood supply to the subcutaneous tissues. Thus it is usually exposure to cold which precipitates the development of the fat necrosis, ulcers and chilblains. All these symptoms are better in summer, except the oedema, which tends to be a little worse in hot weather. These patients are usually very conscious of their legs, and often have other annoying associated symptoms, such as nocturnal cramps in the calf, and a chronic irritation of the skin of the legs. Figure 19.5 shows the typical appearance of the erythrocyanoid limb and the ulcers associated with it.

The next important point is that this type of limb reacts badly to the stress of any sort of venous incompetence. Superficial varicose veins cause more distressing symptoms than in a normal limb. Venous ulcers round the ankle occur more easily, are more painful, and need all the resources and ingenuity of the surgeon to cure them. Moreover, the diagnosis of venous pathology is extremely difficult in these limbs, as large incompetent veins may be so completely hidden in the thick subcutaneous fat as to be invisible and often impalpable. Thus in these people the early diagnosis and treatment of any venous incompetence, superficial or deep, is of great

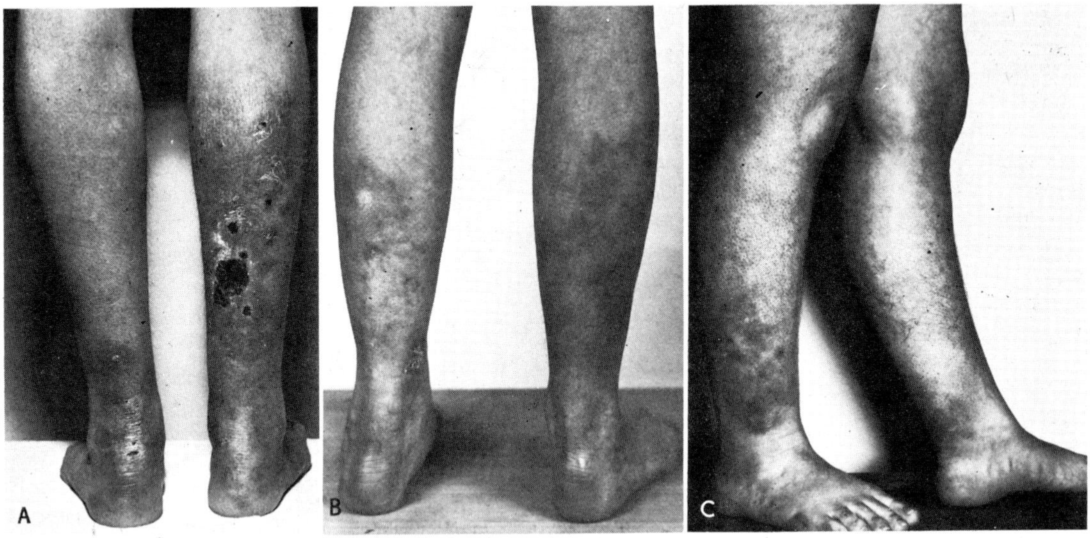

Fig. 19.5 Erythrocyanosis Frigida. Three examples of the necrotic and ulcerative lesions which occur typically over the back, or external surface of these limbs.

importance if chronic and painful sequelae are to be avoided.

The treatment of the erythrocyanoid leg and its complications may be considered under the following headings:

1. General Management. The patients are warned not to expose the leg and toes to extremes of temperature. In winter thick stockings or over-socks and warm ankle boots must be worn. If the patient is very obese a weight-reducing diet will bring some relief.

2. Venous incompetence should be carefully looked for and treated early by adequate operation.

3. Oedema. If there is any venous incompetence in the limb, this symptom is always ameliorated by appropriate surgery. However, in most cases the oedema is not associated with venous incompetence and is best treated by firm support with a webbing-elastic bandage or stout elastic stocking.

4. Ulcers. If recurrent ulceration of the calf tends to occur every winter, then lumbar sympathectomy is indicated, and in this connection it gives good results. The ulcers heal rapidly and pain is relieved, and the patient is grateful for the warm limb. However, it is necessary to warn the patient not to relax the general precautions, because although the immediate results of sympathectomy are good there is a tendency to relapse after a period of about two years. Even so, the ulcers are never so bad, nor so difficult to control, as before sympathectomy. This operation has no effect on the oedema. In fact in the immediate post-operative period (up to two months), during the phase of maximal increase of blood flow, the oedema may be much worse, and the patient may be alarmed. This temporary increase in oedema always settles gradually to what it was before operation. However, a sympathectomy will not maintain healing in ulcers of primarily venous origin unless the appropriate surgery for the defective veins is carried out at the same time.

Post-poliomyelitic ulcers. A leg which has become partly or wholly paralysed as a result of old anterior poliomyelitis (or indeed any other nervous disorder, such as spina bifida) tends to undergo certain changes. The muscles waste and contractures may occur; there is an increased tendency for the deposition of subcutaneous fat in the leg, and owing to its reduced activity the blood flow through it

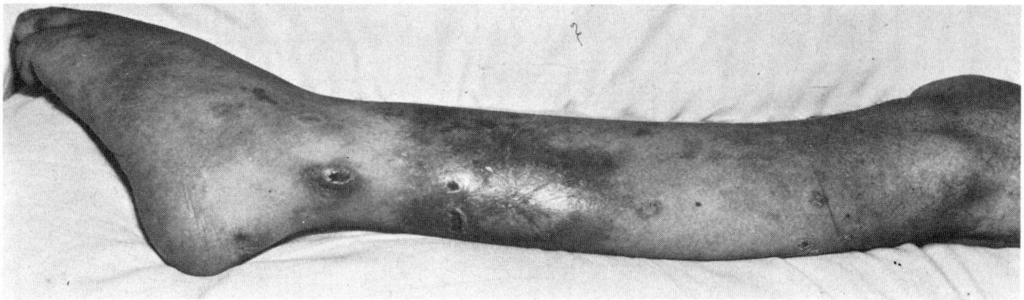

Fig. 19.6 The Post-poliomyelitic Ulcer. The lesions on the wasted leg of a patient who had had poliomyelitis. These are similar in every way to the lesions of erythrocyanosis frigida.

becomes much reduced. The net result of these factors is the cold, blue limb, which approximates closely to the erythrocyanoid leg (Fig. 19.6) and is subject to the same complication, i.e. the development of small painful chronic ulcers in the lower third, which are worse in cold weather. The pathology of these ulcers is exactly the same as that of the ulcers in erythrocyanosis, namely areas of subcutaneous fat necrosis, with a surrounding inflammatory reaction, over which the skin gradually breaks down.

The treatment of this complication follows the same lines as erythrocyanosis. When conservative management fails to control them, lumbar sympathectomy will produce great improvement, although as in the erythrocyanoid persons, minor relapse in the later years must be expected and guarded against.

In the early cases of threatened breakdown of skin over the indurated patches in the legs of both erythrocyanoid and post-poliomyelitic patients—the stage of so-called 'erythema induration'—ulceration may sometimes be arrested and the local symptoms relieved by the local application of 'Trafuril Cream', rubbed in three or four times a day. This cream, which contains histamine, promotes a local vaso-dilatation which lasts for an hour or two. It is useful in the local management of such legs and also is of great use in aborting chilblains. The limb should also be protected by an elastic stocking.

Traumatic and infective ulcers. Any infected abrasion, or insect bite, will take longer to heal when it occurs in the leg or ankle than in the arm or upper part of the body unless the patient is at rest. If, in addition, the limb is of the erythrocyanoid type, or the seat of venous incompetence or of arterial ischaemia, the resultant ulcer may become very chronic.

However, under certain conditions, chronic ulcers may occur in normal legs. Examples of these were the so-called 'desert sores' of the last war. These occurred frequently on the legs, following either a bite or some small abrasion, and the reason for their persistence was chronic, inadequately treated surface infection and repeated trauma, inseparable from the conditions of life on active service. Men were unwilling to report sick for an apparently minor complaint, and so the ulcers tended to persist, get bigger and more obvious. They responded to treatment by simple antiseptics, rest, and dressings. Similar chronic sores may be seen in the legs of the poorer classes in most middle eastern countries.

Occasionally such ulcers become infected with a virulent organism such as the streptococcus, staphylococcus aureus, or even the diphtheria bacillus. In such cases local pain and ulceration increase and the patient may become ill with raised temperature. In cases which became infected with KLB during the last war, the dangerous diphtheritic toxaemia made its appearance and the patients were prostrated with a high pulse rate, and diphtheritic paralysis if the anti-serum was not given.

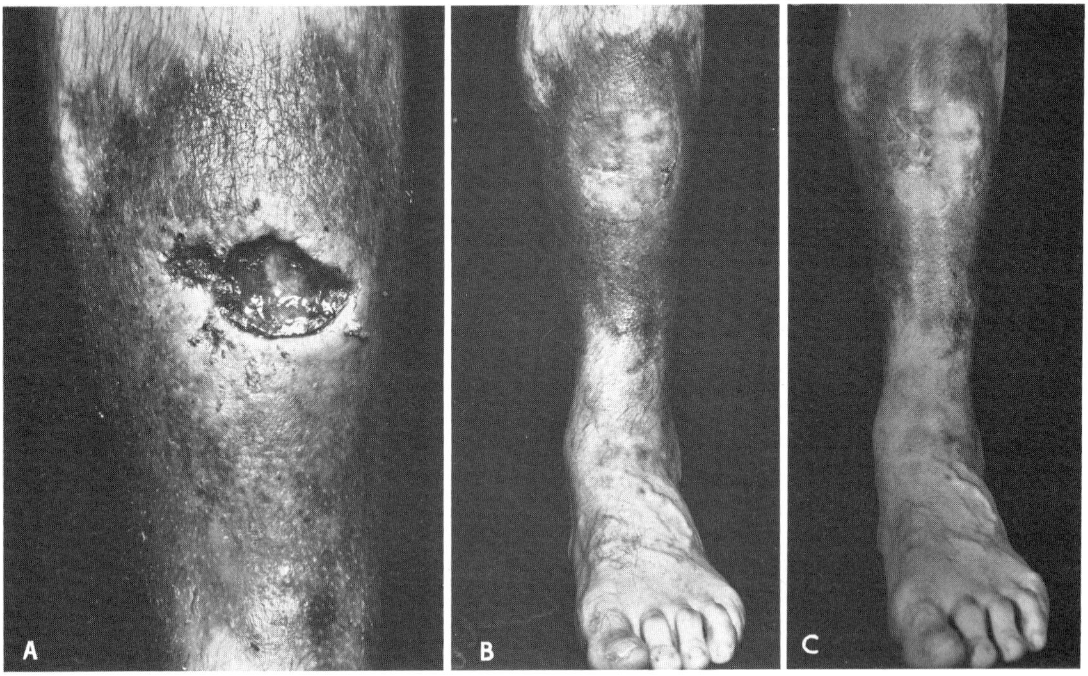

Fig. 19.7 Traumatic Ulcer of the Shin or Footballer's Ulcer. This occurred in a young man of 28 and resisted all attempts at healing for a number of years (including skin grafting). On investigation he was found to have deep vein incompetence. Permanent healing has followed an operation in which the ulcer was *excised* and grafted and the perforating vein in its vicinity removed. After this procedure the pigmentation gradually became less and at the time of writing has almost disappeared. A—Before operation; B—After operation; C—One and a half years after operation.

The commonest traumatic ulcer seen in England in peace time is that of the shin, or 'footballers' ulcer'. This occurs in healthy young men who have received a 'crack on the shin' during a game of football. The resultant sore is allowed to get infected, not properly cared for and the base of the ulcer may get adherent to bone. At this stage the ulcer may be indolent, although control of the sepsis combined with local pad and webbing elastic bandage pressure usually heals them. Occasionally they are associated with unsuspected deep venous pathology in the limb, as was the case depicted in Figure 19.7.

Ulcers due to underlying bone disease

Chronic ulceration of the skin is often associated with and caused by underlying bone disease. The following types of ulceration occur:

1. Ulcer associated with chronic osteomyelitis or 'Brodies' abscess of the tibia (Fig. 19.8).

Such ulcers may occur on either side of the ankle, and are of course associated with chronic sepsis. They may be the source of infection, causing several other septic ulcers often on the other leg. One such patient was treated for chronic ulceration of both ankles for years, before ordinary straight X-ray revealed a chronic 'Brodies' abscess in the right tibia (Fig. 19.8).

Surface ulceration may occasionally be seen in the papery adherent scar following the old fashioned extensive bone-guttering operations for osteomyelitis.

2. Ulceration associated with bone tumours. Figure 19.9 is a fine example of this.

3. Ulcers associated with extensive old compound fractures of the tibia. When there has been an old compound fracture with

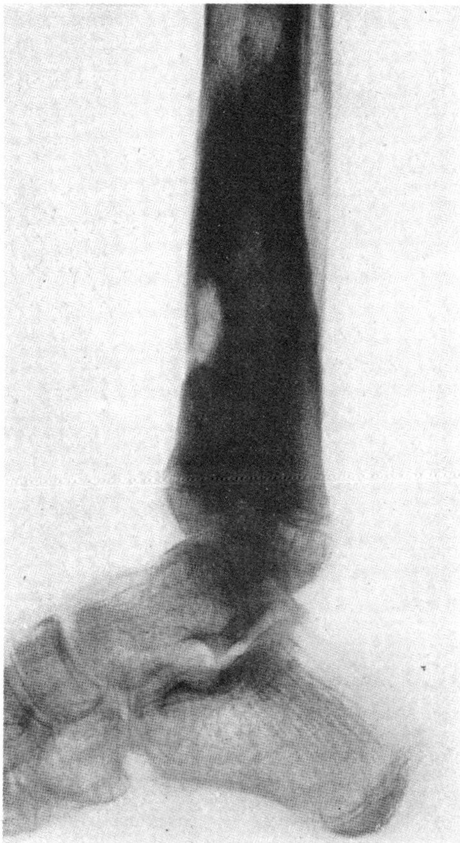

Fig. 19.8 X-ray of a tibia with intransigent eczema of the leg and ulceration at the ankle after osteomyelitis of the tibia. A pure growth of tubercle bacilli was cultured from this Brodie's abscess.

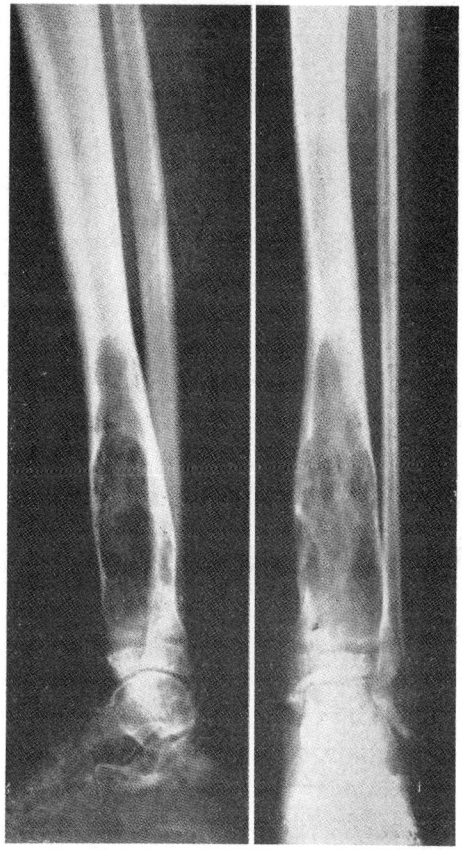

Fig. 19.9 An osteoclastoma of the tibia, which was causing swelling, eczema and ulceration at the ankle.

stripping of the skin over the tibia this skin never quite regains its old vitality as a great deal of its arterial supply may be destroyed. In addition there may be post-traumatic and post-thrombotic venous pathology due to the original accident and infection. There may remain a large area of pigmented skin over the front of the tibia which breaks down and ulcerates if it is not carefully protected and supported. Such cases occasionally need full-thickness skin grafting.

4. Those associated with Paget's disease. Cases of Paget's disease of the tibia may be complicated by a small ulcer, originally traumatic in origin, situated over the bowed edge of the bone. These ulcers rapidly become adherent to the extremely vascular bone and, contrary to what might be expected, are then very resistant to treatment (Fig. 19.10).

Periostitis and chronic ulcers of the leg. The bone adjacent to any chronic ulcer of the leg may develop a periosteal reaction. In very chronic ulcers of the leg the bones may show considerable periostitis. This must not be confused with other bone diseases, particularly syphilitic periostitis (Fig. 19.11 shows a typical X-ray).

Phleboliths. Figure 19.12 shows the X-ray appearances of an old lady with an ulcer of the leg. She had numerous phleboliths in the

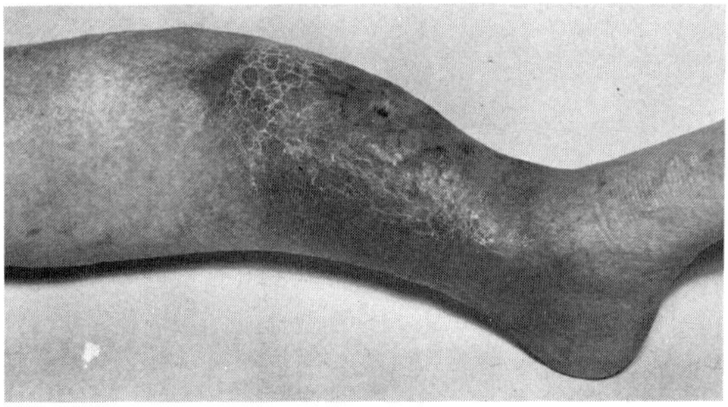

Fig. 19.10 The ulcer associated with Paget's disease of the tibia.

subcutaneous veins—one of which was ulcerating through the skin of the shin and looked exactly like a sequestrum. These phleboliths are not uncommon in the aged, and are the same as the phleboliths which are seen so commonly on X-rays of the pelvis.

Pressure sores. Pressure sores due to badly applied plaster of Paris or webbing elastic bandages too tightly applied in the elderly, are occasionally seen; they tend to occur exactly over the prominent bony points, particularly the malleoli. In normal limbs they heal slowly but satisfactorily after removal of the plaster, but occasionally (particularly if there has been associated deep vein thrombosis or if there is an associated nerve lesion, or they have become badly infected) they may become very chronic; then they may require excision and skin grafting with oral antibiotic to control infection.

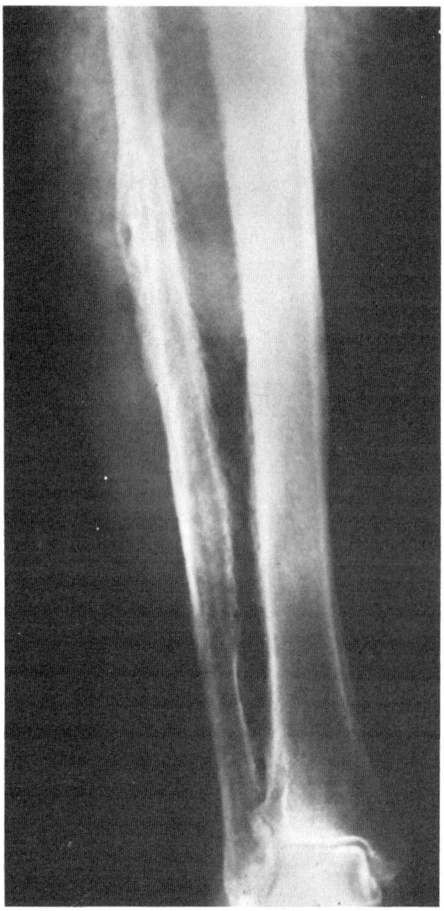

Fig. 19.11 Periostitis of the tibia and fibula under a chronic venous ulcer. The fibula always shows this periostitis reaction first, and it is usually more marked than on the tibia.

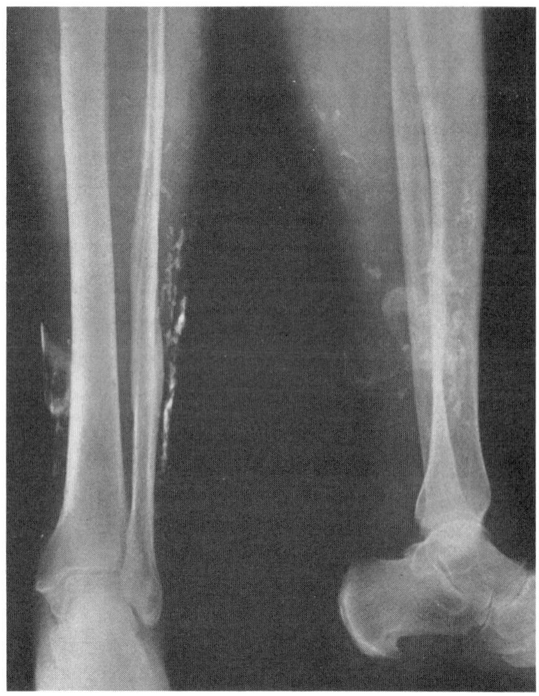

Fig. 19.12 Phleboliths in the subcutaneous tissues of an elderly woman with varicose veins. The calcification occurs within the lumen of the veins. Occasionally a phlebolith will ulcerate through the skin.

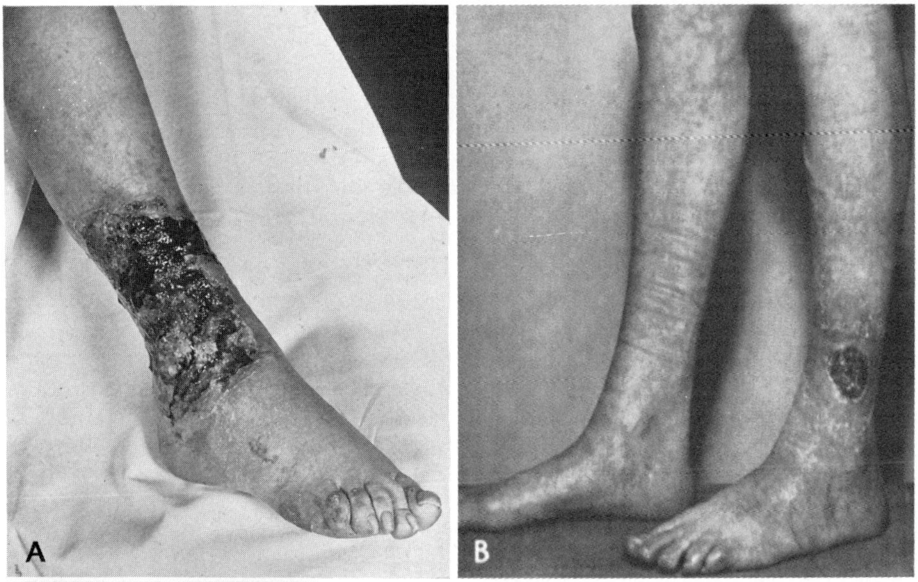

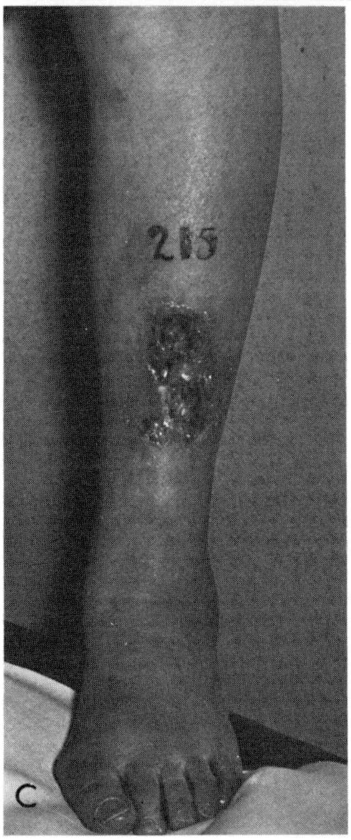

Fig. 19.13 Arterial Ulcers or Martorell's Ulcer. All these ulcers occurred suddenly without obvious trauma, in elderly patients with peripheral arterial disease. They were extremely painful, especially at night. There was no evidence of venous disease. All healed after a period of conservative treatment with supporting bandages.

The so-called 'arterial ulcer', or 'Martorell's Ulcer'. This ulcer is undoubtedly a clinical entity although its exact pathology is disputed. It occurs in older patients who have arteriosclerosis with and without hypertension. It presents usually on the antero-lateral aspect of the lower third of the leg. Some of them start after a specific incident of trauma here, for example a bruise or abrasion. These may be explained on the basis of trauma followed by infection in an ischaemic leg. Such patients usually have arterial thromboses of one or more of the major arteries of the leg. Many such ulcers, however, appear quite suddenly and spontaneously without any obvious predisposing incident. The skin suddenly becomes blue and breaks down. Typically these ulcers are very painful in their early stages and the pain has all the characteristics of ischaemic pain (rest pain). The leg may not show the other signs of arterial ischaemia (i.e. coldness, postural colour changes and absence of the dorsalis pedis, or posterior tibial pulses, or both).

In this connection Learmonth and others have drawn attention to the occasional appearance of isolated areas of skin gangrene in the leg, in patients who have an aortic thrombosis or aortic aneurysm. He attributes the phenomenon to showers of small arterial emboli plugging small arterioles in this region, which is anatomically so ill supplied.

These ulcers, after their initial painful and rather alarming onset, sometimes heal without difficulty on the usual routine dressing and light elastic bandage technique, particularly if the skin only is involved. However, if they are deep and particularly if the tendon sheath or deep fascia becomes exposed, skin grafting and even lumbar sympathectomy may be indicated.

Syphilitic ulcers. Syphilitic ulcers may occur in the secondary or tertiary stages of the disease. Secondary specific eruptions may occur anywhere in the legs, consisting of thin, easily detached scabs covering small shallow ulcers, which heal rapidly unless they become secondarily infected.

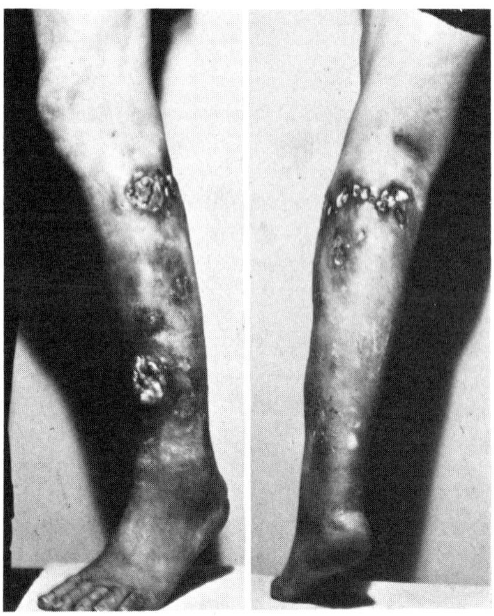

Fig. 19.14 Tertiary Syphilitic Ulcers. These photographs illustrate all the diagnostic features of these ulcers; their multiplicity, their punched-out or serpiginous appearance and their occurrence anywhere on the leg (outside the gaiter area).

In the tertiary stage, gummata may occur anywhere in the leg and may be multiple. These start as dusky red painless nodules which coalesce and break down, forming ulcers which may be circular and clearly punched out, or serpiginous (from the coalescing of a number of single gummatous lesions). The base of these ulcers is formed of yellow necrotic material aptly compared to 'washleather'. These ulcers heal rapidly with antisyphilitic treatment giving white firm scars (the so-called tissue paper scars) the skin of which is surprisingly firm and mobile.

The important diagnostic points about syphilitic ulcers are:

1. They tend to be multiple and painless.
2. They typically occur outside the gaiter area.
3. Their punched out or serpiginous outline and washleather base (when present) are typical.
4. Other signs of specific disease may be present.

Tuberculous ulcers. The term Bazin's disease should be reserved for the rare tuberculide occurring on the calf of the leg. This disease, which is very rare in England, must not be confused with the similar lesions of ulcerating pernio occurring in erythrocyanoid legs which are similar and common. The presence of giant cell systems histologically around the areas of fat necrosis in perniosis has in the past led to much confusion between this disease and the true tuberculide. This was accentuated by the fact that some of the patients had tubercular lesions elsewhere.

Apart from Bazin's disease, primary tubercular ulceration of the skin of the legs with painless enlargement and later caseation of the inguinal lymph glands occurs in children. Miller (1953) collected nineteen cases of primary tuberculosis of the skin in children under twelve in which half the lesions occurred in the leg. These ulcers occur usually after a local abrasion or scratch and there is often a member of the family, or other contact, with open tuberculosis. Similar primary tuberculous ulcers of the skin are occasionally seen as a terminal phenomenon in children with miliary tuberculosis.

A syndrome very similar to the above has recently been described under the name of 'cat scratch fever' (Mollaret et al., 1951). In these cases the local lesion is always due to a cat scratch; the regional glands then enlarge and caseate. These lesions pursue a chronic course with eventual healing. There is an eosinophilia and the intradermal test with the specific antigen is positive.

Occasionally tuberculous ulcers of the skin of the legs are seen which really arise from deep seated tuberculous lesions of bone, joint or tendon sheath. A chronic ulcer of the skin in a boy of eighteen was found to be due to tuberculous tenosynovitis of the extensor sheath in front of the ankle joint. In another boy of fifteen, persistent ulceration occurred in the scar of an incision for old osteomyelitis in the lower part of the tibia. X-ray revealed a Brodie's abscess here. When this was drained tubercle bacilli were grown from the pus. Cold abscesses arising from foci in the greater trochanter, or more rarely in the pelvis or spine, may track down the leg and present as tuberculous ulcers of sinuses on the outer or inner side of the limb.

The essential clinical characteristics of a tuberculous ulcer are a ragged, blue, undermined edge, a base of blue, unhealthy looking granulation tissue, and painless enlargement, with perhaps caseation of the regional lymph nodes. The ulcers may occur anywhere on the legs and the diagnosis should be made clinically and confirmed by biopsy and the demonstration of tubercle bacilli from the surface of the ulcer or in the regional lymph nodes.

Tuberculous ulcers are rare.

Neoplastic ulcers. Occasionally fibro sarcomatous change may occur in a chronic ulcer of twenty to twenty-five years' duration. This malignant transformation, the so-called Marjolin's ulcer, is rarely seen now. It should, however, be suspected when an ulcer which has been present for twenty to twenty-five years or so, becomes more active and increases in size. The edge of such ulcers should always be biopsied. Their malignancy is low. The treatment should be in the first place wide block excision with the deep fascia, and skin graft. The scar and lymph nodes are then observed every three months. We have found that amputation is rarely necessary.

Primary epitheliomata of course occur on the leg, although rare compared with other sites. Old burn scars, or scars of old osteomyelitis occasionally undergo malignant transformation.

Progressive bacterial synergic gangrene of the skin. This comparatively rare condition was first described and investigated by Meleney (1949) and the ulcers when they occur on the legs or elsewhere are often known by his name. The condition is a rapidly spreading necrosis of the subcutaneous tissues and skin. The advancing edge of the lesion is always a centimetre or more in advance of the area of skin necrosis. Meleney claims that it is mainly due to the synergic action of a microaerophilic streptococcus with a haemolytic staphylococcus aureus. These organisms can be obtained from the growing edge of the lesion by special anaerobic culture methods. Many other organisms are found as secondary invaders of the gangrenous tissue. *It occurs particularly in toxaemic patients whose resistance is low*; the classical situation is around an empyema drainage sinus or a colostomy.

The clinical picture is characteristic. The chief symptom is severe pain. Within an advancing zone of erythema, a raised, tender, dusky red area of induration occurs. The skin may become gangrenous in several places over this area, and as it melts away it is seen to be extensively undermined.

Prior to 1945 the only effective treatment of this disease was wide diathermy excision of the area followed by treatment with a special zinc peroxide cream (freshly prepared). The area was then skin grafted. Penicillin and the newer antibiotics have transformed the outlook and prevent spread of the lesion.

Most cases respond rapidly to a wide spectrum antibiotic like Erythromycin.

These ulcers occasionally occur on the legs, usually in association with some severe general disease or anaemia. Sometimes they occur as extensions or complications of an ordinary venous ulcer. In such cases the sudden intense pain, rapid spread and profuse discharge from the lesion is characteristic Whilst the disease is advancing, healing may be occurring from islands of epithelium which have survived the destructive effect of the infection. Such a case is shown in Figure 19.15. The ulcers which are described as a complication of ulcerative colitis may be of this type.

Injection ulcers. When sclerosing solutions such as quinine and urethane and lithium salicylate were in use, the escape of these outside the vein resulted in an area of tissue necrosis, which often ulcerated. Such ulcers were typically round and punched out in appearance, and took about four to six months to heal. These have been much rarer since the introduction of Aethanolamine and the phenol-glycerine solution and also since injection treatment is so much less practised.

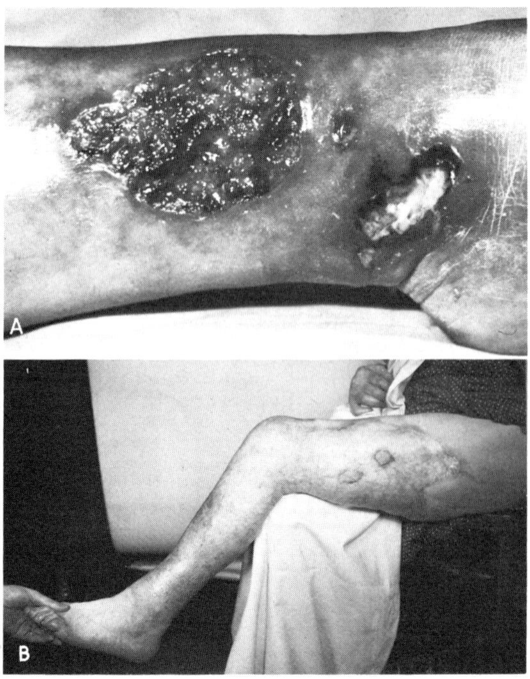

Fig. 19.15 Meleney's Ulcers. (A) Shows the acute painful looking lesions round the ankle of a woman whose haemoglobin was found to be less than 50 per cent. Note the typically undermined edge of the acute lesions. (B) Shows a healed case, demonstrating the great area of skin which may be involved in the lesion.

Ulceration in association with arterio-venous fistulae. (See also Chap. 11.) Eczema or ulceration round the ankle may occur in a leg in which there is an arterio-venous fistula, either congenital or traumatic.

Congenital arterio-venous fistulae may be either very numerous, small and generalised throughout the limb (often in association with cutaneous angiomata) or relatively localised in a peripheral part of the limb. In this latter type ulceration at the ankle may be the presenting complaint and is directly due to the raised local venous pressure. Martorell (1950) states that of nineteen such patients, six had ulceration. An unexplained ulcer of the malleolar region in a young adult should raise the suspicion of this condition. Examination may then reveal any or all of the following signs:

1. Warm skin over and around the ulcer.
2. Excessive pulsation or even a thrill at this point.
3. Pulsating varices.
4. A murmur on auscultation.
5. Increase in length of the affected leg and foot. This is probably the most important and constant sign. Figure 19.16 shows an ulcer occurring in the leg of a young boy. Such ulcers are rarer with traumatic arterio-venous fistulae but Martorell describes four such cases.

These ulcers may heal on the routine compression support with elastic bandages of the local varices, but the final cure lies in the eradication of the arterio-venous fistula. In traumatic cases this is usually possible; in congenital cases it is very difficult and may require several operations and is often manifestly impossible. The more localised peripheral variety is more suitable for this type of surgery (Robertson). Amputation was finally

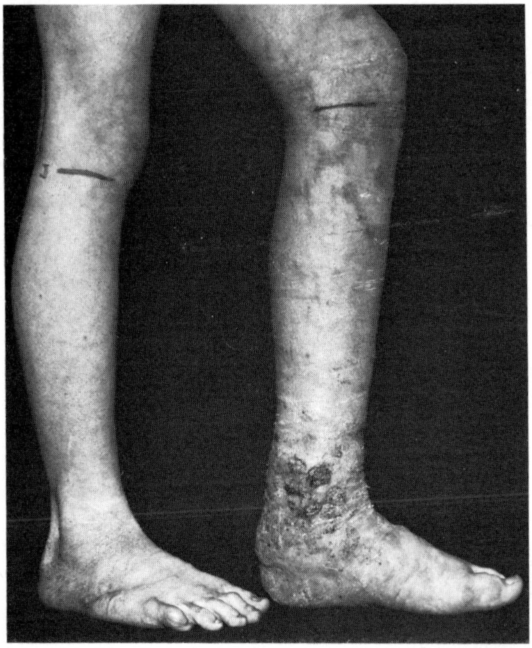

Fig. 19.16 Congenital Arterio-venous Fistula. Appearance of the limb of a boy of 14 with this condition. Note the ulceration, the increase in size and great increase in length of the affected leg.

resorted to in the case of the boy (Fig. 19.16) whose leg was ulcerated; it was 4½ inches longer than the opposite limb, the eczema was intractable, and he bled from punctate spots on it.

Ulceration af the leg related to certain general diseases. Ulceration of the leg has been mentioned as a complication of a large number of diseases in rather a loose manner. Certainly in an ulcer clinic it is a noticeable fact that there is a high incidence of other disease such as cardiac failure, arteriosclerosis, anaemia, and arthritic conditions. Now any patient who has a chronic debilitating disease has spent probably a good deal of time either in hospital or resting. Such people are likely to have had calf vein thrombosis at some time or other, and are therefore likely to develop post-thrombotic ulcers. Their general debilitating condition further favours the appearance and delays the healing of such ulcers. In various blood diseases the haemorrhagic tendency may predispose to the appearance of these lesions. Bearing these remarks in mind, it is possible that many of these leg ulcers at present described as specific complications of certain diseases are in reality no more than post-thrombotic ulcers, whose appearance and course have been particularly determined by the poor general condition of the patient. *It is noticeable that patients who are anaemic from any cause have retarded healing of leg ulcers.*

Ulcerative colitis. Progressive ulceration of the skin of the legs is described as a complication of ulcerative colitis. The lesion is rather similar to the Meleney type of ulcer, and may occur in other parts of the body besides the legs. It usually begins and progresses in the active phase of the disease and gets better as the general disease improves or remits. Its treatment is (1) general—to control the ulcerative colitis and to correct the anaemic and toxic state of the patient; and (2) local—this is as for Meleney's ulcer.

Acholuric jaundice. Some cases of acholuric jaundice are complicated by an ulcerated ankle. In fact the ulcer may be the first symptom which brings the patient to a doctor. It is usually a shallow surface ulceration on the inside or outside of the ankle. It behaves like a venous ulcer, i.e. it heals on adequate support with elastic bandage or rest in bed.

In the same group may be mentioned those ulcers which occasionally complicate the leukaemias.

In any condition in which excessive capillary fragility and general debility or anaemia are combined, a particularly severe extravasation of blood is apt to occur in the area of the body where venous pressure is high, i.e. the ankles. This condition is seen in old people who show the phenomenon of senile purpura. This is usually unassociated with any demonstrable blood disorder or platelet pathology. Such people may present with large ecchymosis in the ankle region, quite spontaneously, which occasionally breaks down and ulcerates. A poor nutritional state, and particularly a lack of Vitamin C may be a contributory factor in such cases.

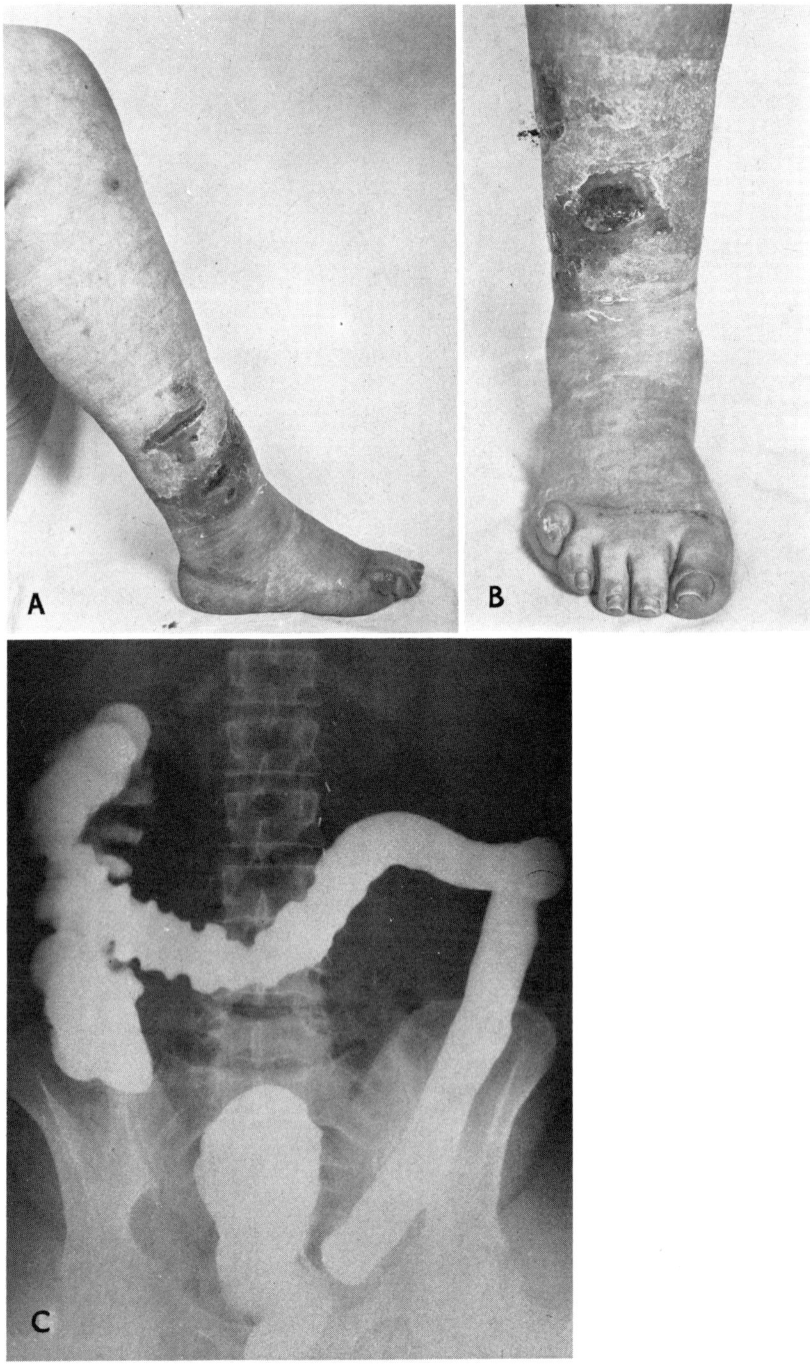

Fig. 19.17 Ulceration of the legs in a case of ulcerative colitis. Note the absence of haustrations in the left colon, the seat of the colitis. The ulcers healed when the ulcerative colitis was controlled.

Gravitational purpura of the legs is not an uncommon phenomenon and occurs in some people for no obvious cause. It may occur in the legs of old people on first getting up after prolonged recumbency (see Fig. 17.8).

Diabetes. One of the rarer manifestations of diabetes is the lesion on the leg known as 'necrobiosis lipoidica diabeticorum'.—This is a definite clinical entity. It may occur anywhere in the lower leg and ankle region. Pathologically it is an area of fat necrosis, as indicated by its name, over which the skin ulcerates. It usually heals on routine pressure bandaging and treatment of the glycosuria.

Chronic diseases of the aged—The senile ulcer. Finally we come to an ill-defined group of patients of advanced age, usually over seventy, who have pigmentation with or without ulceration round the ankles. Many have numerous associated complaints—rheumatoid arthritis, osteo-arthritis and arterio-sclerosis being very common, and nearly all are in a poor nutritional state. Many of the above factors go to the production of such ulcers, but they may be summed up in two words—senility and sepsis.

Ulcers due to self inflicted injuries (artefact or auto-mutilation). Every year, in the average hospital ulcer clinic, a patient attends (usually an adolescent female, although it does occur in older women and men) who has an ulcer on the leg or foot for which no cause is discernible; this lesion may be due to self-mutilation, i.e. it is an 'artefact' ulcer. These sores appear suddenly or at irregular intervals. They are usually situated on the front and outer surface of the leg, i.e. a normally non-ulcerating area, at a point convenient for the patient's particular form of self-abuse. The surroundings pink and clean, but it does not heal. One's attention is ultimately drawn to an oddness of the patient's personality or behaviour, which arouses the suspicion that the sore could be self-inflicted and regularly retraumatised, so explaining its failure to clear up. The stigmata of hysteria may be present, such as anaesthetic palate, pharynx and cornea, glove and stocking anaesthesia, etc. When the limb is dressed in the ordinary way, i.e. frequently changed dressings held by a bandage, the ulcer continues because the patient has access to the wound and can continually apply irritants. If the possibility of the patient interfering with it is considered, then an occlusive casing such as a plaster of Paris bandage is applied over a suitable dressing, thus preventing interference, and healing follows progressively. Recurrence may occur after the dressing is removed, and the procedure has to be repeated. An X-ray may show foreign bodies inserted deeply into the wound; in one such patient numerous gramophone needles were so revealed. There may be family or economic reasons for the maintenance of the ulcer. This is fortunately not so common now as formerly, when the possession of large unhealed ulcer of the leg was part of the stock-in-trade of many beggars.

Cortisone ulcers. Patients who are on large doses of cortisone for various chronic

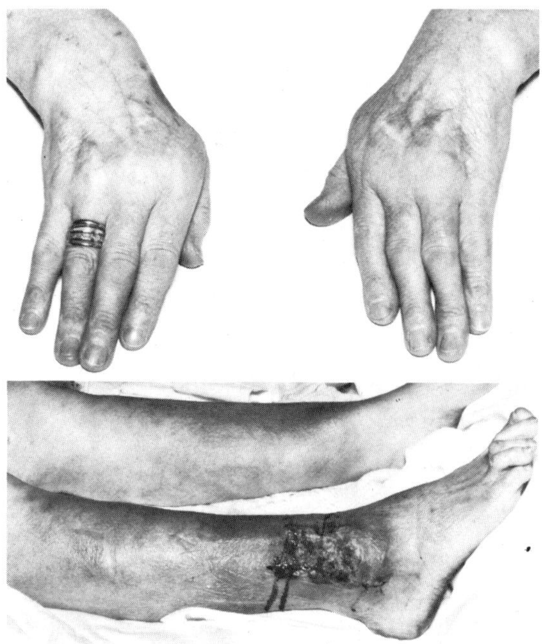

Fig. 19.18 The hands and the legs of a patient with chronic rheumatoid arthritis, on steroids for several years. She now has a large 'cortisone' ulcer.

diseases, particularly rheumatoid arthritis and asthma, develop a typical 'tissue fragility', which is most marked on the lower limb. Quite minor infections or abrasions in such patients may result in large chronic shallow, very indolent looking ulcers. Figure 19.18 shows one such ulcer. They are very difficult to manage, often requiring skin grafting with prolonged after care. Sometimes they fail to heal in spite of everything!

This phenomenon is also seen in patients who apply cortisone containing ointments to small chronic infective ulcers of the ankle, to control pain. These applications are often persisted in by the patients as they control pain, but after six months or a year the result may be a completely unreactive callous ulcer with no healing power!

Tropical ulcers. A detailed consideration of tropical ulcers is excluded from this book, as they are not seen in temperate zones. But in any case of unusual ulcer of the leg with a history of recent sojourn in tropical countries leishmaniasis, moniliasis, and other rare fungus diseases should be considered. Pellagra used to be a common cause of swelling and ulceration of the legs and was so again in the Japanese prisoner of war camps of the 1939–45 war, but in normal peace-time conditions it is very rare.

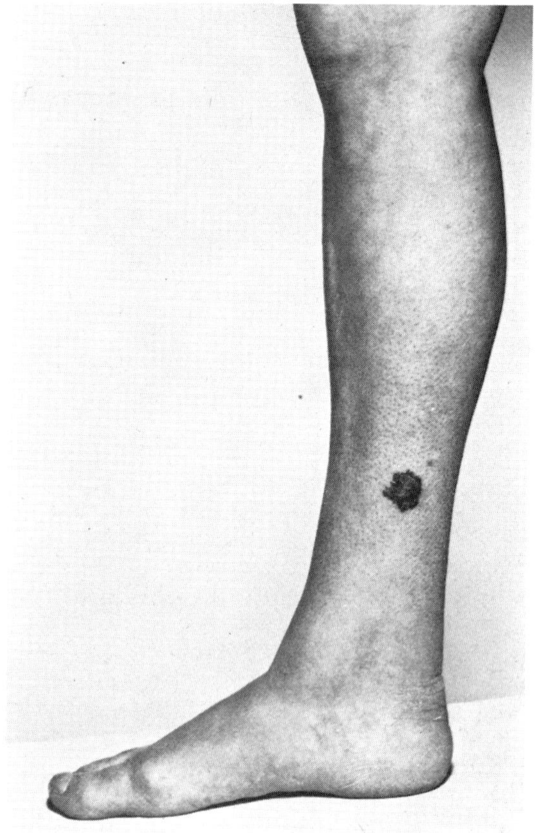

Fig. 19.19 Malignant melanoma of the ankle.

Melanoma. Figure 19.19 is included to remind the reader that malignant melanoma occur not infrequently in the ankle area.

Conclusion

From what has been said in this chapter it is apparent that when a patient presents with an ulcer of the leg the differential diagnosis may require considerable clinical acumen. A detailed history and an examination of the patient as a whole are essential for their diagnosis and treatment.

REFERENCES

Boyd, A. M. (1950) *Proc. R. Soc. Med.*, **43**, 1045.
Gay, J. (1868) On varicose diseases of the lower extremities. *The Lettsomian Lectures of 1867.* London: Churchill.
Learmonth, J. & Burt, C. C. (1952) *Edin. Med. J.*, **59**, 65.
Lynn, R. B. (1954) *Surg. Gynec. Obstet.*, **99**, 720.
Martorell, F. (1950) *Angiology*, **1**, 136.
Meleney, F. L. (1949) *Clinical Aspects and Treatment of Surgical Infections.* London: Saunders.
Miller, F. J. W. (1953) *Lancet*, **1**, 5.
Mollaret, P., Reilley, J., Bartin, R., Tournier, P. (1951) *Pr. med.*, **59**, 681. Ibid. 701.
Rea, W. J., Wyrick, W. J. (1970) *Ann. Surg.*, **172**, 957.
Robertson, D. G. (1954) *Lecture R.C.S. of Eng.*

Author Index

Subject Index

Printed in Great Britain by T. & A. Constable Ltd., Edinburgh